Pelvic Floor, Perineal, and Anal Sphincter Trauma During Childbirth

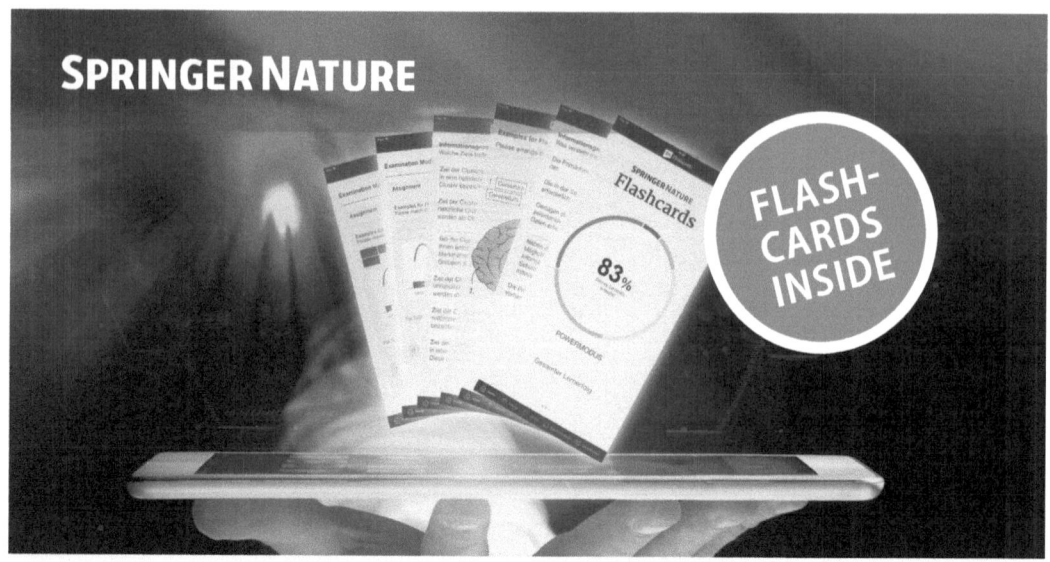

SN Flashcards Microlearning

Quick and efficient studying with digital flashcards –
for work or school!

With SN Flashcards you can:

- **Learn** anytime and anywhere on your smartphone, tablet or computer
- **Master** the content of the book and test your knowledge
- **Get motivated** by using various question types enriched with multimedia components and choosing from three learning algorithms (long-term-memory mode, short-term-memory mode or exam mode)
- **Create** your own question sets to personalise your learning experience

How to access your SN Flashcards content:

1. Go to the **1st page of the 1st chapter** of this book and follow the instructions in the box to sign up for an SN Flashcards account and to access the flashcards content for this book.
2. Download the SN Flashcards mobile app from the Apple App Store or Google Play Store, open the app and follow the instructions in the app.
3. Within the mobile app or web app, select the flashcards content for this book and start learning!

If you have difficulties accessing the SN Flashcards content, please write an email to **customerservice@springernature.com** mentioning "**SN Flashcards**" and the book title in the subject line.

Abdul H. Sultan • Ranee Thakar
Christina Lewicky-Gaupp
Editors

Pelvic Floor, Perineal, and Anal Sphincter Trauma During Childbirth

Diagnosis, Management and Prevention

Second Edition

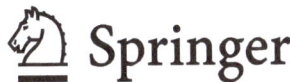 Springer

Editors
Abdul H. Sultan
Croydon University Hospital
London, UK

Ranee Thakar
Croydon University Hospital
London, UK

Christina Lewicky-Gaupp
Obstetrics and Gynecology; Section of
Urogynecology and Reconstructive
Pelvic Surgery
University of Chicago
Chicago, IL, USA

ISBN 978-3-031-43094-7   ISBN 978-3-031-43095-4   (eBook)
https://doi.org/10.1007/978-3-031-43095-4

This Springer imprint is published by the registered company Springer Nature Switzerland AG
The registered company address is: Gewerbestrasse 11, 6330 Cham, Switzerland

Paper in this product is recyclable.

Foreword

Perineal and Anal Sphincter Trauma: Diagnosis and Clinical Management was originally published in 2008, and rapidly became the indispensable resource for midwives, obstetricians, urogynecologists, and colorectal surgeons treating perineal and anal sphincter trauma, as well as raising awareness among all healthcare professionals.

The authors are not only major contributors to the generation of evidence defining best practice in the diagnosis and management of pelvic floor trauma during childbirth, but also global leaders in equipping healthcare providers to treat it. Abdul H. Sultan and Ranee Thakar founded the PROTECT Training program through the International Urogynecological Association. It is a "train the trainer" program that equips midwives and obstetricians from around the world with knowledge to offer optimal management of obstetrical trauma and teach colleagues towards minimizing pelvic floor and perineal morbidity associated with childbirth. This experience in personally teaching colleagues permeates the work making it comfortably accessible to readers from all disciplines.

This second edition expands on this valuable asset through new material on the impact of pregnancy on the pelvic floor, sexual function, and preexisting bowel conditions. It broadens the scope, including obstetrical pelvic floor trauma, neuropathy, and patient-reported outcomes after childbirth. And it informs treatment by exploring prevention through care bundles, physical therapy, and treatments. This broader and deeper scope is reflected in the new title, *Pelvic Floor, Perineal, and Anal Sphincter Trauma During Childbirth.* This interdisciplinary treatise incorporates excellent illustrations supporting the most up-to-date evidence. We have no doubt that it will surpass its predecessor to become an essential resource for healthcare providers in childbirth, with the most up-to-date knowledge to help caregivers around the globe to improve the lives of women who suffer from childbirth trauma by skills of prevention, and best practice of treating it. Nothing short of a must have!

Vancouver, Canada   Geoffrey Cundiff
Delft, Netherlands   Fred Milani
Plymouth, UK   Robert Freeman

Preface

With the recent international renewed push for vaginal over caesarean birth, there is again a need for obstetric providers and trainees to understand how to prevent and manage obstetric perineal and anal sphincter trauma. Over the last decade, more research has emerged in this arena, including the benefit of structured training programs and hands-on workshops to improve understanding of anatomy and repair of perineal and anal sphincter trauma. More studies have emerged supporting early repair of sphincter trauma as well as advantages of early pelvic floor physical therapy in the treatment of symptoms related to the trauma. Similarly, advances have been made in the imaging of obstetric trauma, which have elucidated the anatomic contributions to symptoms that gravely impact a new mother's quality of life.

However, despite these advances, primary and delayed repair of anal sphincter injuries are not universally optimal; continued research on the ideal management is imperative. This also highlights the need to identify women at risk for perineal and anal sphincter trauma in order to prevent it.

Our textbook aims not only to address the above issues, but also to provide detailed education in anatomy, neuroanatomy, and pathophysiology. In addition, we examine pertinent issues such as female genital mutilation, management of fecal incontinence and other pelvic floor disorders, and medicolegal implications of obstetric trauma.

In producing this book, we would like to acknowledge our mentors for their teaching and inspiration, the patients who inspire us question our practices, and the trainees who continue to contribute to the research. We would also like to thank the multidisciplinary authors for their timely submission of chapters, as well as Dr. Dee Fenner for her contribution to the first edition of this book. Lastly, we extend our appreciation to our families for their perseverance and understanding.

London, UK   Abdul H. Sultan
Croydon, UK   Ranee Thakar
Chicago, IL, USA   Christina Lewicky-Gaupp

Contents

Anatomy of the Pelvic Floor, Perineum and Anal Sphincter

1

Ranee Thakar, Dee E. Fenner, and Christopher X. Hong

Overview

Test your learning and check your understanding of this book's contents: use the "Springer Nature Flashcards" app to access questions. To use the app, please follow the instructions below: (1) Go to https://flashcards.springernature.com/login. (2) Create a user account by entering your e-mail address and assigning a password. (3) Use the following link to access your SN Flashcards set: ▶ https://sn.pub/wqrf89. If the link is missing or does not work, please send an e-mail with the subject "SN Flashcards" and the book title to customerservice@springernature.com.

Learning Objectives

- To describe the functional and structural anatomy of the pelvic floor, perineum, and anal sphincter complex.
- To describe anatomical relationships between structures of this region.

R. Thakar
Department of Obstetrics and Gynaecology,
Croydon University Hospital, Surrey, UK

D. E. Fenner · C. X. Hong (✉)
Department of Obstetrics and Gynecology, University of Michigan, Ann Arbor, MI, USA
e-mail: deef@med.umich.edu;
cxhong@med.umich.edu

1.1 Introduction

In this chapter reviewing the anatomy of the pelvic floor, rectum, and anal sphincter complex, anatomical structures are referred to by their accepted terms in *Terminologia Anatomica*, the international standard for human anatomical terminology [1]. Non-preferred terms are stated in parentheses adjacent to accepted terms.

1.2 Embryology

In the early embryo, the allantois, and the hindgut open into a common cavity—the cloaca (Fig. 1.1a). This is an endoderm-lined cavity that is in contact with the surface of the ectoderm. An ectodermal depression develops under the root of the tail of the embryo and sinks in toward the gut until only the thin cloacal membrane remains between the gut and the outside [2]. This ectodermal depression is called the proctodeum. The cloacal membrane is thus comprised of the cloacal endoderm and the ectoderm of the proctodeum, or the anal pit. Partitioning of the cloacal membrane takes place during the fifth to seventh week of development when the urorectal septum, which is mesodermal in origin, expands toward the tail of the embryo between the hindgut and the allantois to fuse with the cloacal membrane (Fig. 1.1b). The area of fusion becomes the perineal body and separates the dorsal anal membrane

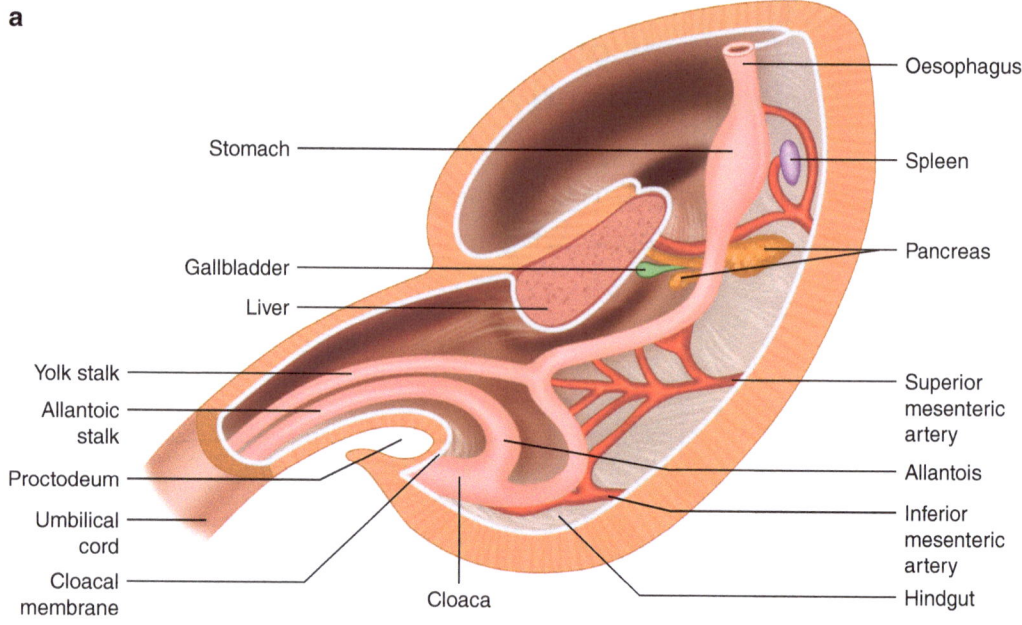

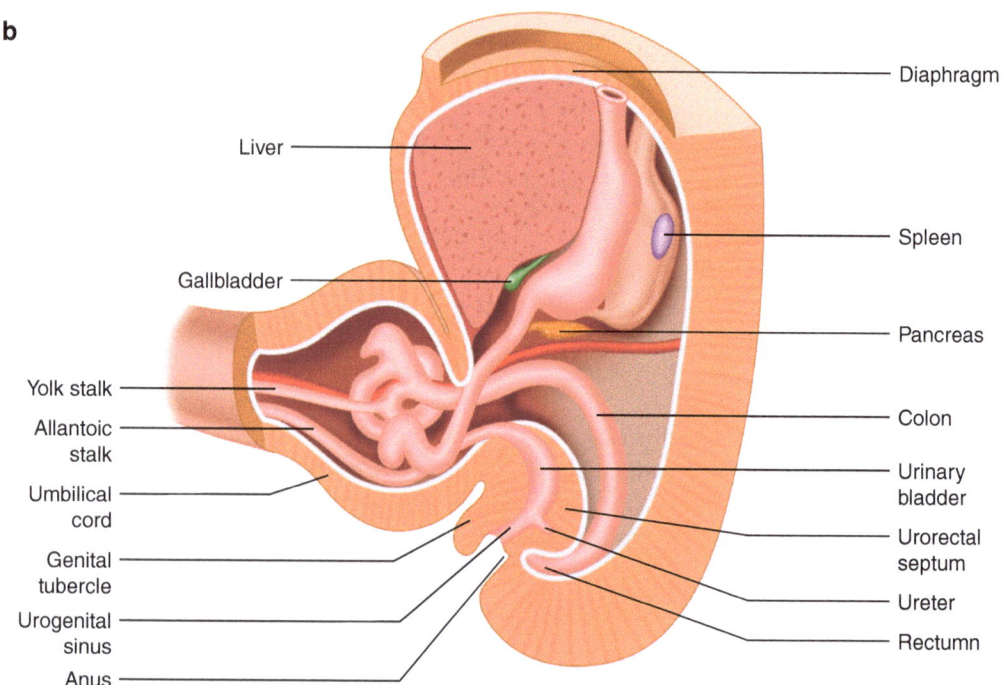

Fig. 1.1 (**a**) Development of the gastrointestinal tract at about 5 weeks. (**b**) Fetus showing development of the ano-rectum after 5 weeks, demonstrating the growth of the urorectum toward the cloacal membrane. (Figure from previous version)

from the larger ventral urogenital membrane. The anal membrane breaks down by the eighth week of gestation, establishing the anal canal. The uro-rectal septum also divides the cloacal musculature into anterior and posterior parts. The posterior portion develops into the EAS, while the anterior portion becomes the superficial transverse perineal muscle, the bulbospongiosus muscle, the ischiocavernosus muscle, and the perineal membrane. This explains why a single nerve—the pudendal nerve—supplies all musculature into which the cloacal membrane divides [3].

Knowledge of embryology is also important to understand the differences in the linings, innervation, vascular supply, and lymphatic drainage of the anal canal. The parts derived from the endoderm are lined by columnar epithelium and innervated by autonomic nerves, with the lymphatics and veins draining toward the abdomen. The parts derived from the ectoderm are lined by stratified squamous epithelium and have a somatic nerve supply, with the veins draining toward the external iliac system and the lymphatics to the inguinal lymph nodes.

The upper two-thirds of the anal canal is derived from the cloaca and the lower third develops from the proctodeum. This junction, about 1–2 cm from the anocutaneous line (anal verge), creates a demarcating line called the pectinate line (dentate line). At this line, the epithelium transitions between stratified squamous and simple columnar cells.

Little is known about the development of the EAS and levator ani muscles. Although closely associated, histologic embryo studies suggest the external sphincter and levator ani arise from two distinct primordia [4]. The puborectalis muscle is a portion of the levator ani and shares primordial cells with the ilio- and pubococcygeous muscles. The EAS begins to take form after 8 weeks of gestation and is clearly distinct from the puborectalis at that time [5].

1.3   Muscles of the Perineum

The perineum corresponds to the outlet of the pelvis and is somewhat lozenge-shaped. Although the area between the vagina and anus is colloquially referred to as the "perineum" in clinical settings, the proper anatomical term for this area is the "perineal body." The anatomic perineum it is bound anteriorly by the pubic arch, posteriorly by the coccyx, and laterally by the ischiopubic rami, ischial tuberosities, and

sacrotuberous ligaments. The deep limit of the perineum is the inferior surface of the pelvic diaphragm and its superficial limit is the skin. The perineum can be divided into two triangular parts by drawing an arbitrary line transversely between the ischial tuberosities [6]. The anterior triangle, which contains the external urogenital organs, is known as the urogenital triangle and the posterior triangle, which contains the termination of the anal canal, is known as the anal triangle.

1.3.1   The Urogenital Triangle

The urogenital triangle (Fig. 1.2a) is bound anteriorly and laterally by the pubic symphysis and the ischiopubic rami. Traditionally, the urogenital triangle has been thought to be divided into two compartments: the superficial and deep perineal spaces, separated by the perineal membrane, which spans the space between the ischiopubic rami [6]. However, more recent studies of this region describe the perineal membrane as a complex structure with many parts [7]. It is composed of two regions: one dorsal and one ventral. The dorsal region consists of bilateral transverse fibrous sheets that attach the lateral wall of the vagina and perineal body to the ischiopubic ramus. The ventral region is a solid three-dimensional tissue mass in which several structures are embedded. It contains the compressor urethrae muscle, the urethrovaginal sphincter muscle of the distal urethra, and the urethra itself with surrounding connective tissue (Fig. 1.3). The ventral margin of this mass is continuous with the insertion of the arcus tendineus fascia pelvis into the pubic bone. The levator ani muscles are attached to the cranial surface of the perineal membrane. The vestibular bulb and clitoral crus lie on the caudal surface of the membrane and are fused with it, with no natural plane of cleavage between these erectile structures and the membrane. Therefore, the structure of the perineal membrane is not a trilaminar sheet with perforating viscera, but a complex three-dimensional structure with two distinctly different dorsal and ventral regions [8].

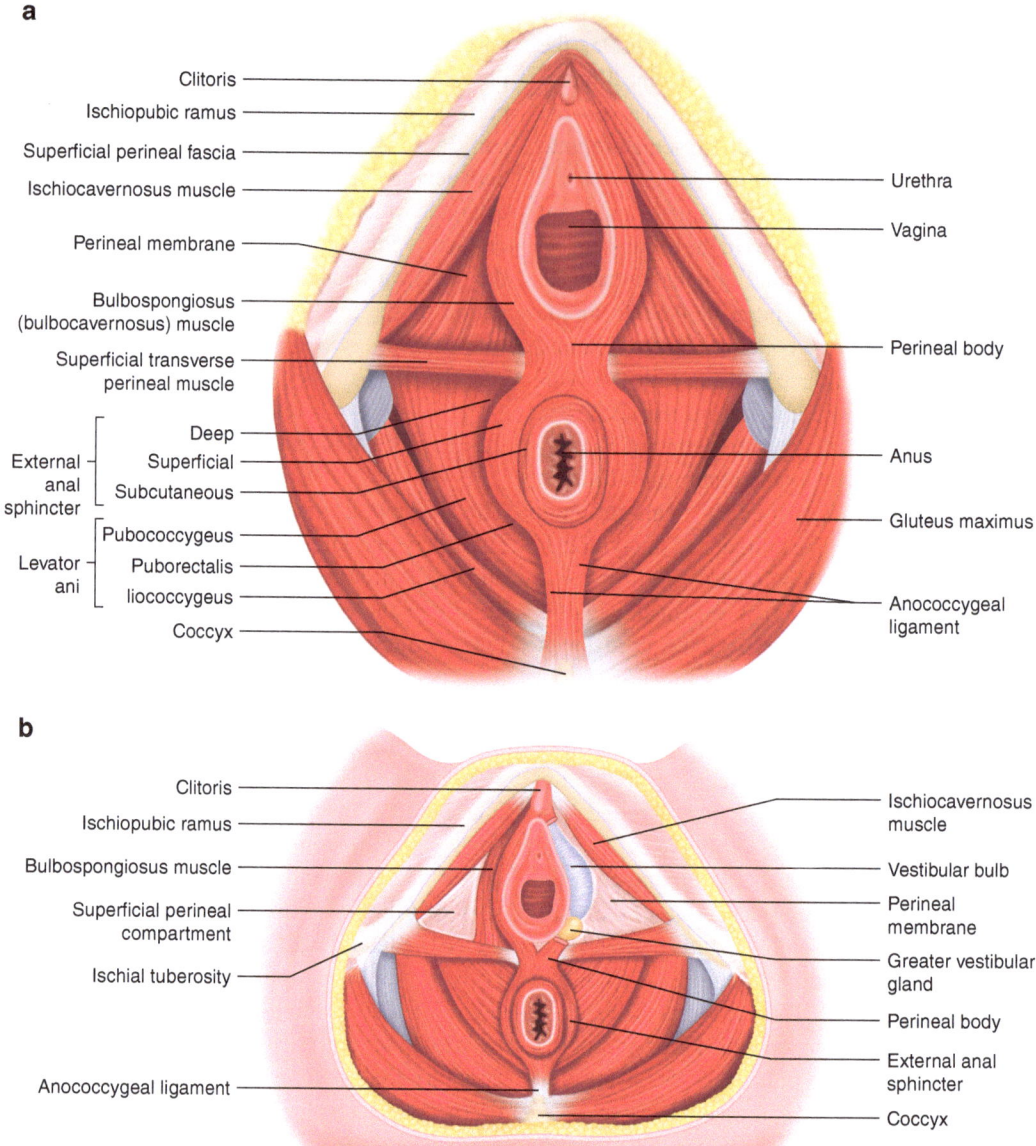

Fig. 1.2 The superficial compartment contains the superficial transverse perineal muscle, the bulbospongiosus muscle, and the ischiocavernosus muscle (**a**). These three muscles form a triangle on either side of the perineum, with a floor formed by the perineal membrane. (**b**) The left bulbospongiosus muscle has been removed to demonstrate the vestibular bulb and greater vestibular gland (Bartholin's gland). (Figure from previous version)

Fig. 1.3 The perineal membrane. The position of the perineal membrane is shown without the overlying erectile tissues (clitoral crura and vestibular bulbs), along with the associated components of the striated urogenital sphincter: the urethrovaginal sphincter (*) and the compressor urethrae muscle (•) © Delancey

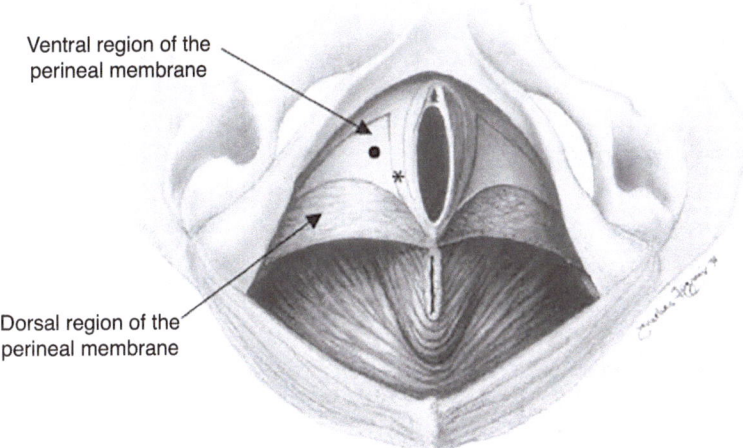

Ventral region of the perineal membrane

Dorsal region of the perineal membrane

Just beneath the skin of the anterior perineum lies the superficial perineal fascia (Colles' fascia). As described above, the erectile tissues are fused to the caudal surface of the perineal membrane complex. The erectile tissues are covered by the bulbospongiosus (bulbocavernosus) and the ischiocavernosus muscles. The superficial transverse perineal muscles attach the perineal body to the ischial tuberosities bilaterally. All of these perineal muscles are innervated by a branch of the pudendal nerve, which is a mixed motor and sensory nerve.

1.3.1.1 Superficial Transverse Perineal Muscle

The superficial transverse muscle is a narrow slip of a muscle, which arises from the inner and forepart of the ischial tuberosity and is inserted into the central tendinous part of the perineal body (Fig. 1.2a). The muscle from the opposite side, the EAS from behind, and the bulbospongiosus in the front all attach to the central tendon of the perineal body [6].

1.3.1.2 Bulbospongiosus Muscle

The bulbospongiosus muscle (bulbocavernosus muscle) runs on either side of the vaginal orifice, covering the lateral aspects of the vestibular bulb anteriorly and the greater vestibular gland (Bartholin's gland) posteriorly (Figs. 1.2b and 1.4). Some fibres merge posteriorly with the superficial transverse perineal

muscle and the EAS in the central fibromuscular perineal body. Anteriorly, its fibres pass forward on either side of the vagina and insert into the corpora cavernosa clitoridis, a fasciculus crossing over the body of the organ that compresses the deep dorsal vein of the clitoris. This muscle diminishes the orifice of the vagina and contributes to the erection of clitoris.

1.3.1.3 Ischiocavernosus Muscle

The ischiocavernosus muscle is elongated, broader at the middle than at either end, and situated on the lateral boundary of the perineum (Figs. 1.2a and 1.4). It arises by tendinous and fleshy fibres from the inner surface of the ischial tuberosity, behind the crus clitoridis, from the surface of the crus and from the adjacent portions of the ischial ramus. The ischiocavernosus compresses the crus clitoridis and retards blood flow through the veins, thus serving to maintain erection of the clitoris.

1.3.2 The Anal Triangle

This area includes the anal canal, the anal sphincters, and the ischioanal fossa.

1.3.2.1 Anal Canal

The rectum terminates in the anal canal (Fig. 1.5a, b). Definitions of the anal canal vary among sur-

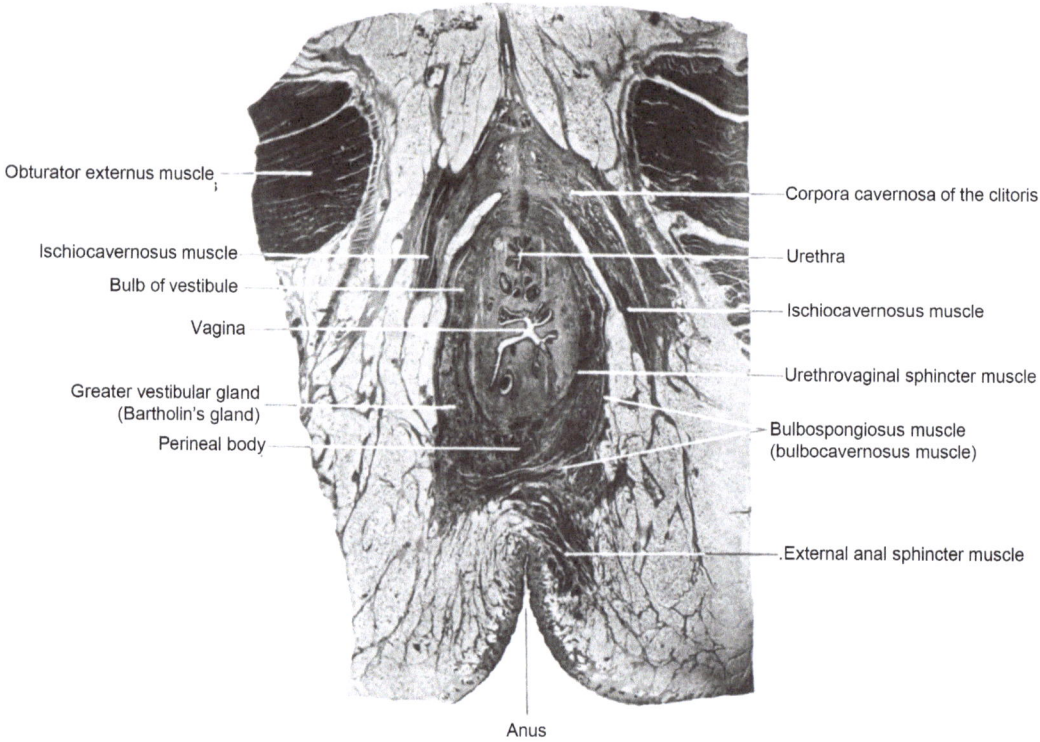

Obturator externus muscle

Ischiocavernosus muscle

Bulb of vestibule

Vagina

Greater vestibular gland
(Bartholin's gland)

Perineal body

Corpora cavernosa of the clitoris

Urethra

Ischiocavernosus muscle

Urethrovaginal sphincter muscle

Bulbospongiosus muscle
(bulbocavernosus muscle)

External anal sphincter muscle

Anus

Fig. 1.4 Histologic cross section of the pelvis perpendicular to the urethra and vagina at the level of the distal vagina (Reproduced from Urogenitalmuskulatur des Dammes by Otto Kalischer, 1900 [9])

geons and anatomists [10]. The surgical anal canal is approximately 4 cm long and extends from the anocutaneous line to the anorectal junction (anorectal ring), which is defined as the proximal level of the levator–EAS complex [11]. This clinical description correlates with a digital or sonographic examination but does not correspond to the histological architecture [12]. The embryological anal canal extends from the anal valves (see below) to the anal margin and is approximately 2 cm long [3].

The anal canal is attached posteriorly to the coccyx by the anococcygeal ligament, a midline fibromuscular structure that runs between the posterior aspect of the EAS and the coccyx (Fig. 1.2). The anus is surrounded laterally and posteriorly by loose adipose tissue within the ischioanal fossa, which is a potential pathway for spread of perianal sepsis from one side to the contralateral side. The pudendal nerves pass over the ischial spines at this point (Fig. 1.6) and can

be accessed digitally at this site for measurement of the pudendal nerve terminal motor latency using a modified electrode [13] (see Chap. 9). The perineum can also be anaesthetised by injection of local anaesthetic into the pudendal nerve at this site. Anteriorly, the perineal body separates the anal canal from the vagina.

The anal canal is surrounded by an inner epithelial lining, a vascular subepithelium, the internal anal sphincter (IAS), the EAS, and fibromuscular supporting tissue. The lining of the anal canal varies along its length due to its embryologic derivation. The proximal anal canal is lined with rectal mucosa (columnar epithelium) and is arranged in vertical mucosal folds called the anal columns (columns of Morgagni) (Fig. 1.5a). Each column contains a terminal radical of the superior rectal artery and vein. The vessels are largest in the left-lateral, right-posterior, and right-anterior quadrants of the wall of the anal canal where the subepithelial tissues

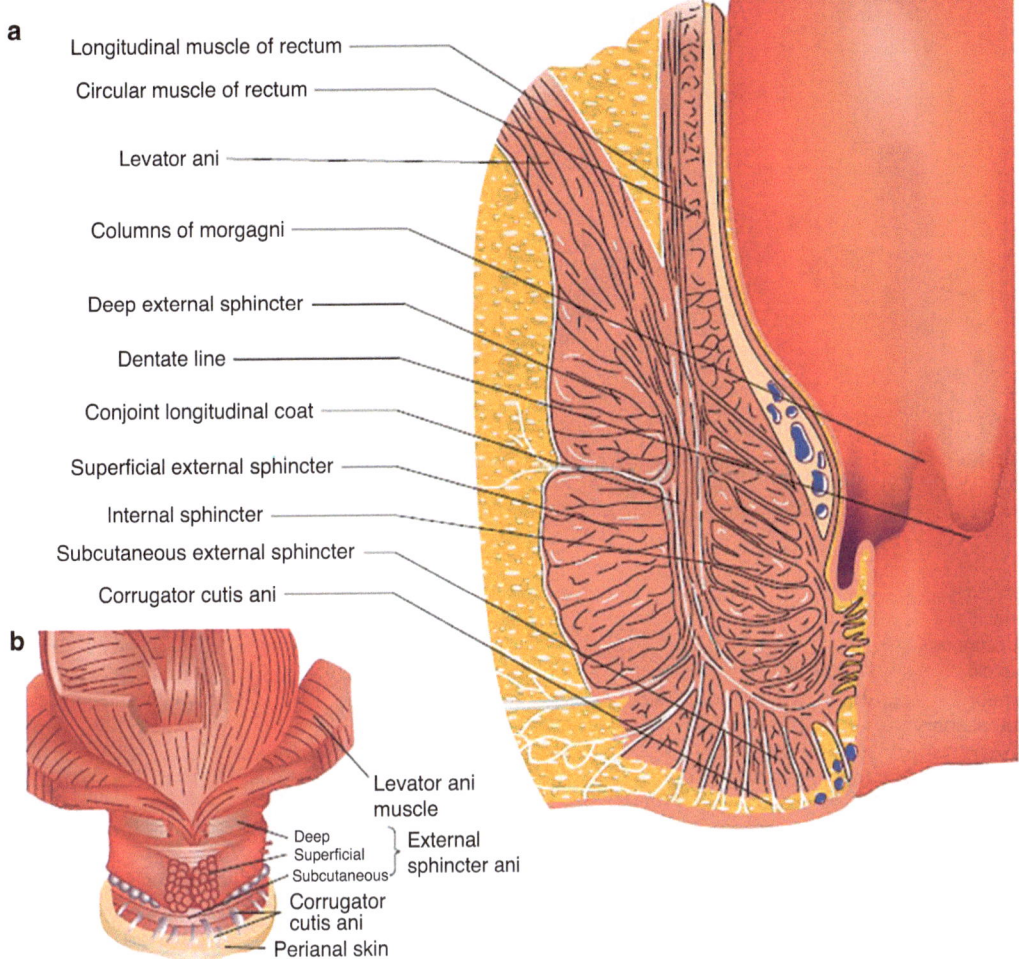

a
- Longitudinal muscle of rectum
- Circular muscle of rectum
- Levator ani
- Columns of morgagni
- Deep external sphincter
- Dentate line
- Conjoint longitudinal coat
- Superficial external sphincter
- Internal sphincter
- Subcutaneous external sphincter
- Corrugator cutis ani

b

Levator ani muscle

Deep
Superficial } External
Subcutaneous } sphincter ani
Corrugator cutis ani
Perianal skin

Fig. 1.5 (**a**) Coronal section of the anorectum. (**b**) Anal sphincter complex and levator ani muscle. (Figure from previous edition)

expand into three anal cushions. These cushions seal the anal canal and help maintain continence of flatus and liquid stools. The columns are joined together at their inferior margin by crescentic folds called anal valves [3]. About 1–2 cm from the anocutaneous line, the anal valves create a demarcation called the pectinate line (dentate line). The anoderm covers the last 1–2 cm of the distal canal below the pectinate line and consists of modified squamous epithelium that lacks skin adnexal tissues such as hair follicles and glands but contains numerous somatic nerve endings. Since the epithelium in the lower canal is well-supplied with sensory nerve endings, acute distension or invasive treatment of hemorrhoids in this area causes profuse discomfort, whereas treatment can be carried out with relatively few symptoms in the upper canal, which is lined by insensate columnar epithelium [13]. As a result of tonic circumferential contraction of the sphincter, the skin is arranged in radiating folds around the anus called the anal margin [12]. These folds appear to be flat or ironed out when there is underlying sphincter damage. The junction between the columnar and squamous epithelia is referred to as the anal transitional zone, which is variable in height and position and often contains islands of squamous epithelium extending into columnar epithelium. Sensory receptors in this zone likely play a role in maintaining continence

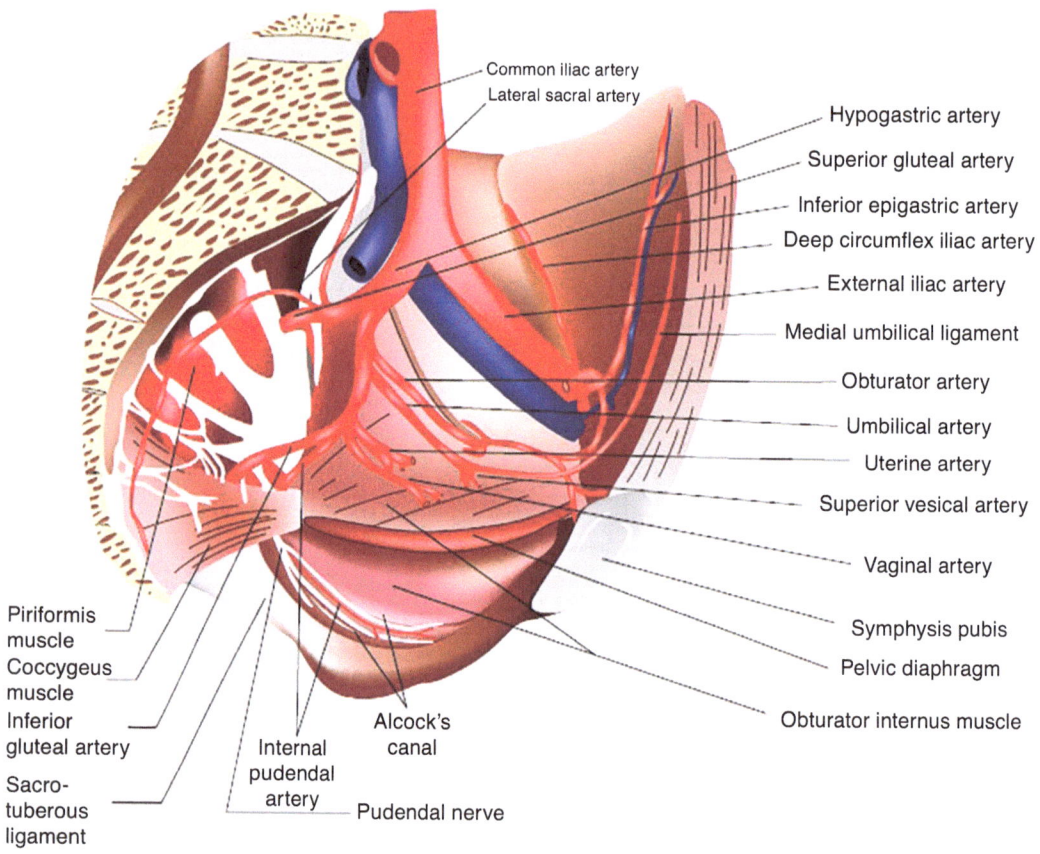

Common iliac artery
Lateral sacral artery
Hypogastric artery
Superior gluteal artery
Inferior epigastric artery
Deep circumflex iliac artery
External iliac artery
Medial umbilical ligament
Obturator artery
Umbilical artery
Uterine artery
Superior vesical artery
Vaginal artery
Symphysis pubis
Pelvic diaphragm
Obturator internus muscle
Piriformis muscle
Coccygeus muscle
Inferior gluteal artery
Sacro-tuberous ligament
Internal pudendal artery
Alcock's canal
Pudendal nerve

Fig. 1.6 Sagittal view of the pelvis demonstrating the pathway of the pudendal nerve and blood supply. (Figure from previous edition)

by providing a highly specialised sampling mechanism (see Chap. 8).

1.3.2.2 Anal Sphincter Complex

The anal sphincter complex consists of the EAS and IAS separated by the conjoint longitudinal coat (Figs. 1.5a and 1.7). Although they form a single unit, they are distinct in structure and function.

External Anal Sphincter

Structurally, the EAS (Figs. 1.5a and 1.7) is subdivided into three parts: subcutaneous, superficial, and deep [14]. Though these subdivisions are not easily demonstrable during anatomical dissection or surgery, they may be of relevance during imaging (see Chap. 10). In females, the EAS is shorter anteriorly (Fig. 1.8) [15]. The deep EAS is intimately related to the puborectalis muscle and does not have posterior attachments [16]. The superficial EAS is fused anteriorly to the perineal body and attached posteriorly to the anococcygeal ligament, which is attached to the tip of the coccyx [13]. The subcutaneous part is circular, but may have attachments to the perineal body anteriorly and the anococcygeal ligament posteriorly. As the only EAS subcomponent that is circular in shape, this is the only part that crosses the midline of the perineum. In females, the bulbospongiosus and the superficial transverse perineal muscles fuse with the EAS in the lower part of the perineum [13].

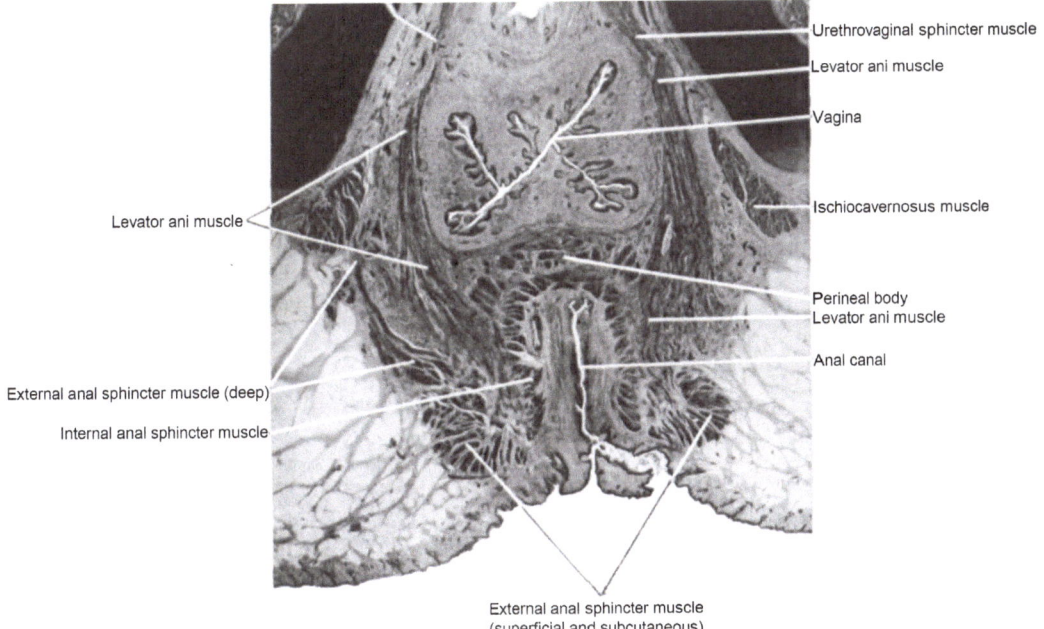

Urethrovaginal sphincter muscle

Levator ani muscle

Vagina

Ischiocavernosus muscle

Perineal body
Levator ani muscle

Anal canal

Levator ani muscle

External anal sphincter muscle (deep)

Internal anal sphincter muscle

External anal sphincter muscle
(superficial and subcutaneous)

Fig. 1.7 Histologic cross section of the pelvis and anal sphincter complex at the level of the anal canal. (Modified from Urogenitalmuskulatur des Dammes by Otto Kalischer, 1900 [9])

Internal Anal Sphincter

The IAS is a thickened continuation of the circular smooth muscle of the bowel and ends with a well-defined rounded edge 6–8 mm above the anal margin at the junction of the superficial and subcutaneous part of the EAS (Fig. 1.5, Fig. 1.7). In contrast to the EAS, which has a reddened appearance due to its striated muscle composition, the IAS has a pale appearance to the naked eye.

The Longitudinal Layer and the Conjoint Longitudinal Coat

The longitudinal layer is situated between the EAS and IAS and consists of a fibromuscular layer, the conjoint longitudinal coat, and the intersphincteric groove (intersphincteric space) with its connective tissue components [17] (Fig. 1.5a). The longitudinal layer has a muscular and fibroelastic component. The muscular component is formed by the fusion of the striated muscle fibres from the puboanalis, the innermost part of the puborectalis, with smooth muscle from the longitudinal muscle of the rectum [13]. Traced downward, it separates opposite the lower border of the IAS, with the fibrous septae fanning out to pass through the EAS and ultimately attach to the skin of the lower anal canal and perianal region [14].

1.3.2.3 Innervation of the Anal Sphincter Complex

As the IAS is a continuation of the circular fibres of the rectum, it shares the same innervation: sympathetic (L5) and parasympathetic nerves (S2–S4). It remains in a state of tonic contraction and accounts for 50–85% of the anal canal resting tone [11]. The conjoint longitudinal coat is innervated by autonomic fibres from the same origin. The EAS is innervated by the inferior rectal branch of the pudendal nerve. In contrast to the other striated muscles, the EAS contributes up to 30% of the unconscious resting tone through a reflex arc at the cauda equine level.

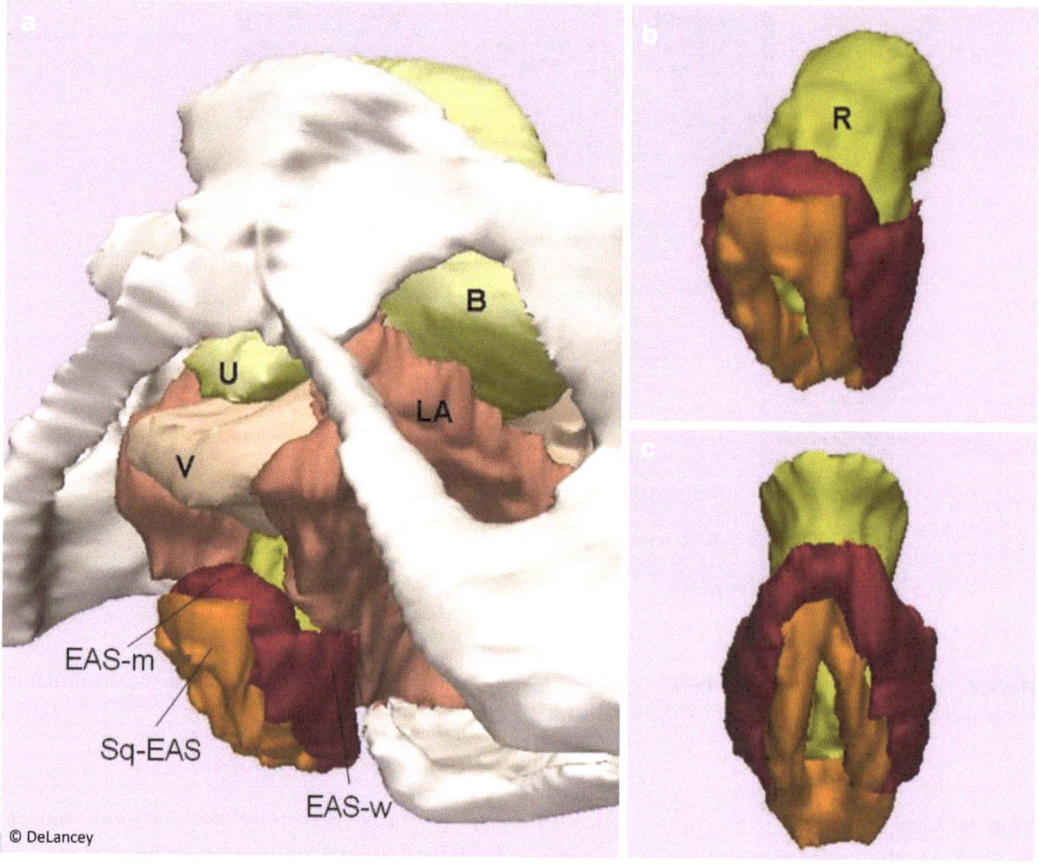

Fig. 1.8 (**a**) Computer reconstruction demonstrating the anal sphincter complex: external anal sphincter (*EAS*), puborectalis muscle (*PRM*), and internal anal sphincter (*IAS**). *Bl* Bladder, *Ut* uterus, *V* vagina, *R* rectum. (**b**) Isometric view of the anal sphincter complex and rectum. (**c**) Midline view of the anal sphincter complex and rectum. (Figure from previous version)

1.3.2.4 Vascular Supply

The anorectum receives its major blood supply from the superior rectal artery (superior haemorrhoidal artery), the terminal branch of the inferior mesenteric artery, and the inferior rectal artery (inferior haemorrhoidal artery), a branch of the internal pudendal artery. To a lesser degree, it also receives blood from the middle rectal artery (middle haemorrhoidal artery), a branch of the internal iliac artery. Together, these arteries form a wide intramural network of collateral vessels [18]. The venous drainage of the upper anal canal mucosa, IAS, and conjoint longitudinal coat passes via the terminal branches of the superior rectal vein into the inferior mesenteric vein. The lower anal canal and the EAS drain via the inferior rectal branch of the internal pudendal vein into the internal iliac vein [13].

1.3.2.5 Lymphatic Drainage

The anorectum has a rich network of lymphatic plexuses. The pectinate line represents the interface between the two different systems of lymphatic drainage. Above the pectinate line (the upper anal canal), the IAS and the conjoint longitudinal coat drain into the inferior mesenteric and internal iliac nodes. Lymphatic drainage below the pectinate line, which consists of the lower anal canal epithelium and the EAS, proceeds to the external inguinal lymph nodes.

1.3.2.6 Ischioanal Fossa

The ischioanal fossa (ischiorectal fossa) extends around the anal canal and is bound anteriorly by the perineal membrane, superiorly by the fascia of the levator ani muscle, and medially by the EAS complex at the level of the anal canal. The lateral border is formed by the obturator fascia and inferiorly by a thin transverse fascia, which separates it from the perianal space. The ischioanal fossa contains fat and neurovascular structures, including the pudendal nerve and the internal pudendal vessels, which enter through the pudendal canal (Alcocks's canal).

1.4   Perineal Body

The perineal body is the central point between the urogenital and anal triangles of the perineum (Fig. 1.2). Its three-dimensional form has been likened to that of the cone of the red pine, with each "petal" representing an interlocking structure, such as a fascia insertion site or a muscle of the perineum [19]. Within the perineal body, there are interlacing muscle fibres from the bulbospongiosus, superficial transverse perineal, and EAS muscles. Above this level there is a con-

tribution from the conjoint longitudinal coat and the medial fibres of the puborectalis muscle. Therefore, the support of the pelvic structures, and to some extent the hiatus urogenitalis between the levator ani muscles, depends on the integrity of the perineal body.

1.5   The Pelvic Floor

The pelvic floor, or pelvic diaphragm, is a musculotendineous sheet that spans the pelvic outlet and consists mainly of the symmetrically paired levator ani muscles (Fig. 1.9). The fasciae investing the muscles are continuous with the visceral pelvic fascia above, perineal fascia below, and obturator fascia laterally. The pelvic floor supports the urogenital organs and the anorectum, exiting the pelvis through their respective foramen. The muscles of the levator ani differ from most other skeletal muscles in that they: (1) maintain constant tone, except during voiding, defaecation, and manoeuvres that cause an increase in intraabdominal pressure (e.g., Valsalva manoeuvre); (2) have the ability to contract quickly in response to an abrupt increase in intraabdominal pressure (such as a cough or

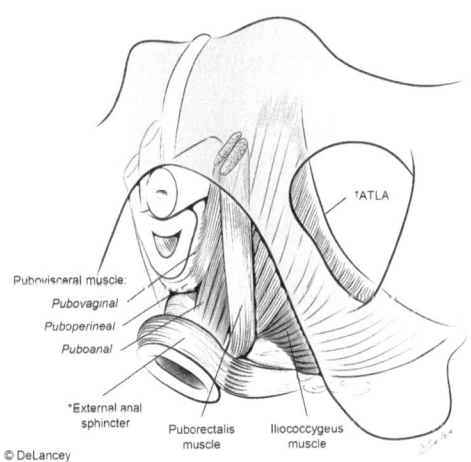
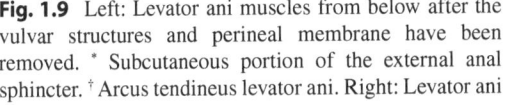
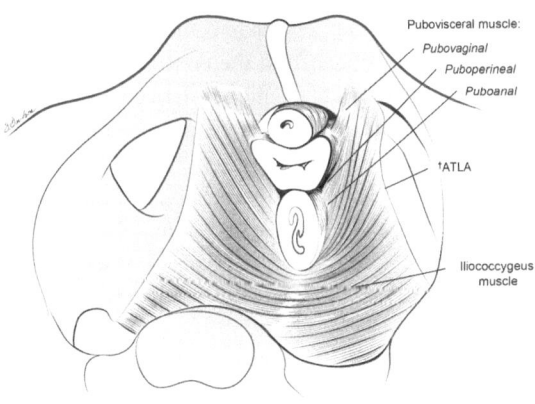

Fig. 1.9 Left: Levator ani muscles from below after the vulvar structures and perineal membrane have been removed. * Subcutaneous portion of the external anal sphincter. † Arcus tendineus levator ani. Right: Levator ani muscle seen from above. The internal obturator muscles have been removed to clarify levator muscle origins. © DeLancey (modified from Kearney, 2004)

sneeze) to maintain continence; and (3) distend considerably during parturition to allow the passage of the term infant and then contract after delivery to resume normal functioning [20].

The levator ani (Fig. 1.9) is a broad muscular sheet of variable thickness attached to the internal surface of the true pelvis and is subdivided into three portions: iliococcygeus, pubococcygeus, and puborectalis [6]. These portions were historically named based on pelvic structures to which they were thought to be attached. However, it is important to note that while "pubococcygeus" is the accepted *Terminologia Anatomica* term for this portion based on historic nomenclature, most of the muscle inserts to the walls of the vagina and the anorectum rather than the coccyx. As such, some anatomists have recommended the alternative term "pubovisceral" to better capture the origin and insertion of the muscle in its nomenclature [21, 22]. Although referred to as separate muscles, the boundaries between the different parts cannot be easily distinguished and they perform many similar physiological functions.

The iliococcygeus muscle is the lateral component of the levator ani muscle and arises from the ischial spine inferior and anterior to the attachment of the ischiococcygeus and to the obturator fascia as far anterior as the obturator canal; this area constitutes the tendinous arch of the levator ani muscle. The most posterior fibres are attached to the coccyx and the sacrum, but most join with fibres from the contralateral side to form a raphe, which is more or less continuous with the fibroelastic anococcygeal ligament and is attached to the coccyx.

The pubococcygeus muscle, also referred to as the pubovisceral muscle, is often subdivided into three parts according to the pelvic viscera to which they relate: puboperinealis, pubovaginalis, and puboanalis [21]. While all three parts originate from the pubis, their insertions differ; the puboperinealis part inserts into the perineal body, the pubovaginalis part inserts into the vaginal wall at the level of the mid-urethra, and the puboanalis inserts into the intersphincteric groove between the EAS and IAS (Fig. 1.9). Together, the three parts of the pubococcygeal muscle elevate the perineal body, vagina (at the level of the mid-urethra), and anus toward the pubis.

The puborectalis, which originates from the pubis and forms a sling around the rectum, is the most caudal component of the levator ani complex. It is situated cephalad to the deep component of the EAS, from which it is almost inseparable (Figs. 1.4a, b and 1.8). Thus the puborectalis serves both functions, as part of the sphincter mechanism and of the pelvic floor. The U-shaped sling of striated muscle pulls the anorectal junction anteriorly to the posterior aspect of the pubis [11], resulting in an angulation between the rectal and anal canal called the anorectal angle. There is considerable controversy as to the importance of this angle in the maintenance of continence [23]. Between the two arms of the puborectalis lies the levator hiatus, through which the rectum, vagina, and urethra pass.

The coccygeus muscle (ischiococcygeus muscle) may be considered as a separate muscle. It is a narrow triangular sheet of muscular and tendinous fibres, with its apex arising from the spine of the ischium and sacrospinous ligament and its base inserting into the margin of the coccyx and into the side of the lowest piece of the sacrum. It assists the levator ani and piriformis in closing the posterior portion of the pelvic outlet.

In the female, the anterior fibres of the levator ani descend upon both sides of the vagina. These fibres have been called the puboperineal muscle and appear to undergo the greatest stretch during vaginal delivery [24]. They have been found to be damaged in women with urinary incontinence and pelvic organ prolapse following delivery [25, 26].

1.5.1   Innervation of the Levator Ani

Although it is widely believed that the levator ani is innervated by the sacral nerve roots (S2–S4) on its superior surface and by the perineal branch of the pudendal nerve on its inferior surface, recent cadaveric dissections along with nerve staining studies have shown that the female levator ani is not innervated by the pudendal nerve, but rather by innervation that originates in the sacral nerve roots (S3–S5) and travels on the superior surface of the pelvic floor (levator ani nerve) [20].

The most common arrangement appears to be that the pubococcygeus is supplied by second and third sacral spinal segments via the pudendal nerve, and the puborectalis and iliococcygeus by direct branches from third and fourth sacral spinal segments [6].

1.5.2 Vascular Supply

The levator ani is supplied by branches of the inferior gluteal artery, the inferior vesical artery, and the internal pudendal artery.

1.6 The Pudendal Nerve

The pudendal nerve derives its fibres from the ventral branches of the second, third, and fourth sacral nerves and leaves the pelvis through the lower part of the greater sciatic foramen (Fig. 1.6). It then crosses the ischial spine and re-enters the pelvis through the lesser sciatic fora-men. It accompanies the internal pudendal vessels superiorly and anteriorly along the lateral wall of the ischioanal fossa, contained in a sheath of the obturator fascia termed the pudendal canal (Alcock's canal) (Fig. 1.6). It is presumed that during a prolonged second stage of labour, the pudendal nerve is vulnerable to stretch injury due to its relative immobility at this site.

The inferior rectal nerve (inferior haemorrhoidal nerve) then branches off posteriorly from the pudendal nerve to innervate the EAS (Fig. 1.10). The pudendal nerve then divides into two terminal branches: the perineal nerve and the dorsal nerve of the clitoris. The perineal nerve, the inferior and larger of the two terminal branches of the pudendal, is located inferior to the internal pudendal artery. It divides into posterior labial and muscular branches. The posterior labial branches supply the labium majora. The muscular branches are distributed to the superficial transverse perineal, bulbospongiosus, ischio-

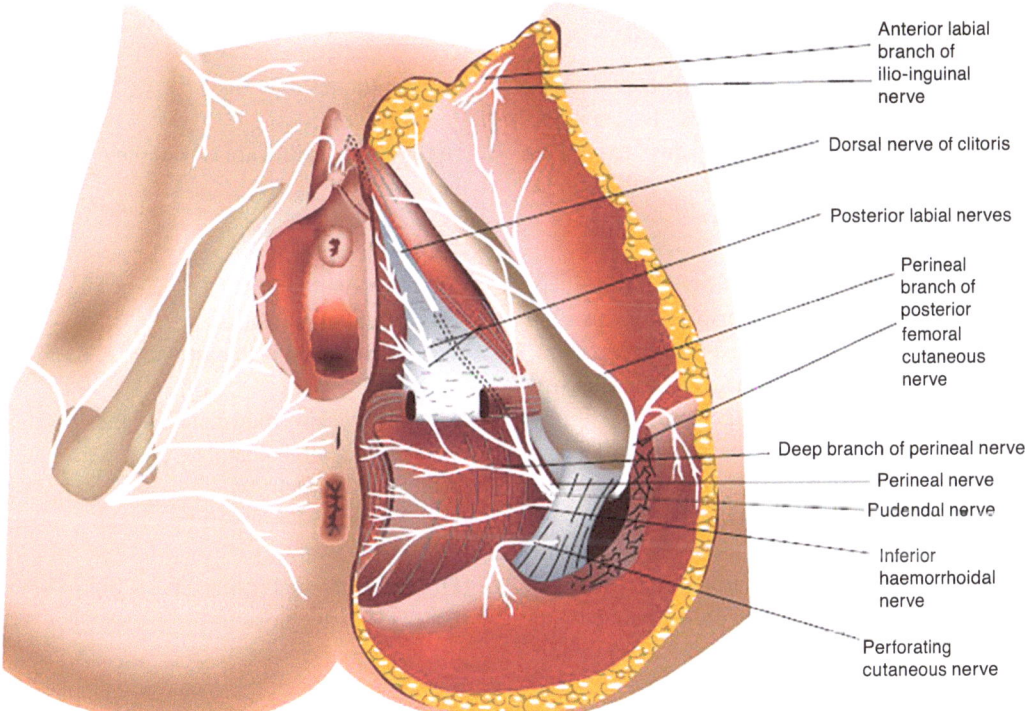

Fig. 1.10 Terminal branches of the pudendal nerve. (Figure from previous edition)

cavernosus, and compressor urethrae muscles. Branches from the perineal division frequently innervate the anterior EAS as well. The dorsal nerve of the clitoris, which innervates the clitoris, is the deepest division of the pudendal nerve (Fig. 1.10).

1.7   Conclusion

An understanding of the anatomy of the pelvic floor, anal sphincter complex, and perineum is essential for health care providers to care for patients during and after vaginal delivery. Proper perineal laceration and anal sphincter repair requires clear visualisation of structures comprising the perineal body and anal sphincter complex. When trauma occurs, the practitioner must be aware of the relationships between nerves, muscles, and vessels in order to restore, at best, normal anatomy and function.

Take Home Messages

- The anatomy of the pelvic floor, perineum, and anal sphincter complex is complex. Anatomical knowledge in this region is derived from surgical dissection, radiographic imaging, and tissue histology.
- The anatomic perineum corresponds to the outlet of the pelvis. It is bound anteriorly by the pubic arch, posteriorly by the coccyx, and laterally by the ischiopubic rami, ischial tuberosities, and sacrotuberous ligaments. In contrast, the perineal body refers to the area between the vagina and anus.
- The perineum can be divided into two triangular parts, the urogenital triangle and the anal triangle. The urogenital triangle includes the urethra with its associated surrounding structures, perineal membrane, superficial transverse perineal muscle, and bulbospongeosus muscle, among other structures. The anal triangle includes the anal canal, anal sphincter muscles, and ischioanal fossa.

- The anal sphincter complex consists of the external anal sphincter (EAS) and internal anal sphincter (IAS). Structurally, the EAS is subdivided into three parts: subcutaneous, superficial, and deep.
- The pelvic floor, or pelvic diaphragm, is a musculotendineous sheet that spans the pelvic outlet and consists mainly of the symmetrically paired levator ani muscles. The levator ani muscle is subdivided into three portions: iliococcygeus, pubococcygeus, and puborectalis.

Appendix: MCQ

Mark each item TRUE or FALSE

Questions

1. Which muscles comprise the levator ani?
   - (A)   Iliococcygeus
   - (B)   Coccygeus
   - (C)   Pubococcygeus (pubovisceral)
   - (D)   Puborectalis
   - (E)   Obturator internus

2. The anatomic perineum is bound by: Select all that apply.
   - (A)   Pubic arch
   - (B)   Coccyx
   - (C)   Ischiopubic rami
   - (D)   Ischial tuberosities
   - (E)   Sacrotuberous ligaments

3. Which muscles contribute to the perineal body? Select all that apply.
   - (A)   Bulbospongiosus
   - (B)   Superficial transverse perineal
   - (C)   Puborectalis
   - (D)   External anal sphincter
   - (E)   Ischiocavernosus

4. What is the name of the demarcation in the anal canal marking the transition between stratified squamous and simple columnar cells?
   - (A)   Anocutaneous line
   - (B)   Anal margin

(C) Pectinate line (dentate line)

(D) Anorectal junction

(E) Anal column

5. What is the origin of the pudendal nerve? Select all that apply.
   (A) S1
   (B) S2
   (C) S3
   (D) S4
   (E) S5

Answers

1. Which muscles comprise the levator ani?
   (A) TRUE
   (B) FALSE
   (C) TRUE
   (D) TRUE
   (E) FALSE

2. The anatomic perineum is bound by: Select all that apply.
   (A) TRUE
   (B) TRUE
   (C) TRUE
   (D) TRUE
   (E) TRUE

3. Which muscles contribute to the perineal body? Select all that apply.
   (A) TRUE
   (B) TRUE
   (C) FALSE
   (D) TRUE
   (E) FALSE

4. What is the name of the demarcation in the anal canal marking the transition between stratified squamous and simple columnar cells?
   (A) FALSE
   (B) FALSE
   (C) TRUE
   (D) FALSE
   (E) FALSE

5. What is the origin of the pudendal nerve? Select all that apply.
   (A) FALSE
   (B) TRUE
   (C) TRUE
   (D) TRUE
   (E) FALSE

References

1. Federative Committee on Anatomical Terminology. Terminologia Anatomica: International Anatomical Terminology. 2nd ed. Stuttgart: Thieme Stuttgart; 2019.
2. Lunsman HH, Robertson EG. Evolution of the pelvic floor. In: Benson JT, editor. Female pelvic floor disorders. Scranton: W.W. Norton & Co.; 1992.
3. Cook TA, Mortensen N. Colon, rectum, anus, anal sphincters and the pelvic floor. In: Pemberton JH, Swash M, Henry MM, editors. The pelvic floor: its function and disorders. London: W.B. Saunders; 2001.
4. Levi AC, Borghi F, Garavoglia M. Development of the anal canal muscles. Dis Colon Rectum. 1991;34(3):262–6.
5. Moore KL. The urogenital system. In: Moore KL, editor. The developing human. 2nd ed. London: W.B. Saunders; 1977.
6. Karram M, Yuen HTH. Lesser pelvis and perineum. In: Standring S, editor. Gray's anatomy. 42nd ed. Amsterdam: Elsevier; 2020.
7. Brandon CJ, Lewicky-Gaupp C, Larson KA, Delancey JO. Anatomy of the perineal membrane as seen in magnetic resonance images of nulliparous women. Am J Obstet Gynecol. 2009;200(5):583.e581–6.
8. Stein TA, DeLancey JO. Structure of the perineal membrane in females: gross and microscopic anatomy. Obstet Gynecol. 2008;111(3):686–93.
9. Kalischer O. Die Urogenitalmuskulatur des Dammes. Berlin: Verlag von S. Karger; 1900.
10. Wendell-Smith CP. Anorectal nomenclature: fundamental terminology. Dis Colon Rectum. 2000;43(10):1349–58.
11. Carmichael JC, Mills S. Anatomy and embryology of the colon, rectum, and anus. In: Steele SR, Hull TL, Read TE, Saclarides TJ, Senagore AJ, Whitlow CB, editors. The ASCRS textbook of colon and rectal surgery. 3rd ed. Cham: Springer International Publishing; 2016.
12. Kaiser AM, Ortega AE. Anorectal anatomy. Surg Clin North Am. 2002;82(6):1125–38. v
13. Bhullar JS. Large intestine. In: Standring S, editor. Gray's anatomy. 42nd ed. Amsterdam: Elsevier; 2020.
14. Milligan ETC, Morgan CN. Surgical anatomy of the anal canal with special reference to anorectal fistulae. Lancet. 1934;224(5804):1150–6.

15. Sultan AH, Kamm MA. Ultrasound of the anal sphincter. In: Schuster MM, Crowell MD, Koch KL, editors. Schuster atlas of gastrointestinal motility in health and disease. Baltimore: Williams & Wilkins; 1993.

16. Oh C, Kark AE. Anatomy of the external anal sphincter. Br J Surg. 1972;59(9):717–23.

17. Lunniss PJ, Phillips RK. Anatomy and function of the anal longitudinal muscle. Br J Surg. 1992;79(9):882–4.

18. Lund JN, Binch C, McGrath J, Sparrow RA, Scholefield JH. Topographical distribution of blood supply to the anal canal. Br J Surg. 1999;86(4):496–8.

19. Woodman PJ, Graney DO. Anatomy and physiology of the female perineal body with relevance to obstetrical injury and repair. Clin Anat. 2002;15(5):321–34.

20. Barber MD, Bremer RE, Thor KB, Dolber PC, Kuehl TJ, Coates KW. Innervation of the female levator ani muscles. Am J Obstet Gynecol. 2002;187(1):64–71.

21. Kearney R, Sawhney R, DeLancey JO. Levator ani muscle anatomy evaluated by origin-insertion pairs. Obstet Gynecol. 2004;104(1):168–73.

22. Lawson JO. Pelvic anatomy. I. Pelvic floor muscles. Ann R Coll Surg Engl. 1974;54(5):244–52.

23. Bartolo DCC, Macdonald ADH. Faecal incontinence and defecation. In: Pemberton JH, Swash M, Henry MM, editors. The pelvic floor: its function and disorders. London: W.B. Saunders; 2001.

24. Lien KC, Mooney B, DeLancey JO, Ashton-Miller JA. Levator ani muscle stretch induced by simulated vaginal birth. Obstet Gynecol. 2004;103(1):31–40.

25. Hoyte L, Schierlitz L, Zou K, Flesh G, Fielding JR. Two- and 3-dimensional MRI comparison of levator ani structure, volume, and integrity in women with stress incontinence and prolapse. Am J Obstet Gynecol. 2001;185(1):11–9.

26. DeLancey JO, Kearney R, Chou Q, Speights S, Binno S. The appearance of levator ani muscle abnormalities in magnetic resonance images after vaginal delivery. Obstet Gynecol. 2003;101(1):46–53.

Pathophysiology and Effects of Pregnancy on the Pelvic Floor

John O. L. DeLancey and Fernanda Pipitone

Overview

Test your learning and check your understanding of this book's contents: use the "Springer Nature Flashcards" app to access questions using ▶ https://sn.pub/wqrf89. To use the app, please follow the instructions in Chap. 1.

Learning Points

- What are the inciting factors for pelvic floor disorders and their separate injury mechanisms.
- What is the prevalence of childbirth-related pelvic floor injury and how they are related to the failure of the hiatal closure mechanism and to the development of prolapse later in life.
- What hypotheses have been considered to explain levator ani muscle injury and what is our current understanding of its mechanism.

- How delivery may impact urethral function and support.
- In which ways childbirth can lead to anal incontinence.

2.1 Introduction

Vaginal birth is one of the most important causes of pelvic organ prolapse, as well as urinary and anal incontinence—problems collectively known as pelvic floor disorders (PFDs) [1–4]. For vaginal delivery to occur, the pelvic floor must rapidly undergo changes unprecedented in the human body (Fig. 2.1). In considering the role of childbirth in causing different PFDs, it is important to emphasize that the pelvic floor is not a single entity, but an intricately interconnected, complex collection of structures. Each element might be affected in unique ways, while at the same time, injury to one aspect of the complex may be associated with adjacent structure damage or may affect the normal function of others. Our ability to prevent birth-related injuries—and to understand management of the disorders that result when they do occur—depends on a *precise* understanding of the structural anatomy, interactions among different anatomic elements, mechanism of injury to those elements, and how these injuries can ultimately relate to pelvic floor disorders.

J. O. L. DeLancey (✉)
Pelvic Floor Research Group, Departments of Obstetrics and Gynecology and Urology, University of Michigan, Ann Arbor, MI, USA
e-mail: delancey@med.umich.edu

F. Pipitone
University of São Paulo, São Paulo, Brazil

a

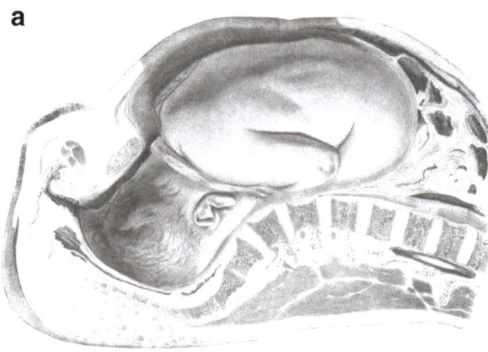

b

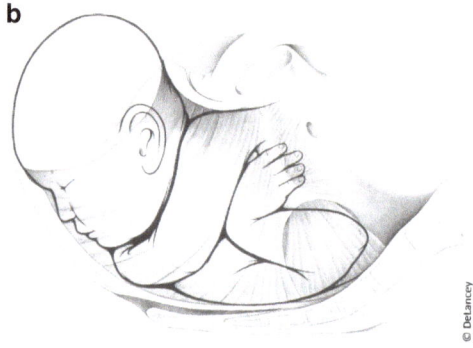

© DeLancey

Fig. 2.1 Discrepancy between the large fetal size and small pelvic floor opening (**a**) and the situation during the late second stage of birth (**b**) showing the remarkable pelvic floor changes required during birth. (**a**, from Bumm, 1921 [5]; **b**, ©DeLancey)

2.2   Pelvic Floor Anatomy

During vaginal birth, the primary changes that are related to pelvic floor disorders are those occurring in the lower birth canal involving DeLancey Level III of support and closure mechanisms [6–9]. We refer to the structures that close the lower vaginal canal as the "perineal complex," which is comprised of (1) the levator ani muscles, (2) the perineal membrane, and (3) the perineal body and associated connective tissues (Fig. 2.2).

The levator ani muscle consists of three portions: the pubovisceral (also known as the pubococcygeal), the iliococcygeal, and the puborectal (Fig. 2.3). The pubovisceral, in turn, has three portions: the pubovaginal, the puboperineal, and the puboanal [11, 12]. The three components of the pubovisceral muscle lift the perineal structures and close the hiatuses in the pelvic floor. The names of its subdivisions indicate the structures to which it is attached (vagina, perineal body, and anus). The puborectal muscle arises lateral to the pubovisceral muscle and passes dorsally to the anorectal junction. Whereas both the pubovisceral and puborectal muscles can act to close the pelvic floor, only the pubovisceral muscle can lift perineal structures because of its more vertical orientation. The iliococcygeal muscle is a thin sheet of muscle that spans the pelvic canal from the tendinous arch of the levator ani to the midline iliococcygeal raphe, where it interdigitates with the muscle of the other side and connects with the superior surface of the sacrum and coccyx. Pelvic floor closure in Level III is provided by the pubic portions of the levator ani muscles and their connections to the perineal membrane and perineal body in the perineal complex. Damage to any one of the three components (levator, perineal membrane, perineal body) can affect the others, since they all work in consonance to maintain perineal closure.

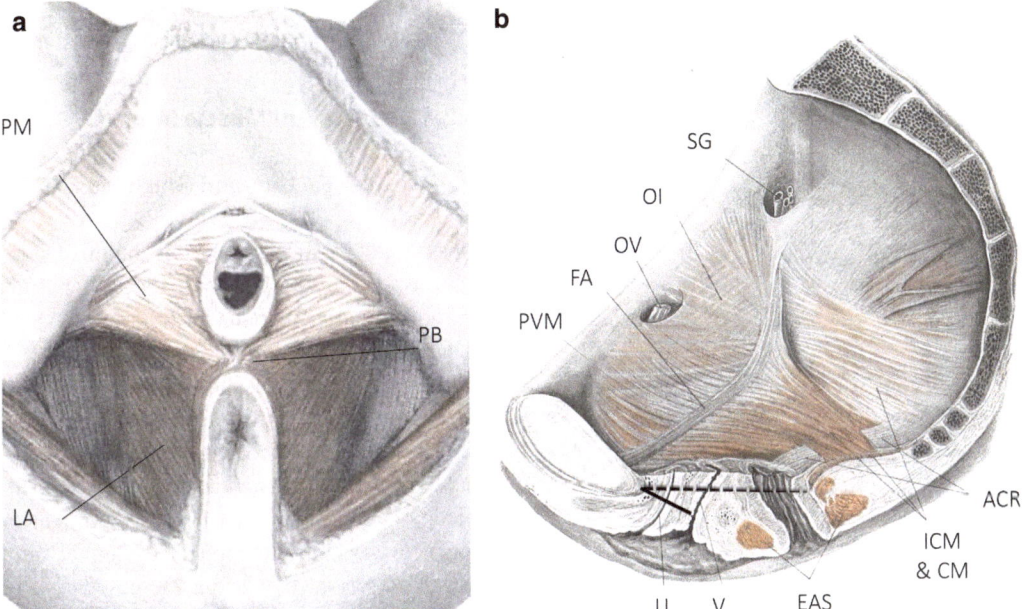

Fig. 2.2 Perineal complex seen in dissections as viewed from below (**a**) showing the levator ani (LA), perineal body (PB), and perineal membrane (PM). (**b**) Left lateral view of the pelvis after removal of the upper pelvic organs, showing antero-posterior diameter of urogenital hiatus (solid line) and levator hiatus (dotted line). *CM* coccygeus muscle, *ICM* iliococcygeal muscle, *OC* obturator canal, *OI* obturator internus muscle, *OV* obturator vessels, *SG* superior gluteal vessels, *PVM* pubovisceral muscle, *FA* fascial arch (=arcus tendinous fascia pelvis), *R* rectum, *U* urethra, *V* vagina, *EAS* external anal sphincter, *ACR* ano-coccygeal raphe. Dotted lines, levator hiatus; solid line, urogenital hiatus. (From Halban and Tandler (1907) [10])

2.3 Pelvic Floor Changes

2.3.1 Pelvic Floor Changes in Preparation for Birth

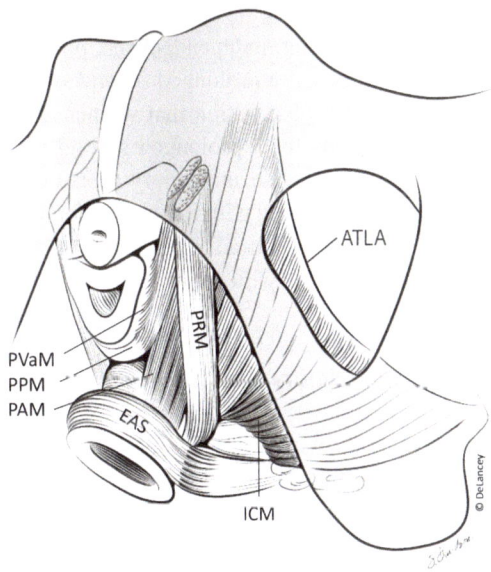

Fig. 2.3 Levator ani muscles viewed from below after the vulvar structures and perineal membrane have been removed. *ATLA* arcus tendineus levator ani, *EAS* external anal sphincter, *ICM* iliococcygeal muscle, *PAM* puboanal muscle, *PB* perineal body, *PPM* puboperineal muscle, *PRM* puborectal muscle, *PVaM* pubovaginal muscle. (© DeLancey; modified from Kearney (2004) [11])

Accommodation of a 10 cm fetal head through a 2.5 cm diameter opening in the pelvic floor is one of the most remarkable phenomena in all human biology (Fig. 2.4). It would not be possible without the major changes that happen to the pelvic floor in preparation for delivery. For example, between 21 and 37 weeks of gestation, there is a 17–29% increase in the size of the levator hiatus area at rest and a 13–26% increase during maximal contraction force [13]. In addition, studies in rats have shown that muscles around the birth canal add sarcomeres late in pregnancy, allowing for 20–30% fibre elongation [14]. Connective tissue in the extracellular matrix also increases 50–140% in these muscles. Some hypothesize that these changes could reduce how much the

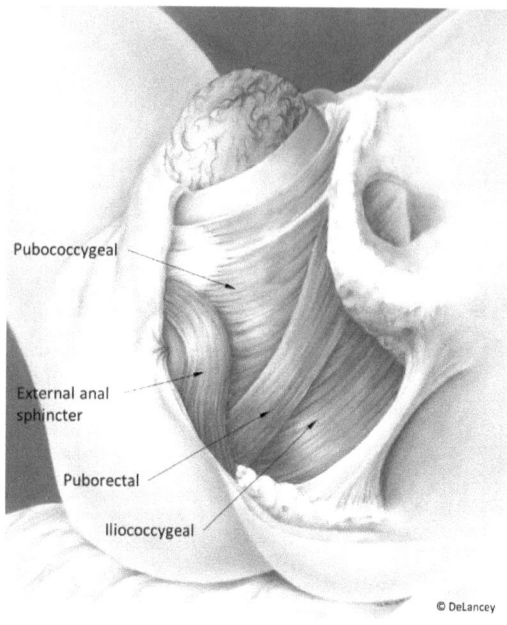

Fig. 2.4 Levator ani muscle subdivisions and external anal sphincter at crowning of the fetal head (pubococcygeal = pubovisceral). (© DeLancey 2002)

muscles would have to lengthen and how that plays a role in decreasing stretch-induced injury. Yet perhaps the most remarkable changes occur in the viscoelastic properties ("stretchiness") of the connective tissues and muscles of the birth canal. Biomechanical studies have documented these changes [15], but the hormonal factors responsible for this phenomenon have not yet been established. How this happens before birth and how the connective tissue recovers after birth remain a mystery.

2.3.2 Pelvic Floor Injury During Birth

Vaginal birth increases the likelihood that a woman will develop a pelvic floor disorder [2–4] and has also been identified as a cause of levator ani muscle damage. Understanding how and what type of levator injury can occur and how recovery does or does not proceed are central both to optimizing postpartum care for new mothers and to ultimately developing preventive

strategies in the delivery room to decrease the risk of these injuries.

2.3.2.1 Levator Ani Muscle Injury

Incidence, Risk Factors, and which Muscle Is Injured

Injury to the levator ani muscle is the most studied birth-related injury to the pelvic floor aside from obstetrical anal sphincter injuries (OASIS) and has been reported in 13% of women [16]. These levator injuries usually involve the pubovisceral portion of the muscle (Fig. 2.5) and occasionally the iliococcygeal muscle [17].[1] Dietz et al. have presented an overview of birth-related pelvic muscle injury [19]. Several factors associated with more complicated vaginal birth were also associated with an increased risk of levator injury. These included the use of forceps, a longer second stage of labor, and a larger head circumference. In several studies, forceps delivery is associated with levator injury rates as high as 63% [20–23], with an odds ratio of 3.8 for muscle avulsion in the study by Krofta et al. [20]. Similarly, a longer second stage of labor has been associated with an increased levator hiatus area (OR 1.01 per minute; 95% CI 1.0–1.02) [16]. However, the greater, independent risk posed by forceps compared to a prolonged second stage is supported by the observation that women delivered with forceps for a prolonged second stage have a higher rate of levator injury (63%) compared to those delivered with forceps for fetal distress (42%) [23]. A head circumference over 35.5 cm is associated with an odds ratio of 3.3 for levator injury [24].

Mechanism of Injury and Concept of Injury Spectrum

Among women with pubovisceral muscle injuries, the amount of muscle damage varies. Some of these injuries involve complete, bilateral loss

---

[1] Ultrasound literature frequently uses the term puborectal muscle for the pubovisceral muscle. Studies that have examined what the anatomists call the puborectal muscle as described earlier in this chapter show that it is the pubovisceral muscle that is injured [18].

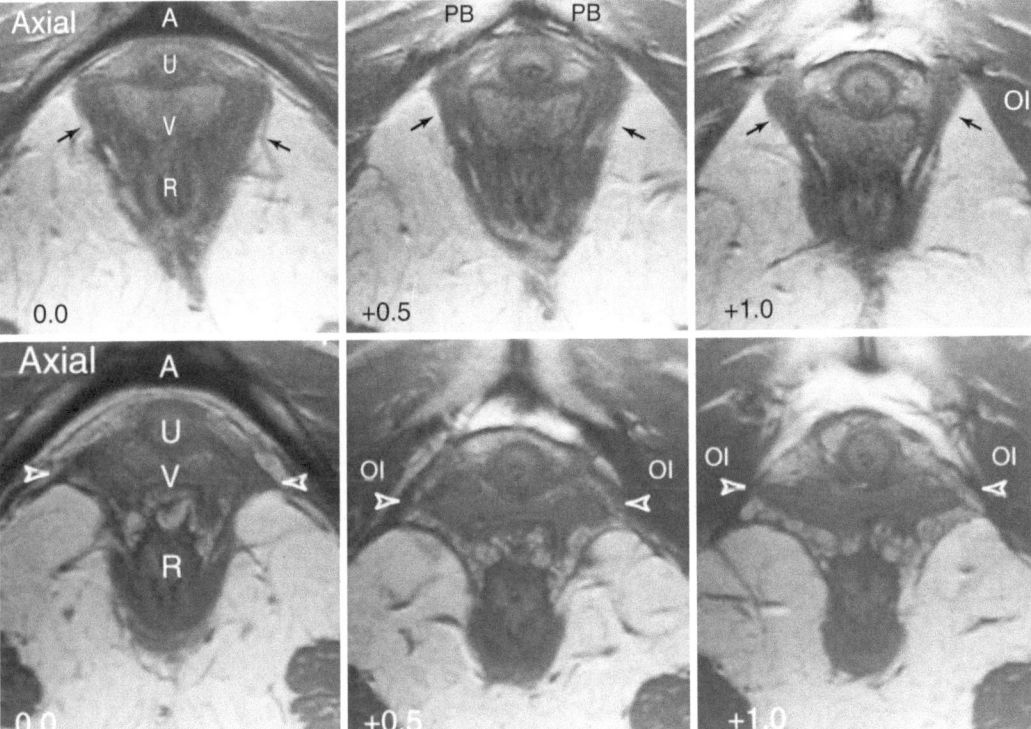

Fig. 2.5 Top row shows axial MRI from primiparous woman with normal levator ani muscles (arrows). Lower row shows an individual with a complete pubovisceral muscle tear. The location of the missing muscle is indicated (open arrowheads). The vagina protrudes laterally into the defects to lie close to the obturator internus muscle (OI). Locations relative to the arcuate ligament (+ indicates cephalad to the ligament) shown in the lower left corner in cm. *A* arcuate pubic ligament, *R* rectum, *PB* pubic bone, *U* urethra, *V* vagina. (Modified from DeLancey (2003) [17])

of pubovisceral muscle bulk (Fig. 2.5), while others have only unilateral loss (Fig. 2.6). There is also variation in the amount of architectural distortion [25] that occurs, as seen in Fig. 2.5, views +0.5 and +1.0 where the vagina extends laterally to reach the obturator internus muscle.

What Is the Cause of Levator Ani Injury?

Several injury mechanisms have been hypothesized, namely (1) neuropathy/nerve injury, (2) muscle tearing or stretching, and (3) compression. Techniques used in musculoskeletal MRI to determine injury mechanisms have been applied to study the muscle in women at high risk for injury after vaginal birth [26]. The injury mechanisms were evaluated using fluid-sensitive and anatomical sequences made in the early (1 month) and late (7 months) postpartum periods. Levator

injuries were seen in seven of 19 women, all of whom experienced focal tears at the muscle's insertion into the pubic bone. Interestingly, delayed atrophy, where the muscle is relatively normal early and shows loss of muscle bulk late (consistent with nerve injury), was not seen in any of the women. It is known that tissue edema is radiographically present both with muscle compression and muscle stretching or tearing. In these cases, if the resulting muscle edema was due to compression, it would be expected to involve the internal obturator muscle that shares the space between the fetal head and pubic bone. While all subjects were found to have edema in the levator ani muscle, none exhibited it in the obturator muscle—indicating that edema was caused by muscle stretch/tear rather than compression. Subsequent studies in a larger study

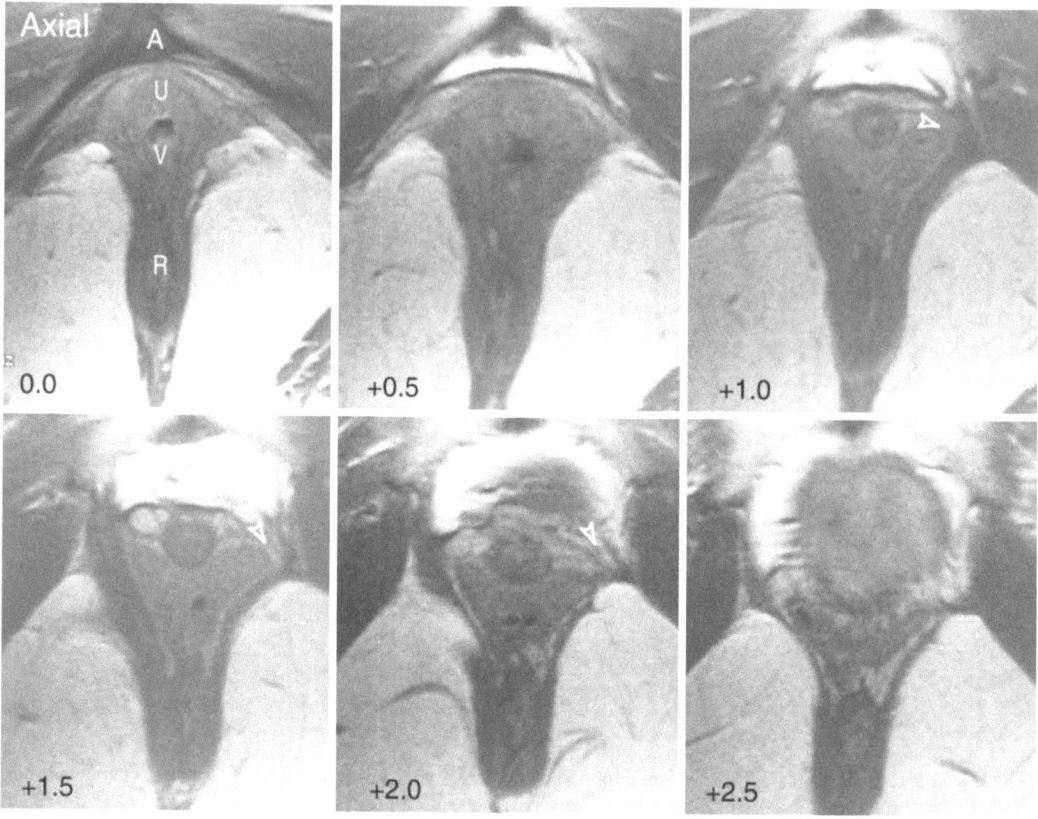

Fig. 2.6 Axial MRI scans from a 34-year-old incontinent primiparous woman showing a unilateral defect in the left pubovisceral portion of the levator ani muscle. The arcuate pubic ligament (A), urethra (U), vagina (V), rectum (R), and bladder (B) are shown. The location normally occupied by the pubovisceral muscle is indicated by the open arrowhead in images 1.0, 1.5, and 2.0. (From DeLancey (2003) [17])

sample (n = 69) have confirmed these findings and have shown the associated bony injuries that also occur [27]. While the earliest studies of muscle injury used electrodiagnostic techniques that demonstrated that birth causes changes in mean motor unit duration after vaginal birth [28], as well as neuropathic changes outside the normal range in turns/amplitude data in 29% of women at 6 months postpartum [29], it is not this injury that causes loss of levator bulk seen on MRI.

Stretching and Tearing Is the Cause of Injury

Biomechanical simulation helps explain the muscle stretching that occurs during vaginal birth. Using a computer model of the levator ani muscle based on anatomy from a nulliparous woman, Lien et al. studied the degree to which individual muscle bands are stretched (Fig. 2.7) [31]. This analysis revealed that the portion of muscle that was injured most often, the pubovisceral (pubococcygeal), was the one that underwent the greatest degree of stretch. Not surprisingly, the second most common area of observed injury, the iliococcygeal muscle, was the second most stretched portion. Furthermore, when the portion of the muscle at risk was identified in cross-sections cut in the same orientation as axial MRI scans, the pattern of predicted injury matched the injury seen in MRI (Fig. 2.8). Further studies that include the viscoelastic properties of the muscle have revealed that the pubovisceral muscle enthesis and the muscle near the perineal body are the regions of greatest strain, thereby placing them at highest risk for stretch-related injury. Decreasing perineal body

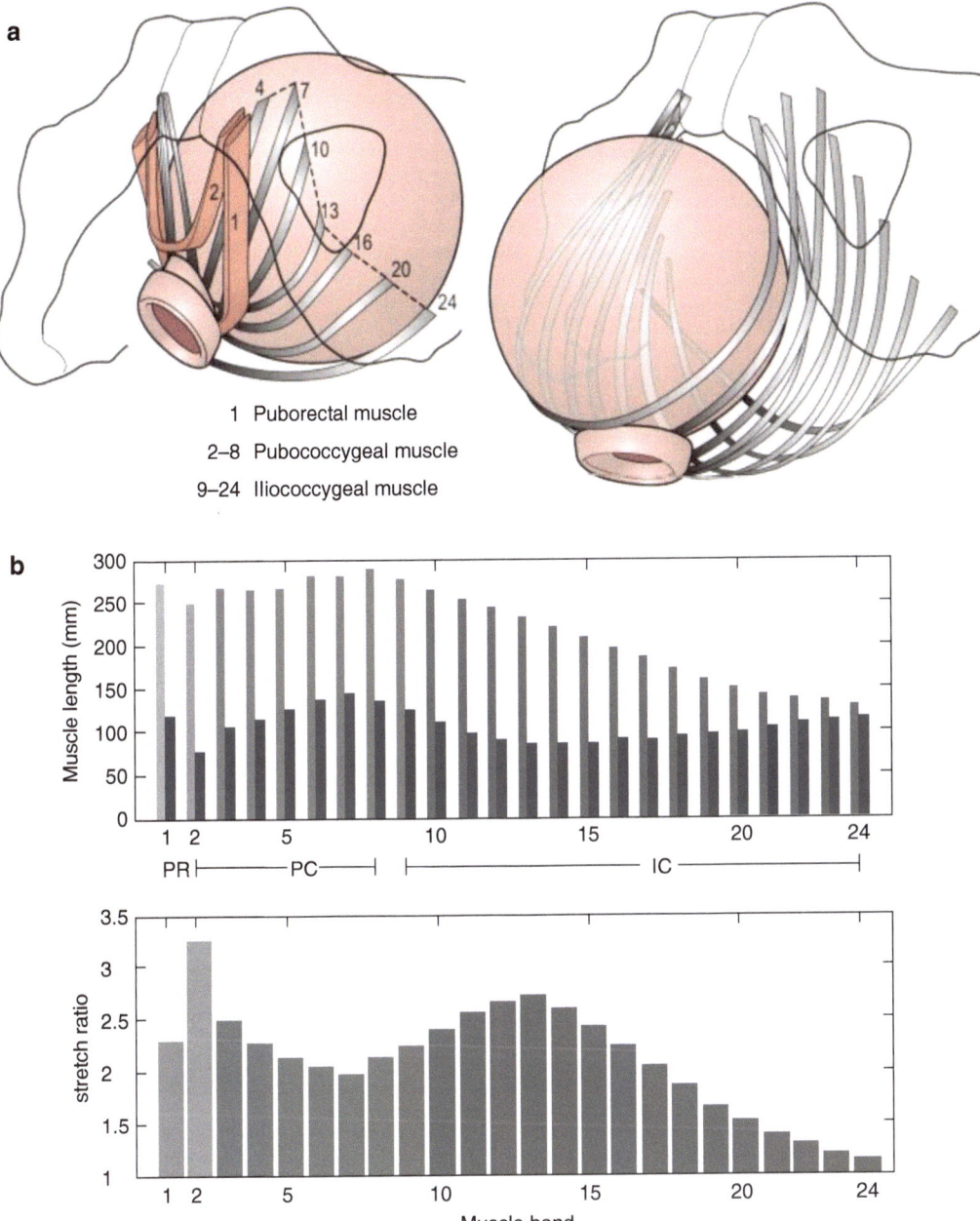

a

1 Puborectal muscle
2–8 Pubococcygeal muscle
9–24 Iliococcygeal muscle

b

Fig. 2.7 (**a**) Computer model of selected levator ani muscle bands before birth, with muscle fibers numbered and the muscle groups identified (left); the figure on the right demonstrates muscle band lengthening present at the end of the second stage of labor. (**b**) Original and final muscle lengths (top graph) and the stretch ratio (bottom graph), indicating the degree to which each muscle band must lengthen to accommodate a normal-sized fetal head. Note that the pubococcygeal muscle fascicles labeled band 2 undergo the greatest degree of stretch and would be the most vulnerable to stretch-induced injury. (Modified from Lien, 2004 [30] © DeLancey 2016)

tissue stiffness significantly reduced tissue stress and strain—and therefore injury risk—in those regions [32–34]. Reducing perineal tissue stiffness by hot compresses and perineal massage may be a mechanism that reduces perineal trauma at vaginal delivery.

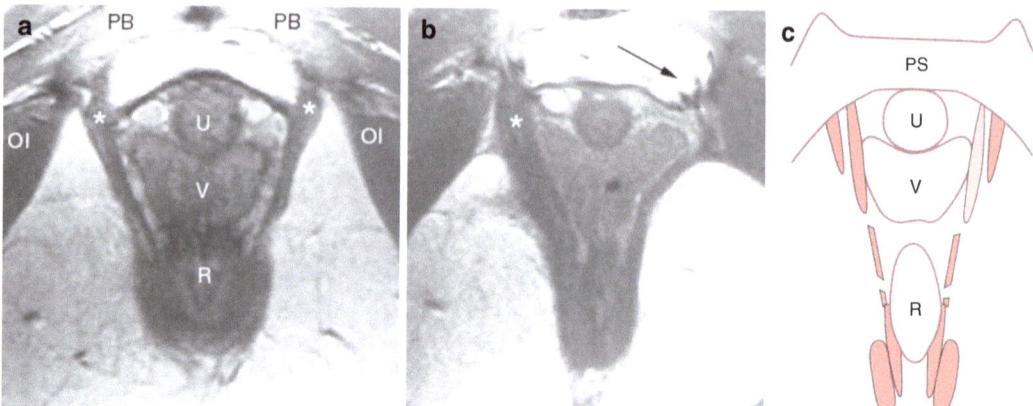

Fig. 2.8 (a) Normal anatomy in an axial mid-urethra proton density MRI showing the pubovisceral muscle (*). (b) Woman who has lost a part of the left pubovisceral muscle (displayed on the right side of the image, according to standard medical imaging convention) with lateral displacement of the vagina into the area normally occupied by the muscle. The arrow points to the expected location of the missing muscle. The puborectalis is left intact bilaterally. (c) Axial, mid-urethral section of the model through the arch of the pubic bone (see pubic symphysis [PS], top) and the model levator ani muscles corresponding to those from the patients shown in (a) and (b). Intact muscles are shown in dark shading. Simulated pubococcygeal muscle loss (equivalent to band 2 from Fig. 2.7) is illustrated by the light shading of the left-side muscle. *OI* obturator internus muscle, *PB* pubic bone, *R* rectum, *U* urethra, *V* vagina. (Modified from Lien, 2004 [30] ©DeLancey)

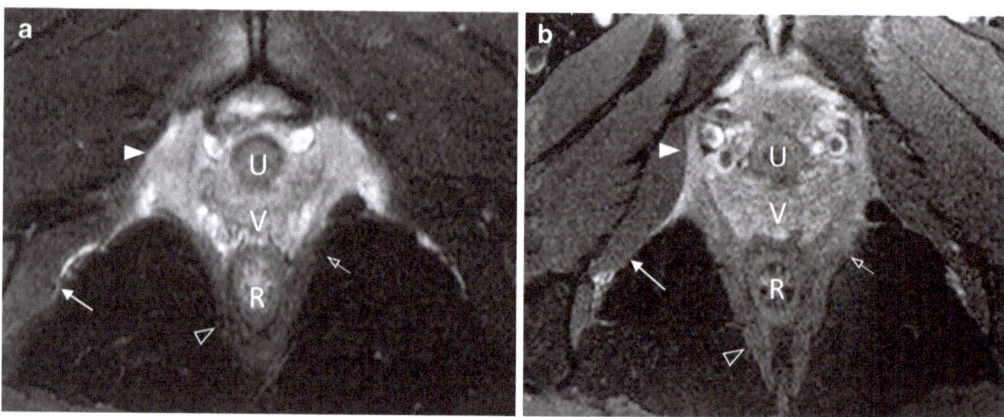

Fig. 2.9 Fluid-sensitive axial MRI scans 6–8 weeks postpartum of two women (a and b) at the level where the pubovisceral (closed arrowhead) and the puborectal (open arrowhead) fibers diverge. Open arrow indicates transition between edema in the pubococcygeal and lack of edema in the puborectal muscles. Obturator internus muscle is indicated (closed arrow). *U* urethra, *V* vagina, *R* rectum. (From Pipitone, 2021 [35])

Computer simulations indicating that the pubovisceral muscle is subject to the largest stretch are now confirmed clinically with information about edema patterns within the muscle (Fig. 2.9). Edema in the injured levator is localized; the location of these changes in MR signals can be mapped to show areas of stretch-induced injury in the absence of full muscle disruption [35]. In a group of 78 women at high risk for levator ani muscle injury during delivery, 51% showed muscle edema in the pubovisceral muscle, while only 5% had involvement of the puborectal and 5% of the iliococcygeal muscles. The pubovisceral muscle was seven times more likely than other muscles to show the edema, adding further evidence that muscle stretching, and tearing is an important mechanism of injury because it occurs in the parts of the muscle that are, in fact, stretched the most.

2.3.3 Recovery After Vaginal Birth

Childbirth represents a biomechanical overload to the pelvic floor, and after being stretched to 3–4 times its original fiber length [30, 36], the levator muscles and birth canal connective tissue must go through a period of recovery. Imaging has allowed us to study the process of normal recovery and provided insights into changes the muscle must undergo to return to its healthy state.

2.3.3.1 How Do the Hiatuses Recover?

Soon after delivery, the urogenital hiatus is wider than at baseline [20, 37–39] (Fig. 2.10). The decrease in hiatus size after vaginal delivery mostly happens in the first 4–6 months postpartum and is most rapid in the first 2 weeks. Increased fluid from edema in certain muscle parts early in recovery reveals the chemical changes in muscular tissue during the healing process [35]. In most women, muscle recovery

results in resumption of the near-baseline position over the course of the first 6 months—the time when pelvic muscle strength also returns to baseline [40].

Current evidence shows that while levator hiatus size (similar to urogenital hiatus size) decreases gradually after vaginal delivery, it does not return to first trimester size or nulliparous metrics in all women. The decrease in levator hiatus size after vaginal delivery also mostly happens in the first 4–6 months postpartum [38, 41] and is also most rapid in the first 2 weeks [37]. When compared to nulliparous women, the levator hiatus antero-posterior diameters at 4.5 months postpartum were larger by 30% at rest and 36% with Valsalva [42]. To the contrary, in a study including women who underwent caesarean delivery before the second stage of labor, levator hiatus area at rest 4–6 months postpartum was not significantly different from that in the first trimester, but it was significantly smaller during Valsalva and Kegel (9% and 6%, respectively) than in the first trimester [43]. This implies that levator hiatus size in women following caesarean delivery might be able to recover back to pre-pregnancy values, especially when it occurred before the second stage labor.

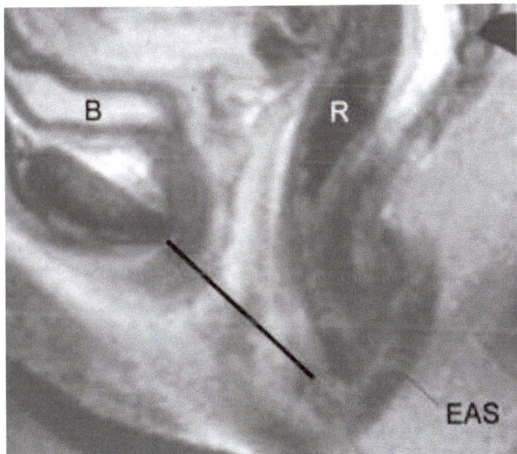
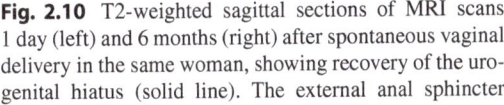
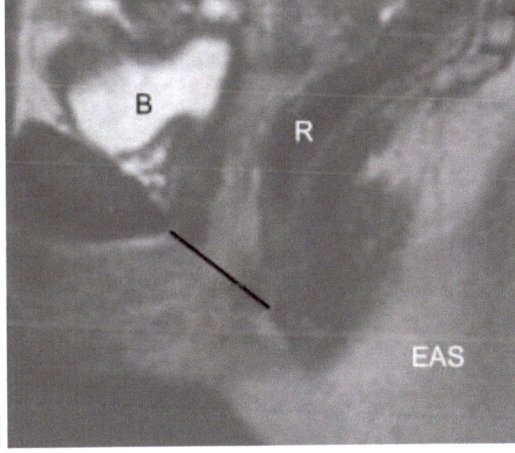

Fig. 2.10 T2-weighted sagittal sections of MRI scans 1 day (left) and 6 months (right) after spontaneous vaginal delivery in the same woman, showing recovery of the urogenital hiatus (solid line). The external anal sphincter (EAS) and perineal body that lies ventral to it are much lower on the first day after delivery compared with the anatomy 6 months later. (From Tunn, 1999 [37])

2.4   The Hiatus and Pelvic Floor Disorders

2.4.1   How Does High Pressure Zone Contribute to Providing Support?

Injury to the levator ani muscles has been the most extensively studied birth-induced injury associated with pelvic floor disorders—namely, pelvic organ prolapse and widened genital hiatus. However, more recently, it has been recognized that levator injury is not the only factor involved in hiatal enlargement.

The openings in the pelvic floor through which birth occurs, the urogenital and levator hiatuses, are the largest hiatuses in the body (Fig. 2.2) and can become enlarged and "gaping" with pelvic floor disorders (Fig. 2.11). Effectively maintaining closure of these hiatuses is altered by vaginal birth, and knowledge of the consequences of those injuries is essential to the understanding of the causes and prevention of pelvic floor disorders. The ability to maintain successful closure is dependent on the creation of a vaginal "high-pressure zone" [44, 45], much like those created by the anal and urethral sphincter muscles to maintain continence. The perineal complex that creates this area of increased vaginal pressure is dependent on intricate interactions between the levator ani muscles and their neural control mechanism, the perineal membrane, and the perineal body (Fig. 2.2). Women with levator defects have a lower vaginal closure force (2.0 N) compared to women without defects (3.1 N, $p < 0.001$) [46–48]. The levator hiatus area also increases in 28% of women with injury compared to 6% in those without injury [7].

2.4.2   An Enlarged Hiatus Is One Cause of Pelvic Organ Prolapse

It is well known that an enlarged genital hiatus (distance from the urethra to the perineal body on physical exam) is associated with pelvic organ prolapse [48–51] (Fig. 2.11). In addition, hiatal enlargement precedes the occurrence of prolapse, indicating a potentially causal relationship [52]. In a study by Handa et al., during the first 20 years after birth, approximately 25% of women with an enlarged hiatus followed prospectively developed prolapse at least 1 cm below the hymenal ring. For a woman with a 3 cm hiatus, the estimated median time to develop prolapse was 33 years, while for a woman with a 4.5 cm hiatus, it would be only 6 years [47]. Prolapse also is more common with reduced muscle strength (OR 0.9 per 5 cmH_2O). Prolapse was associated with

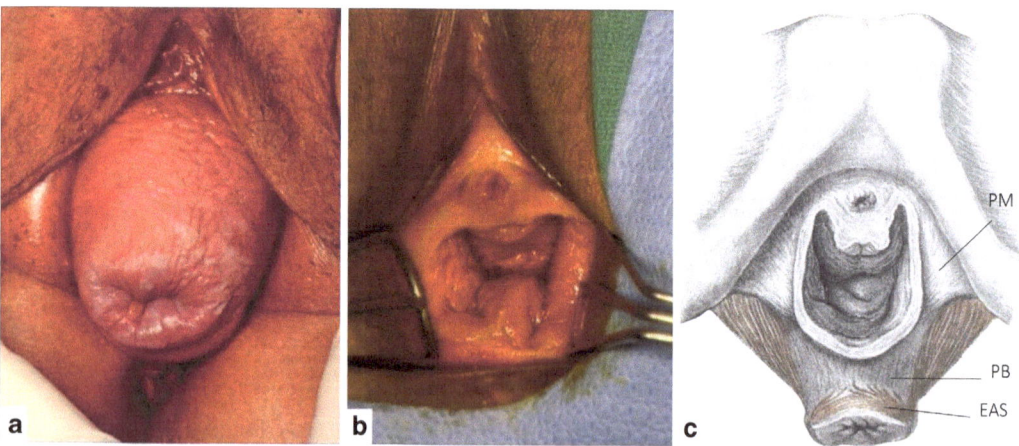

Fig. 2.11 (**a**) Uterine prolapse and (**b**) the enlarged hiatus seen when the prolapse is reduced. (**c**) Structural alterations responsible for the open hiatus seen in dissection of a cadaver with prolapse. *EAS* external anal sphincter, *LA* levator ani muscle, *PB* perineal body. (**c**, from Halban and Tandler (1907) [10])

levator avulsion (OR 4.2), and hiatus area and strength mediated 61% of the association between avulsion and prolapse.

2.4.3 Factors Affecting Hiatus Size

Recent studies have shown that, as important as the levator ani muscle is to maintaining hiatal size, it is not the only factor responsible for hiatal closure. For example, Nandikanti et al. showed that less than 25% of variation in hiatus size is attributable to the degree of muscle injury present on MRI [53]. When several aspects of pelvic floor hiatus closure are examined (muscle strength, perineal elevation with muscle contraction, descent during Valsalva, and visible muscle on MRI), they are each found to be independent contributing factors [51]. Correlations between these factors revealed that no one factor explains more than 20% of the variation in others. For example, only 4% of hiatus size was explained by muscle contraction strength. The only significant association was between levator defect status, and both resting urogenital hiatus and change in urogenital hiatus with straining. However, these were weak associations, only explaining 13% of variation in hiatus size [51].

2.4.4 The Perineal Complex

The other two components of the perineal complex, the perineal membrane and perineal body, are also abnormal in women with prolapse (Fig. 2.11) and are altered by pregnancy and childbirth. These structural alterations have been demonstrated using a recently-developed MRI-based reconstruction technique [54]. Preliminary analysis shows a caudal rotation of the membrane as a pregnancy effect, as well as separation of the two sides of the membrane from the midline as the most prominent childbirth-related structural change. The clinical consequences of these changes and their relationship to other Level III abnormalities have yet to be determined.

The connective tissues in the perineal body and lower birth canal are also greatly susceptible to the impact of childbirth. Experienced clinicians have observed that differences in these tissues among different ethnic groups may be related to pelvic floor injury during birth. Epidemiologic studies show, for instance, a higher prevalence of stress urinary incontinence in white women and suggest Black race as being protective for obstetric anal sphincter injury [55–57]. Since connective tissues are involved in supporting the urethra and the anal sphincter is intimately embedded in the connective tissues of the perineal body, differences in the vulnerability of these tissues based on racial differences might be important for a full understanding of birth and pelvic floor disorders. Specific mechanistic research has not yet been conducted to clarify the nature of these differences.

2.5 Pelvic Floor Dysfunctions in Relation to Birth Injuries

2.5.1 Pelvic Organ Prolapse

2.5.1.1 Levator Ani Injury at Birth and Prolapse

It is well known that levator injury at birth is a major factor in the development of pelvic floor disorders, especially pelvic organ prolapse. In a case-control study comparing the occurrence of major levator ani muscle defects that involve loss of more than 50% of the pubovisceral portion of the levator ani muscle, major defects were found in 16% of women with normal support and 55% of women with prolapse [46]. The women with prolapse also generated 37% less vaginal closure force during pelvic muscle contraction than controls (2.0 vs 3.2 N), and those with major levator defects generated 35% less force than women without defects. Among women attending a clinic for pelvic floor disorders, prolapse was seen in 150/181 (83%) women with avulsion and in only 265/600 (44%) women without avulsion [58].

2.5.1.2 Load Sharing Between Levator Ani and Connective Tissue

Understanding how birth contributes to the development of prolapse requires an understand-

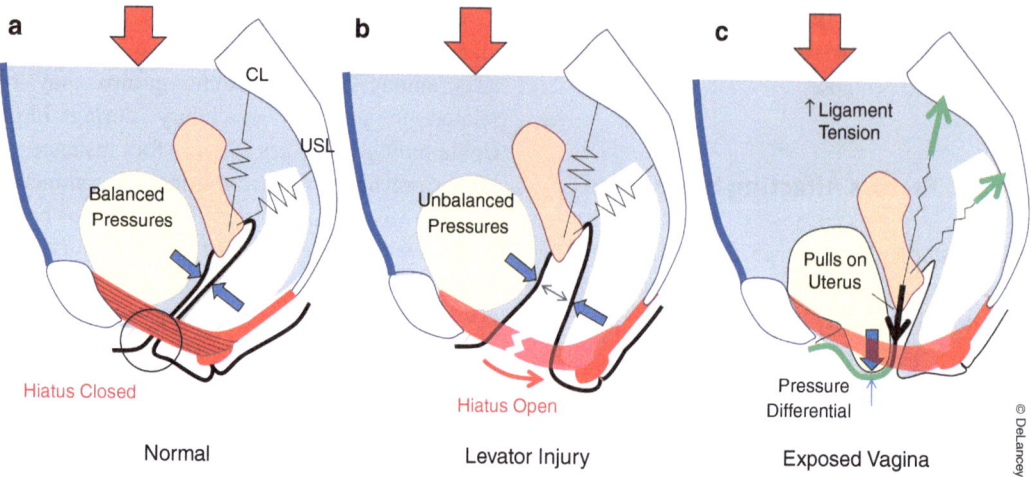

Fig. 2.12 Diagrammatic representation of interactions between levator ani muscle (red), anterior vaginal wall prolapse and cardinal/uterosacral ligament suspension. Red arrows represent the force created by gravity and abdominal pressure. With normal levator function (**a**), the hiatus is closed, and the vaginal walls are in apposition; the anterior and posterior pressures are equal and cancel each other (blue arrows). Levator damage (**b**) results in hiatal opening, and the vagina becomes exposed to a pressure differential between abdominal and atmospheric pressures. This pressure differential (**c**) makes the vaginal wall protrude (green) and creates a traction force on the cardinal ligament and uterosacral ligament. (©DeLancey)

ing of the basic mechanism of prolapse. To provide pelvic support, the muscles and ligaments must resist the downward force applied on the pelvic floor by the abdominal organs and the forces that arise from increases in abdominal pressure during cough, sneeze, or from inertial loads placed on them, such as when landing from a jump (Fig. 2.12). This normal load-sharing between the adaptive action of the muscles and the energy-efficient action of static connective tissues is part of the elegant load-bearing design of the pelvic floor. When injury to one of these two components occurs, the other must carry the increased demands placed on it. For example, when the muscle is injured, the connective tissue is subjected to increased load. If this load exceeds the strength of the pelvic tissues, they may be stretched or broken and prolapse may result. This forms a causal chain of events by which pelvic muscle injury may influence pelvic organ prolapse or urinary incontinence. In addition, there is accumulating evidence that women operated on for pelvic organ prolapse or urinary incontinence have higher postoperative failure rates if they have levator ani muscle impairment assessed by biopsy [59], muscle function testing [60], and ultrasound [61] than women who have undamaged muscles. There are also early differences in pelvic organ support seen after surgery depending on whether a levator defect is present [62]. Similarly, muscle avulsion is seen more commonly in women with anatomical recurrence at 2 years after reconstructive surgery compared to women with no avulsion [63].

2.5.2 Urinary Incontinence

2.5.2.1 Urethral Support and Birth

Vaginal birth is also associated with the development of stress urinary incontinence in many women [64]. In studies, primiparous women with new stress incontinence that persisted for at least 9 months had 25% lower urethral closure pressures (63 cmH$_2$O) than women who did not (84 cmH$_2$O, d = 0.91) [65]. Vesical neck movement on ultrasound during cough was 16 mm in incontinent women compared with only 11 mm in primiparous continent women (p < 0.001, d = 0.76). Major injuries to the levator ani muscles may have contributed to this incontinence, as they were twice as common (28%) in the incontinent group compared with the continent group (12%). Longitudinal studies show that there is an increase in urethral mobility 4 months after delivery when compared with support assessed in the third trimester [16]. Interestingly, the women who developed *de novo* stress incontinence did not have more mobility than those who did not. The cause for this increased mobility after birth may be related to levator ani muscle injury. Women studied 9 months after vaginal birth who had a major levator defect had similar urethral closure pressures at that timepoint than women who had intact muscles both at rest and during maximal contraction, indicating the independent nature of levator injury and urethral function [66].

There is useful evidence about whether pregnancy alters urethral function. A longitudinal study in healthy primigravidae showed that urethral function did not change throughout pregnancy and was similar to values seen in nulligravid women. Additionally, values in women who delivered by caesarean section were similar to pre-pregnancy values [67]. This would indicate that women who leak during pregnancy inherently have weaker urethral closure pressures, and that their sphincter weakness is likely attributed to the increased mechanical loads of the pregnant uterus. This hypothesis also could explain why women who experience stress incontinence during pregnancy are more prone to persistent incontinence. As vaginal birth often results in worse urethral support (which injury to the levator ani muscles contributes to), it determines, in association with the woman's inherited urethral function, whether she is going to be persistently incontinent after delivery. It should be noted that in middle-aged women presenting for treatment of stress urinary incontinence, there is no difference in levator injury and the difference in urethral function is greater [68]—indicating that the well-known decrease in urethral pressure over time [69, 70] becomes the dominant factor later in life.

2.5.2.2 Levator Ani Injury Associated Urethral Sphincter Dysfunction

When one pelvic floor structure is injured, other adjacent structures may be injured or affected as well. For example, birth-induced levator ani muscle injury may, or may not, be accompanied by changes in urethral function during pelvic muscle contractions. Overall, women with damaged levator muscles had a 24% lower urethral closure pressure during a maximal pelvic muscle contraction than women without damage (65.9 vs 86.8 cmH_2O, P = 0.004) [71]. However, levator injury does not necessarily affect urethral sphincter contraction in all women. Of 28 women with normal levator muscles on MRI and 17 women with complete bilateral pubovisceral muscle loss, those with intact muscles generated a greater increase in urethral pressure during a maximal pelvic muscle contraction than those with absent pubovisceral muscles (14 ± 11 vs 6 ± 9 cmH_2O) [72]. More of the women with intact muscles (86%) were able to elicit a measurable increase (>5 cmH_2O) in urethral closure than those with missing muscles (41%). Interestingly, however, among women in both groups who could increase urethral closure pressure, the increase in pressure was the same. This indicates that some women who are unable to contract their levator ani muscles (due to muscle or nerve injury) escape injury to the urethral sphincter and pudendal nerve and can therefore still volitionally elevate urethral pressure. Others, unfortunately, sustain injuries to both levator and urethral sphincter muscles and cannot.

2.5.3 Anal Incontinence

Fecal incontinence and obstetrical anal sphincter injury (OASI) will be covered extensively in other sections of this book, but a few comments here may be helpful. Although less strongly associated than urinary incontinence and pelvic organ prolapse, anal incontinence is certainly linked to childbirth [73, 74]. Two separate yet overlapping aetiologies have been discussed: (1) direct injury to the anal sphincter complex, and (2) damage to the pudendal nerve. OASI occurs in 3% of vaginal births, with primiparous women at 3.6-fold higher risk than multipara [75] for this trauma. Of these, 10–50% will develop fecal incontinence symptoms later in life [76–79]. There is also evidence that levator defects are associated with fecal incontinence. In a study of women with OASI at birth, women who had a levator tear seen in association with the sphincter tear trended toward more fecal incontinence (35.3%) compared to women who had sphincter laceration but intact levator ani muscles (16.7%, p = 0.10) [80]. This association is likely due to the common denominator of a complicated birth and the ability of the intact levator muscles to compensate for a torn sphincter.

2.5.3.1 Ultrasound Studies and Anal Incontinence

Ultrasound studies done 15–24 years after delivery reported odds ratios of 2.5 and 4 for fecal incontinence if external anal sphincter and internal anal sphincter defects were seen [81]. Pudendal nerve damage is probably attributable to the fact that the inferior rectal branch of the pudendal nerve is stretched the most during vaginal birth [31]. This is furthered by the findings that pudendal terminal motor latency is increased in women who delivered vaginally when compared to nullipara and those delivered by caesarean section [82, 83].

2.6   Summation

The historical concept that birth causes pelvic floor disorders because "everything gets stretched out" is giving way to a growing body of evidence concerning the specific pelvic floor failures that can occur due to vaginal birth. This expanding knowledge can help guide efforts toward injury prevention, more specific treatments for pelvic floor disorders, and, hopefully, a reduction in the problems some women experience due to their unique role in reproduction.

Take Home Messages

- Pelvic floor disorders, although grouped under the same name, should be considered separate entities that have different causes and therefore different injury mechanisms.
- In-depth knowledge of each injury mechanism is key to developing prevention strategies and individualized treatment plans.
- Pelvic organ prolapse is highly related to levator ani muscle injury and failure of the hiatal closure mechanism and the injury mechanism is muscle tearing rather than compression or neuropathy.
- Vaginal delivery only causes minor changes in urethral function. But does affect urethral support and therefore contributes to stress urinary incontinence.
- Although less strongly associated than urinary incontinence and pelvic organ prolapse, anal incontinence is certainly linked to childbirth. Symptoms seem to arise due to direct injury to the anal sphincter complex and/or damage to the pudendal nerve.

Funding Dr. DeLancey's effort for this work is supported by NIH grant RC2 DK122379.

Appendix: MCQ

Questions

1. Regarding pelvic floor anatomy, which of the following statements is false:
   - (A) The levator ani muscle is comprised of three portions: the pubovisceral (also known as the pubococcygeal), the iliococcygeal, and the puborectal portions.
   - (B) Although both the pubovisceral and puborectal muscles can act to close the pelvic floor, only the pubovisceral muscle can lift perineal structures due its more vertical orientation.

(C) Pelvic floor closure in Level III is provided by the pubic portions of the levator ani muscles and their connections to the perineal membrane and perineal body in the perineal complex.

(D) The iliococcygeal muscle is a thin sheet of muscle that spans the pelvic canal from the tendinous arch of the levator ani to the midline iliococcygeal raphe, and has a line of action similar to the puborectal muscle.

2. Regarding levator ani muscle injury during childbirth, which of the following statements is false:

(A) Different injury mechanisms have been hypothesized, namely (1) neuropathy/nerve injury, (2) muscle tearing or stretching, and (3) compression.

(B) The compression mechanism was not confirmed, as imaging methods show no edema in adjacent pelvic muscles also subject to compression by the fetal head—e.g. obturator internus muscle.

(C) Late postpartum MRI scans show muscle atrophy when compared to early postpartum imaging, which corroborates the nerve injury hypothesis.

(D) Biomechanical studies back up stretching and tearing as cause of levator ani muscle injury since the portion that shows the greatest degree of stretch in simulations—e.g. pubovisceral– is the most common area of observed injury.

3. Regarding pelvic organ prolapse, which of the following statements is false:

(A) Recent data shows that an enlarged urogenital hiatus precedes the development of pelvic organ prolapse.

(B) Levator ani muscle is the primary factor in maintaining hiatus size and other pelvic floor structures have lesser roles in the hiatal closure mechanism.

(C) Women with prolapse are more likely to have major levator ani muscle defects and to generate less vaginal closure force during pelvic floor muscle contraction than controls.

(D) There is accumulating evidence that women operated on for pelvic organ prolapse have higher postoperative failure rates if they have an enlarged urogenital hiatus preoperatively.

4. Regarding urinary incontinence, which of the following statements is false:

(A) Vaginal birth can potentially result in worse urethral support. However, there is no evidence that it affects urethral function.

(B) Women who leak during pregnancy might have an inherently weaker urethra that is unmasked by the increased mechanical loads of the pregnant uterus.

(C) Increased urethral mobility is strongly associated with stress urinary incontinence and is proven to be the major factor in determining whether a woman leaks or not.

(D) Major injuries to the levator ani muscle 9 months after vaginal delivery are twice as common in incontinent woman than in their continent counterparts.

5. Regarding anal incontinence, which of the following statements is false:

(A) Childbirth-related anal incontinence can have two separate yet overlapping etiologies: (1) direct injury to the anal sphincter complex, and (2) damage to the pudendal nerve.

(B) Pudendal nerve damage is probably attributable to the fact that the inferior rectal branch of the pudendal nerve is the branch that is stretched the most during vaginal birth.

(C) Obstetric anal sphincter injury is 3- to 4-fold more common in nulliparous than parous women and is often associated with levator ani avulsion.

(D) Nearly all woman who sustain obstetric anal sphincter injuries will develop anal incontinence symptoms later in life.

Answers

1. Regarding pelvic floor anatomy, which of the following statements is false:
   (A) FALSE
   (B) FALSE
   (C) FALSE
   (D) TRUE

2. Regarding levator ani muscle injury during childbirth, which of the following statements is false:
   (A) FALSE
   (B) FALSE
   (C) TRUE
   (D) FALSE

3. Regarding pelvic organ prolapse, which of the following statements is false:
   (A) FALSE
   (B) TRUE
   (C) FALSE
   (D) FALSE

4. Regarding urinary incontinence, which of the following statements is false:
   (A) FALSE
   (B) FALSE
   (C) TRUE
   (D) FALSE

5. Regarding anal incontinence, which of the following statements is false:
   (A) FALSE
   (B) FALSE
   (C) FALSE
   (D) TRUE

References

1. Lopez-Lopez AI, Sanz-Valero J, Gomez-Perez L, Pastor-Valero M. Pelvic floor: vaginal or caesarean delivery? A review of systematic reviews. Int Urogynecol J. 2021;32(7):1663–73. https://doi.org/10.1007/s00192-020-04550-8.
2. Mant J, Painter R, Vessey M. Epidemiology of genital prolapse: observations from the Oxford Family Planning Association Study. Br J Obstet Gynaecol. 1997;104(5):579–85.
3. Nygaard I, Barber MD, Burgio KL, Kenton K, Meikle S, Schaffer J, Spino C, Whitehead WE, Wu J, Brody DJ, Pelvic Floor Disorders N. Prevalence of symptomatic pelvic floor disorders in US women. JAMA. 2008;300(11):1311–6. https://doi.org/10.1001/jama.300.11.1311.
4. Rortveit G, Daltveit AK, Hannestad YS, Hunskaar S, Norwegian ES. Urinary incontinence after vaginal delivery or cesarean section. N Engl J Med. 2003;348(10):900–7. https://doi.org/10.1056/NEJMoa021788.
5. Bumm E. Grundriss zum Studium der Geburtschifte. J. F. Bergmann, München und Weisbaden; 1921.
6. van Delft K, Sultan AH, Thakar R, Schwertner-Tiepelmann N, Kluivers K. The relationship between postpartum levator ani muscle avulsion and signs and symptoms of pelvic floor dysfunction. BJOG. 2014;121(9):1164–71; discussion 1172. https://doi.org/10.1111/1471-0528.12666.
7. Shek KL, Dietz HP. The effect of childbirth on hiatal dimensions. Obstet Gynecol. 2009;113(6):1272–8. https://doi.org/10.1097/AOG.0b013e3181a5ef23.
8. Toozs-Hobson P, Balmforth J, Cardozo L, Khullar V, Athanasiou S. The effect of mode of delivery on pelvic floor functional anatomy. Int Urogynecol J Pelvic Floor Dysfunct. 2008;19(3):407–16. https://doi.org/10.1007/s00192-007-0455-0.
9. DeLancey JO. Anatomic aspects of vaginal eversion after hysterectomy. Am J Obstet Gynecol. 1992;166(6 Pt 1):1717–24; discussion 1724–1718.
10. Halban J, Tandler J. Anatomie und Atiologie der Genital prolapse biem Weibe. Wilhelm Braumüller, Vienna and Leipzig; 1907.
11. Kearney R, Sawhney R, DeLancey JO. Levator ani muscle anatomy evaluated by origin-insertion pairs. Obstet Gynecol. 2004;104(1):168–73. https://doi.org/10.1097/01.AOG.0000128906.61529.6b.
12. Lawson JO. Pelvic anatomy. I. Pelvic floor muscles. Ann R Coll Surg Engl. 1974;54(5):244–52.
13. Bo K, Hilde G, Tennfjord MK, Sperstad JB, Engh ME. Pelvic floor muscle function, pelvic floor dysfunction and diastasis recti abdominis: prospective cohort study. Neurourol Urodyn. 2017;36(3):716–21. https://doi.org/10.1002/nau.23005.
14. Alperin M, Lawley DM, Esparza MC, Lieber RL. Pregnancy-induced adaptations in the intrinsic structure of rat pelvic floor muscles. Am J Obstet Gynecol. 2015;213(2):191.e191–7. https://doi.org/10.1016/j.ajog.2015.05.012.
15. Jing D. Experimental and theoretical biomechanical analyses of the second stage of labor. Ann Arbor: University of Michigan; 2010. https://hdl.handle.net/2027.42/76013
16. Shek KL, Dietz HP, Kirby A. The effect of childbirth on urethral mobility: a prospective observational study. J Urol. 2010;184(2):629–34. https://doi.org/10.1016/j.juro.2010.03.135.

17. DeLancey JO, Kearney R, Chou Q, Speights S, Binno S. The appearance of levator ani muscle abnormalities in magnetic resonance images after vaginal delivery. Obstet Gynecol. 2003;101(1):46–53.

18. DeLancey JO, Sorensen HC, Lewicky-Gaupp C, Smith TM. Comparison of the puborectal muscle on MRI in women with POP and levator ani defects with those with normal support and no defect. Int Urogynecol J. 2012;23(1):73–7. https://doi.org/10.1007/s00192-011-1527-8.

19. Dietz HP. Ultrasound imaging of maternal birth trauma. Int Urogynecol J. 2021;32(7):1953–62. https://doi.org/10.1007/s00192-020-04669-8.

20. Krofta L, Otcenasek M, Kasikova E, Feyereisl J. Pubococcygeus-puborectalis trauma after forceps delivery: evaluation of the levator ani muscle with 3D/4D ultrasound. Int Urogynecol J Pelvic Floor Dysfunct. 2009;20(10):1175–81. https://doi.org/10.1007/s00192-009-0837-6.

21. Heliker BD, Kenton K, Leader-Cramer A, Brown O, Bochenska K, Geynisman-Tan J, Mueller M, Lewicky-Gaupp C. Adding insult to injury: levator ani avulsion in women with obstetric anal sphincter injuries. Female Pelvic Med Reconstr Surg. 2021;27(7):462–7. https://doi.org/10.1097/SPV.0000000000000954.

22. Memon HU, Blomquist JL, Dietz HP, Pierce CB, Weinstein MM, Handa VL. Comparison of levator ani muscle avulsion injury after forceps-assisted and vacuum-assisted vaginal childbirth. Obstet Gynecol. 2015;125(5):1080–7. https://doi.org/10.1097/AOG.0000000000000825.

23. Kearney R, Fitzpatrick M, Brennan S, Behan M, Miller J, Keane D, O'Herlihy C, DeLancey JO. Levator ani injury in primiparous women with forceps delivery for fetal distress, forceps for second stage arrest, and spontaneous delivery. Int J Gynaecol Obstet. 2010;111(1):19–22. https://doi.org/10.1016/j.ijgo.2010.05.019.

24. Valsky DV, Lipschuetz M, Bord A, Eldar I, Messing B, Hochner-Celnikier D, Lavy Y, Cohen SM, Yagel S. Fetal head circumference and length of second stage of labor are risk factors for levator ani muscle injury, diagnosed by 3-dimensional transperineal ultrasound in primiparous women. Am J Obstet Gynecol. 2009;201(1):91.e91–7. https://doi.org/10.1016/j.ajog.2009.03.028.

25. Huebner M, Margulies RU, DeLancey JO. Pelvic architectural distortion is associated with pelvic organ prolapse. Int Urogynecol J Pelvic Floor Dysfunct. 2008;19(6):863–7. https://doi.org/10.1007/s00192-007-0546-y.

26. Miller JM, Brandon C, Jacobson JA, Low LK, Zielinski R, Ashton-Miller J, Delancey JO. MRI findings in patients considered high risk for pelvic floor injury studied serially after vaginal childbirth. AJR Am J Roentgenol. 2010;195(3):786–91. https://doi.org/10.2214/AJR.09.3508.

27. Miller JM, Low LK, Zielinski R, Smith AR, DeLancey JO, Brandon C. Evaluating maternal recovery from labor and delivery: bone and levator ani injuries. Am J Obstet Gynecol. 2015;213(2):188.e181–11. https://doi.org/10.1016/j.ajog.2015.05.001.

28. Allen RE, Hosker GL, Smith AR, Warrell DW. Pelvic floor damage and childbirth: a neurophysiological study. Br J Obstet Gynaecol. 1990;97(9):770–9.

29. Weidner AC, Jamison MG, Branham V, South MM, Borawski KM, Romero AA. Neuropathic injury to the levator ani occurs in 1 in 4 primiparous women. Am J Obstet Gynecol. 2006;195(6):1851–6. https://doi.org/10.1016/j.ajog.2006.06.062.

30. Lien KC, Mooney B, DeLancey JO, Ashton-Miller JA. Levator ani muscle stretch induced by simulated vaginal birth. Obstet Gynecol. 2004;103(1):31–40. https://doi.org/10.1097/01.AOG.0000109207.22354.65.

31. Lien KC, Morgan DM, Delancey JO, Ashton-Miller JA. Pudendal nerve stretch during vaginal birth: a 3D computer simulation. Am J Obstet Gynecol. 2005;192(5):1669 76. https://doi.org/10.1016/j.ajog.2005.01.032.

32. Jing D, Ashton-Miller JA, DeLancey JO. A subject-specific anisotropic visco-hyperelastic finite element model of female pelvic floor stress and strain during the second stage of labor. J Biomech. 2012;45(3):455–60. https://doi.org/10.1016/j.jbiomech.2011.12.002.

33. Aasheim V, Nilsen ABV, Reinar LM, Lukasse M. Perineal techniques during the second stage of labour for reducing perineal trauma. Cochrane Database Syst Rev. 2017;6:CD006672. https://doi.org/10.1002/14651858.CD006672.pub3.

34. Beckmann MM, Stock OM. Antenatal perineal massage for reducing perineal trauma. Cochrane Database Syst Rev. 2013;(4):CD005123. https://doi.org/10.1002/14651858.CD005123.pub3.

35. Pipitone F, Miller JM, DeLancey J. Injury-associated levator ani muscle and anal sphincter ooedema following vaginal birth: a secondary analysis of the EMRLD study. BJOG. 2021;128(12):2046–53. https://doi.org/10.1111/1471-0528.16760.

36. Svabik K, Shek KL, Dietz HP. How much does the levator hiatus have to stretch during childbirth? BJOG. 2009;116(12):1657–62. https://doi.org/10.1111/j.1471-0528.2009.02321.x.

37. Tunn R, DeLancey JO, Howard D, Thorp JM, Ashton-Miller JA, Quint LE. MR imaging of levator ani muscle recovery following vaginal delivery. Int Urogynecol J Pelvic Floor Dysfunct. 1999;10(5):300–7. https://doi.org/10.1007/s001929970006.

38. Shek KL, Kruger J, Dietz HP. The effect of pregnancy on hiatal dimensions and urethral mobility: an observational study. Int Urogynecol J. 2012;23(11):1561–7. https://doi.org/10.1007/s00192-012-1795-y.

39. Fairchild PS, Low LK, Kowalk KM, Kolenic GE, DeLancey JO, Fenner DE. Defining "normal recovery" of pelvic floor function and appearance in a high-risk vaginal delivery cohort. Int Urogynecol J. 2020;31(3):495–504. https://doi.org/10.1007/s00192-019-04152-z.

40. Sampselle CM, Miller JM, Mims BL, Delancey JO, Ashton-Miller JA, Antonakos CL. Effect of pel-

vic muscle exercise on transient incontinence during pregnancy and after birth. Obstet Gynecol. 1998;91(3):406–12. https://doi.org/10.1016/s0029-7844(97)00672-8.

41. Yousuf AA, DeLancey JO, Brandon CJ, Miller JM. Pelvic structure and function at 1 month compared to 7 months by dynamic magnetic resonance after vaginal birth. Am J Obstet Gynecol. 2009;201(5):514.e511–7. https://doi.org/10.1016/j.ajog.2009.06.048.

42. Wang XM, Chang X, Ding Y, Wang SZ, Zhen Y, Ding JX, Kong FB. Translabial three-dimensional ultrasound investigation of the levator hiatus in postpartum women. J Med Ultrason (2001). 2015;42(3):373–8. https://doi.org/10.1007/s10396-014-0609-x.

43. Sanozidis A, Mikos T, Assimakopoulos E, Athanasiadis A, Tantanassis T, Tarlatzis BC, Papameletiou V. Changes in levator hiatus dimensions during pregnancy and after delivery in nulliparas: a prospective cohort study using 3D transperineal ultrasound. J Matern Fetal Neonatal Med. 2018;31(11):1505–12. https://doi.org/10.1080/14767058.2017.1319926.

44. Raizada V, Bhargava V, Jung SA, Karstens A, Pretorius D, Krysl P, Mittal RK. Dynamic assessment of the vaginal high-pressure zone using high-definition manometery, 3-dimensional ultrasound, and magnetic resonance imaging of the pelvic floor muscles. Am J Obstet Gynecol. 2010;203(2):172.e171–8. https://doi.org/10.1016/j.ajog.2010.02.028.

45. Guaderrama NM, Nager CW, Liu J, Pretorius DH, Mittal RK. The vaginal pressure profile. Neurourol Urodyn. 2005;24(3):243–7. https://doi.org/10.1002/nau.20112.

46. DeLancey JO, Morgan DM, Fenner DE, Kearney R, Guire K, Miller JM, Hussain H, Umek W, Hsu Y, Ashton-Miller JA. Comparison of levator ani muscle defects and function in women with and without pelvic organ prolapse. Obstet Gynecol. 2007;109(2 Pt 1):295–302. https://doi.org/10.1097/01.AOG.0000250901.57095.ba.

47. Handa VL, Blomquist JL, Carroll MK, Munoz A. Genital hiatus size and the development of prolapse among parous women. Female Pelvic Med Reconstr Surg. 2021;27(2):e448–52. https://doi.org/10.1097/SPV.0000000000000960.

48. Handa VL, Roem J, Blomquist JL, Dietz HP, Munoz A. Pelvic organ prolapse as a function of levator ani avulsion, hiatus size, and strength. Am J Obstet Gynecol. 2019;221(1):41.e41–7. https://doi.org/10.1016/j.ajog.2019.03.004.

49. Delancey JO, Hurd WW. Size of the urogenital hiatus in the levator ani muscles in normal women and women with pelvic organ prolapse. Obstet Gynecol. 1998;91(3):364–8. https://doi.org/10.1016/s0029-7844(97)00682-0.

50. Sammarco AG, Nandikanti L, Kobernik EK, Xie B, Jankowski A, Swenson CW, DeLancey JOL. Interactions among pelvic organ protrusion, levator ani descent, and hiatal enlargement in women with and without prolapse. Am J Obstet Gynecol.

2017;217(5):614.e611–7. https://doi.org/10.1016/j.ajog.2017.07.007.

51. English EM, Chen L, Sammarco AG, Kolenic GE, Cheng W, Ashton-Miller JA, DeLancey JO. Mechanisms of hiatus failure in prolapse: a multifaceted evaluation. Int Urogynecol J. 2021;32:1545–53. https://doi.org/10.1007/s00192-020-04651-4.

52. Handa VL, Blomquist JL, Carroll M, Roem J, Munoz A. Longitudinal changes in the genital hiatus preceding the development of pelvic organ prolapse. Am J Epidemiol. 2019;188(12):2196–201. https://doi.org/10.1093/aje/kwz195.

53. Nandikanti L, Sammarco AG, Kobernik EK, DeLancey JOL. Levator ani defect severity and its association with enlarged hiatus size, levator bowl depth, and prolapse size. Am J Obstet Gynecol. 2018;218(5):537–9. https://doi.org/10.1016/j.ajog.2018.02.005.

54. Pipitone F, Swenson CW, DeLancey JOL, Chen L. Novel 3D MRI technique to measure perineal membrane structural changes with pregnancy and childbirth: technique development and measurement feasibility. Int Urogynecol J. 2021;32(9):2413–20. https://doi.org/10.1007/s00192-021-04795-x.

55. Kim S, Harvey MA, Johnston S. A review of the epidemiology and pathophysiology of pelvic floor dysfunction: do racial differences matter? J Obstet Gynaecol Can. 2005;27(3):251–9. https://doi.org/10.1016/s1701-2163(16)30518-7.

56. Williams A, Gonzalez B, Fitzgerald C, Brincat C. Racial/ethnic differences in perineal lacerations in a diverse urban healthcare system. Female Pelvic Med Reconstr Surg. 2019;25(1):15–21. https://doi.org/10.1097/SPV.0000000000000517.

57. Chiu K, McKay E, Fazzari M, Leegant A. Risks and associations of third- and fourth-degree lacerations: an urban single center experience. Female Pelvic Med Reconstr Surg. 2021;27(1):e146–51. https://doi.org/10.1097/SPV.0000000000000867.

58. Dietz HP, Simpson JM. Levator trauma is associated with pelvic organ prolapse. BJOG. 2008;115(8):979–84. https://doi.org/10.1111/j.1471-0528.2008.01751.x.

59. Hanzal E, Berger E, Koelbl H. Levator ani muscle morphology and recurrent genuine stress incontinence. Obstet Gynecol. 1993;81(3):426–9.

60. Vakili B, Zheng YT, Loesch H, Echols KT, Franco N, Chesson RR. Levator contraction strength and genital hiatus as risk factors for recurrent pelvic organ prolapse. Am J Obstet Gynecol. 2005;192(5):1592–8. https://doi.org/10.1016/j.ajog.2004.11.022.

61. Oversand SH, Staff AC, Volloyhaug I, Svenningsen R. Impact of levator muscle avulsions on Manchester procedure outcomes in pelvic organ prolapse surgery. Acta Obstet Gynecol Scand. 2019;98(8):1046–54. https://doi.org/10.1111/aogs.13604.

62. Morgan DM, Larson K, Lewicky-Gaupp C, Fenner DE, DeLancey JO. Vaginal support as determined by levator ani defect status 6 weeks after primary surgery for pelvic organ prolapse. Int J Gynaecol Obstet. 2011;114(2):141–4. https://doi.org/10.1016/j.ijgo.2011.02.020.

63. Weemhoff M, Vergeldt TF, Notten K, Serroyen J, Kampschoer PH, Roumen FJ. Avulsion of puborectalis muscle and other risk factors for cystocele recurrence: a 2-year follow-up study. Int Urogynecol J. 2012;23(1):65–71. https://doi.org/10.1007/s00192-011-1524-y.

64. Handa VL, Blomquist JL, Knoepp LR, Hoskey KA, McDermott KC, Munoz A. Pelvic floor disorders 5-10 years after vaginal or cesarean childbirth. Obstet Gynecol. 2011;118(4):777–84. https://doi.org/10.1097/AOG.0b013e3182267f2f.

65. DeLancey JO, Miller JM, Kearney R, Howard D, Reddy P, Umek W, Guire KE, Margulies RU, Ashton-Miller JA. Vaginal birth and de novo stress incontinence: relative contributions of urethral dysfunction and mobility. Obstet Gynecol. 2007;110(2 Pt 1):354–62. https://doi.org/10.1097/01.AOG.0000270120.60522.55.

66. Brincat CA, Delancey JO, Miller JM. Urethral closure pressures among primiparous women with and without levator ani muscle defects. Int Urogynecol J. 2011;22(12):1491–5. https://doi.org/10.1007/s00192-011-1458-4.

67. van Geelen JM, Lemmens WA, Eskes TK, Martin CB Jr. The urethral pressure profile in pregnancy and after delivery in healthy nulliparous women. Am J Obstet Gynecol. 1982;144(6):636–49. https://doi.org/10.1016/0002-9378(82)90431-8.

68. DeLancey JO, Trowbridge ER, Miller JM, Morgan DM, Guire K, Fenner DE, Weadock WJ, Ashton-Miller JA. Stress urinary incontinence: relative importance of urethral support and urethral closure pressure. J Urol. 2008;179(6):2286–90; discussion 2290. https://doi.org/10.1016/j.juro.2008.01.098.

69. Rud T. Urethral pressure profile in continent women from childhood to old age. Acta Obstet Gynecol Scand. 1980;59(4):331–5. https://doi.org/10.3109/00016348009154090.

70. Trowbridge ER, Wei JT, Fenner DE, Ashton-Miller JA, Delancey JO. Effects of aging on lower urinary tract and pelvic floor function in nulliparous women. Obstet Gynecol. 2007;109(3):715–20. https://doi.org/10.1097/01.AOG.0000257074.98122.69.

71. Sheng Y, Liu X, Low LK, Ashton-Miller JA, Miller JM. Association of pubovisceral muscle tear with functional capacity of urethral closure: evaluating maternal recovery from labor and delivery. Am J Obstet Gynecol. 2020;222(6):598.e591–7. https://doi.org/10.1016/j.ajog.2019.11.1257.

72. Miller JM, Umek WH, Delancey JO, Ashton-Miller JA. Can women without visible pubococcygeal muscle in MR images still increase urethral closure pressures? Am J Obstet Gynecol. 2004;191(1):171–5. https://doi.org/10.1016/j.ajog.2004.03.082.

73. Sultan AH, Kamm MA, Hudson CN, Thomas JM, Bartram CI. Anal-sphincter disruption during vaginal delivery. N Engl J Med. 1993;329(26):1905–11. https://doi.org/10.1056/NEJM199312233292601.

74. Blomquist JL, Munoz A, Carroll M, Handa VL. Association of delivery mode with pelvic floor disorders after childbirth. JAMA. 2018;320(23):2438–47. https://doi.org/10.1001/jama.2018.18315.

75. Thiagamoorthy G, Johnson A, Thakar R, Sultan AH. National survey of perineal trauma and its subsequent management in the United Kingdom. Int Urogynecol J. 2014;25(12):1621–7. https://doi.org/10.1007/s00192-014-2406-x.

76. Mous M, Muller SA, de Leeuw JW. Long-term effects of anal sphincter rupture during vaginal delivery: faecal incontinence and sexual complaints. BJOG. 2008;115(2):234–8. https://doi.org/10.1111/j.1471-0528.2007.01502.x.

77. Pollack J, Nordenstam J, Brismar S, Lopez A, Altman D, Zetterstrom J. Anal incontinence after vaginal delivery: a five-year prospective cohort study. Obstet Gynecol. 2004;104(6):1397–402. https://doi.org/10.1097/01.AOG.0000147597.45349.e8.

78. Samarasekera DN, Bekhit MT, Wright Y, Lowndes RH, Stanley KP, Preston JP, Preston P, Speakman CT. Long-term anal continence and quality of life following postpartum anal sphincter injury. Color Dis. 2008;10(8):793–9. https://doi.org/10.1111/j.1463-1318.2007.01445.x.

79. Sangalli MR, Floris L, Faltin D, Weil A. Anal incontinence in women with third or fourth degree perineal tears and subsequent vaginal deliveries. Aust N Z J Obstet Gynaecol. 2000;40(3):244–8. https://doi.org/10.1111/j.1479-828x.2000.tb03330.x.

80. Heilbrun ME, Nygaard IE, Lockhart ME, Richter HE, Brown MB, Kenton KS, Rahn DD, Thomas JV, Weidner AC, Nager CW, Delancey JO. Correlation between levator ani muscle injuries on magnetic resonance imaging and fecal incontinence, pelvic organ prolapse, and urinary incontinence in primiparous women. Am J Obstet Gynecol. 2010;202(5):488.e481–6. https://doi.org/10.1016/j.ajog.2010.01.002.

81. Guzman Rojas R, Wong V, Shek KL, Dietz HP. Impact of levator trauma on pelvic floor muscle function. Int Urogynecol J. 2014;25(3):375–80. https://doi.org/10.1007/s00192-013-2226-4.

82. Snooks SJ, Setchell M, Swash M, Henry MM. Injury to innervation of pelvic floor sphincter musculature in childbirth. Lancet. 1984;2(8402):546–50. https://doi.org/10.1016/s0140-6736(84)90766-9.

83. Snooks SJ, Swash M, Henry MM, Setchell M. Risk factors in childbirth causing damage to the pelvic floor innervation. Int J Color Dis. 1986;1(1):20–4. https://doi.org/10.1007/BF01648831.

Diagnosis of Obstetric Anal Sphincter Injuries (OASIs)

Abdul H. Sultan and Ranee Thakar

Overview

Test your learning and check your understanding of this book's contents: use the "Springer Nature Flashcards" app to access questions using ▶ https://sn.pub/wqrf89. To use the app, please follow the instructions in Chap. 1.

Learning Objectives

- Understand the anatomy of the perineum and anal sphincter
- Learn new tips and tricks to diagnose OASIs
- Classify OASIs according to the international convention
- Avoid overdiagnosis and underdiagnosis of OASIs

3.1 Introduction

Prior to the advent of endoanal ultrasound, clinically diagnosed OASIs had been reported in 0.6% of vaginal deliveries [1]. However prospective studies using endoanal ultrasound have shown that the majority of OASIs were being undiagnosed [2]. This was attributed to confusion with and lack of knowledge, wrong classification and training [3–5]. Using endoanal ultrasound, it has subsequently been shown that with adequate training, nearly all of these injuries can be diagnosed clinically [6]. This chapter aims to provide tips and tricks to avoid missing the diagnosis of OASIs, using a structured clinical examination.

3.2 Classification of Perineal Trauma

Previous classifications of perineal trauma, particularly in the UK, have been inconsistent. Sultan and Thakar systematically reviewed all relevant obstetric textbooks in the Library of The Royal College of Obstetricians & Gynaecologists (RCOG) and found that 17% did not mention any classification, while 22% misclassified anal sphincter injury as "second degree" [5].

Fernando et al. in 2002 surveyed 672 consultants in active obstetric practice and found that 33% similarly misclassified a complete or partial external sphincter tear as a "second degree" tear [4]. There was up to a ten-fold regional variation in the "misclassification" with a distinct increasing trend towards the Northern parts of the UK, whereby a complete external anal sphincter tear was considered to be a second degree tear. This may reflect the original teachings of Ian Donald from Glasgow, who defined a third degree as one in which both the anal sphincter and anal mucosa was torn [7].

A. H. Sultan (✉) · R. Thakar
Croydon University Hospital, London, UK

© The Author(s), under exclusive license to Springer Nature Switzerland AG 2024
A. H. Sultan et al. (eds.), *Pelvic Floor, Perineal, and Anal Sphincter Trauma During Childbirth*,
https://doi.org/10.1007/978-3-031-43095-4_3

First degree: laceration of the vaginal epithelium or perineal skin only.

Second degree: involvement of the perineal muscles but not the anal sphincter

Third degree: disruption of the anal sphincter muscles subdivided into:
    3a: <50% thickness of external sphincter torn.
    3b: >50% thickness of external sphincter torn.
    3c: internal sphincter also torn.

Fourth degree: a third degree tear with disruption of the anorectal epithelium

Rectal Buttonhole tear: Isolated tear of the rectal mucosa extending into vagina*

*Can occur concomitantly with a third/fourth degree tear when there is an intervening island of anorectal mucosa[17]

Fig. 3.1 Sultan classification of perineal trauma [8]

In order to standardise the classification of perineal trauma, Sultan [8] proposed the following classification in 1999 (Fig. 3.1) that has been subsequently adopted globally [9] by most Institutions [10] including the RCOG [11] and the American College of Obstetricians and Gynecologists [12]. The Sultan classification is demonstrated in a schematic representation of the anal sphincter complex and highlights that the classification hinges on the thickness of the injury (Fig. 3.2). The intact anal sphincter appears as a circular band of muscle (Fig. 3.3a) that can be demonstrated by insertion of a finger in the anal canal (Fig. 3.3b). However, in order to identify OASIs (while avoiding overdiagnosis of OASIs) [13], it is important for doctors and midwives to be aware of the clinical extent of the injury as compared to the mean length of the anterior anal sphincter. It should be noted that in the female, the anterior anal sphincter is usually no more than 2.5–3 cm, which corresponds to the distal digit of the finger (Fig. 3.3b). Without this knowledge, OASIs can be missed or over-diagnosed, as it is known that compared to males, the anterior anal sphincter is shorter in the female [14]. In Fig. 3.3c, it can be seen that if the length of the anal sphincter is not known, rectal wall muscle tears can be mistaken for third degree tears. These tears may cause posterior vaginal wall weakness, as it is likely that the overlying rectovaginal fascia is also torn; this, in turn, could result in posterior vaginal prolapse (rectocele). Previously, we conducted a study in which we took measurements of the fingers of doctors and midwives and found that both have poor accuracy in estimating the length of their index finger, cervical dilatation and anal sphincter length [15]. In the first edition of this textbook [16], Sultan described, the technique of pill-rolling to identify the integrity of the anal sphincter during a rectal examination, which involves rolling the anal sphincter between the index finger (up to the distal crease) in the anal canal and the thumb on the perineum or vaginal tear (Fig. 3.4). An intact anal sphincter would flick off the thumb during rolling; after identification of the sphincter ring, a full assessment would enable grading of the tear.

An isolated tear of the rectal mucosa (rectal buttonhole) and vagina [17] (Fig. 3.5) can also occur. When an OASI is in continuity with a rectal tear it should be called a fourth-degree tear (see below). However, when a third- or fourth degree tear occurs concomitantly with an isolated

Fig. 3.2 A schematic representation of the Sultan Classification of third and fourth degree tears. Note that the longitudinal muscle of the rectum continues as the conjoint longitudinal muscle. The lowermost images demonstrate the grade of tear according to the thickness of the injury to the external sphincter (brown) and any involvement of the internal sphincter (pink)

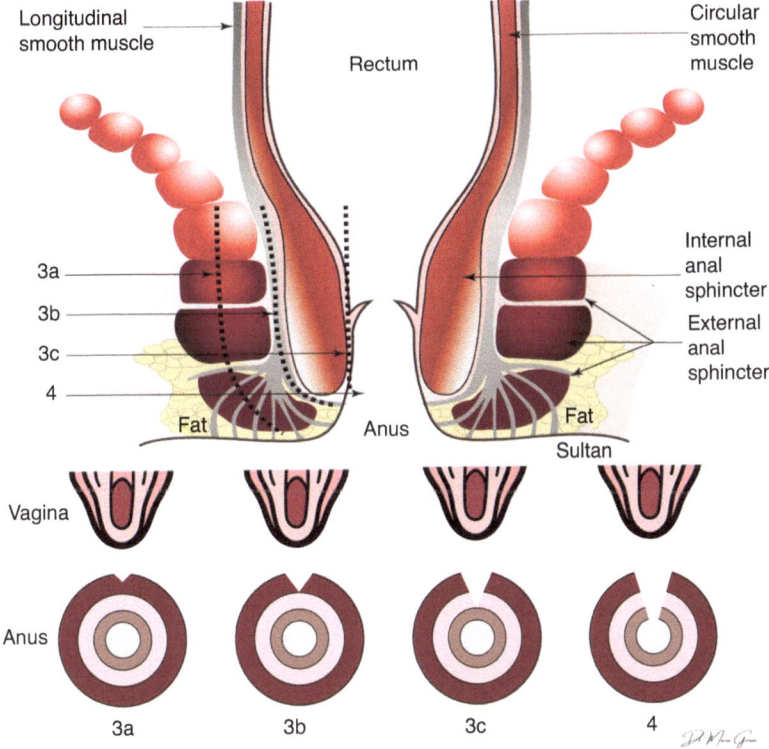

rectal buttonhole tear (an island of intact rectal mucosa between the third/fourth-degree tear and the isolated rectal buttonhole tear), it is classified and described as such namely, rectal buttonhole tear plus the OASI grade [17].

A grade 3a tear involves less than 50% of the thickness of the external anal sphincter (EAS), irrespective of the length of the injury (Fig. 3.6); likewise, a grade 3b tear involves more than 50% of the thickness (Fig. 3.7). It is also possible to sustain a full thickness third degree tear that only involves part of the length of the anal sphincter (Fig. 3.8). In such circumstances or when the clinician is doubtful, the higher classification should be selected (e.g., if there is uncertainty between a 3a and 3b tear, the tear should be classified as 3b). If there is a partial length defect, it should still be graded according to thickness of the defect, because the management would remain the same (see Chap. 5).

Some refer to Grade 3a and 3b as minor OASI (only EAS injury) as opposed to major OASI for grade 3c and fourth degree tears (EAS and IAS injury) [18].

3.2.1 Steps to Making an Accurate Clinical Diagnosis of OASIS

1. Informed consent should be obtained for a vaginal and rectal examination.
2. Adequate exposure of the injury is imperative; if this is not possible, lithotomy position should be assumed.
3. Good lighting is essential.
4. If the examination is limited due to pain, adequate analgesia must be obtained.
5. Following a visual examination of the external genitalia, the labia should be parted with the thumb and index finger of one hand, and a vaginal examination should be performed with the index and middle fingers of the other (Fig. 3.9). When multiple or deep tears are present, it is best to examine and repair in lithotomy. The apex of the vaginal laceration should always be identified before repair commences.
6. In the absence of regional anaesthesia, the perineum should be visualised, and the

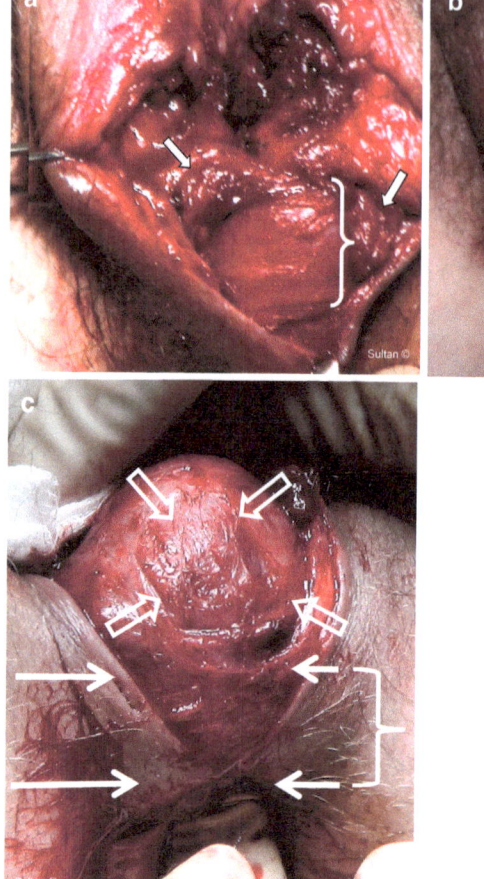

Fig. 3.3 (**a**) An intact anal sphincter (bracket). The arrows show the torn Superficial Transverse Perineal Muscles. (**b**) Following a rectal examination, the torn perineal skin can be seen extending to the anal verge with the proximal and distal border of the intact external sphincter (bracket). This is the normal length of the exter-nal sphincter corresponding to the distal crease of the index finger (2.5–3 cm). (**c**) Demonstrating how a third degree tear can be overdiagnosed if the anal sphincter length (brackets) is not known. The open arrows point to a tear of the rectal wall muscles corresponding to 4–5 cm of the inserted finger (second crease)

woman should be asked to squeeze the anal sphincter muscles. Any asymmetry, particularly of the perianal skin overlying the corrugator cutis ani should be noted, as this could indicate disruption of the subcutaneous EAS.

7. A structured rectal examination should then be performed (Fig. 3.5) to exclude injury to the anorectal mucosa and anal sphincter. The vagina should be exposed as noted above (Fig. 3.9). Every woman must have a rectal examination after vaginal birth prior to sutur-ing, in order to avoid missing an OASI or an isolated rectovaginal buttonhole tear (Fig. 3.5). The whole index finger should be inserted into the rectum and elevated whilst moving from side to side; this is continued down to the anal verge. For example, as can be seen in Fig. 3.5, there is a rectal laceration with an intact anal sphincter. Furthermore, a third or fourth degree tear may be present beneath what appears to be intact perineal skin (Fig. 3.10a, b) with a tear extending behind the fourchette. These examples fur-

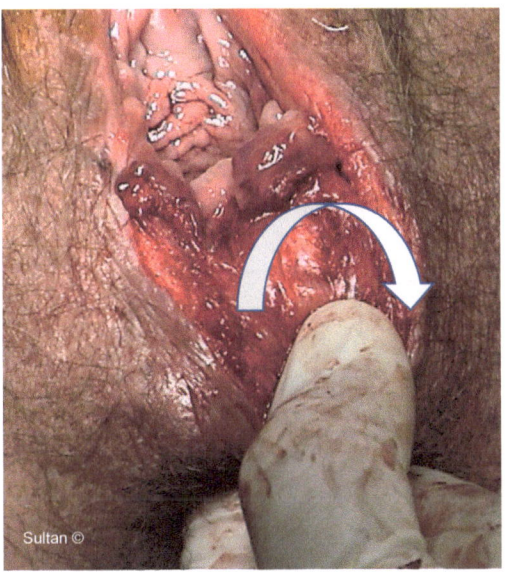

Fig. 3.4 Pill-rolling motion between the distal digit of the index finger in the anal canal and the thumb in the perineal wound commencing at 9 o'clock and rotating to 3 o'clock

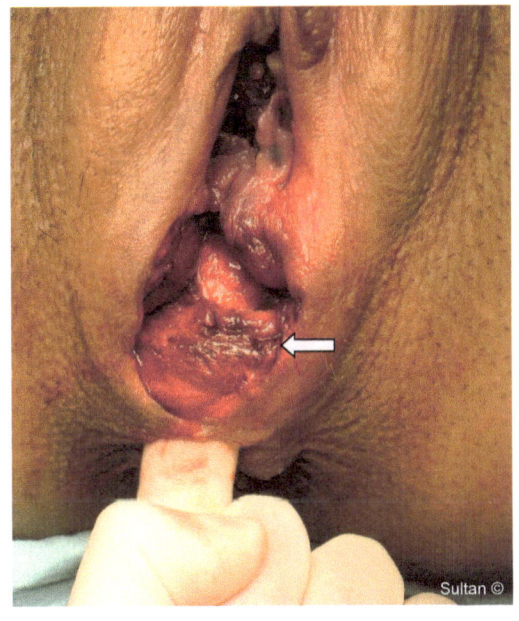

Fig. 3.6 Grade 3a tear (less than 50% of the thickness of the external sphincter)

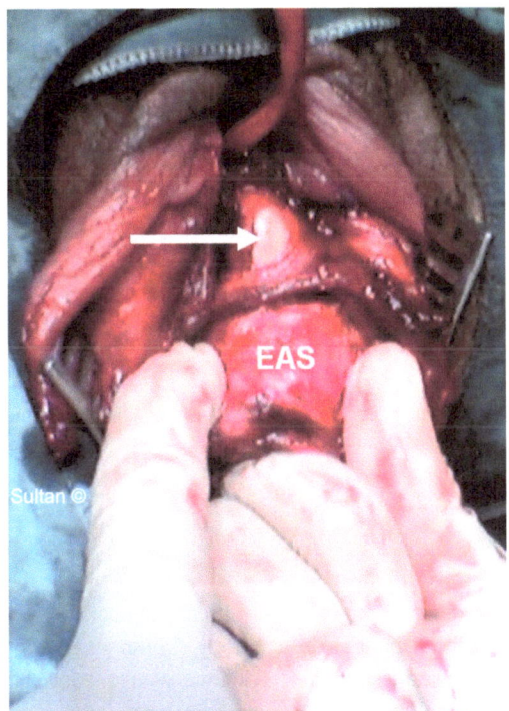

Fig. 3.5 Buttonhole tear of the rectal mucosa (arrow) with an intact external anal sphincter (EAS) demonstrated during a digital rectal examination

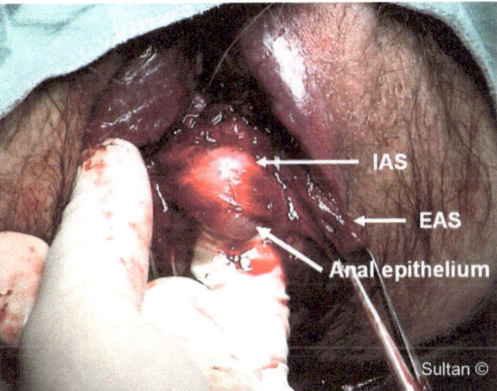

Fig. 3.7 Photograph demonstrating a Grade 3b tear with an intact IAS. The EAS is being grasped with Allis forceps. Note the difference in appearance of the grey anal epithelium, the pink IAS and the dark red EAS

ther highlight the need to perform a recto-vaginal examination after *every* vaginal delivery in order to exclude an OASI. While not common practice, an episiotomy may need to be performed if visibility and exposure are limited; Fig. 3.10c depicts a grade 3b tear that would otherwise have been

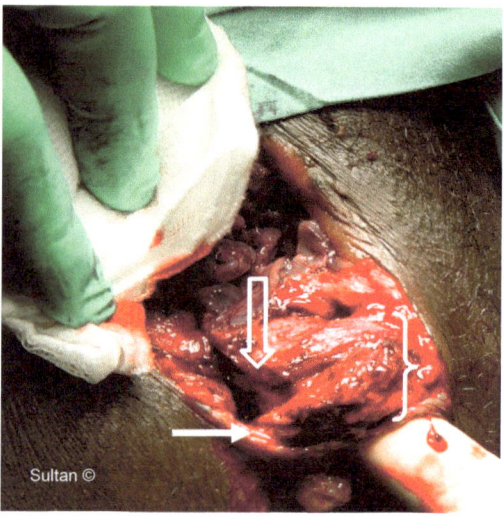

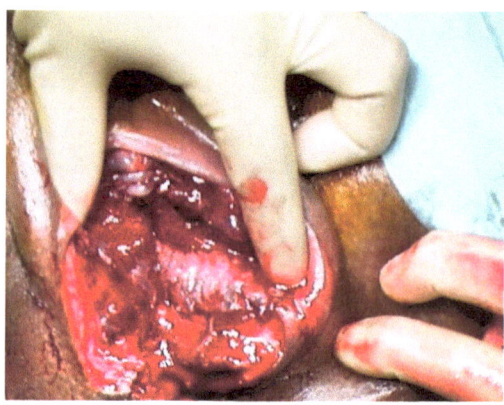

Fig. 3.9 Good exposure of the perineal wound being demonstrated by using the thumb and index finger of one hand

Fig. 3.8 Partial tear of the external anal sphincter (bracket) demonstrating a Grade 3b tear (open arrow) and a grade 3a tear (closed arrow)

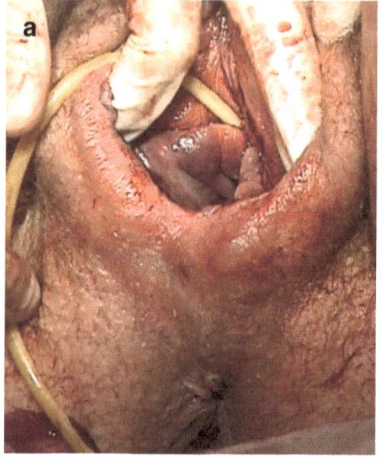
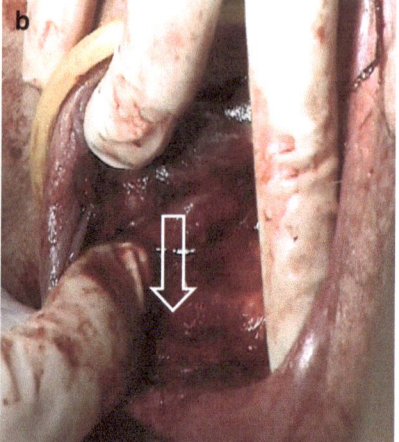
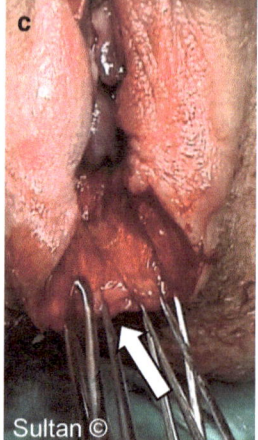

Fig. 3.10 Perineum immediately after delivery (**a**) demonstrating an apparently intact perineum. (**b**) Deep 'bucket handle' tear just behind the posterior fourchette (open arrow). (**c**) Grade 3b tear (arrow) following incision of the perineum and exploration

missed. Again, while rupture of the anal sphincter is unlikely to occur if there is no laceration involving the vagina and perineum, it can only be excluded by performing a proper rectal examination.

8. The presence or absence of sphincter injury should be confirmed not only with visualisation but also with palpation. The woman should be asked to contract her anal sphincter. If the anal sphincter is disrupted, a gap can be felt anteri-

orly. If the perineal skin is intact above the defect, there will be an absence of puckering on the perianal skin anteriorly (in the absence of anaesthesia); this is known as the "dovetail sign" usually seen with chronic sphincter injuries. Palpation should be thoroughly performed by inserting the index finger in the anal canal and the thumb in the vaginal outlet. This will allow for the anal sphincter to be palpated in a "pill-rolling" motion commencing at the 9 o'clock position and rotating circumferentially to the 3 o'clock position (Fig. 3.4). As the EAS is in a state of tonic contraction, complete disruption results in retraction of the sphincter ends. Therefore, the sphincter ends need to be grasped with Allis tissue forceps and retrieved prior to repair, as shown in Chap. 5.

9. Identification of the IAS is critical. The IAS is a circular smooth muscle that appears paler (similar to uncooked fish or chicken breast) (Fig. 3.7) than the striated EAS (similar to uncooked red meat) (Figs. 3.5, 3.6, 3.7, and 3.8). As the IAS is a thickened continuation of the circular muscle of the rectum, no transition is seen. The distal end of the IAS lies a few millimetres proximal to the distal end of the EAS. However, if the EAS is relaxed (for example, following regional or general anaesthesia), the distal end of the IAS will appear to be at a lower level. If the IAS (Fig. 3.11) or anal epithelium is torn (Fig. 3.12), the EAS will invariably be torn and therefore careful examination is mandatory.

10. Identification of the Superficial Transverse Perineal Muscles (STPM) is imperative. The EAS is closely related to the STPM lying at its proximal borders. However, when the STPM is torn, the upper border of the EAS comes into clear view (Figs. 3.3a, 3.5, 3.6, and 3.7).

11. Care needs to be taken to avoid mistaking the STPM for the EAS. As can be seen in Fig. 3.13, the STPM can be a substantial muscle and of a similar colour as the EAS. The crucial difference, however, between the two muscles is the direction of attachment laterally towards the pubic rami (Fig. 3.14). Failure to recognise this could result in either an overdiagnosis of an OASI,

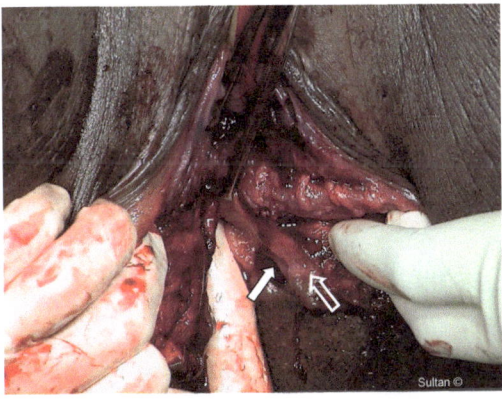

Fig. 3.12 A fourth degree tear with the closed arrow demonstrating the anal mucosa and the internal anal sphincter (open arrow)

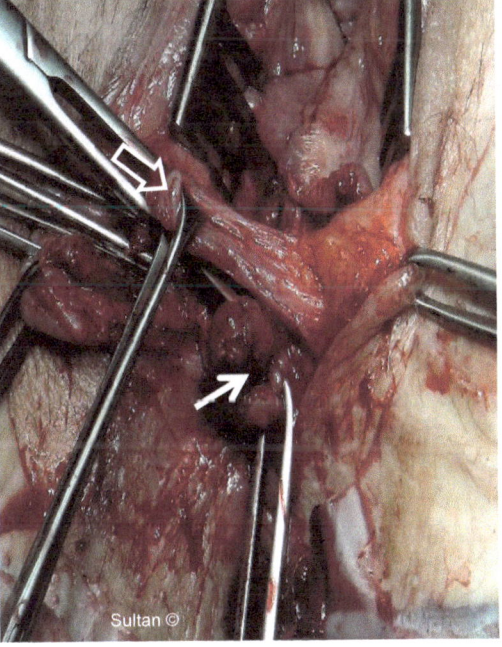

Fig. 3.13 A Grade 3b tear (closed arrow) alongside the Superficial Transverse Perineal Muscle (open arrow) which can easily be mistaken for the EAS

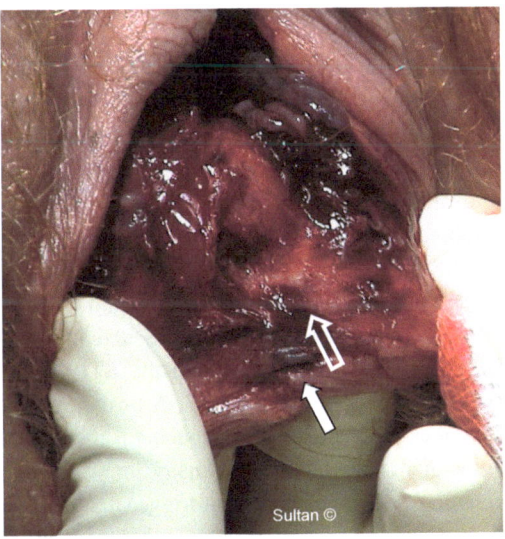

Fig. 3.11 Grade 3c tear demonstrating a torn internal sphincter (open arrow) and anal skin (closed arrow)

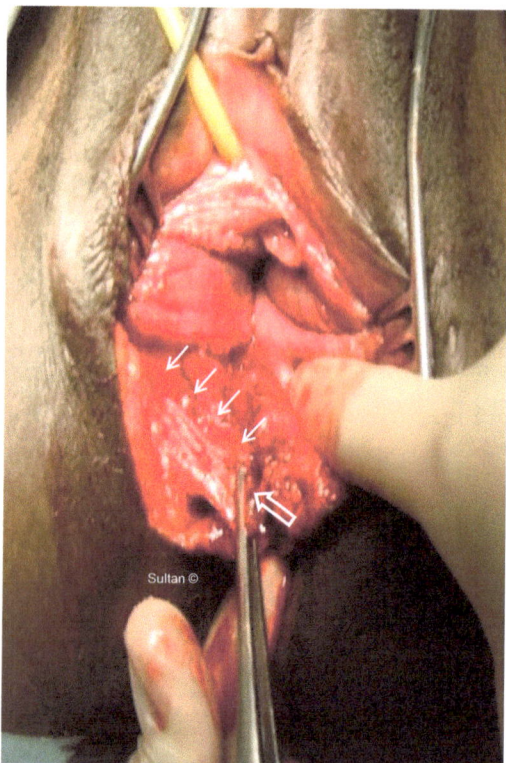

Fig. 3.14 The Superficial Transverse Perineal Muscle (arrows) being grasped by Allis forceps (open arrow) can easily be mistaken for the external sphincter but for the direction of insertion towards the right pubic ramus

or if the STPM was repaired on the assumption that it was a disrupted EAS, an OASI could be missed; this would be associated potentially with the development of anal incontinence [19]. For this reason, Sultan described the 'finger-lift test' such that a finger in the anal canal should elevate as the ends of the torn EAS muscles are grasped and pulled anteriorly (see Chap. 5).

3.3 Undiagnosed OASIs

Following the advent of endoanal ultrasound (see Chap. 10) Sultan et al. [2] demonstrated that 33% of women sustained OASIs that had not been identified at delivery (See Chap. 15 on imaging). At that time, these were labelled as "occult" because it was assumed that these injuries seen on ultrasound could not be seen clinically. Older prospective studies [9, 16] have identified "occult" injuries occurring between 20 [20] and

41% [21] of the time. However, it has now been established that these injuries were, in fact, unrecognised at delivery. Andrews et al. [6] reported a study in which 241 primiparous women had their perineum re-examined by an experienced research fellow after vaginal delivery, and endoanal ultrasound was performed immediately after delivery and repeated 7 weeks postpartum. When OASIs were identified by the research fellow, the injuries were confirmed and repaired by the duty registrar or consultant. The prevalence of clinically diagnosed OASIs increased from 11 to 25% (n = 59). Every clinically diagnosed injury was identified by postpartum endoanal ultrasound. However, there were three women with sonographic defects in whom the injury was not identified clinically. Two of these had only small IAS defects (with an intact EAS); one would not expect to detect these clinically. The other was a defect of both the IAS and EAS and while this could represent an occult injury, it was most probably, an undiagnosed tear. At 7 weeks, no *de novo* defects were identified by ultrasound. This study concluded that most sphincter defects that have previously been designated as "occult" injuries were, in fact, injuries that were missed clinically at vaginal birth.

It was alarming to find that 87% and 27% of OASIS were not identified by midwives and doctors respectively [6]. Although it is likely that some of these would have been detected at the time of suturing the tear, it was concerning that clinical recognition of OASIS was suboptimal. This finding is not unique, as Groom and Patterson [22] found that the rate of third degree tears doubled to 15% when all "second degree tears" were re-examined by a second experienced person.

Roper et al. [23] studied 1056 women with OASIS and found that 11% of the injuries were underclassified; Sioutis et al. [13] found that 7% of women diagnosed with OASIS actually sustained second degree tears and the STPM was probably mistaken for the EAS. A further reason for under-reporting by the accoucher is the stigma associated with OASIS. In many units, OASIS constitute a risk management trigger that may be regarded as punitive and there is therefore a disincentive to accurate reporting.

These studies [6, 22] pointed to a need for more focused and intensive training in the identification of OASIS. In 1995, Sultan et al. [3] conducted an interview of 75 doctors and 75 midwives and reported that 91% and 60%, respectively, believed they had inadequate training in perineal anatomy; 84% and 61%, respectively, reported inadequate training in identifying third degree tears. Fortunately, the introduction of hands-on workshops and audiovisual material (perineum. net) has made a remarkable difference to the detection of OASIs [24]. Using Transperineal Ultrasound, Wong et al. [25] repeated the study performed by Andrews et al. [6], and have shown that 15 years later (after the introduction of hand-on workshops), the rate of missed OASIs had halved. Unfortunately, as there is no such program for midwives, their rate of undiagnosed OASI has remained changed. (See Chap. 23).

If OASIs are being missed, one would expect to see more women with anal incontinence after only having an episiotomy or second-degree tear. Lal et al. [26] showed that significantly more women develop anal incontinence following a second degree tear than with an intact perineum 23% vs 3% (p = 0.01). Benifla et al. [27] identified a 16 fold increase in anal incontinence following a second degree tear (p < 0.05). Both these studies support the findings of Andrews et al. [6], in which they found that a large number of OASIs were undiagnosed and wrongly classified as second degree tears. Not surprisingly, it has been shown that missed injuries have a worse outcome compared to women in whom OASIs was diagnosed and repaired at the time of delivery [19].

3.4   Can Routine Anal Sonography Immediately After Delivery Improve Accuracy of Detection of OASIs?

Faltin et al. [28] randomised 752 primiparous women with second degree lacerations to conventional examination (control group) and additional postpartum endoanal ultrasound (experimental group) and demonstrated that a considerable number of women have full thickness OASIS that are not recognised at delivery. However, they excluded partial thickness sphincter tears from their study. On identifying new injuries in the experimental group, a formal sphincter repair was performed. Overall, severe faecal incontinence was significantly reduced from 8.7% in the control group to 3.3% in the experimental group.

Despite its utility in diagnosis of OASIs, endoanal ultrasound is a technique that requires specific expertise. This is particularly true in the immediate postpartum period when the anal canal is relaxed (even more with anaesthesia). Ultimately, the diagnosis of OASIs rests on clinical assessment and a rectal examination because even if a defect is seen on ultrasound, it has to be clinically apparent to be repaired. As Faltin et al. [28] found in their study, when routine postpartum anal endosonography was used as the gold standard of diagnosing OASIs, five women had an unnecessary intervention; the sonographic defect was not clinically visible despite exploration of the anal sphincter. As a result of this unnecessary exploration based solely on anal endosonography, 20% developed severe faecal incontinence.

Wong et al. [25] were the first to use transperineal ultrasound immediately after vaginal birth to detect OASIs. They found no significant difference between clinical detection and ultrasound detection. We therefore believe that with improvement in clinical diagnostic skills, detection of OASIs immediately after delivery can be significantly improved [6] and in practice, postpartum anal sonography is of limited value. Huber et al. [29] performed a study of 554 postpartum women where the obstetrician was blinded to the scan and found that endoanal ultrasound added no convincing diagnostic power to clinical examination in the diagnosis of OASI immediately after birth. Ultimately, in order to repair an OASI, the injury needs to be identified clinically before it can be repaired. It would therefore be prudent to divert resources towards clinical training instead of attempting to teach new trainees the art of postpartum anal endosonography with its attendant limitations [30]. This strategy regarding training has also been highlighted by Young et al. [31] and is described in great detail in Chap. 22.

3.5   Conclusions

While every effort must be made to prevent an OASI, causing a third or fourth degree tear is rarely culpable; missing the diagnosis of OASIs however, is usually regarded as negligent. Postpartum endoanal ultrasound is an invasive and expensive alternative that requires expertise and may result in overdiagnosis of OASIs. Instead, the keystone to diagnosis of OASIs lies in improved clinical training of doctors and midwives. To minimise the risk of undiagnosed OASIs, a structured digital vaginal and anorectal examination should be performed in every woman following vaginal birth, especially prior to any suturing.

Take Home Messages

- Obstetricians and midwives must be trained to diagnose OASIs
- Failure to recognise OASIs can have a dramatic effect on quality of life
- Implementing the tips and tricks taught in this chapter will minimise the risk of missing OASIs
- A structured vaginal and rectal examination must be performed after each vaginal birth to exclude OASIs and rectal buttonhole tears

Appendix: MCQ

Questions

1. In terms of classification of OASIs, which of the following statements are true?
    (A)   A diagnosis of a third degree tear should only be made if the anal mucosa has been breached.
    (B)   A superficial tear of the EAS is a second degree tear.
    (C)   When the internal sphincter is torn it is classified as a Grade 3c tear.
    (D)   When it is uncertain whether more than 50% of the EAS thickness has been breached, the tear should be classified as a Grade 3b.

    (E)   An isolated button-hole tear of the rectum is a fourth degree tear.

2. Concerning the clinical diagnosis of OASIs which of the following statements are true?
    (A)   OASIs cannot occur when the vaginal and perineal skin is intact.
    (B)   Any tear of the perineal skin that extends to the anal verge should be considered a third/fourth degree tear until proven otherwise.
    (C)   OASIs cannot be excluded without a digital rectal examination.
    (D)   When doing a rectal examination, the thumb plays an essential role in confirming the diagnosis of an OASIs.
    (E)   Asking the woman to contract her sphincters will clearly demarcate any injury to the anal sphincter.

3. Regarding the clinical diagnosis of OASIs, which of the following statements are true?
    (A)   A full thickness grade 3b tear is always obvious and easy to diagnose.
    (B)   If the IAS is clinically visible, the EAS is inevitably torn.
    (C)   The ruptured conjoint longitudinal muscle appears as a bright pink sheet between the anal mucosa and the IAS.
    (D)   The superficial transverse perineal muscle can be easily confused with the EAS.
    (E)   There is evidence of clinical under and over diagnosis of OASIs.

4. With regards to the landmarks during diagnosis of OASIs, which of the following statements is/are correct?
    (A)   The proximal margin of the IAS margin is better demarcated than the EAS.
    (B)   The distal margin of the IAS is always proximal to the subcutaneous EAS.
    (C)   The ischioanal fat lies lateral to the EAS.
    (D)   When a 3a tear occurs the EAS can retract completely within its capsule.
    (E)   The anal sphincter length in the female measures 5 cm in length.

5. With regards to imaging of the anal sphincter, which of the following statements is/are true?
   (A) The best way to diagnose a rectal buttonhole tear is using ultrasound.
   (B) Endoanal ultrasound performed during pregnancy is not a risk for preterm labour.
   (C) Most OASIs are occult and can only be diagnosed by anal ultrasound.
   (D) Postpartum anal ultrasound is superior to digital rectal and vaginal examination in the detection of acute OASIs and should be used as first line when available.
   (E) All women who have had a vaginal birth should have endoanal scans performed within 3 months of delivery to diagnose missed OASIs.

Answers

1. In terms of classification of OASIs, which of the following statements are true?
   (A) FALSE
   (B) FALSE
   (C) TRUE
   (D) TRUE
   (E) FALSE

2. Concerning the clinical diagnosis of OASIs which of the following statements are true?
   (A) TRUE
   (B) TRUE
   (C) TRUE
   (D) TRUE
   (E) FALSE

3. Regarding the clinical diagnosis of OASIs, which of the following statements are true?
   (A) FALSE
   (B) TRUE
   (C) FALSE
   (D) TRUE
   (E) TRUE

4. With regards to the landmarks during diagnosis of OASIs, which of the following statements is/are correct?
   (A) FALSE
   (B) FALSE
   (C) TRUE
   (D) FALSE
   (E) FALSE

5. With regards to imaging of the anal sphincter, which of the following statements is/are true?
   (A) FALSE
   (B) TRUE
   (C) FALSE
   (D) FALSE
   (E) FALSE

References

1. Sultan AH, Kamm MA, Hudson CN, Bartram CI. Third degree obstetric anal sphincter tears: risk factors and outcome of primary repair. BMJ. 1994;308:887–91.
2. Sultan AH, Kamm MA, Hudson CN, Thomas JM, Bartram CI. Anal sphincter disruption during vaginal delivery. N Engl J Med. 1993;329:1905–11.
3. Sultan AH, Kamm MA, Hudson CN. Obstetric perineal tears: an audit of training. J Obstet Gynaecol. 1995;15:19–23.
4. Fernando RJ, Sultan AH, Radley S, Jones PW, Johanson RB. Management of obstetric anal sphincter injury: a systematic review and national practice survey. BMC Health Serv Res. 2002;2:9.
5. Sultan AH, Thakar R. Lower genital tract and anal sphincter trauma. Best Pract Res Clin Obstet Gynaecol. 2002;16:99–116.
6. Andrews V, Thakar R, Sultan AH, Jones PW. Occult anal sphincter injuries—myth or reality? BJOG. 2006;113:195–200.
7. Donald I. Practical obstetric problems. 5th ed. London: Lloyd-Luke; 1979. p. 811–24.
8. Sultan AH. Editorial: obstetric perineal injury and anal incontinence. AVMA Med Legal J (Clinical Risk). 1999;5:193–6. https://doi.org/10.1177/135626229900500601.
9. Norton C, Christiansen J, Butler U, Harari D, Nelson RL, Pemberton J, Price K, Rovnor E, Sultan A. Anal incontinence. In: Abrams P, Cardozo L, Khoury WA, editors. Incontinence. 2nd ed. Plymouth: Health Publication; 2002. p. 985–1044.

10. Roper JC, Amber N, Wan OYK, Sultan AH, Thakar R. Review of available national guidelines for obstetric anal sphincter injury. Int Urogynecol J. 2020;31(11):2247–59.

11. Royal College of Obstetricians and Gynaecologists. Management of third and fourth degree perineal tears following vaginal delivery. London: RCOG Press; 2015. RCOG green-top guideline no. 29.

12. American College of Obstetricians and Gynecologists. Practice bulletin no. 198: prevention and management of obstetric lacerations at vaginal delivery. Obstet Gynecol. 2018;132(3):e87–e102.

13. Sioutis D, Thakar R, Sultan AH. Overdiagnosis and rising rate of obstetric anal sphincter injuries (OASIS): time for reappraisal. Ultrasound Obstet Gynecol. 2017;50(5):642–7.

14. Thakar R, Sultan AH. Anal endosonography and its role in assessing the incontinent patient. Best Pract Res Clin Obstet Gynaecol. 2004;18:157–73. https://doi.org/10.1016/j.bpobgyn.2003.09.007.

15. Roper JC, Naidu M, Thakar R, Sultan AH. Getting the size right: are clinicians ready for it? Eur J Obstet Gynecol Reprod Biol. 2023;280:154–9.

16. Sultan AH, Kettle C. Diagnosis of perineal trauma. In: Sultan AH, Thakar R, Fenner D, editors. Perineal and anal sphincter trauma. London: Springer; 2007. p. 33–5.

17. Roper JC, Thakar R, Sultan AH. Isolated rectal buttonhole tears in obstetrics: case series and review of the literature. Int Urogynecol J. 2021;32(7):1761–9.

18. Roos A-M, Thakar R, Sultan AH. Outcome of primary repair of obstetric anal sphincter injuries (OASIS): does the grade of tear matter? Ultrasound Obstet Gynecol. 2010;36(3):368–74.

19. Taithongchai A, Veiga SI, Sultan AH, Thakar R. The consequences of undiagnosed obstetric anal sphincter injuries (OASIS) following vaginal delivery. Int Urogynecol J. 2020;31:635–41.

20. Zetterstrom J, Mellgren A, Jensen LJ, Wong WD, Kim DG, Lowry AC, Madoff RD, Congilosi SM. Effect of delivery on anal sphincter morphology and function. Dis Colon Rectum. 1999;42:1253–60.

21. Rieger N, Schloithe A, Saccone G, Wattchow D. A prospective study of anal sphincter injury due to childbirth. Scand J Gastroenterol. 1998;33:950–5.

22. Groom KM, Paterson-Brown S. Can we improve on the diagnosis of third degree tears? Eur J Obstet Gynecol Reprod Biol. 2002;101:19–21.

23. Roper JC, Thakar R, Sultan AH. Under-classified obstetric anal sphincter injuries. Int Urogynecol J. 2022;33(6):1473–9.

24. Andrews V, Thakar R, Sultan AH. Structured hands-on training in repair of obstetric anal sphincter injuries (OASIS): an audit of clinical practice. Int Urogynecol J. 2009;20(2):193–9.

25. Wong KW, Thakar R, Sultan AH, Andrews V. Can transperineal ultrasound improve the diagnosis of obstetric anal sphincter injuries? Int Urogynecol J. 2022;33(10):2809–14.

26. Lal M, Mann CH, Callender R, Radley S. Does cesarean delivery prevent anal incontinence? Obstet Gynecol. 2003;101:305–12.

27. Benifla JL, Abramowitz L, Sobhani I et al. [Postpartum sphincter rupture and anal incontinence: prospective study with 259 patients]. Gynecol Obstet Fertil. 2000;28(1):15–22.

28. Faltin DL, Boulvain M, Floris LA, Irion O. Diagnosis of anal sphincter tears to prevent fecal incontinence: a randomized controlled trial. Obstet Gynecol. 2005;106(1):6–13.

29. Huber M, Larsson C, Harrysson M, Strigård K, Lehmann JP, Nordin P, Tunón K. Use of endoanal ultrasound in detecting obstetric anal sphincter injury immediately after birth. Acta Obstet Gynecol Scand. 2023;102:389–95. https://doi.org/10.1111/aogs.14514. Epub ahead of print. PMID: 36683208.

30. Sultan AH, Thakar R. Diagnosis of anal sphincter tears to prevent fecal incontinence: a randomized controlled trial. Obstet Gynecol. 2005;106:1108–9.

31. Young R, Nippita TAC. Training in obstetric anal sphincter injuries in Australia and New Zealand: a survey of Royal Australian and New Zealand College of Obstetricians and Gynaecologists trainees. Aust N Z J Obstet Gynaecol. 2022;62(2):250–4. https://doi.org/10.1111/ajo.13437. Epub 2021 Sep 29. PMID: 34585741.

Episiotomy, First and Second Degree Tears

4

Sara Webb and Ranee Thakar

Overview
Test your learning and check your understanding of this book's contents: use the "Springer Nature Flashcards" app to access questions using ▶ https://sn.pub/wqrf89. To use the app, please follow the instructions in Chap. 1.

Learning Points

- To learn the definition and classification of perineal trauma
- To understand the type of episiotomies performed
- To understand the established evidence for various repair techniques and materials used in repair of a second-degree tear or episiotomy
- To understand the basic surgical principles of suturing perineal tears
- To learn the technique of perineal repair

S. Webb (✉)
Royal College of Midwives, London, UK
e-mail: sara.webb@rcm.org.uk

R. Thakar
Department of Obstetrics and Gynaecology, Croydon University Hospital, Croydon, Surrey, UK

4.1 Introduction

The morbidity associated with perineal injury related to childbirth constitutes a major health problem, affecting millions of women worldwide. The majority of women following vaginal delivery will suffer some degree of perineal pain or discomfort during the early postpartum period [1]. Pain associated with perineal trauma can be very distressing for a new mother and may interfere with her ability to breastfeed and cope with the daily tasks of motherhood [2–4]. It also appears to have a clear causal association with sexual dysfunction, which ultimately may affect the woman's relationship with her partner [5].

A cohort study in Spain demonstrated that, irrespective of parity, there were clear differences in perineal pain and dyspareunia depending on which perineal muscle was injured and the complexity of damage sustained [6]. This study found that significantly more women with more complex muscle trauma reported dyspareunia at 3 months postpartum compared with women with less complex muscle trauma; when perineal muscle trauma encompassed >50% of the bulbospongiosus ± the superficial transverse perineal muscle, perineal pain and dyspareunia persisted until 10 days and 6 months postpartum, respectively.

There are several key factors that may have a direct effect on the extent of morbidity experienced by women following perineal repair and include the degree of perineal damage, the technique and materials used for suturing, and the skill of the person performing the procedure. If the suturing is performed perfunctorily, it may have a major impact on women's health, as well as significant implications for health service resources. It is important that practitioners ensure that routine procedures such as perineal repair are evidence-based in order to provide quality care that is effective, appropriate and cost-efficient.

4.2   Definition

Perineal trauma during vaginal birth may occur either spontaneously or when the midwife or obstetrician facilitates delivery by making a surgical incision (episiotomy) to increase the diameter of the vulval outlet. The standard obstetric and midwifery texts usually describe only two types of episiotomy (median and mediolateral), although seven different incisions have been described in the literature [7]. The term 'episiotomy' refers to cutting the pudenda (external genitalia), whereas the term 'perineotomy' is defined as an incision of the perineum and is thus the more accurate term [8].

Anatomically, the perineum extends from the pubic arch to the coccyx and is divided into the anterior urogenital and posterior anal triangle. Anterior perineal trauma is defined as injury to the labia, anterior vagina, urethra or clitoris. Trauma in this area is associated with less morbidity, however, little is known about the long-term effects of anterior perineal trauma. Posterior perineal trauma is defined as any injury to the posterior vaginal wall, perineal muscles or anal sphincters (external and internal) and may include disruption of the rectal mucosa [9].

4.3   Prevalence

Although maternity care has vastly improved over the past decade, perineal trauma is one aspect of childbirth that women appear to be unprepared for. Findings from a large randomised controlled trial (RCT) indicate that 85% of women who have a vaginal birth will sustain some form of perineal trauma and up to 69% of

these lacerations will require stitches [10] However, these rates vary considerably according to the policies of individuals and institutions throughout the world. It is difficult to ascertain global rates of spontaneous perineal trauma requiring suturing and episiotomy due to classification inconsistencies and a lack of reporting of perineal trauma. For example, compared to high-income settings, a systematic review identified that episiotomy rates are significantly higher in low-middle income country (LMIC) medical facilities. This review also highlighted an urgent need to improve reporting of birth related perineal trauma in LMICs, particularly with regards to births taking place in community settings [11].

4.4   Episiotomy Rates: Is There an 'Ideal'?

A comprehensive review of available data by Graham et al. highlighted that despite episiotomy being a common surgical procedure, there is difficulty in ascertaining the rates at which it is performed, both across and within countries, due to the way the data are collected and reported [12].

Based on data from a RCT, the World Health Organization recommends an episiotomy rate of 10% as "a good goal to pursue", and strongly advocates for all countries to adhere to a selective episiotomy practice [13, 14]. Within the United Kingdom, the mean rate of episiotomy has grown from 21.9% in 2015/2016 to 25.1% in 2018/2019 [15]. On the other hand,

Freidman et al. demonstrated that use of episiotomy in the United States (US) has declined over time, possibly reflecting the adoption of some recommendations [16]. There was a temporal decline in rates of episiotomy between 2006 (17.3%; 95% CI, 17.2–17.4%) and 2012 (11.6%; 95% CI, 11.5–11.7%). The analysis demonstrated substantial between-hospital variation in episiotomy not accounted for by demographic, obstetric, and hospital characteristics. In addition, demographic and hospital factors, such as insurance, race, rurality, and hospital teaching status, were associated with the rates of episiotomy. These observations suggest nonmedical factors influence the use of episiotomy.

4.5 Classification of Perineal Trauma

Spontaneous perineal trauma can be sub-divided into the following classifications according to the extent of the tissue damage:

- First degree, which may involve:
  - skin and subcutaneous tissue of the anterior or posterior perineum
  - vaginal mucosa
  - a combination of the above resulting in multiple superficial lacerations
- Second degree, which is deeper and may involve:
  - superficial perineal muscles (bulbospongiosus, transverse perineal)
  - perineal body

Second degree trauma usually extends downwards from the posterior and/or lateral vaginal walls, through the hymenal remnants, towards the anal margin; it usually occurs in the weakest part of the stretched perineum. Less frequently, the tear extends in a circular direction, behind the hymenal remnants, bilaterally upwards towards the clitoris causing the lower third of the vagina to detach from underlying structures [17]. This type of complex trauma causes vast disruption to the perineal body and muscles, but the perineal skin may remain intact making it difficult to repair.

An episiotomy usually involves the same structures as a second-degree tear, but occasionally spontaneous trauma may occur simultaneously resulting in more complex perineal injury.

4.6 Indications for Episiotomy

The wide variation in episiotomy rates globally suggests that the indications for episiotomy are not evidence-based. A Cochrane review which included 12 studies concluded that for women where an unassisted vaginal birth was anticipated, a policy of selective episiotomy may result in 30% fewer women experiencing severe perineal/vaginal trauma [18]. This evidence-based review thus demonstrates that routine episiotomy does not reduce perineal/vaginal trauma. On the other hand, the evidence for performing episiotomy during an assisted birth is covered in Chap. 12. A recent meta-analysis, which included only two studies, showed no significant difference between non-episiotomy and selective episiotomy regarding OASIS. This raises important questions as to whether episiotomy should be performed in a setting of labour [19].

The main indications for performing an episiotomy are to:

- Aid in the birth if the perineal tissue is very rigid and is delaying the second stage.
- Reduce prolonged maternal 'pushing' in cases of severe maternal cardiac disease or hypertension.
- Accelerate spontaneous vaginal birth in cases of suspected fetal compromise.
- Prevent severe perineal trauma during instrumental birth (forceps or ventouse)
- Facilitate maneuvers necessary in cases of shoulder dystocia and breech vaginal birth.

4.7 Non-suturing of First and Second Degree Tears

The controversy regarding the best management of perineal trauma relating to suturing following childbirth has continued throughout the centuries.

Non-suturing of first and second degree tears is becoming widespread in the UK, despite the dearth of evidence to support this practice [20–23]. Metcalfe and colleagues [23] reported that up to 50% of first and second degree tears were not sutured in some hospitals within the West Midlands, UK. Midwives who advocate for this practice claim that women experience less pain and infection and the wound heals at a faster rate. However, those who support suturing question what effects non-suturing may have on wound healing, aesthetics, sexual function, pelvic floor muscle strength, incontinence and prolapse. In the United States, suturing remains the primary management of perineal trauma following childbirth.

There is limited evidence available from RCTs to guide the choice between surgical or non-surgical repair of first- or second-degree perineal tears sustained during childbirth [19].

Two RCTs compared the effects of non-suturing versus suturing of first and second degree tears [24, 25]. A Swedish RCT (n = 78 primiparous women) found a non-significant increase in short-term discomfort (burning sensation and soreness) associated with non-suturing and no difference in rates of wound healing between groups; however, it is unclear how healing was defined and assessed [24]. Similarly, a Scottish RCT (n = 74 primiparous women) [25], found no significant difference in McGill pain scores at 10 days and 6 weeks between non-suturing and suturing.

As there is little evidence of good methodological quality to support this controversial practice of non-suturing, practitioners must be cautious about leaving trauma unsutured, unless it is the explicit wish of the woman [26].

4.8 Suturing Methods

Perineal trauma is conventionally repaired in three layers. First, a continuous 'locking' stitch is used to close the vaginal trauma, commencing at the apex of the wound and finishing at the level of the fourchette with a loop knot. Traditional, a 'locking' stitch is used, as a continuous 'running' stitch may cause shortening of the vagina if it is pulled too tight. However, no controlled studies have investigated this theory. Next, the deep and superficial perineal muscles are re-approximated using a continuous running stitch. Sometimes, interrupted sutures may be necessary. Finally, the skin is closed using continuous subcutaneous or interrupted transcutaneous techniques when necessary [27].

A Cochrane review that included 16 studies involving 8184 women showed that continuous suture techniques compared with interrupted sutures for perineal closure (all layers or perineal skin only) are associated with less pain for up to 10 'days' postpartum. There was also an overall reduction in analgesia use associated with the continuous subcutaneous technique for repair of the perineal skin. A reduction in suture removal in the continuous suturing groups was also observed, and no significant differences were

seen in the need for re-suturing of wounds or long-term pain [28].

This difference in pain between suturing methods is thought to be due to increasing suture tension caused by oedema. With the continuous technique of repair, tension is transferred throughout the whole length of the single knotless suture; this differs from interrupted stitches, which are placed transversely across the wound. Also, continuous skin sutures are inserted into the subcutaneous tissue, thus avoiding nerve endings in the skin surface whereas interrupted transcutaneous sutures are inserted through the skin. Given that the benefits of the technique are apparent in 2 days, this explanation seems most plausible [27]. Another advantage of the continuous technique is that only one packet of suture material is usually required to complete the repair (as compared to two or three packets used for the interrupted method), thus reducing the overall expenditure for hospitals.

4.9 Suture Materials

Throughout the ages, many techniques have used to close wounds. Between 50,000 and 30,000 B.C., 'eyed' needles were invented [29]. Other references indicate that linen strips coated with an adhesive mixture of honey and flour (similar to steri-strips), were used to close wounds. In the late nineteenth and twentieth centuries, catgut was favoured to repair perineal tears because stitches dissolved, whereas silkworm gut sutures usually had to be removed on the seventh day. Other materials that have been used for perineal repair over the past 50 years include silk, nylon, polyamide, prolene, chromic catgut, softgut and tissue adhesive.

Sutures are inserted to maintain wound closure, control bleeding, minimise the risk of infection and expedite healing. Well-aligned perineal wounds heal by primary intention with minimal complications, usually within 2 weeks of suturing. Wound edges must be re-approximated without tension, otherwise the tissue may become devascularised resulting in disruption of the healing process [30]. Suture materials should cause minimal tissue reaction and be absorbed once the wound has healed [31]. Most skin requires suture support for approximately 8 to 14 days to achieve adequate healing.

Polyglycolic acid (*Dexon®*, Davis & Geck Ltd. UK) and polyglactin 910 (*Vicryl®*, Ethicon Ltd., Edinburgh, UK), introduced in 1970 and 1974, respectively, were the two most common absorbable, synthetic sutures used for perineal repair. Standard polyglactin 910 sutures (*Vicryl®*) are prepared from a copolymer of glycolide and lactide in a ratio of 90/10, and the substances are derived from glycolic and lactic acids [30]. The material is braided to improve handling and is coated with a mixture of a copolymer of lactide and glycolide in the ratio of 65/35 and an equal ratio of calcium stearate to reduce bacterial adherence and tissue drag [32, 33]. During the manufacturing process, the material is dyed a bright violet colour to improve visualisation during surgical procedures [34]. It is attached to various sized stainless steel needles terilizatised by ethylene oxide gas. On the other hand, polyglycolic acid sutures (*Dexon®*) are produced from a homopolymer of glycolide without dye, so the resulting material is a light tan colour. The polymer is converted into a braided suture, which is very similar in composition to standard polyglactin 910 [33]. This material is designed to maintain wound support for up to 30 days and is not completely absorbed from the tissue until approximately 90 to 120 days [34]. The suture material is retained in the tissue beyond the required healing time, whereby it becomes a potential source of infection, defeating the purpose of using absorbable stitches [33].

Since 1996, absorbable polyglactin 910 material (*Vicryl rapide®*) but has been available in both the US and United Kingdom (UK) (Data on file at Ethicon Research Foundation). This suture is identical to standard polyglactin 910 (*coated Vicryl®*) in chemical composition, but it is undyed and is absorbed in less time. Its tensile strength is reduced in 10–14 days and it is completely absorbed by tissue in 42 days [35]. The more rapid absorption characteristics are achieved by exposing the material to gamma irradiation during terilizationtion process, resulting in a suture

with a lower molecular weight that is more readily hydrolysed [35]. Hydrolysis is the absorption mechanism whereby water penetrates the implanted sutures and causes breakdown of the fibrous? polymer chain with minimal inflammatory response. The degraded lactide and glycolide acid material is then eliminated from the body mainly in urine and faeces (Data on file at Ethicon Research Foundation [36]).

A Cochrane review of 18 trials (10,171 women) assessed the effects of different suture materials on short- and long-term morbidity following perineal repair after vaginal birth [36]. Compared with catgut, standard synthetic sutures were associated with less pain up to 3 days after birth and less analgesia up to 10 days postpartum. More women with catgut sutures required re-suturing and more women with standard synthetic sutures required the removal of unabsorbed suture material. Comparing standard synthetic with rapidly absorbing sutures, short- and long-term pain were similar, although in one trial fewer women with rapidly absorbing sutures reported using analgesics at 10 days. More women in the standard synthetic suture group required suture removal compared with those in the rapidly absorbed group. There were no significant differences between groups in long-term pain (3 months after delivery) or dyspareunia at three, or at six to 12 months [36].

Therefore, in the light of current evidence, more rapidly absorbed polyglactin 910 (*Vicryl rapide®*) is the most appropriate suture material for perineal repair [1].

4.10 Management of Perineal Trauma

4.10.1 Basic Surgical Principles

Carefully sutured perineal trauma following childbirth generally heals within 2 weeks by primary intention. This is probably because immediately after parturition, the perineum provides optimal conditions for quality healing. Some of these include moisture, warmth, increased vascularity, reduced exposure, and a favourable acidic pH in which organisms are usually unable to grow. The most common local factor associated with delayed perineal wound healing and dehiscence is infection, which causes reduced collagen synthesis. This adversely causes the wound edges to be softened, which may result in sutures 'cutting out' of the tissue with subsequent wound breakdown.

The following basic surgical principles should be followed when performing primary perineal repairs:

- Suture as soon as possible after childbirth to prevent excessive blood loss and to minimise the risk of infection.
- Check equipment and count cotton swabs and sponges prior to commencing the perineal repair and repeat following completion of the procedure.
- Ensure use of a good light source to enable full visualialization of the extent of the trauma and to identify the structures involved.
- Repair complex trauma in an operating room under regional or general anaesthesia. An indwelling urinary catheter should be inserted for 24 hours to prevent urinary retention.
- Ask for more experienced assistance if the trauma is beyond the operator's scope of practice.
- Close dead space and ensure haemostasis to prevent haematoma formation.
- Do not over-tighten sutures; this might cause tissue hypoxia, which subsequently may delay the healing process.
- Tie sutures securely using square surgeon's knots.
- Ensure good anatomical alignment of the wound and also give consideration to the cosmetic results.

4.10.2 First Degree Tears and Labial Lacerations

First degree tears must be sutured if there is excessive bleeding or if there is any uncertainty regarding alignment of the traumatised tissue which may affect healing. If the tear is left unsutured, the midwife or doctor must discuss the potential implications of this and obtain the patient's informed consent. Details regarding the discussion and consent must be fully documented in the woman's case notes.

Labial lacerations are usually very superficial but may be very painful. Some practitioners do not recommend suturing, but if the trauma is bilateral, the lacerations can sometimes adhere together over the urethra and the woman may present with voiding difficulties. It is important to advise the patient to part the labia daily during bathing to prevent adhesions from occurring. If suturing is performed, this is best done using 3-0 polyglactin (Vicryl®).

4.10.3 Repair of Episiotomy and Second Degree Tears

Prior to performing the perineal repair, the practitioner must prepare the equipment according to practice policies and guidelines. Safety glasses and gloves must be worn during all obstetric procedures to protect the operator against infection. The woman should be placed in a comfortable position, so that the trauma can easily be visualized. Second degree perineal tears and episiotomies are repaired under aseptic conditions, and the area should be cleaned prior to commencing the suturing according to local policy. A rectal examination should be performed routinely when assessing perineal injury to avoid missing an obstetric anal sphincter injury. This should be repeated once the repair is complete to ensure that suture material has not been accidentally inserted through the rectal mucosa.

As long as adequate visualisation is possible, it is not always necessary to use lithotomy poles or stirrups to support the woman's legs during the repair, especially if she is a survivor of abuse, as this may be triggering [37]. Furthermore, leg restraints (high stirrups or lithotomy poles) cause flexion and abduction of the hips and may result in excessive stretching of the perineum and tearing or gapeing of the laceration. This may make the trauma more difficult to realign and suture. Furthermore, a tampon may obscure visualisation of the apex of the vaginal trauma, so excessive uterine bleeding should be managed appropriately prior to commencing the perineal suturing.

It is imperative that the wound is adequately anaesthetised prior to commencing the repair. Ten to twenty millilitres of Lignocaine 1% should be injected evenly into the perineal wound. We recommend this even if the woman has an epidural, as it may be used to block perineal pain during suturing.

4.10.4 The Continuous Suturing Technique

As noted above, current evidence suggests that perineal trauma should be repaired using a continuous, non-locking technique to re-approximate all layers (vagina, perineal muscles and skin) with absorbable polyglactin 910 material (*Vicryl rapide®*).

4.10.4.1   Suturing the Vagina

The first stitch is inserted above the apex of the vaginal trauma to secure any bleeding points that might not be visible. The vaginal trauma is closed with a loose, continuous, non-locking technique ensuring that each stitch is not inserted too widely, thus potentially narrowing the vagina. Suturing is continued down to the hymenal remnants. The needle is inserted through the skin at the fourchette to emerge in the centre of the perineal muscle trauma (Fig. 4.1).

4.10.4.2   Suturing the Muscle Layer

Next, the depth of the trauma is determined and the perineal muscles (deep and superficial) are approximated again using continuous, non-locking stitches without tension. If the trauma is deep, the perineal muscles can be closed using two layers of continuous stitches. It is important to ensure that the stitches are not inserted through the rectum or anal canal (Fig. 4.1).

4.10.4.3   Suturing the Perineal Skin

At the inferior margin of the wound, the needle is brought out just under the skin surface, reversing the stitching direction. The skin sutures are placed in a subcuticular fashion, thus avoiding the profusion of nerve endings. The wound edges are reapproximated serially to the level of the hymenal remnants. The finished repair is secured with a loop or Aberdeen knot placed in the vagina behind the hymenal remnants (Fig. 4.2).

At the completion of the repair:

- Check that there is no excessive bleeding and that the repair is anatomically correct.
- Document a detailed account of the repair in the woman's case notes, including suture method and materials used. It is also useful to include a simple diagram illustrating the structures involved.
- Inform the patient regarding the use of appropriate analgesia, hygiene and the importance of a good diet and daily pelvic floor exercises.
- Detail for the patient a full explanation of the injury sustained and contact information if she has any problems during the postnatal period. Specially designated clinics should be available for women with perineal complications to ensure appropriate, sensitive and effective treatment.

4.10.5 Training

It is current practice in the UK for the attending midwife to suture an episiotomy, undertake repair of first and second degree perineal tears as necessary, and refer if additional trauma has occurred [39]. However, there are wide variations between hospitals and practitioners in suturing techniques and materials chosen for perineal repair.

A recent survey in the UK and Spain found that 91% of UK students completed their training without cutting or repairing an episiotomy [40]. This compares to only 39% of registered midwives, who did not cut an episiotomy during their period of training. Only 20% of Spanish and 10% of UK registered midwives felt confident undertaking these techniques. In the US, McClellan [41] surveyed senior obstetrics and gynaecology house officers concerning their experience and knowledge of perineal repairs. Sixty percent of

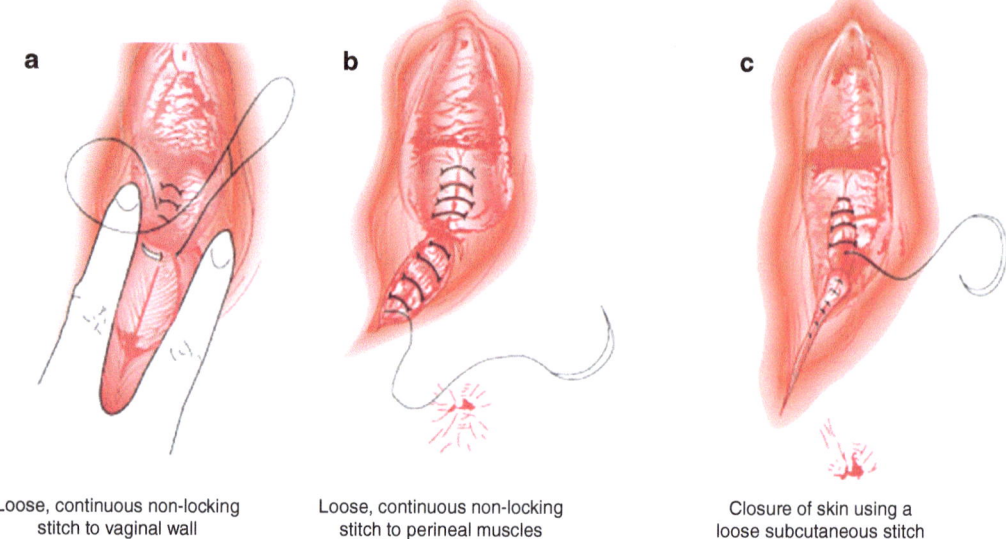

a	b	c
Loose, continuous non-locking stitch to vaginal wall	Loose, continuous non-locking stitch to perineal muscles	Closure of skin using a loose subcutaneous stitch

Fig. 4.1 The continuous suturing technique for mediolateral episiotomy. (Adapted with permission from an illustration in Cunningham et al. (1993) by Kettle [27])

residents reported receiving no didactics or formal training on episiotomy techniques. Only 7% had repaired more than 20 fourth-degree lacerations and 40% reported repairing more than 20 third-degree lacerations. This research highlights the discontent amongst trainee doctors and midwives with their training in perineal repair; clearly more intense and focused training in this arena is warranted. A more recent cross-sectional US national survey of certified nurse-midwives assessing the classification and identification of OASI and other birth related perineal lacerations, demonstrated a wide range (49–99%) of overall accuracy for classification and identification of perineal lacerations [42].

Similarly, midwifery patients have expressed dissatisfaction following their personal experiences of perineal repair. Most concerns were directly related to training issues; these included the operator being inexperienced, unsupervised or having to learn by trial and error [43, 44]. A further consideration is that most practitioners have no means of observing the long-term effects of the perineal suturing in order to audit their own practice [45]. Furthermore, there continue to be wide variations in the way the procedure is taught, supervised and assessed, as there are no national guidelines relating to the training of operators. Practitioners who are appropriately trained and assessed will be more likely to consistently provide a high standard of perineal repair which likely has a direct effect on the short- and long-term reduction of morbidity associated with this procedure.

4.11 Conclusion

Mismanagement of perineal trauma has a major impact on women's health and significant implications on health service resources. Health professionals must base their practice on current evidence-based medicine and be aware of complications associated with perineal trauma and repair. Careful identification and repair of trauma by a skilled practitioner likely decreases short and long-term complications. Furthermore, it is important that prompt and sensitive treatment is provided for those women with complications in order to reduce the morbidity associated with perineal injury following childbirth.

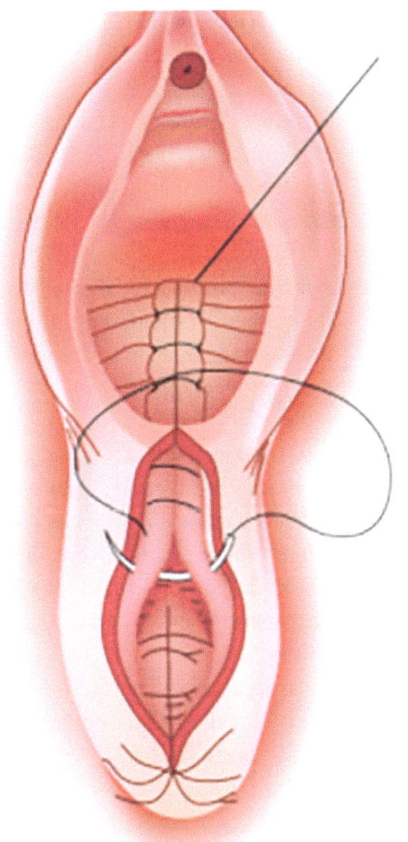

There is no evidence to support the use of routine episiotomy during unassisted vaginal birth.

• Continuous suture techniques compared with interrupted sutures for perineal closure (all layers or perineal skin only) are associated with less pain and a reduction in the need for suture removal.

• Current evidence suggests that the more rapidly absorbed polyglactin 910 (*Vicryl rapide*®) is the most appropriate suture material for perineal repair.

• Health professionals must be aware of complications associated with perineal trauma and repair, as the majority of women will experience pain in the early postnatal period that may interfere with daily activities, breastfeeding and sexual relationships.

• It is important that prompt and sensitive treatment is provided for women with complications during the postnatal period in order to reduce the morbidity associated with perineal injury following childbirth.

• There is a need for more focused training on perineal repair for both obstetricians and midwives.

Fig. 4.2 Continuous suturing technique for midline episiotomyOnce the vaginal mucosa has been closed to the hymenal ring, the needle is passed from the midline to the perineal body and a crown stitch reapproximating the bulbospongiosus muscles is performed. A subcuticular stitch is carried from the inferior perineal margin to the hymen and tied [38]

Take Home Messages

• Up to 85% of women giving birth vaginally will sustain perineal trauma and 69% of these tears will require suturing.

• As there is little evidence to support non-suturing of first and second-degree tears, practitioners must be cautious about leaving trauma un-sutured, unless it is the explicit wish of the woman.

Appendix: MCQ

Mark each item TRUE or FALSE

Questions

1. In terms of the classification of OASIS:
   (A) A diagnosis of a third degree tear should only be made if the anal mucosa has been breached.
   (B) A superficial tear of the EAS is a second degree tear.
   (C) When the internal sphincter is torn it is classified as a Grade 3c tear.
   (D) When it is uncertain whether more than 50% of the EAS thickness has been breached, the tear should be classified as a Grade 3b.

(E)   An isolated button-hole tear of the rectum is a fourth degree tear.

2. In terms of the classification of perineal trauma:
   (A)   A lateral episiotomy should be classified as a first degree tear.
   (B)   A second degree perineal tear involves the superficial perineal muscles (bulbospongiosus, transverse perineal).
   (C)   A first degree perineal tear only involves the vaginal mucosa.
   (D)   An episiotomy only involves the same structures as a second degree tear.
   (E)   Second degree tears can extend to damage the levator ani muscles.

3. With respect to complications of perineal trauma:
   (A)   The majority of women will not suffer pain or discomfort during the early postnatal period.
   (B)   Pain associated with perineal trauma can be very distressing for the new mother and may interfere with her ability to breast feed and cope with the daily tasks of motherhood.
   (C)   It is important that practitioners ensure that perineal repair is evidence-based in order to provide quality care which is effective, appropriate and cost-efficient.
   (D)   The rates of complications reported by women do not depend on the severity of perineal trauma or on the effectiveness of treatment.
   (E)   Perineal trauma appears to have a clear causal association with sexual dysfunction and ultimately may affect the woman's relationship with her partner.

4. The following are a primary indication for an episiotomy:
   (A)   To maintain integrity of the perineal muscles particularly in a primigravid woman

   (B)   To decrease the risk of OASIS if the woman has previously sustained a third degree tear
   (C)   To reduce severe perineal trauma during an instrumental birth
   (D)   To decrease the complications of a shoulder dystocia

5. With respect to perineal repairs:
   (A)   The Surgeon's square knot is preferable for securing the apex of the vaginal wall in the perineal repair.
   (B)   If there is good anatomical alignment, the cosmetic results are not important.
   (C)   Providing the layers are sutured, closing of dead space is not necessary.
   (D)   Sutures must not be over-tightened as this might cause tissue hypoxia, which subsequently may delay the healing process.
   (E)   All aspects of the perineal repair must be explained to the woman both prior and following repair.

Answers

1. In terms of the classification of OASIS:
   (A)   FALSE
   (B)   FALSE
   (C)   TRUE
   (D)   TRUE
   (E)   FALSE

2. In terms of the classification of perineal trauma:
   (A)   FALSE
   (B)   TRUE
   (C)   FALSE
   (D)   FALSE
   (E)   TRUE

3. With respect to complications of perineal trauma:
   (A)   FALSE
   (B)   TRUE

(C) TRUE
(D) FALSE
(E) TRUE

4. The following are a primary indication for an episiotomy:
   (A) FALSE
   (B) FALSE
   (C) TRUE
   (D) TRUE

5. With respect to perineal repairs:
   (A) TRUE
   (B) FALSE
   (C) FALSE
   (D) TRUE
   (E) TRUE

References

1. Macarthur AJ, Macarthur C. Incidence, severity, and determinants of perineal pain after vaginal delivery: a prospective cohort study. Am J Obstet Gynecol. 2004;191(4):1199–204.

2. O'Malley D, Higgins A, Smith V. Postpartum sexual health: a principle-based concept analysis. J Adv Nurs. 2015;71(10):2247–57.

3. Sleep J. Postnatal perineal care revisited. In: Alexander J, Levy V, Roch S, editors. Aspects of midwifery practice. A research based approach. 1st ed. London: Macmillan Press; 1995. p. 132–53.

4. Sleep J. Perineal care: a series of five randomized controlled trials. In: Robinson S, Thomson A, editors. Midwives, research and childbirth, vol. 2. 1st ed. London: Chapman and Hall; 1991. p. 199–251.

5. O'Malley D, Higgins A, Begley C, Daly D, Smith V. Prevalence of and risk factors associated with sexual health issues in primiparous women at 6 and 12 months postpartum; a longitudinal prospective cohort study (the MAMMI study). BMC Pregnancy Childbirth. 2018;18(1):196.

6. Manresa M, Pereda A, Goberna-Tricas J, Webb SS, Terre-Rull C, Bataller E. Postpartum perineal pain and dyspareunia related to each superficial perineal muscle injury: a cohort study. Int Urogynecol J. 2020;31(11):2367–75.

7. Kalis V, Laine K, de Leeuw J, Ismail K, Tincello D. Classification of episiotomy: towards a standardisation of terminology. BJOG. 2012;119:522–6.

8. Thacker SB, Banta HD. Benefits and risks of episiotomy: an interpretative review of the English language literature 1860–1980. Obstet Gynecol Surv. 1983;38(6):322–34.

9. Kettle C, O'Brien S. Methods and materials used in perineal repair. London: Royal College of Obstetricians and Gynaecologists Guideline No 23, Revised July 2004.

10. McCandlish R, Bowler U, Van Asten H, Berridge G, Winter C, Sames L, Garcia J, Renfrew M, Elbourne D. A randomised controlled trial of care of the perineum during second stage of normal labour. Br J Obstet Gynaecol. 1998;105:1262–72.

11. Aguiar M, Farley A, Hope L, Ami A, Shah P. Birth-related perineal trauma in low- and middle-income countries; A systematic review and meta-analysis. Semira Manaseki Published online: 26 Mar 2019.

12. Graham ID, Carroli G, Davies C, Medves JM. Episiotomy rates around the world: an update. Birth. 2005;32(3):219–23. https://doi.org/10.1111/j.0730-7659.2005.00373.x.

13. World Health Organization Division of Family Health Maternal Health and Safe Motherhood. Care in normal birth: a practical guide. Report of a technical working group. Geneva: World Health Organization; 1996.

14. Sleep J, Grant A, Garcia J, Elbourne D, Spencer J, Chalmers I. West Berkshire perineal management trial. Br Med J (ClinRes Ed). 1984;289:587–90. https://doi.org/10.1136/bmj.289.6445.587.

15. Organisational Surveys, National maternity and Perinatal Audit, Royal College of Obstetricians and Gynaecologists. Accessed online 13th July 2022.

16. Friedman AM, Ananth CV, Prendergast E, D'Alton ME, Wright JD. Variation in and factors associated with use of episiotomy. JAMA. 2015;313(2):197–9. https://doi.org/10.1001/jama.2014.14774.

17. Sultan AH, Kamm MA, Bartram CI, Hudson CN. Perineal damage at delivery. Contemp Rev Obstet Gynaecol. 1994;6:18–24.

18. Jiang H, Qian X, Carroli G, Garner P. Selective versus routine use of episiotomy for vaginal birth. Cochrane Database Syst Rev. 2017;2(2):CD000081. https://doi.org/10.1002/14651858.CD000081.pub3. PMID: 28176333; PMCID: PMC5449575

19. Pereira GMV, Hosoume RS, de Castro Monteiro MV, Juliato CRT, Brito LGO. Selective episiotomy versus no episiotomy for severe perineal trauma: a systematic review with meta-analysis. Int Urogynecol J. 2020;31(11):2291–9. https://doi.org/10.1007/s00192-020-04308-2. Epub 2020 Apr 24

20. McCandlish R, Brocklehurst P, King V, Kettle C. Midwives should offer perineal repair. Pract Midwife. 1999;2(7):14–5.

21. Wood T. Not suturing is safe. Pract Midwife. 1999;2(7):15.

22. Gilpin-Blake D, Elliot S. A natural alternative to suturing. Midwifery Today (Winter). 2001;6:32.

23. Metcalfe A, Tohill S, Williams A, Haldon V, Brown L, Henry L. A pragmatic tool for the measurement of perineal tears. Br J Midwifery. 2002;10(7):412–7.

24. Lundquist M, Olsson A, Nissen E, Norman M. Is it necessary to suture all lacerations after a vaginal delivery? Birth. 2000;27(2):79–85.

25. Fleming EM, Hagan S, Niven C. Does perineal suturing make a difference? The SUNS trial. Br J Obstet Gynaecol. 2003;110:684–9.

26. Lewis P. Poor science makes poor practice. Mod Midwife. 1997;7(6):4–5.

27. Kettle C. Perineal repair: a randomised controlled trial of suturing techniques and materials following spontaneous vaginal birth. PhD thesis, Keele University, UK. 2002.

28. Kettle C, Dowswell T, Ismail KM. Continuous and interrupted suturing techniques for repair of episiotomy or second-degree tears. Cochrane Database Syst Rev. 2012;11(11):CD000947. https://doi.org/10.1002/14651858.CD000947.pub3. PMID: 23152204; PMCID: PMC7045987.

29. Kettle C, Johanson RB. Absorbable synthetic versus catgut suture material for perineal repair (Cochrane Review). In: The Cochrane Library, Issue 3. Oxford: Update Software; 2003.

30. Cuschieri A, Steele RJC, Moossa AR. Essential surgical practice. 4th ed. Oxford: Butterworth-Heinmann; 2000.

31. Taylor I, Karran SJ. Surgical principles. 1st ed. London: Oxford University Press; 1996.

32. Ethicon. Coated Vicryl Polyglactin 910: the gentle approach. Edinburgh: Ethicon Limited; 1992.

33. McCaul LK, Bagg J, Jenkins WMM. Rate of loss of irradiated polyglactin 910 (Vicryl Rapide) from the mouth: a prospective study. Br J Oral Maxillofacial Surg. 2000;38:328–30.

34. Craig PH, Williams JA, Davis KW, Magoun AD, Levy AJ, Bogdansky S, Jones JP. A biologic comparison of polyglactin 910 and polyglycolic acid synthetic absorbable sutures. Surg Gynecol Obst. 1975;141:1–10.

35. Mackrodt C, Gordon B, Fern E, Ayers S, Truesdale A, Grant A. The Ipswich childbirth study: 2. A randomised comparison of polyglactin 910 with chromic catgut for postpartum perineal repair. Br J Obstet Gynaecol. 1998;105(4):441–5.

36. Kettle C, Dowswell T, Ismail KMK. Absorbable suture materials for primary repair of episiotomy and second degree tears. Cochrane Database Syst Rev. 2010;(6):Art. No.: CD000006. https://doi.org/10.1002/14651858.CD000006.pub2. Accessed 13 July 2022.

37. Walton I. Sexuality and motherhood. Hale: Books for Midwives Press; 1994. p. 125.

38. Ethicon. A unique new product completes the family: VICRYL rapide. Edinburgh: Ethicon Limited; 1991.

39. NMC. Standards of proficiency for midwives. London: NMC; 2019.

40. Webb SS, Skene ER, Manresa M, Percy EK, Freeman RM, Tincello DG. Evaluation of midwifery pelvic floor education and Training across the UK and Spain. Eur J Obst Gynecol Reprod Biol. 2021;256:140–4.

41. McClellan MT, Melick CF, Clancy SL, Artel R. Episiotomy and perineal repair. An evaluation of resident education and experience. J Reprod Med. 2002;47(12):1025–30.

42. Diko S, Sheeder J, Guiah M, Nacht A, Reeves S, Connell KA, Joseph Hurt K. Identification of obstetric anal sphincter injuries (OASIs) and other lacerations: a national survey of nurse-midwives. Received: 19 Feb 2020/Accepted: 21 Mar 2021.

43. Rix JA. Painful and perineal problem, vol. 14. London: Daily Telegraph; 1992.

44. Brimacombe J. Reaping the pain which others have sewn. The Independent (14th March). 1995:21.

45. Lewis L. Are you sitting comfortably? The development of a perineal audit system to enable midwives to follow their perineal management up to 13 months postnatally. Midwives Chron. 1994:226–7.

Management of Acute Obstetric Anal Sphincter Injuries (OASIs)

Abdul H. Sultan and Ranee Thakar

Overview

Test your learning and check your understanding of this book's contents: use the "Springer Nature Flashcards" app to access questions using ▶ https://sn.pub/wqrf89. To use the app, please follow the instructions in Chap. 1.

Learning Objectives

- To appreciate that under-diagnosis and improper repair techniques of OASIs are associated with poor outcomes including anal incontinence
- To understand how to properly repair a torn internal and external sphincter as well as rectal "buttonhole" tears
- To understand evidence-based counseling of women who sustained OASIs regarding the mode of subsequent delivery

classification of OASIs (initially described by Sultan in 1999 [1]) is now widely adopted, in which third degree tears are subdivided into grade 3a, 3b and 3c tears. This is described in more detail in Chap. 3. The importance of this classification is highlighted by the fact that a network analysis of studies that used the Sultan Classification has shown that the outcome of a repair is related to the grade of that tear [2].

Apart from injuries to the anal sphincter, isolated rectal "buttonhole" tears can occur with or without a concomitant third degree tear [3]. Accurate assessment of these injuries (See Chap. 3) and proper repair are paramount to minimise the risk of anal incontinence and other complications [4]. Lastly, the ideal mode of subsequent birth is largely based on expert opinion and recommendations based on anal manometry and anal endosonography findings [5–9]. This chapter aims to describe the best repair techniques, post-partum management of these tears, and discuss the optimal mode of birth following OASIs.

5.1 Introduction

Acute Obstetric Anal Sphincter Injuries (OASIs) includes third and fourth degree perineal tears sustained during vaginal birth. A more nuanced

5.2 Historical Perspective

The earliest evidence of severe perineal injury sustained during childbirth is from the mummy of Henhenit, an Egyptian woman approximately 22 years of age from the harem of King Mentuhotep II of Egypt in 2050 BC [10]. Henhenit's pelvis was of abnormal shape and

A. H. Sultan (✉) · R. Thakar
Croydon University Hospital, London, UK

© The Author(s), under exclusive license to Springer Nature Switzerland AG 2024
A. H. Sultan et al. (eds.), *Pelvic Floor, Perineal, and Anal Sphincter Trauma During Childbirth*,
https://doi.org/10.1007/978-3-031-43095-4_5

showed evidence of vaginal rupture into the bladder and large bowel was found protruding from the anus. These severe perineal injuries may have been due to cephalo-pelvic disproportion that probably resulted in her early death.

The first mention of the surgical management of severe perineal injury appears in Avicenna's famous Arabic book, "Al Kanoun". In this text, he recommended a form of a crossed or "bootlace" suture for the repairs of perineal injuries. This was unlike Celsus, who offered only bedrest with legs secured together. Others, including Abroise Pare, Mauriceau and Smellie disagreed with this approach and recommended the use of sutures. Yet, the first recorded case of perineal suture use was around 1610 when Guillemeau attempted to repair a fourth degree tear using a suture twisted around a straight needle. Unfortunately, this attempt was unsuccessful [10]. In 1834, Roux described a technique of approximating the torn edges of perineal tissue with a quilted suture, reinforced by interrupted sutures [10]. Subsequently, there have been various reports in which materials such as carbolised catgut, silk, silkworm gut, and silver wire were used for suturing. However, success with primary wound union of perineal wounds were only about 50–60% [11].

In 1930, Royston [12] described a commonly practised technique in which the ends of the torn anal sphincter were approximated by inserting a deep catgut suture through the inner third of the sphincter muscle and a second set (mattress or interrupted) through the outer third of the sphincter. Ingraham et al. [13] mention the Royston technique as their method of repair, but their description differs in that sutures are only inserted in the fascial sheath or "capsule" of the anal sphincter. Fulsher and Fearl [14] also described this technique and emphasised that no sutures should pass through the sphincter muscle. More specifically, Cunningham and Pilkington [15] inserted 4 interrupted sutures in the capsule of the external anal sphincter (EAS) at the anterior, posterior, superior and inferior points. However, as early as 1948, Kaltreider and Dixon [16] described their series of women since 1935 in whom only one mattress or figure-of-eight suture was used to approximate the sphincter ends during primary repair.

The end-to-end approximation type of repair is still used widely. However, in 1999, Sultan et al. described the overlap technique of primary repair of the EAS [17]. This technique was previously described by Parks and McPartlin for secondary sphincter repair in patients presenting with faecal incontinence [18]. In addition, Sultan et al. highlighted the importance of recognition and separate repair of the acutely torn internal anal sphincter (IAS), as it is largely responsible for maintaining the resting tone of the anal sphincter. Damage to the IAS is associated with incontinence to flatus and passive soiling of stool (Chap. 14).

5.3 Prevalence

The reported rates of OASIS vary not only amongst hospitals within the same country [19] but also from one country to the next [20]. This seems to be secondary to variation in obstetric practice, namely the type of episiotomy practised. In centres where midline episiotomy is practised, OASIs has been reported to occur in 19% of primiparous women [21] compared to 6.1% in centres practising mediolateral episiotomy [19]. In the UK, the overall median rate of OASIs in all vaginal births is 2.9% (6.1% in nulliparous and 1.7 in multiparous women) [19]. In the past, midline episiotomies have been favoured in North American practice, while mediolateral episiotomies are favoured in Europe and other countries. However, it has become well known that restricted use of episiotomy in non-instrumented vaginal birth is preferred over routine use and results in over 30% fewer women having more severe perineal trauma (Chap. 3). Analysis of Hospital Episode Statistics in England from 2000 to 2012 showed an increase of reported third- or fourth-degree perineal tears have tripled in primiparous women from 1.8% to 5.9% [22]. However, this apparent increase probably reflects improvements in diagnosis and classification of OASIs rather than an increase in the incidence.

Following the introduction of the Sultan Classification of OASIs in 1999, Okeahialam performed a network analysis of all studies using this classification ($n = 2647$) and reported on the prevalence of the grade of tears: grade 3a = 42.2%;

grade 3b tears = 36.8%; grade 3c = 13.9% and fourth degree = 7.1% [2]. By contrast, prior to this classification, the overall rates of OASIs were as low as 0.6%; interestingly, in this study, 40 percent of OASIs were fourth degree tears [23]. This low rate of OASIs (combined with such a high rate of fourth degree tears) seems to indicate that previously, a large number of third degree tears had been missed or classified as second degree tears.

Although training workshops have been shown to have a beneficial impact in education and a change of practice [24, 25], there are no validated assessment tools of clinical competence for the diagnosis of acute OASIs. The limited value of the use of ultrasound immediately postpartum [26] and the argument for a second rectal examination following every vaginal delivery is compelling (Chap. 23).

5.4 Repair Techniques

For decades, the most popular technique of primary repair following OASIs has been by "end-to-end" approximation of the torn sphincters with either interrupted or "figure-of-eight" sutures (Fig. 5.1, b) [23]. By contrast, when faced with patients with faecal incontinence, colorectal and trained gynaecologic surgeons favour the "overlap technique" of sphincter repair (secondary) as described by Parks and McPartlin [18]. (see Chap. 20). Jorge and Wexner reported on 21 studies using the overlapping technique, with good results ranging from 74% to 100% [27]. Unfortunately, as already alluded to above, there are similar limitations in performing a meta-analysis to look at outcomes regarding studies relating to secondary sphincter repair (Chap. 20). Engel et al. pro-

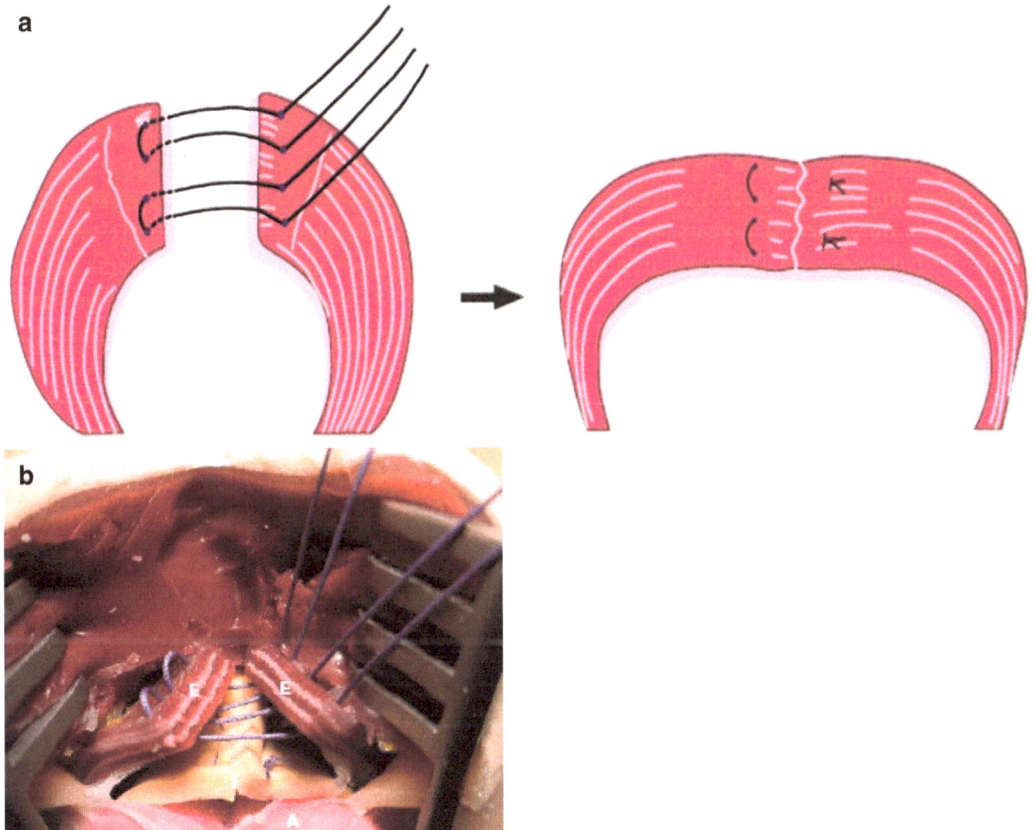

Fig. 5.1 (**a**) Diagrammatic representation of end-to-end repair with mattress sutures. (**b**) End-to-end repair of the external sphincter (*E*) demonstrated on a model using two mattress sutures (*I* internal sphincter, *A* anal epithelium)

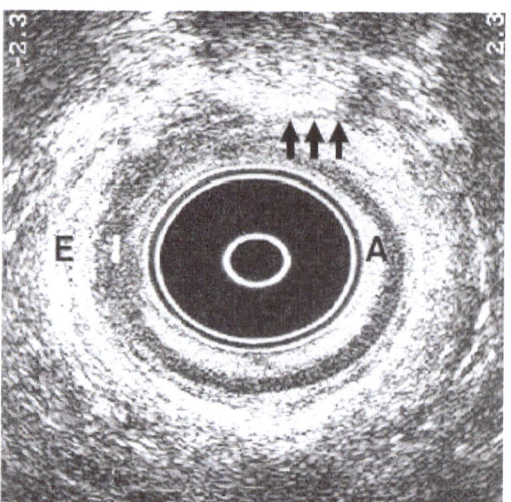

Fig. 5.2 Endoanal ultrasound image at 6 months after repair (*E* external sphincter, *I* internal sphincter, *A* anal epithelium) with arrows indicating site of overlap repair of the external anal sphincter

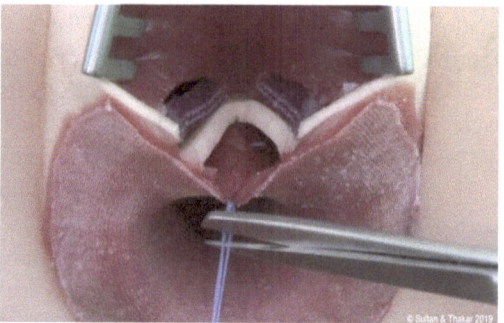

Fig. 5.3 Anal mucosal repair performed transvaginally using a continuous non-locking suture from the apex of the tear to outside the anal verge

spectively studied 55 patients with faecal incontinence undergoing overlapping anterior anal sphincter repair and reported a good clinical outcome in 80% at 15 months [28]. A poor result was found to be associated with an EAS defect, while demonstration of an overlap by anal endosonography (Fig. 5.3) correlated with a favourable outcome. At 5-years, however, 46 of the 55 patients were followed up and only 50% remained continent [29]. However, at least one third of these women had more than one attempt at sphincter repair [29].

Despite scepticism from surgeons that overlapping friable torn muscle as a primary procedure may not be possible, Sultan et al. demonstrated that EAS overlap repair as well as identification and end-to-end repair of the IAS was possible following acute OASI in 27 women [17]. They observed that compared to matched historical controls who had an end-to-end repair, anal incontinence could be reduced from 41% to 8% using the overlap technique and separate repair of the internal sphincter [30]. Based on this, they recommended a randomised trial between end-to-end and overlap repair (Fig. 5.2).

Several randomized trials have been published. Fitzpatrick et al. in Dublin published the first randomised trial and found no significant difference

between the two methods of repair, although there appeared to be trend towards more symptoms in the end-to-end group [31]. There were methodological differences in that the torn IAS was not identified and repaired separately, and a constipating agent was used for 3 days after the repair. Moreover, partial EAS tears were included; needless to say, a true overlapping repair is not possible if the sphincter ends are not completely divided. It would also be expected that if an overlap is attempted, the residual intact sphincter muscle would have to curl up resulting in undue tension on the remaining torn ends of muscle that would be overlapped [17, 18]. This technique would therefore go against the general surgical principle of deliberately placing tissue under avoidable tension. Nevertheless, the authors concur, a better outcome would be expected with both techniques as a consequence of focused education and training in anal sphincter repair.

Garcia et al. also performed a randomised trial of the two techniques; only complete ruptures of the EAS were included (full thickness 3b, 3c and fourth degree tears) [32]. There were 23 women in the end-to-end group and 18 in the overlap group. Unfortunately, only 15 and 11 women, respectively, returned for follow-up at 3 months. No significant differences was found between the groups in terms of symptoms of faecal incontinence or transperineal ultrasound findings. However, the authors acknowledged that the major limitations of their study were that randomisation was inaccurate and that their study was underpowered.

Williams et al. performed a factorial randomised controlled trial ($n = 112$); women were randomised into four groups: overlap with polyglactin (Vicryl; Ethicon, Edinburgh, UK); end-to-end repair with Vicryl; overlap repair with polydiaxanone (PDS; Ethicon, Edinburgh, UK); end-to-end repair with PDS [33]. This trial was specifically designed to test the hypothesis regarding suture-related morbidity (need for suture removal due to pain, suture migration or dyspareunia) using the two techniques. At 6 weeks post repair, there were no differences in suture-related morbidity. Similarly, the authors claimed that there were no differences in outcome based on repair technique. Unfortunately, the majority of patients included in this trial had only partial EAS tears (3a tears) and as mentioned above, a true overlap likely was not performed [17, 18]. Furthermore, a power calculation was not performed for this outcome and the follow-up rate at 12 months was only 54%. This data therefore needs to be interpreted with caution.

Fernando et al. performed a randomised trial of end-to-end vs overlap technique [34]. This study had adequate power ($n = 64$), and the primary outcome was faecal incontinence at 1 year. All repairs were performed by two trained operators and 3a EAS tears were excluded. At 12 months (81% follow-up rate), 24% in the end-to-end and none in the overlap group reported faecal incontinence ($P = 0.009$). Faecal urgency was reported by 32% in the end-to-end group and 3.7% in the overlap group ($P = 0.02$). There were no significant differences in dyspareunia and quality of life between the groups. At 12 months, 20% reported perineal pain in the end-to-end group and none in the overlap group ($P = 0.04$). During 12 months, 16% in the end-to-end group and none in the overlap group reported deterioration of defaecatory symptoms ($P = 0.01$). Further calculation revealed that four women need to be treated with the overlap technique to prevent one woman with OASIs developing faecal incontinence.

In yet another randomised study, with the primary outcome measure "of at least weekly solid stool incontinence" [35] Rygh and Korner [87] ($n = 101$) concluded that the overlap technique was not superior to the end-to-end repair. However, there were more women with symptoms of anal incontinence in the end-to-end repair group (34% vs. 20%).

In a study with longer-term outcomes, Farrell et al. randomized end-to-end ($n = 62$) and overlapping ($n = 63$) EAS repairs in primiparous women [36]. They reported significantly higher rates of flatal but not faecal incontinence in the overlap group. However, there were more fourth-degree tears in the overlap group and therefore more IAS injury that could explain the increased flatal incontinence in this group. At a 3-year follow-up, there was no significant difference in anal incontinence between the groups, but the rate of fecal incontinence in the end-to-end group doubled while it remained static in the overlap group [37]. These findings support the findings of Fernando et al. who demonstrated a significantly higher risk of deterioration in anal incontinence over time in the end-to-end group [34]. This study highlights the importance of longer term follow-up, as one technique may prove to be more robust.

In the most recent Cochrane review concluded that, compared with immediate primary end-to-end repair of OASIS, immediate primary overlapping repair appears to be associated with a reduced risk for fecal urgency, anal incontinence severity score, and deterioration of anal incontinence symptoms at 12 months [38]. At 36 months (based on only two small trials), there appeared to be no difference in flatus or fecal incontinence between the two techniques. They concluded that either an end-to-end or overlap repair of the EAS may be performed at the discretion of the clinician. It is important, however, to emphasise that the overlap technique has only been described for full-thickness EAS tears [17].

Lastly, Kairaluoma et al. reported on 31 consecutive women who sustained OASIs (3b and fourth degree). All had an EAS overlap repair immediately after delivery performed by two colorectal surgeons [39]. In addition to end-to-end repair of the IAS, they also performed a levatorplasty with two sutures. At a median follow-up of 2 years, 23% complained of anal incontinence,

23% developed wound infection, 27% complained of dyspareunia and one developed a rectovaginal fistula. Levatorplasty therefore should be avoided during primary anal sphincter repair.

5.4.1 Principles and Technique of Repair

1. Repair of OASIs should be conducted by a doctor who has been formally trained and certified in primary anal sphincter repair (of all grades of third degree and fourth degree tears) or under the supervision of a certified trainer.
2. Repair should be conducted in the operating theatre where there is access to good lighting, appropriate equipment and aseptic conditions. An instrument tray containing a Weitlander self-retaining retractor, four Allis tissue forceps, McIndoe scissors, tooth forceps, two artery forceps, stitch scissors and a needle holder (www.perineum.net) is helpful [40]. In addition, deep retractors (e.g. Deavers retractor) can be useful when there are associated paravaginal tears.
3. A general or regional (spinal, epidural, caudal) anaesthetic provides analgesia and muscle relaxation, which are important pre-requisites to enable proper evaluation of the full extent of the injury. The inherent tone of the EAS can result in retraction of the torn muscle ends within its capsular sheath, and adequate muscle relaxation allows these to be grasped and retrieved, enabling a tension-free repair.
4. The full extent of the injury should be evaluated by a careful vaginal and rectal examination in lithotomy and graded according to the recommended Sultan classification (see Chap. 3). If there is any ambiguity about the grading of the EAS injury, the next higher grade should be selected, e.g. if there is a discrepancy between grade 3a and 3b, the injury should be classified as 3b.

5. In the presence of a fourth degree tear, the torn anal epithelium should be repaired with continuous non-locking Vicryl 3/0 sutures (Fig. 5.3). Previously, the teaching was that the repair should be performed with the knots tied in the anal lumen [41], theoretically reducing the quantity of foreign body within the tissue and thus minimising the risk of infection. However, this concern probably applies to catgut (which dissolves by proteolysis/phagocytosis) rather than the newer synthetic materials such as Vicryl or Dexon (polyglycolic acid), which dissolve by hydrolysis. Catgut made from submucosa of sheep gastrointestinal tract has now been withdrawn from the UK and other European countries. A subcuticular repair of the anal epithelium via the transvaginal approach has also been described but given that the anal epithelium is less than 1 mm thick and adherent to the IAS, we believe that it would be difficult to secure a robust repair that would withstand distention during the passage of stool. We therefore perform a full thickness anorectal epithelium repair and ensure that the suturing is continued distally to outside the anal verge (Fig. 5.3).
6. The sphincter muscles are repaired with 3/0 PDS dyed sutures. Compared to a braided suture material, monofilamentous sutures are believed to lessen the risk of infection [42]. Non-absorbable monofilament sutures such as nylon or Prolene (polypropylene) are preferred by some colorectal surgeons when performing secondary sphincter repair. However, non-absorbable sutures can cause stitch abscesses and the sharp ends of the suture can migrate and cause discomfort, necessitating removal. Complete absorption of PDS takes significantly longer than Vicryl, with 50% tensile strength lasting more than 3 months compared to 3 weeks, respectively [33]. To minimise suture migration, care should be taken to cut suture ends short and

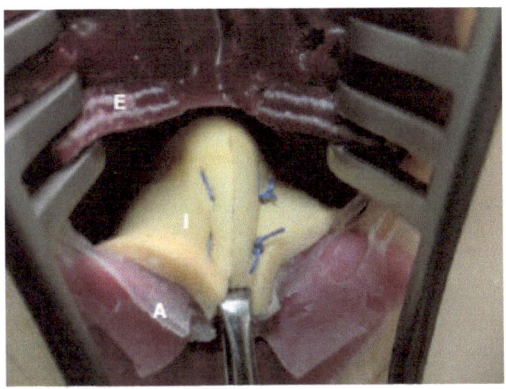

Fig. 5.4 Internal anal sphincter (*I*) repair using mattress sutures demonstrated on a model (*E* external sphincter, *A* anal epithelium)

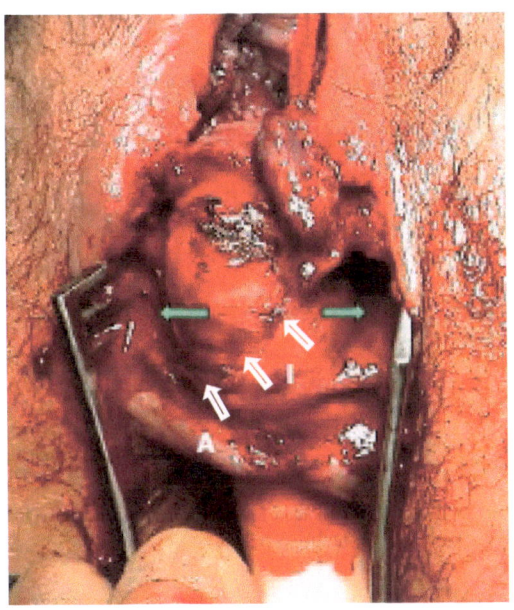

Fig. 5.5 Third degree tear (grade 3c) with two arrows demonstrating retraction of the torn ends of the external sphincter on each side. The internal sphincter (*I*) is also partially torn (3 white arrows) and tear extends to the anal verge (*A*) with the anal epithelium being intact

ensure that they are covered by the overlying superficial perineal muscles. Of note, however, a randomised controlled trial revealed no differences in suture-related morbidity between Vicryl and PDS at 6 weeks postpartum [33] (Fig. 5.4).

7. The IAS lies between the EAS and conjoint longitudinal muscle and would not usually be visible unless there is a full thickness EAS tear. It should be identified and, if torn, repaired separately from the EAS. It is thinner (2–4 mm) and paler than the striated EAS (7–8 mm) (see Chap. 3). The appearance of the IAS can be described as being analogous to the flesh of uncooked fish, as opposed to the red meat appearance of the EAS. The ends of the torn muscle are grasped with Allis forceps and an end-to-end repair is performed with mattress 3/0 PDS sutures (Fig. 5.3). No attempt should be made to overlap the IAS. There is an increasing awareness of the role of the IAS in maintaining continence. In a recent blinded randomised study of repair after OASIs, all nine women who had a repair of an IAS tear (grade 3c or fourth degree) were found to have a largely intact IAS at follow-up using anal endosonography [43].

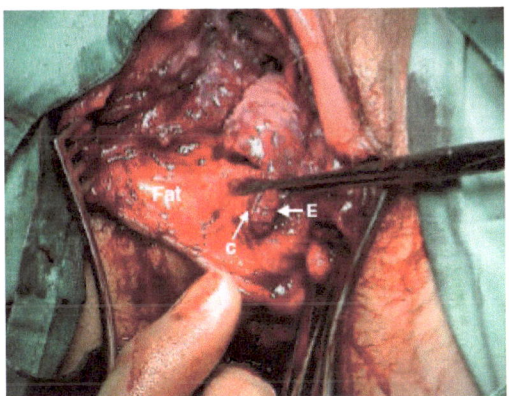

Fig. 5.6 The external sphincter (*E*) grasped with Allis forceps is surrounded by the capsule (*C*) and lies medial to the ischio-anal fat

8. As the EAS is normally under tonic contraction, it tends to retract when torn as noted above (Fig. 5.5). The torn ends of the EAS therefore need to be identified and grasped with Allis tissue forceps (Fig. 5.6). To per-

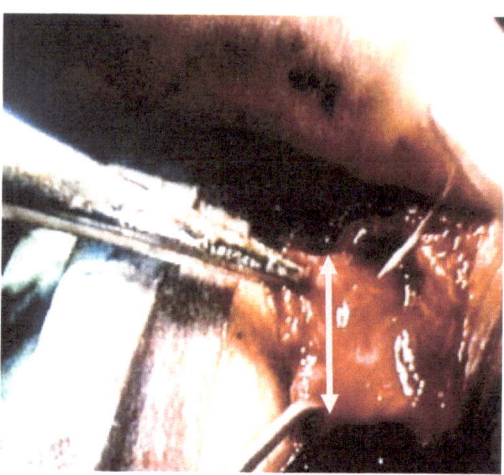

Fig. 5.7 The full length of the external sphincter (arrow) must be identified before repair is attempted

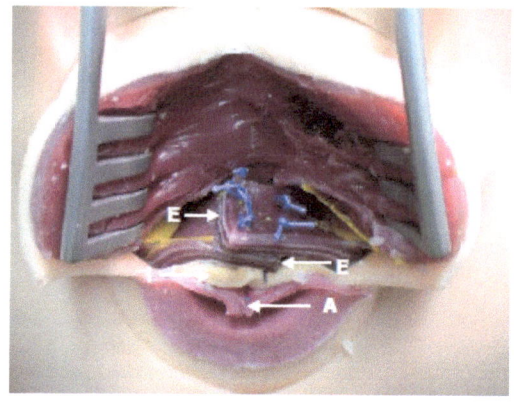

Fig. 5.8 Repair of a fourth degree tear (demonstrated on a model) using the overlap repair technique of the external sphincter (*E*). The anal epithelium (*A*) and the internal sphincter (*I*) have also been repaired

form an overlap, the muscle may need mobilisation by dissection with a pair of McIndoe scissors separating it from the ischioanal fat laterally (Fig. 5.6). A proper overlap is possible only when the full thickness and full length of the torn ends of the EAS are identified (Fig. 5.7). The torn ends of the EAS can then be overlapped in a "double-breasted" fashion (Fig. 5.8) using PDS 3/0 (Ethicon) sutures.; overlapping allows for a greater surface area of contact between the muscle ends (Fig. 5.8). By contrast, it is possible to perform an end-to-end repair without identifying the full length of the EAS, giving rise to incomplete apposition (Fig. 5.9). Consequently, the woman may remain continent temporarily but would be at an increased risk of developing faecal urgency and incontinence later in life. A shorter anal length has been reported following end-to-end primary

repair of the EAS and anal sphincter length was inversely correlated with the degree of incontinence [44]. It has also been shown that a shorter anal length is the best predictor of faecal incontinence following secondary sphincter surgery [45]. Unlike end-to-end repair, if further retraction of the overlapped muscle ends were to occur, it is highly probable that muscle continuity would be maintained. However, if the operator is not familiar with the overlap technique or if the EAS is only partially torn (grade 3a/3b), an end-to-end repair must be performed using two or three mattress sutures similar to IAS repair (Fig. 5.4). As "figure-of-eight" sutures are haemostatic and can cause strangulation of tissue, they should never be used to repair the anorectal epithelium or the sphincters.

9. After repair of the sphincter, the perineal muscles (Superficial Transverse Perineal and Bulbospongiousus muscles) should be

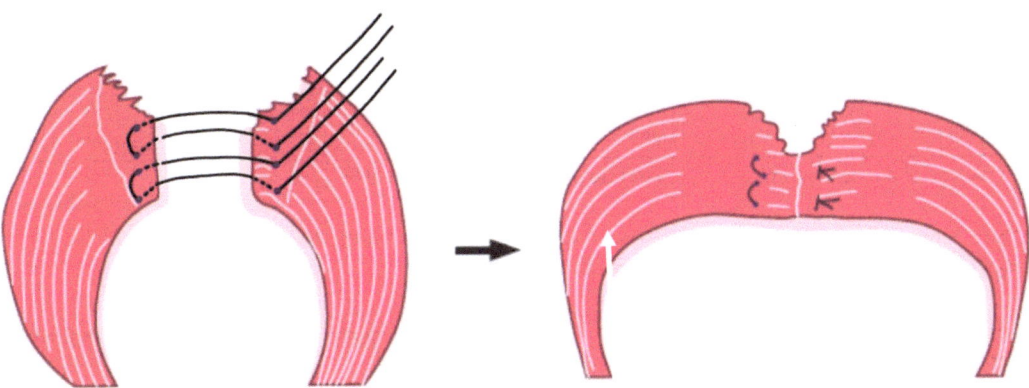

Fig. 5.9 If the full length of the EAS is not exposed and grasped (left drawing), apposition may be incomplete, leading to subsequent functional compromise

sutured to reconstruct the perineal body in order to provide support to the repaired anal sphincter. A short and thus deficient perineum is a known risk factor for a subsequent OASIS. It is important to ensure that the PDS knots are covered by the perineal muscles to avoid suture migration through the overlying skin. Finally, the vaginal skin should be sutured, and the perineal skin approximated with a Vicryl rapide 2/0 subcuticular suture. Alternatively, if the torn Transverse Perineal and Bulbospiogiosus muscle are readily visible, the vaginal skin can be repaired commencing at the apex of the vaginal laceration. These muscles can then be sutured in continuity with a single suture followed by the perineal skin repair as during repair of an episiotomy (Chap. 4).

10. A rectovaginal examination should be performed to confirm complete repair and ensure that (unless there is a fourth degree tear), no sutures have been passed inadvertently through the rectal mucosa. If so, the repair would need to be undone and the offending suture removed to minimise the risk of a rectovaginal fistula. Also it is imperative to ensure that all tampons or swabs have been removed from the vagina.

11. Detailed notes should be made of the findings and repair. Completion of a pre-designed proforma and a pictorial representation of the tears prove very useful when notes are being reviewed following complications, audit or litigation (Fig. 5.10).

DETAILS OF PERINEAL TRAUMA REPAIR___May University Hospital

Patient Name: ....   Number .... Date: ....

Tick type of perineal trauma   **First degree** ☐   **Second degree** ☐

Third degree ☐   *, if third degree please specify* **3a / 3b /3c   Fourth degree** ☐
Episiotomy ☐   **If yes, Please state indication** ....

Extent of trauma **tick ALL relevant boxes)   Unilateral vaginal tear**   ☐   **Bilateral vaginal
tear** ☐

Labial trauma   ☐   **Perineal skin edges down ot anal margin**

Anaesthetic for repair   **None** ☐   **Epidural** ☐   **Spinal** ☐   **Lignocaine** ☐_____ **mls**

Repair details
Time of delivery .... **Time repair commenced** ....**Time repair finished** ....

Method of repair
Vagina   Interrupted / Continuous
Perineal muscles   Interrupted / Continuous   Suture used Vicryl / Vicryl Rapide
Perineal skin   Interrupted / Continuous   Suture used Vicryl / Vicryl Rapide
Anal mucosa   Interrupted / Continuous   Suture used Vicryl / Vicryl Rapide
Internal anal sphincter   Interrupted / Mattress   Suture used Vicryl / Vicryl Rapide
External anal sphincter   Overlap / End to end   Suture used PDS / Vicryl
                                                                                     Suture used PDS / Vicryl

Additional information
....

Please complete diagram, mark lacertions an suture repair
Urethra   → → →

Vagina   → →

Anal sphincter   → → →

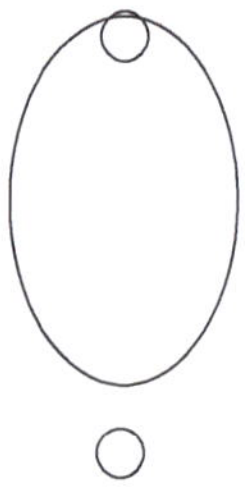

Rectal exmination done before repair   **Yes / No**   Rectal exmination done after repair   **Yes / No**
Vaginal exmination done   **Yes / No**   Tampon Removed   **Yes / No**
Needle count correct   **Yes / No**   Swab count correct   **Yes / No**

Estimated blood loss   **After delivery** .... **mls**   **After suturing** .... **mls**   **Total** .... **mls**

Repaired by
(Print Name) ....   **Midwife / Doctor**
If midwife: grade ....   **If doctor: Consultant / Staff Grade / SpR/**
SHO

Fig. 5.10 An example of a proforma that can be used for documentation of perineal trauma and repair

5.5   Rectal Buttonhole Tears

As described in Chap. 3, a rectal buttonhole tear is an isolated tear of the rectal mucosa and vagina [46]. When an OASI is in continuity with a rectal mucosal tear, it should be called a fourth-degree tear (see below). However, when a third- or fourth degree tear occurs concomitantly with an isolated rectal buttonhole tear (with an island of intact rectal mucosa between the third/fourth-degree tear and the isolated rectal buttonhole tear), it should be classified and described as such: namely, rectal buttonhole tear plus the OASI grade [46].

Prior to repair of the rectal buttonhole tear, it is important to ensure that both the proximal end and distal ends of the tear are clearly visualised (Fig. 5.11). The repair should then be performed via the transvaginal approach in three layers (open access video available) [46].

1. First, the mucosal tear should be sutured similarly to the anorectal mucosal repair of a fourth degree tear with a full thickness continuous Vicryl 3-0 suture.

2. Second, the intervening rectovaginal fascia must be approximated using interrupted or continuous PDS 2-0 or 3-0 sutures (Fig. 5.11). This is an essential step to minimise the risk of developing a rectovaginal fistula.

3. Third, the vaginal skin should be closed using a continuous Vicryl or Vicryl rapide 2-0 suture.

On rare occasions, an isolated rectal buttonhole tear can occur in association with a third degree tear (see Chap. 3), in which case it should be classified as such and the repair should be done separately for each [46]. A colostomy is rarely indicated but should be considered following discussion with the colorectal surgeon in the presence of a large rectal tear (±7 cm) extending above the pelvic floor or if there is gross faecal contamination of the wound. There is a risk of requiring a colostomy following a wound breakdown as well, but in our experience, this is uncommon (occurring in less than 5–10% of cases). Still, this information should be included during counselling of a woman undergoing a rectal buttonhole tear repair [46].

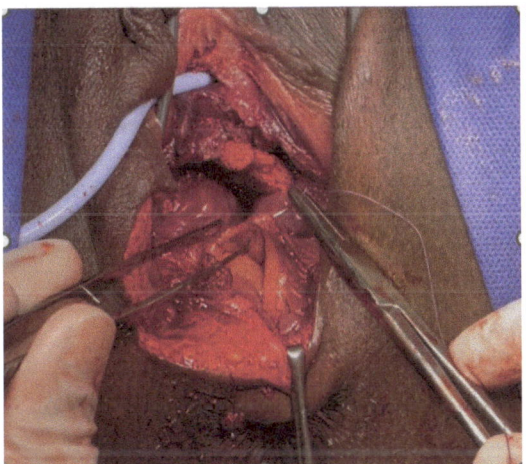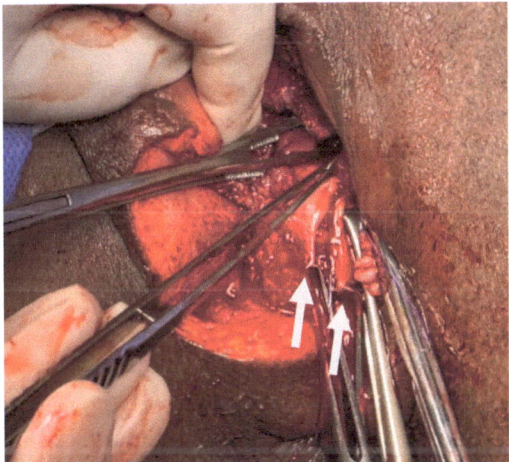

Fig. 5.11 Repair of a rectal buttonhole tear. The photograph on the left demonstrates the mucosa is being sutured while the photograph indicates the rectovaginal fascia being grasped (arrows)

5.6 Outcome of Primary Repair of OASIs

A meta-analysis of the outcomes of primary repair of OASIs is difficult to establish due to considerable variability in study design classification and data collection. Similarly, there are variations in repair techniques (anaesthesia used, suture material, repair techniques, antibiotic use, stool softeners etc.), a wide range of follow-up periods, and discrepancies exist in subjective and objective assessments. Most older studies have used non-validated structured questionnaires, while others have used different scoring systems. Given these limitations, the outcomes of older studies where end-end to end repair of the EAS had been performed and where the IAS had not been repaired have been published in the first edition and updated in the seventh edition of this text. Based on 42 studies identified following a Medline search between 1980 and 2010, a mean of 37% of women suffered anal incontinence (12% faecal incontinence) despite a primary repair of their OASIS.

Okeahialam et al. [2] performed a network meta-analysis to establish the incidence of anal incontinence in all studies that used the Sultan Classification of grading OASIs [1]. This allowed for consistency in reporting outcomes according to the severity of injury and appropriate repair. The ten studies are shown in in Table 5.1. The mean incidence of anal incontinence according to grade of tear is shown in Fig. 5.11. These results indicate that 3a tears have the best outcome, with 3b tears ranking second, 3c tears ranking third and fourth degree tears having the worst clinical outcome [2]. Overall, on analysis of the raw data of all studies using the Sultan Classification, the mean rate of anal incontinence was 18% compared to the 42 older studies before 2010 where the reported rate was 37% as noted above [47].

It is known that faecal urgency with or without anal incontinence can be very debilitating with greater impact on quality of life when compared to passive incontinence [49]. This is shown in Table 5.2. Compared to grade 3a and grade 3b tears, faecal urgency was found to be worse in women who sustained fourth degree tears [2] (Fig. 5.12).

In addition, faecal urgency can affect 16 to 37% depending on the grade of tear (Table 5.2).

Despite repair, persistent sonographic anal sphincter defects were identified in 16 [52] to 30% [50] of primarily-repaired OASIs. One study reported persistent sphincter defects in

Table 5.1 Anal incontinence according to grade of tear in the 10 studies that used the Sultan classification [2]

Author[c]	Follow-up in months	Country	Study[b] design	Sample size	Anal Incontinence Incidence			
					3a	3b	3c	4th
Bagade [37]	6	UK	R	75	16.10%	6.90%	10.00%	20.00%
Everist [23]	6	Australia	P	122	17.20%	29.70%	55.50%	71.40%
Gommesen [33]	12	Denmark	P	189	13.60%	15.20%	35.00%	33.30%
Joris [34]	6	Switzerland	P	88	27.90%	43.80%	37.50%	40.00%
Linneberg [38]	60	Denmark	R	82	51.20%	38.50%	0%	53.30%
Ménard [39]	2	France	R	79	41.50%	46.70%	55.60%	0%
Ramage [36]	3–24	UK	R	161	[a]	[a]	[a]	[a]
Ramalingam [35]	6	UK	P	255	6.10%	8.60%	11.10%	33.30%
Roos [20]	9	UK	R	531	18.80%	18.50%	23.80%	10.00%
Wan [40]	3	UK	R	1065	9%	16.20%	13.10%	30.60%

[a]Overall incidence of anal incontinence not reported, but incidence of faecal incontinence and flatal incontinence reported
[b]Study design (*P* prospective, *R* retrospective)
[c]The references in this Table can be found in the publication [2]

Table 5.2 The rates of defaecatory symptoms in all the studies that have provided this information [4, 50–52]

Defaecatory Symptoms	Mean rates (%)			
	3a	3b	3c	4th
Urgency	16	19	29	37
Flatus	11	16	14	25
Faecal	3	4	9	13

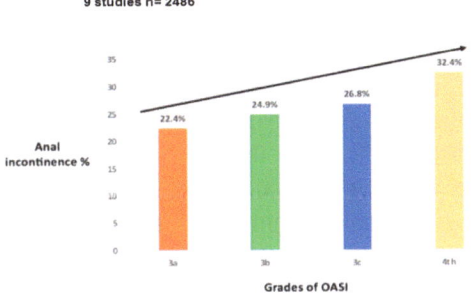

9 studies n= 2486

Fig. 5.12 Rates of anal incontinence according to grade of tear in the 9 studies ($n = 2486$) [2]

11.5% of minor OASIs (grade 3a/b) and 38.5% of major (Grade3c/4) OASIs [52]. Another distressing symptom following OASIs that is not frequently volunteered because of embarrassment is the development of anal incontinence during coitus, affecting about 17% of women [42]. Risk factors for the development of OASIs are discussed in detail in Chap. 12.

5.7 Post-Operative Management

5.7.1 Antibiotics

Antibiotics are commonly prescribed [53] especially during and after repair of fourth degree tears [41]. In this only prospective, randomised placebo-controlled study [54] of it's kind, in 147 women who sustained OASIs, women who received a single dose of intravenous second generation cephalosporin had a significantly lower risk of perineal complications compared to a placebo (8% compared to 24%) at 2 weeks following birth. This was the only study in a Cochrane review addressing antibiotic prophylaxis following OASIs, although the data suggested that pro-

phylactic antibiotics help prevent perineal wound complications loss to follow-up was very high. Infection and wound breakdown could jeopardise the outcome of repair and lead to incontinence or fistula formation. We prescribe intravenous broad-spectrum antibiotics at the time of repair such as Co-amoxiclav 1.2 g (an alternative regime for true Penicillin allergy are Cefuroxime 1.5 g + Metronidazole 500 mg for mild allergy or Clindamycin 900 mg + Ciprofloxacin 400 mg for severe allergy). In case of MRSA positive patients, Teicoplanin 400 mg + Gentamicin 160 mg + Metronidazole IV 500 mg is given. Similarly, again based on expert opinion, oral antibiotics can be continued for 3 days, but the regime should be based on local microbiological advice.

5.7.2 Bladder Catheterisation

Severe perineal discomfort, particularly following instrumental birth, is a known risk factor for urinary retention. Similarly, following regional anaesthesia, it can take up to 12 hours before bladder sensation returns. A Foley catheter should be inserted for about 24 hours unless midwifery staff can ensure that spontaneous voiding occurs at least every 3–4 hours without undue bladder overdistension.

5.7.3 Post-Operative Analgesia

The degree of pain following perineal trauma is related to the extent of the injury and by definition, OASIs are more extensive injuries. In a systematic review, Hedayati et al. [55] found that rectal analgesia such as diclofenac reduces pain from perineal trauma within the first 24 hours after birth and results in less additional analgesia needed within the first 48 hours after birth. Diclofenac is almost completely protein bound and excretion in breast milk is negligible [56]. In women who have had a repair of a fourth degree tear, Diclofenac should be administered orally, as insertion of suppositories may be uncomfortable; there is also a theoretical risk of poor healing associated with local anti-inflammatory agents [57]. Codeine-based preparations are best avoided, as they may cause constipation, leading to excessive straining, faecal impaction and possible disruption of the repair. Similarly, dependence on opiods is a risk.

5.7.4 Dietary Advice and Stool Softeners

Management of postpartum constipation is paramount, as passage of constipated stool or faecal impaction requiring manual evacuation may disrupt the repair. Although there are conflicting practices described in the literature, the majority consensus is that stool softeners should be prescribed [41]. Mahony et al. [58] performed a randomised trial ($n = 105$) of constipating versus laxative regimens and found that use of laxatives was associated with a significantly earlier and less painful first bowel motion, as well as earlier discharge from hospital. Nineteen per cent of women in the constipated regimen group experienced troublesome constipation (two required hospital admission for faecal impaction) compared to only 5% in the laxative group. There were no significant differences in continence scores, anal manometry findings or endoanal scan findings. Bulking agents such as Ispaghula husk (Fybogel) should be avoided, as another randomised study [59] found that incontinence occurred significantly more often (33% versus 18%) when lactulose was combined with Fybogel. Similarly, another prospective, randomised surgeon-blinded study [59] of patients undergoing anorectal reconstructive surgery ($n = 46$) reported a faecal impaction rate of 26% in the group given constipating agents till the third postoperative day compared to 7% in the group allowed a regular diet.

As a bowel movement is not necessary prior to discharging the woman from hospital, i is important that the community midwife/healthcare provider checks that bowel action had occurred within 3 days. If not, early interven-

tion with mineral oil, milk of magnesia, or another oral bowel stimulant should be given. Glycerine suppositories are also useful alternatives.

5.7.5 Patient Information

Williams et al. [60] performed a qualitative study of six women who sustained OASIs, and four who had a subsequent pregnancy after OASIs. Some of the themes identified in these women were: apprehension about the consequences of the injury in terms of incontinence, body image and sexual functioning, poor communication and emotional support and unresolved anxieties in partners. In fact, there is a body of literature addressing symptoms of post-traumatic stress disorder in women who undergo operative vaginal birth [61, 62]. A patient information sheet is available from the RCOG website [63]. that addresses some of these issues. Ideally, these women should be under the care of a specialist team who run the perineal clinic (see Chap. 10 and below). The perineal/maternity clinic is viewed as a supportive environment and women feel confident about the information provided by the team [60]. Providers practice trauma-informed care. Following discharge from hospital women should have open access to this type of clinic if possible, until their postnatal appointment, usually between 6 and 8 weeks after birth. Pelvic floor and anal sphincter exercises can be initiated when the discomfort resolves and the woman feels comfortable (Chap. 18)

If a perineal/maternal recovery clinic is not available, women with OASIs should be given clear instructions, preferably in writing, before leaving the hospital. In the first 6 weeks following delivery, they should look for signs of infection or wound dehiscence and seek help with any increase in pain or swelling, rectal bleeding, or purulent discharge. Any incontinence of stool or flatus should be enquired about at every postnatal visit, documented and appropriate action taken.

5.7.6 Follow-Up

All women who sustain OASIs should be assessed in hospital by a senior obstetrician and again soon after delivery. Many women in the UK have access to a perineal clinic for follow-up care (Chap. 10) and in the United States, maternal recovery clinics are becoming the standard of care for follow-up as well [64–66]. In these specialty clinics, objective and validated measures are used to assess patient symptoms and their impact on quality of life. Targeted physical examination is also performed, specifically assessing for scarring, residual granulation tissue and tenderness. Women may undergo anal manometry and endosonography (see Chaps. 5 and 10). Providers are trained to counsel patients about the circumstances surrounding the delivery and provide an explanation if there are concerns to the woman and her partner. The women are advised to continue pelvic floor exercises while others with minimal sphincter contractility may need electrical stimulation (see Chaps. 18 and 19) or sacral nerve modulation in the longer term (see Chap. 20).

5.8 Management of Subsequent Pregnancies After OASIs

Women who sustain OASIs need careful counselling regarding their management in a subsequent pregnancy. It is important to build evidence-based recommendations in order for counseling and advice to be consistent and unbiased, especially in a population which is vulnerable [60]. For example, forty nine percent of women with a history of OASIs report experiencing anxiety regarding subsequent pregnancy [67]. In one survey, 71% of colorectal surgeons recommended caesarean birth CB (a further 19% admitted they were uncertain), compared to fewer than 22% of obstetricians [53]. These figures are similar (about 60%) to that obtained from Colorectal surgeons who were members of the UK Pelvic Floor Society (Roper J. Colorectal Disease, accepted). Unfortunately, the data currently available to develop evidence-based guidelines are limited and therefore we have to rely largely on recommended practice. There are two major issues that concern most women following OASIs when contemplating birth in a subsequent pregnancy: namely, the risk of recurrence and the risk of developing anal incontinence.

5.8.1 What Is the Risk of Sustaining a Recurrent OASIs (rOASIs)?

While there are various risk factors for a recurrent OASI, one important consideration is whether and what type of episiotomy is used. Peleg et al. [63] studied 4,015 consecutive primiparae who had a singleton, cephalic presentation at term and found 704 sustained OASIs (19%). The risk of recurrence of OASIs in these women was 2.1% when no episiotomy was performed, 11% when a midline episiotomy was performed and 21% when a midline episiotomy was accompanied by instrumental delivery. In another study where only midline episiotomies were practised, the recurrence rate of OASIs was reported to be 11% [68]. Harkin et al. [69] studied 20,111 consecutive vaginal births in a unit that practised only mediolateral episiotomies and OASIs occurred in 342 women (2.9% in primiparae and 0.8% in multiparae). OASIs recurred in two (4.4%) of the 45 women who had sustained OASIs previously. Although risk of OASIs was increased fivefold in a subsequent pregnancy, 95% of women who had sustained previous sphincter injury did not sustain a recurrence.

Table 5.3 outlines the rates of recurrent OASIs as reported in different studies. The highest risk of sustaining an OASI is still in primiparous women. Therefore, the multicentre study by D'Souza et al. [77] involving 2272 primiparous women provides the most representative rates of a homogenous cohort in centres where mediolateral episiotomy is practised. All OASIs in this study were also analysed according to the Sultan classification [1, 2, 4, 47, 79]. They found that the rOASI rate was 10.2%. Other factors independently associated with risk of rOASI were increased maternal age, babyweight >4 kg, instrumental delivery particularly forceps and increasing degree of OASIs severity at index delivery [77].

Table 5.3 Reported rates of recurrent OASIs

Author	Rate
Yogev [70]	2%
Webb [71]	3.8%
Harkin [69]	4.4%
Reid [72]	4.4%
Fitzpatrick [7]	5.1%
Young [73]	5.4%
Bagestan [74]	5.6%
Scheer [5]	6.8%
Jango [75]	7.1%
Edozien [76]	7.2%
Jordan [6]	9.8%
DeSouza [77]	10%
Ali [78]	13.4%
Mean	**6.5%**

5.8.2 What Is the Risk of Anal Incontinence After Another Vaginal Birth?

Poen et al. [80] identified 43 women (out of original cohort of 117) who had subsequent vaginal births following previous OASIs. The rate of anal incontinence was 56% compared to 34% in those who did not subsequently give birth (relative risk 1.6; 95% confidence interval 1.1–2.5). There was no comparable CB group.

Sangalli et al. [81] studied 177 women about 13 years after OASIs (48 fourth degree tears altogether). Anal incontinence was significantly more common in women who had sustained fourth degree tears compared with those with third degree tears (25 vs. 11.5%; $P = 0.049$). Unlike women with previous fourth degree tears, those who had sustained a previous third degree tear did not demonstrate an increase in anal incontinence symptoms after a subsequent vaginal birth. This is in keeping with the findings of Fenner et al. [82], who found that worse bowel control was 10 times more prevalent in women who sustained fourth as opposed to third degree tears. This could be attributed to persistent injury of the IAS that had not been repaired at birth. Taithongchai et al. performed the first and largest study to investigate fourth-degree tears using validated anal incontinence scores, endoanal ultrasound and manometry to evaluate outcomes and assess variations in different pro-

tocols regarding the management of subsequent births ($n = 74$) [83]. They concluded that as there are only a few units that offer specialist investigations to their OASI cohort, it would be reasonable to offer CB to all women who have sustained a fourth-degree tear. However, in centres where endoanal ultrasound and anal manometry are available, clinicians should offer these investigations for more individualised counselling.

Webb et al. performed a systematic review and meta-analysis of 14 studies (977 women) and concluded that due to sample size, quality and heterogeneity of the studies, the optimal birth route for women with OASIs remains to be established [84]. The difficulty regarding using the outcome of anorectal symptoms based on mode of birth is that most women randomised to CB already have anal incontinence symptoms; therefore the analysis after a subsequent birth may show no difference between CB and vaginal birth [77, 84, 85]. Abramowitz et al. published a multicentre randomised controlled trial in which 222 women who sustained a third degree tear and/or a forceps delivery in their first pregnancy but without any symptoms of anal incontinence were randomised to a planned CB or vaginal birth [9]. They concluded that a CB had no significant impact on anal continence 6 months after the second delivery in women with asymptomatic OASI lesions diagnosed by ultrasound. However, in this study only 29 of 222 (15%) women had OASIs diagnosed and repaired at the time of birth. In addition, the patients did not undergo anal manometry and the definition of a sphincter defect has been questioned [86]. The value of anal manometry alone in identification of women at risk for anal incontinence has been highlighted by Badri et al. in which only one third of women with a previous OASI had isolated abnormal manometry [87]. Therefore, the conclusions of Abramowitz et al. [9] do not fit in to the criteria recommended by the RCOG [79] (see below) and it is therefore difficult to incorporate into clinical practice.

The aetiology of anal incontinence is multifactorial and has been reported in upwards of 17% of all women during the first year after birth.

Hence, in these cases, anal ultrasound and manometry could help to determine if the symptoms are due to a sphincteric cause or other cause [87, 88]. For example, if the ultrasound findings are normal, but the squeeze pressures are low, this would indicate a pudendal neuropathy or a pelvic neuropathy. In this scenario, a CB could be recommended because if an OASI is sustained in the presence of this neuropathy, the outcome is expected to be worse. Women would need to understand the short- and long-term risks, including the recovery period of each mode of delivery, as well as the fact that a CB would be a recurring indication for all subsequent pregnancies with its attendant risks.

5.8.3 What Is Recommended Practice?

All women who are symptomatic with anal incontinence should be referred to a centre with facilities for anorectal assessment and should be counselled about the risks of subsequent vaginal and CB. If facilities for anal manometry and endosonography (Fig. 5.13) are unavailable, the management of a subsequent pregnancy will depend on symptomatic and clinical evaluation. Although studies are lacking, it would be reasonable to allow asymptomatic women without any clinical evidence of sphincter compromise (good resting tone and squeeze contraction on digital

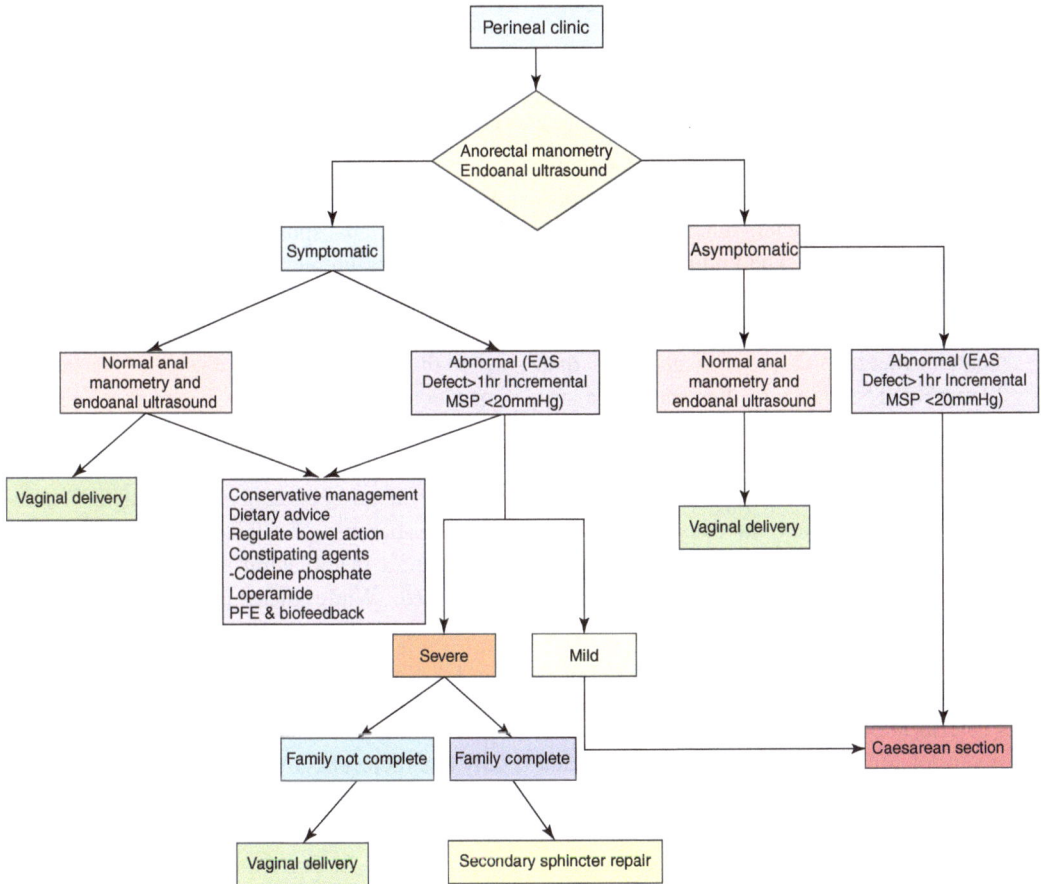

Fig. 5.13 Flow diagram demonstrating the management of OASIs for subsequent pregnancies [6]. *EAS* External anal sphincter, *MSP* maximum squeeze pressure, *PFE* Pelvic floor exercises

rectal exam) to proceed with vaginal birth. This should be part of a shared decision process with the woman. It should, however, be acknowledged that compared to manometry, digital rectal examination has poor sensitivity for detecting sphincter defects [89]. The RCOG recommends 'If the woman is symptomatic or shows abnormally low anorectal manometric pressures and/or endoanal ultrasonographic defects, an elective caesarean section may be considered'. [79]

Scheer et al. [5] performed the first prospective study ($n = 59$) after OASIs evaluating the effect of subsequent childbirth using objective validated methods (questionnaires, endoanal ultrasound and manometry). Using set criteria (Fig. 5.13) recommendations regarding mode of birth and a management protocol were proposed as follows:

- Women who were found to have an EAS defect >1 hour (i.e. 30° and a maximum squeeze pressure increment of <20 mmHg) were considered to have substantial compromise of anal sphincter function and were offered planned CB. The finding of no defect or a defect <1 hour was considered a substantially compromised anal sphincter if the incremental squeeze pressure was also less than 20 mmHg. The reason for this was that a suspected defect of <1 hour could also reflect healing of the wound and therefore we did not wish to over-diagnose a defect. Any IAS defects were not taken into consideration.
- A vaginal delivery was recommended to all other women.

In this study, 70% of women underwent a vaginal delivery. Compared to CB, there was no significant deterioration in bowel or bladder symptoms or quality of life. There were also no significant differences in ultrasound findings. In a larger study ($n = 122$) using the same criteria as Scheer et al., Jordan et al. [6] found similar results except that the squeeze pressure was significantly reduced in the vaginal delivery group at 3 months postpartum. However, there were no significant differences among groups in symptoms or anal sphincter defects. Internal sphincter defects had

no impact on symptoms or pressures supporting its exclusion in Scheer's study.

Lastly, two other studies used similar criteria to determine mode of subsequent birth and both had similar findings. Karmarkar et al. studied 50 women (26 vaginal delivery and 24 CB) and found no deterioration in symptoms or defects in either group on ultrasound or manometry [8]. Lastly, Fitzpatrick et al. looked at 197 women but not all had endoanal scans and anal manometry [7], 70% of whom underwent a vaginal birth. They too found no significant change in continence following either mode of birth. Cassis et al. performed a retrospective study of 233 women who sustained OASIs and applied the algorithm of other studies to calculate the rate of CB [90]. However, as they did not look at outcomes after a subsequent pregnancy, no conclusions can be drawn.

5.8.3.1 Asymptomatic Women Post OASIs

Asymptomatic women with minimal compromise of their anal sphincter function (satisfactory pressure measurements and ultrasound images) are the best candidates for a subsequent vaginal birth (Fig. 5.13). These women should be counselled that they have a 94% chance of not sustaining a recurrent OASI (Table 5.3) or developing de novo anal incontinence [70]. However, their birth should be attended to by an experienced doctor or midwife. If an episiotomy is considered necessary, e.g. because of a thick inelastic or scarred perineum, a mediolateral episiotomy should be performed. While there is reducing evidence from one observational study of primiparous women that a prophylactic episiotomy reduced the risk of recurrent OASIs by 80% [77], eight episiotomies need to be performed to prevent only one recurrent OASI.

On the other hand, in women with compromised anal sphincters, counseling may differ and lean toward CB. For example, in a prospective study ($n = 539$) using anal ultrasound and anal manometry at 9 weeks postpartum and 3 years, 10% of women developed de novo, symptomatic anal incontinence for the first time within three years. All of these women had compromised anal sphincters at the 9 week visit [77]. This provides justification to offer CB to asymptomatic women with compromised anal sphincters (Fig. 5.13). In fact, the threshold at which these women may be considered for a CB may be lowered even further if a traumatic delivery is anticipated, e.g. in the presence of one or more additional relative risk factors such as a big baby, shoulder dystocia, prolonged labour, or difficult instrumental delivery. However, in deciding the mode of birth, counselling (and its clear documentation) is extremely important. Some of these women who have sustained OASIs may be scarred both physically and emotionally and may find it difficult to cope with the thought of another vaginal delivery. These women will require sympathy, psychological support and consideration to their request for CB.

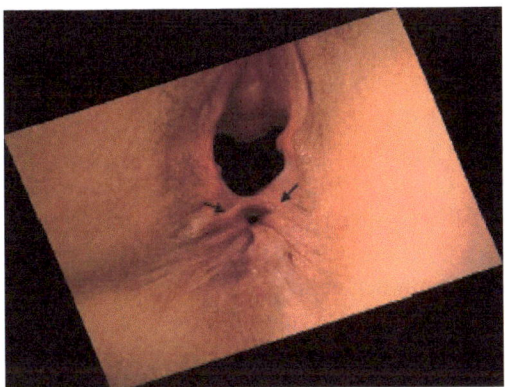

Fig. 5.14 Demonstration of a cloacal defect following a missed third degree tear. The perineal body is absent and the external sphincter is deficient between 10 and 2 o'clock (between arrows) as noted by the absence of the corrugator cutis ani

5.8.3.2 Symptomatic Women Post OASI

All symptomatic women are first treated conservatively (see Chaps. 18 and 19) depending on their main symptoms and findings at investigation. Women whose symptoms are adequately controlled by conservative measures (Chaps. 18 and 19) are offered CB in any subsequent delivery pregnancy, so as to minimise the risk of further compromise to anal sphincter function. On the other hand, women with faecal incontinence in whom conservative measures have failed should be considered for anal sphincter surgery (provided there is contractility of the residual sphincter), while others may need sacral nerve modulation or other advanced surgical techniques (Chap. 20). All pregnant women who have undergone successful incontinence surgery should be delivered by CB.

A management dilemma arises in women who suffer from persistent faecal incontinence but who wish further pregnancies. These women could undergo a vaginal delivery followed by a secondary sphincter repair at a later date. The only rationale behind this is that most of the damage that occurs during childbirth occurs with the first vaginal birth [91, 92] and therefore the risk of further damage during a subsequent vaginal birth is relatively small. However, there are certainly exceptions to this. For example, women who have a cloacal like defect with a thin anovaginal septum

and completely deficient perineum (Fig. 5.14) are at a very high risk of recurrent OASI with another vaginal birth. These cases are best individualised and discussed in a multidisciplinary meeting and informed consent is obtained according to the patient's wishes. However, there is a potentially unquantified risk of deteriorating pudendal neuropathy. By contrast, CB is not without major morbidity and mortality [93] (Chap. 6) and therefore, counselling plays an important role in the shared decision-making process.

Of note, women who suffer from varying degrees of irritable bowel syndrome will need evaluation and appropriate dietary advice depending on whether their bowel pattern is diarrhoea or constipation predominant. It has been shown that in women who have pre-existing irritable bowel syndrome, symptoms of defaecatory urgency and/or flatus incontinence deteriorate significantly following vaginal birth, independent of anal sphincter injury [94].

5.8.4   What Is the Risk of Worsening anal Incontinence Symptoms After Recurrent OASIs?

Jha and Parker performed a systematic review of risk factors for recurrent OASI (rOASI) and found that that the risk of recurrence was between 2 and

13.4% [95]. Recurrent OASIs shared similar risk factors as the index OASI, namely instrumental delivery with forceps [OR 3.12, 95% confidence interval (CI) 2.42–4.01] or ventouse (OR 2.44, 95% CI 1.83–3.25), birth weight ≥ 4 kg (OR 2.29, 95% CI 2.06–2.54). Maternal age ≥ 35 years marginally increased the risk (OR 1.16, 95% CI 1–1.35). As shown by Taithongchai et al., a previous fourth-degree tear (OR 1.7, 95% CI 1.24–2.36) also increased the subsequent risk [83].

In women who have suffered a rOASIs, compared to one OASI, Sze et al. found no significant difference in the prevalence and severity of anal incontinence among women who sustained two OASIs at 10 years; this study, however, did not evaluate anal sphincter integrity and anorectal function [96]. Okeahialam et al. performed a nested controlled study ($n = 84$) comparing women who had no sphincter damage after a previous OASI to a matched group of women who sustained a rOASI. Using validated tools (St. Mark's score, anal endosonography, Stark Score and anal manometry), they found no significant difference in anorectal symptoms, however, there was a significant reduction in resting and squeeze pressures on manometry as well as a worsening Stark score [97]. This data would suggest that women with rOASI who have compromised anal sphincters may be more likely to develop anal incontinence symptoms in later life [72]. Moreover, there are other uncontrolled mitigating factors at the time of a recurrent OASI birth such as the experience of the accoucheur, underestimation or incorrect diagnosis of OASIs (Chap. 3), and experience of the doctor performing the rOASI repair. It should also be noted that scoring algorithms to predict OASIs have been explored [98], others specifically after vaginal birth after CB [99, 100] and some for pelvic floor dysfunction [101, 102] with some success but they need to be tested prospectively and in randomized controlled trials.

5.8.5   How Safe Is Caesarean Birth?

One of the biggest concerns for women who have sustained OASIs and their providers is a recurrence of the injury and associated risk of faecal incontinence. While CB may decrease the risk of this, it is important to consider the morbidity and mortality associated with the procedure. In particular, CB is associated with an increased risk of maternal mortality, higher blood loss, peripartum hysterectomy, urinary tract injury, and thromboembolic disease. Furthermore, there are implications for future pregnancies, as there is an increased risk of placenta praevia, uterine rupture, antepartum stillbirth and infertility [103]. In an analytical model looking at elective CB for women with a previous OASIs [104], McKenna reported that a woman who undergoes CB has an 11.3% risk of morbidity compared to 4.2% following vaginal birth (relative risk 2.7); the relative risk of maternal death was 2.6 following CB. It is therefore important that women are made fully aware of the associated risks of both vaginal and CB (Chap. 6). In order to make a balanced informed decision, women need to be made aware of the short and long-term outcomes of both vaginal and CB; more importantly, women need to understand the most serious complications of both modes of birth.

5.8.6   Can Objective Assessments Predict Who Will Develop Incontinence?

There are limited prospective studies to address this issue. Fynes et al. [92] performed a prospective study of 59 women at three time points: at 34 weeks gestation during their first pregnancy and again at 6–12 weeks after two consecutive vaginal births. Of all the asymptomatic women after the first vaginal birth who had a large "occult" sonographic anal sphincter defect (>one quadrant) or anal squeeze pressures of less than 20 mmHg, 75% (six of eight) developed anal incontinence symptoms after their second vaginal birth. By contrast, only 5% (two of the 43) with less extensive defects became symptomatic ($P < 0.0001$).

There is an increasing awareness of the role of the IAS in maintaining continence. Nichols et al. [105] followed up 56 women who sustained

OASIs and found that combined defects of the IAS and EAS were associated with the highest risk of bowel symptoms compared to an intact sphincter (odds ratio 18.7; CI 3–101, $P < 0.001$) and isolated defects of the EAS (odds ratio 15.7; 95% CI 3–76; $P = 0.003$). Reid et al. found that 10% of women who were asymptomatic at 9 weeks following OASIs but did have anal sphincter defects, developed symptoms within 3 years [72]. Okeahialam et al. performed a prospective study ($n = 146$) to establish which women who undergo postpartum (usually 8 to 12 weeks) anal ultrasound and manometry may require these tests to be repeated in a subsequent pregnancy [106]. They determined that asymptomatic women with normal findings on ultrasound and monometry do not need to have the investigations repeated; a significant improvement in anal pressures was noted when the studies were repeated during pregnancy. Based on this study more than half the women would not have needed to be seen in a subsequent pregnancy. Thus, the decision regarding mode of birth could have been based on symptomatic postpartum assessment alone. However, symptomatic women or women with compromised sphincters should be re-evaluated in a subsequent pregnancy to establish recovery and counselled regarding the preference for a CB [106].

5.9 Who Should Be Performing Acute Primary Obstetric Sphincter Repairs?

In view of the observed, sometimes suboptimal, outcomes associated with primary OASI repair by obstetricians with varying degrees of experience, it has been suggested that perhaps colorectal surgeons' repairs may be associated with a better outcome [107]. However, as shown above [49], this has not borne out. Furthermore, in a survey of colorectal practice in the UK [53], the following was noted:

- Only 6.7% of colorectal surgeons reported that they performed more than ten acute repairs per year

- 60% of colorectal surgeons had never performed an acute sphincter repair and
- 30% of colorectal surgeons performed fewer than five repairs per year.

It is therefore not surprising that only 19% of colorectal surgeons believed that they should be involved in the acute management of OASIs. Yet, 30% of colorectal surgeons recommended a covering colostomy for OASIs, confirming that while they may have expertise in dealing with women presenting with faecal incontinence (Fig. 5.12), very few have any experience with acute OASIs [53].

There is also known scepticism by colorectal surgeons that the IAS cannot be repaired as a secondary procedure, as obstetricians do in the acute situation. However, there is recent evidence that separate repair of the IAS is associated with a better long-term outcome [108]. Thus, it is imperative that the most experienced clinician performs the repair as soon as possible after the injury. Ideally, this should be an obstetrician who would be easily accessible at any time. Furthermore, women who sustain OASIs often have concomitant vaginal lacerations (some multiple and deep) that will need to be repaired by an obstetrician (as well as reconstruction of the perineal body) Some have suggested that repair be delayed until a colorectal surgeon becomes available to perform the repair [30]. We believe this is suboptimal for numerous reasons. For example, the patient may be actively bleeding, the tissues may become oedematous, wound contamination is more likely to occur and therefore there is an increased risk of infection. Similarly, a delay in care can create unnecessary anxiety. Only in exceptional circumstances should a delay in care occur: when an experienced obstetrician may not be available. In such cases, we can be reassured that outcomes may still be very successful. However, Nordenstam et al. performed a randomised controlled study ($n = 161$) of immediate repair vs delayed repair (8 to 12 hours) with a team of 3 obstetricians and 3 colorectal surgeons and found no difference in outcome [109].

5.10   Education and Training

Physician and midwife training programmes and their deficiencies have been alluded to and are discussed in Chap. 23, while strategies for prevention of OASIs are discussed in Chap. 12. One explanation for the inadequate training in anatomy and pathophysiology can be attributed to the compartmentalisation of the pelvic floor such that many specialities (obstetricians, colorectal surgeons, urologists, gastroenterologists, etc.) deal with conditions that are in close proximity to each other. The territorial effects have been well illustrated by Wall and DeLancey [110] in an excellent article on the "politics of the pelvic floor". Unfortunately, as Sultan has highlighted in 1991, the "bottom line" is that politics also exist on the perineum, where an arbitrary dividing line has been drawn separating the territory of the obstetrician from that of the colorectal surgeon (Fig. 5.15). Unfortunately, the exact location of this line is undefined. Consequently, there is a large grey zone on either side of this line that each speciality believes belongs to the other specialty … leaving a chasm in education and training that this book endeavours to fill.

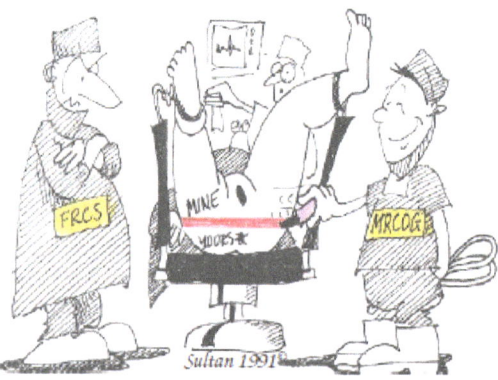

Fig. 5.15 Political interaction between the obstetrician (MRCOG) and the surgeon (FRCS) regarding the "bottom line"

5.11   Conclusions

OASIs can have a devastating effect on the physical, emotional and social wellbeing of a woman. Although there has been a notable increase in the prevalence of OASIs, this could be largely attributed to improvements in detection and classification of such injuries. Recognition of the full extent of the injury and appropriate repair by a trained obstetrician can provide an optimal outcome. A good understanding of perineal and anal sphincter anatomy and adherence to sound principles (described above) are essential. Postpartum care should be standardized according to the local or RCOG guidelines. Duty of candour and debriefing should be ensured in a dedicated clinic such as the Perineal Clinic/Maternal Recovery Clinic. It is important to recognise that many woman may be traumatised by the birth and OASI to the extent that they may be reticent to have another vaginal birth. Counselling regarding the mode of subsequent birth must follow a full explanation and shared decision making.

Take Home Messages

- Before repair of an OASI, a careful vaginal and rectal examination must be performed to establish the full extent and classification of the injury.
- Repair should be performed in layers with good apposition, especially of the IAS and EAS
- Mandatory steps should include clear documentation of the injuries, intra-operative antibiotics, stool softeners, duty of candour, physiotherapy and follow-up plans.
- Women need to be provided with the best available evidence regarding outcomes of vaginal birth and CB to enable them to make an informed decision about mode of subsequent birth.

Appendix: MCQ

Mark each item TRUE or FALSE

Questions

1. Regarding the primary repair of OASIs:
   (A) Repair conducted under regional anaesthesia in the operating theatre has advantages over repair under local anaesthesia.
   (B) Intra-operative antibiotics significantly reduce the risk of perineal wound infection.
   (C) On average about one third of women who undergo a primary anal sphincter repair of OASIs develop anal incontinence.
   (D) A rectal examination should only be performed after the repair to avoid wound contamination by the glove.
   (E) Colorectal surgeons have more experience in primary repair of the anal sphincter and therefore should be called to repair acute OASIs.

2. Regarding the repair technique of OASIs:
   (A) The torn anorectal epithelium should always be repaired with interrupted sutures and the knots should be tied within the anal canal.
   (B) Figure-of–eight sutures are ideal as they provide a secure and tight repair.
   (C) The thickness of the anal sphincter muscle after repair is not the single independent predictive factor of continence.
   (D) Overlap repair of the external anal sphincter (EAS) has been shown to be consistently superior to the end-to-end technique.
   (E) Delayed absorbable monofilament sutures are contraindicated because they can migrate and cause discomfort to the woman.

3. With further regard to sphincter repair:
   (A) The torn internal sphincter will heal not spontaneously if a proper overlap repair of the EAS is performed.
   (B) Levator plication at the time of primary repair of OASIs has been shown to improve quality of life.
   (C) When there is wound breakdown after repair of OASIs it is best to wait 3 months before secondary repair is attempted.
   (D) The outcome of secondary repair conducted by a colorectal surgeon is as good as a primary repair usually performed by obstetricians.
   (E) The development of fecal incontinence after primary repair of OASIS is invariably considered to be negligent.

4. With regards to the post operative care following repair of OASIS:
   (A) Post-operative catheterisation of the bladder is recommended.
   (B) Stool softeners, as opposed to bowel confinement for 3 days with codeine phosphate, are associated with significantly earlier and less painful bowel motion.
   (C) The addition of fibre supplements to stool softeners has been shown to improve the success of repair.
   (D) Women are less likely to complain or institute litigation if follow up is arranged in a dedicated specialist perineal clinic.
   (E) Diclofenac rectal suppositories should be avoided in women who have sustained a fourth degree tear.

5. Regarding subsequent pregnancy and birth:
   (A) The risk of recurrent OASIs is dependent on the type of episiotomy practised in that unit.
   (B) The recurrence rate of OASIs following a subsequent vaginal delivery is 15%.
   (C) Caesarean birth prevents the development of anal incontinence.
   (D) Recommendations on the mode of subsequent birth based on endoanal ultrasound and manometry findings have been shown to be beneficial.
   (E) Woman who have undergone a successful secondary sphincter repair should be advised to have future births by caesarean birth.

Answers

1. Regarding the primary repair of OASIs:
   - (A) TRUE
   - (B) TRUE
   - (C) TRUE
   - (D) FALSE
   - (E) FALSE

2. Regarding the repair technique of OASIs:
   - (A) FALSE
   - (B) FALSE
   - (C) TRUE
   - (D) FALSE
   - (E) FALSE

3. With further regard to sphincter repair:
   - (A) TRUE
   - (B) FALSE
   - (C) FALSE
   - (D) FALSE
   - (E) FALSE

4. With regards to the post operative care following repair of OASIS:
   - (A) TRUE
   - (B) TRUE
   - (C) FALSE
   - (D) TRUE
   - (E) TRUE

5. Regarding subsequent pregnancy and birth:
   - (A) TRUE
   - (B) FALSE
   - (C) FALSE
   - (D) TRUE
   - (E) TRUE

References

1. Sultan AH. Obstetric perineal injury and anal incontinence. AVMA Med Legal J. 1999;5:193–6. https://doi.org/10.1177/135626229900500601.
2. Okeahialam NA, Taithongchai A, Thakar R, Sultan AH. The incidence of anal incontinence following obstetric anal sphincter injury graded using the Sultan classification: a network meta-analysis. Am J Obstet Gynecol. 2023;228(6):675–688.e13. https://doi.org/10.1016/j.ajog.2022.11.1279. Epub 2022 Nov 13. PMID: 36379266.
3. Roper JC, Thakar R, Sultan AH. Isolated rectal buttonhole tears in obstetri: case series and review of the literature. Int Urogynecol J. 2021;32(7):1761–9. https://doi.org/10.1007/s00192-020-04502-2. Epub 2020 Sep 15. PMID: 32930849; PMCID: PMC8295104.
4. Wan OYK, Taithongchai A, Veiga SI, et al. A one-stop perineal clinic: our eleven-year experience. Int Urogynecol J. 2020;31:2317–26. https://doi.org/10.1007/s00192-020-04405-2.
5. Scheer I, Thakar R, Sultan AH. Mode of delivery after previous obstetric anal sphincter injuries (OASIS) – A reappraisal? Int Urogynecol J Pelvic Floor Dysfunct. 2009;20(9):1095–101. https://doi.org/10.1007/s00192-009-0908-8. Epub 2009 May 28. PMID: 19475329.
6. Jordan PA, Naidu M, Thakar R, Sultan AH. Effect of subsequent vaginal delivery on bowel symptoms and anorectal function in women who sustained a previous obstetric anal sphincter injury. Int Urogynecol J. 2018;29(11):1579–88. https://doi.org/10.1007/s00192-018-3601-y. Epub 2018 Mar 29. PMID: 29600403; PMCID: PMC6208957
7. Fitzpatrick M, Cassidy M, Barassaud ML, Hehir MP, Hanly AM. Does anal sphincter injury preclude subsequent vaginal delivery? Eur J Obstet Gynaecol Reprod Biol. 2016;198:30–4.
8. Karmarkar R, Bhide A, Digesu A, Khullar V, Fernando R. Mode of delivery after obstetric anal sphincter injury. Eur J Obst Gynecol Reprod Biol. 2015;194:7–10.
9. Abramowitz L, Mandelbrot L, Bourgeois Moine A, Le Tohic A, de Carne CC, Poujade O, et al. Cesarean section in the second delivery to prevent anal incontinence after asymptomatic obstetrical anal sphincter injury: the EPIC multicenter randomized trial. BJOG: Int J Obstet Gy. 2020;128:685. https://doi.org/10.1111/1471-0528.16452.
10. Magdi I. Obstetric injuries of the perineum. J Obstet Gynaecol Br Commonw. 1949;49:687–700.
11. Garrigues HJ. The obstetric treatment of the perineum. Am J Obstet Gynecol. 1880;13(2):231–64.
12. Royston GD. Repair of complete perineal laceration. Am J Obstet Gynecol. 1930;19:185–95.
13. Ingraham HA. A report on 159 third degree tears. Am J Obstet Gynecol. 1949;57:730–5.
14. Fulsher RW, Fearl CL. The third-degree laceration in modern obstetrics. Am J Obstet Gynecol. 1955;69:786–93.
15. Cunningham CB, Pilkington JW. Complete perineotomy. Am J Obstet Gynecol. 1955;70:1225–31.
16. Kaltreider DF, Dixon DM. A study of 710 complete lacerations following central episiotomy. South Med J. 1948;41(9):814–20. https://doi.org/10.1097/00007611-194809000-00011. PMID: 18879671
17. Sultan AH, Monga AK, Kumar D, Stanton SL. Primary repair of obstetric anal sphincter rupture

using the overlap technique. Br J Obstet Gynaecol. 1999;106:318–23.

18. Parks AG, McPartlin JF. Late repair of injuries of the anal sphincter. Proc R Soc Med. 1971;64(12): 1187–9.

19. Thiagamoorthy G, Johnson A, Thakar R, Sultan AH. National survey of perineal trauma and its subsequent management in the United Kingdom. Int Urogynecol J. 2014;25:1621–7. https://doi.org/10.1007/s00192-014-2406-x.

20. Health at a glance: OECD indicators. 2019. https://www.oecd-ilibrary.org/sites/c2a6b2da-en/index.html?itemId=/content/component/c2a6b2da-en

21. Fenner DE, Genberg B, Brahma P, Marek L, DeLancey JOL. Fecal and urinary incontinence after vaginal delivery with anal sphincter disruption in an obstetrics unit in the United States. Am J Obstet Gynecol. 2003;189:1543–50.

22. Gurol-Urganci I, Cromwell DA, Edozien LC, Mahmood TA, Adams EJ, Richmond DH, et al. Third- and fourth-degree perineal tears among primiparous women in England between 2000 and 2012: time trends and risk factors. BJOG. 2013;120:1516–25.

23. Sultan AH, Kamm MA, Hudson CN, Bartram CI. Third degree obstetric anal sphincter tears: risk factors and outcome of primary repair. Br Med J. 1994;308:887–91.

24. Andrews V, Thakar R, Sultan AH. Structured hands-on training in repair of obstetric anal sphincter injuries (OASIS): an audit of clinical practice. Int Urogynecol J. 2009;20:193–9.

25. Zimmo K, Laine K, Vikanes Å, Fosse E, Zimmo M, Ali H, Thakar R, Sultan AH, Hassan S. Diagnosis and repair of perineal injuries: knowledge before and after expert training – a multicentre observational study among Palestinian physicians and midwives. BMJ Open. 2017;7:e014183.

26. Wong KW, Thakar R, Andrews V, Sultan AH. Is there a role for transperineal ultrasound imaging of the anal sphincter immediately after primary repair of third degree tears? Eur J Obstet Gynecol Reprod Biol. 2022;271:260–4. https://doi.org/10.1016/j.ejogrb.2022.02.182. Epub 2022 Mar 2. PMID: 35255362.

27. Jorge JM, Wexner SD. Etiology and management of fecal incontinence. Dis Colon Rectum. 1993;36(1):77–97.

28. Engel AF, Kamm MA, Sultan AH, Bartram CI, Nicholls RJ. Anterior anal sphincter repair in patients with obstetric trauma. Br J Surg. 1994;81(8):1231–4.

29. Malouf AJ, Norton CS, Engel AF, Nicholls RJ, Kamm MA. Long-term results of overlapping anterior anal-sphincter repair for obstetric trauma. Lancet. 2000;355(9200):260–5.

30. Sultan AH. Third degree tear repair. In: MacClean AB, Cardozo L, editors. Incontinence in women. London: RCOG Press; 2002. p. 379–90.

31. Fitzpatrick M, Behan M, O'Connell PR, O'Herlihy C. A randomised controlled trial comparing primary overlap with approximation repair of third-degree obstetric tears. American J Obstet Gynecol. 2000;183(5):1220–4.

32. Garcia V, Rogers RG, Kim SS, Hall RJ, Kammerer-Doak DN. Primary repair of obstetric anal sphincter laceration: a randomized trial of two surgical techniques. Am J Obstet Gynecol. 2005;192(5):1697–701.

33. Williams A, Adams EJ, Tincello DG, Alfirevic Z, Walkinshaw SA, Richmond DH. How to repair an anal sphincter injury after vaginal delivery: results of a randomised controlled trial. BJOG. 2006;113(2):201–7.

34. Fernando R, Sultan AH, Kettle C, Radley S, Jones P, O'Brien S. Repair techniques for obstetric anal sphincter injuries: a randomized trial. Obstet Gynecol. 2006;107:1261–8.

35. Rygh AB, Korner H. The overlap technique versus end-to-end approximation technique for primary repair of obstetric anal sphincter rupture: a randomized controlled study. Acta Obstet Gynecol Scand. 2010;89(10):1256–62.

36. Farrell SA, Gilmour D, Turnbull GK, Schmidt MH, Baskett TF, Flowerdew G, Fanning CA. Overlapping compared with end-to-end repair of third- and fourth-degree obstetric anal sphincter tears: a randomized controlled trial. Obstet Gynecol. 2010;116(1):16–24.

37. Farrell SA, Flowerdew G, Gilmour D, Turnbull GK, Schmidt MH, Baskett TF, Fanning CA. Overlapping compared with end-to-end repair of complete third-degree or fourth-degree obstetric tears: three-year follow-up of a randomized controlled trial. Obstet Gynecol. 2012;120(4):803–8. (Erratum: Obstet Gynecol December 2012;120(6):1482).

38. Fernando RJ, Sultan AH, Kettle C, Thakar R. Methods of repair for obstetric anal sphincter injury. Cochrane Database Syst Rev. 2013;(12):CD002866.

39. Kairaluoma MV, Raivio P, Aarnio MT, Kellokumpu IH. Immediate repair of obstetric anal sphincter rupture: medium-term outcome of the overlap technique. Dis Colon Rectum. 2004;47:1358–63.

40. https://www.perineum.net/gallery/repair

41. Sultan AH, Thakar R. Lower genital tract and anal sphincter trauma. Best Pract Res – Clin Obstet Gynaecol. 2002;16:99–116.

42. Katz S, Izhar M, Mirelman D. Bacterial adherence to surgical sutures. A possible factor in sutures induced infection. Annals Surg. 1981;194(1):35–41.

43. Fernando RJ. Obstetric anal sphincter injury and its management. Doctor of Medicine thesis, Keele University. 2005. p. 184.

44. Norderval S, Oian P, Revhaug A, Vonen B. Anal incontinence after obstetric sphincter tears: outcome of anatomic primary repairs. Dis Colon Rectum. 2005;48(5):1055–61. https://doi.org/10.1007/s10350-004-0887-2. PMID: 15785888

45. Hool GR, Lieber ML, Church JM. Postoperative anal canal length predicts outcome in patients having sphincter repair for fecal incontinence. Dis Colon Rectum. 1999;42(3):313–8.

46. Roper JC, Thakar R, Sultan AH. Isolated rectal buttonhole tears in obstetrics: case series and review of the literature. Int Urogynecol J. 2021;32(7):1761–9.

47. Salvatore S, et al. Pathophysiology of urinary incontinence, pelvic organ prolapse and faecal Incontinence. In: Abrams P, Cardozo L, Wagg A, Wein A, editors. Incontinence. 7th ed. Bristol: ICI-ICS. International Continence Society; 2023. ISBN: 978-0956960733.

48. Okeahialam NA, Thakar R, Sultan AH. Early secondary repair of obstetric anal sphincter injuries (OASIs): experience and a review of the literature. Int Urogynecol J. 2021;32(7):1611–22. https://doi.org/10.1007/s00192-021-04822-x. Epub 2021 May 15. PMID: 33991222

49. Samarasekera DN, Bekhit MT, Wright Y, et al. Long-term anal continence and quality of life following postpartum anal sphincter injury. Colorectal Disease. 2008;10:793–9. https://doi.org/10.1111/j.1463-1318.2007.01445.x.

50. Ramalingam K, Monga AK. Outcomes and follow-up after obstetric anal sphincter injuries. Int Urogynecol J. 2013;24:1495–500. https://doi.org/10.1007/s00192-013-2051-9.

51. Ramage L, Yen C, Qiu S, et al. Functional and quality of life outcomes following obstetric anal sphincter injury (OASI): does the grade of injury affect outcomes? Int Urogynecol J. 2017;28:1709–17. https://doi.org/10.1007/s00192-017-3334-3.

52. Roos A-M, Thakar R, Sultan AH. Outcome of primary repair of obstetric anal sphincter injuries (OASIS): does the grade of tear matter? Ultrasound Obstet Gynecol. 2010;36:368–74. https://doi.org/10.1002/uog.7512.

53. Fernando RJ, Sultan AH, Radley S, Jones PW, Johanson RB. Management of obstetric anal sphincter injury: a systematic review and national practice survey. BMC Health Serv Res. 2002;2(1):9.

54. Duggal N, Mercado C, Daniels K, Bujor A, Caughey AB, El-Sayed Y. Antibiotic prophylaxis for the prevention of postpartum wound infections. Obstet Gynecol 2008;111:1268–73.

55. Hedayati H, Parsons J, Crowther CA. Rectal analgesia for pain from perineal trauma following childbirth. Cochrane Database Syst Rev. 2003;3:CD003931.

56. Kettle C, Hills RK, Jones P, Darby L, Gray R, Johanson R. Continuous versus interrupted perineal repair with standard or rapidly absorbed sutures after spontaneous vaginal birth: a randomised controlled trial. Lancet. 2002;359(9325):2217–23.

57. Abdul-Wahid FS, Qureshi A, Soon-Keng C. Indomethacin-induced rectovaginal fistula in a postpartum patient. Dis Colon Rectum. 2002;45(6):843–4. PMID: 12072643

58. Mahony R, Behan M, O'Herlihy C, O'Connell PR. Randomized, clinical trial of bowel confinement vs. laxative use after primary repair of a third-degree obstetric anal sphincter tear. Dis Colon Rectum. 2004;47(1):12–7.

59. Nessim A, Wexner SD, Agachan F, Alabaz O, Weiss EG, Nogueras JJ, et al. Is bowel confinement necessary after anorectal reconstructive surgery? A prospective, randomized, surgeon-blinded trial. Dis Colon Rectum. 1999;42(1):16–23.

60. Williams A, Lavender T, Richmond DH, Tincello DG. Women's experiences after a third-degree obstetric anal sphincter tear: a qualitative study. Birth. 2005;32(2):129–36.

61. Ayers S, Bond R, Bertullies S, Wijma K. The aetiology of post-traumatic stress following childbirth: a meta-analysis and theoretical framework. Psychol Med. 2016;46(6):1121–34.

62. Carter J, Bick D, Gallacher D, Chang YS. Mode of birth and development of maternal postnatal post-traumatic stress disorder: a mixed-methods systematic review and meta-analysis. Birth. 2022;49(4):616–627.0.

63. Peleg D, Kennedy CM, Merrill D, Zlatnik FJ. Risk of repetition of a severe perineal laceration. Obstet Gynecol. 1999;93(6):1021–4.

64. Brincat C, Crosby E, McLeod A, Fenner DE. Experiences during the first four years of a postpartum perineal clinic in the USA. Int J Gynaecol Obstet. 2015;128(1):68–71. https://doi.org/10.1016/j.ijgo.2014.07.026. Epub 2014 Sep 6. PMID: 25262441.

65. Hickman LC, Propst K, Swenson CW, Lewicky-Gaupp C. Subspecialty care for peripartum pelvic floor disorders. Am J Obstet Gynecol. 2020;223(5):709–14.

66. Madsen AM, Hickman LC, Propst K. Recognition and management of pelvic floor disorders in pregnancy and the postpartum period. Obstet Gynecol Clin North Am. 2021;48(3):571–84.

67. Keighley MR, Perston Y, Bradshaw E, Hayes J, Keighley DM, Webb S. The social, psychological, emotional morbidity and adjustment techniques for women with anal incontinence following Obstetric Anal Sphincter Injury: use of a word picture to identify a hidden syndrome. BMC Pregnancy Childbirth. 2016;16(1):275. https://doi.org/10.1186/s12884-016-1065-y. PMID: 27654450; PMCID: PMC5031357

68. Payne TN, Carey JC, Rayburn WF. Prior third- or fourth-degree perineal tears and recurrence risks. Int J Gynecol Obstet. 1999;64:55–7.

69. Harkin R, Fitzpatrick M, O'Connell PR, O'Herlihy C. Anal sphincter disruption at vaginal delivery: is recurrence predictable? Eur J Obstet Gynecol Reprod Biol. 2003;109(2):149–52.

70. Yogev Y, Hiersch L, Maresky L, Wasserberg N, Wiznitzer A, Melamed N. Third and fourth degree perineal tears – the risk of recurrence in subsequent pregnancy. J Matern Fetal Neonatal Med. 2014;27(2):177–81. https://doi.org/10.3109/14767058.2013.806902. Epub 2013 Jun 14. PMID: 23682932.

71. Webb SS, Sitch A, MacArthur C. The impact of mode of subsequent birth after obstetric anal

sphincter injury on bowel function and related quality of life: a cohort study. Int Urogynecol J. 2020;31(11):2237–45.

72. Reid AJ, Beggs AD, Sultan AH, Roos AM, Thakar R. Outcome of repair of obstetric anal sphincter injuries after three years. Int J Gynaecol Obstet. 2014;127(1):47–50. https://doi.org/10.1016/j.ijgo.2014.04.013.

73. Young R, Bates L, The S, King J. Mode of delivery following obstetric anal sphincter injury: a 7-year retrospective review and follow-up cohort survey. Int Urogynecol J. 2022;33(12):3365–9.

74. Baghestan E, Irgens LM, Børdahl PE, Rasmussen S. Risk of recurrence and subsequent delivery after obstetric anal sphincter injuries. BJOG. 2012;119(1):62–9. https://doi.org/10.1111/j.1471-0528.2011.03150.x. Epub 2011 Oct 10. PMID: 21985470.

75. Jango H, Langhoff-Roos J, Rosthoj S, Sakse A. Risk factors of recurrent anal sphincter ruptures: a population-based cohort study. BJOG. 2012;119(13):1640–7.

76. Edozien LC, Gurol-Urganci I, Cromwell DA, Adams EJ, Richmond DH, Mahmood TA, van der Meulen JH. Impact of third- and fourth-degree perineal tears at first birth on subsequent pregnancy outcomes: a cohort study. BJOG. 2014;121(13):1695–703. https://doi.org/10.1111/1471-0528.12886. Epub 2014 Jul 9. PMID: 25040835.

77. D'Souza JC, Monga A, Tincello DG, Sultan AH, Thakar R, Hillard TC, et al. Maternal outcomes in subsequent delivery after previous obstetric anal sphincter injury (OASI): a multi-centre retrospective cohort study. Int Urogynecol J. 2020;31(3):627–33.

78. Ali A, Glennon K, Kirkham C, Yousif S, Eogan M. Delivery outcomes and events in subsequent pregnancies after previous anal sphincter injury. Eur J Obstet Gynecol Reprod Biol. 2014;174:51–3. https://doi.org/10.1016/j.ejogrb.2013.12.004. Epub 2013 Dec 12. PMID: 24398029.

79. Royal College of Obstetricians and Gynaecologists. Management of third and fourth degree perineal tears following vaginal delivery. RCOG Guideline No. 29. London: RCOG Press; 2015.

80. Poen AC, Felt-Bersma RJ, Strijers RL, Dekker GA, Cuesta MA, Meuwissen SG. Third-degree obstetric perineal tear: long-term clinical and functional results after primary repair. Br J Surg. 1998;85(10):1433–8.

81. Sangalli MR, Floris L, Faltin D, Weil A. Anal incontinence in women with third or fourth degree perineal tears and subsequent vaginal deliveries. Aust N Z J Obstet Gynaecol. 2000;40(3):244–8.

82. Fenner DE, Genberg B, Brahma P, Marek L, DeLancey JOL. Fecal and urinay incontinence after vaginal delivery with anal sphincter disruption in an obstetrics unit in the United States. Am J Obstet Gynecol. 2003;189:1543–50.

83. Taithongchai A, Thakar R, Sultan A. Management of subsequent pregnancies following fourth-degree obstetric anal sphincter injuries (OASIS). Eur J Obst Gynecol Reprod Biol. 2020;250:80–5.

84. Webb SS, Yates D, Manresa M, Parsons M, MacArthur C, Ismail KM. Impact of subsequent birth and delivery mode for women with previous OASIS: systematic review and meta-analysis. Int Urogynecol J. 2017;28(4):507–14. https://doi.org/10.1007/s00192-016-3226-y. Epub 2016 Dec 26. PMID: 28025682.

85. Fradet-Menard C, Deparis J, Gachon B, Sichitiu J, Pierre F, Fritel X, Desseauve D. Obstetrical anal sphincter injuries and symptoms after subsequent deliveries: a 60 patient study. Eur J Obstet Gynecol Reprod Biol. 2018;226:40–6. https://doi.org/10.1016/j.ejogrb.2018.05.007. Epub 2018 May 21. PMID: 29804027.

86. Okeahialam NA, Wong KW, Roper J, Thakar R, Sultan AH. Re: Cesarean section in the second delivery to prevent anal incontinence after asymptomatic obstetrical anal sphincter injury: the EPIC multicentre randomised trial. BJOG. 2021;128(4):770–1. https://doi.org/10.1111/1471-0528.16578. Epub 2020 Nov 20. PMID: 33215820.

87. Badri H, Fowler G, Lane S. Follow up of women after obstetric anal sphincter injuries (OASI)-What is the role of anorectal testing? Neurourol Urodyn. 2023;42(6):1374–80. https://doi.org/10.1002/nau.25220. Epub 2023 Jun 3. PMID: 37269480.

88. Brown SJ, Gartland D, Donath S, MacArthur C. Fecal incontinence during the first 12 months postpartum: complex causal pathways and implications for clinical practice. Am J Obstet Gynecol. 2012;119(2):240–9.

89. Roos AM, Abdool Z, Thakar R, Sultan AH. Predicting anal sphincter defects: the value of clinical examination and manometry. Int Urogynecol J. 2012;23(6):755–63. https://doi.org/10.1007/s00192-011-1609-7. Epub 2011 Nov 18. PMID: 22095551.

90. Cassis C, Giarenis I, Mukhopadhyay S, Morris E. Mode of delivery following an OASIS and caesarean section rates. Europ J Obstet Gynecol Rep Biol. 2018;230:28–31.

91. Sultan AH, Kamm MA, Hudson CN, Thomas JM, Bartram CI. Anal sphincter disruption during vaginal delivery. New Engl J Med. 1993;329:1905–11.

92. Fynes M, Donnelly V, Behan M, O'Connell PR, O'Herlihy C. Effect of second vaginal delivery on anorectal physiology and faecal continence: a prospective study [see comments]. Lancet. 1999;354(9183):983–6.

93. Sultan AH, Stanton SL. Preserving the pelvic floor and perineum during childbirth – elective caesarean section? Br J Obstet Gynaecol. 1996;103(8):731–4.

94. Donnelly V, Fynes M, Campbell D, Johnson H, O'Connell PR, O'Herlihy C. Obstetric events leading to anal sphincter damage. Obstet Gynecol. 1998;92(6):955–61.

95. Jha S, Parker V. Risk factors for recurrent obstetric anal sphincter injury (rOASI): a systematic review and meta-analysis. Int Urogynecol J. 2016;27:849–57.

96. Sze EHM. Anal incontinence among women with one versus two complete third-degree perineal lacerations. Int J Gynecol Obst. 2005;90:213–7. https://doi.org/10.1016/j.ijgo.2005.04.017.

97. Okeahialam NA, Thakar R, Naidu M, Sultan AH. Outcome of anal symptoms and anorectal function following two obstetric anal sphincter injuries (OASIS)-a nested case-controlled study. Int Urogynecol J. 2020;31(11):2405–10. https://doi.org/10.1007/s00192-020-04377-3. Epub 2020 Jun 16. PMID: 32556846; PMCID: PMC7561534

98. McPherson KC, Beggs AD, Sultan AH, Thakar R. Can the risk of obstetric anal sphincter injuries (OASIs) be predicted using a risk-scoring system? BMC Research Notes. 2014;7:471.

99. Brown O, Luchristt D, Miller ES, Pidaparti M, Geynisman-Tan J, Kenton K, Lewicky-Gaupp C. Is there an association between vaginal birth after cesarean prediction and obstetric anal sphincter injury? Am J Perinatol. 2022;39(7):750–8.

100. Luchristt D, Brown O, Pidaparti M, Kenton K, Lewicky-Gaupp C, Miller ES. Predicting obstetrical anal sphincter injuries in patients who undergo vaginal birth after cesarean delivery. Am J Obstet Gynecol. 2021;225(2):173.e1–8.

101. Bugge C, Strachan H, Pringle S, Hagen S, Cheyne H, Wilson D. Should pregnant women know their individual risk of future pelvic floor dysfunction? A qualitative study. BMC Pregnancy Childbirth. 2022;22(1):161. https://doi.org/10.1186/s12884-022-04490-9. PMID: 35220939; PMCID: PMC8883628.

102. Jelovsek JE, Piccorelli A, Barber MD, Tunitsky-Bitton E, Kattan MW. Prediction models for postpartum urinary and fecal incontinence in primiparous women. Female Pelvic Med Reconstr Surg. 2013;19(2):110–8.

103. National Institute for Health and Clinical Excellence. Caesarean birth. London: NICE; 2023. www.nice.org.uk/guidance/ng192

104. McKenna DS, Ester JB, Fischer JR. Elective cesarean delivery for women with a previous anal sphincter rupture. Am J Obstet Gynecol. 2003;189(5):1251–6.

105. Nichols CM, Lamb EH, Ramakrishnan V. Differences in outcomes after third- versus fourth-degree perineal laceration repair: a prospective study. Am J Obstet Gynecol. 2005;193(2):530–4.

106. Okeahialam NA, Thakar R, Sultan AH. Effect of a subsequent pregnancy on anal sphincter integrity and function after obstetric anal sphincter injury (OASI). Int Urogynecol J. 2021;32(7):1719–26. https://doi.org/10.1007/s00192-020-04607-8. Epub 2020 Dec 2. PMID: 33263781; PMCID: PMC8295136

107. Cook TA, Mortensen NJ. Management of faecal incontinence following obstetric injury. Br J Surg. 1998;85(3):293–9.

108. Berg MR, Gregussen H, Sahlin Y. Long-term outcome of sphincteroplasty with separate suturing of the internal and the external anal sphincter. Tech Coloproctol. 2019;23(12):1163–72. https://doi.org/10.1007/s10151-019-02122-7. Epub 2019 Nov 26. PMID: 31773346; PMCID: PMC6890595

109. Nordenstam J, Mellgren A, Altman D, López A, Johansson C, Anzén B, Li ZZ, Zetterström J. Immediate or delayed repair of obstetric anal sphincter tears-a randomised controlled trial. BJOG. 2008;115(7):857–65. https://doi.org/10.1111/j.1471-0528.2008.01726.x. PMID: 18485164.

110. Wall LL, DeLancey JO. The politics of prolapse: a revisionist approach to disorders of the pelvic floor in women. Perspect Biol Med. 1991;34(4):486–96.

Short and Long-term Maternal and Neonatal Outcomes of Caesarean Section

6

Clare Richards and Mairead Black

Overview
Test your learning and check your understanding of this book's contents: use the "Springer Nature Flashcards" app to access questions using ▶ https://sn.pub/wqrf89. To use the app, please follow the instructions in Chap. 1.

Learning Objectives

- Understand the short-term implications of Caesarean birth, including frequent, less severe risks and rare, life-threatening risks
- Understand the evidence around long-term implications of Caesarean birth, and where evidence is lacking
- Understand the implications of Caesarean birth to future pregnancy, including complications in delivery

C. Richards (✉)
Aberdeen Maternity Hospital, Aberdeen, UK
e-mail: Clare.richards@nhs.scot

M. Black
NHS, Aberdeen Maternity Hospital,
Aberdeen, Scotland
e-mail: ogy474@abdn.ac.uk

6.1 Introduction

Caesarean birth (CB) is one of the oldest, most frequently performed operations globally. Although it has evolved slowly over time, it remains remarkably unchanged [1]. However, over the past few years, the rate and indication of use have changed massively [2].

The procedure is usually performed by a low transverse abdominal incision, entry into the peritoneal cavity, and a uterine incision to allow delivery of the fetus. For the sake of simplicity, caesarean birth (CB) will here refer to a lower uterine segment incision, as it is the most common method performed, with the lowest rate of complications [3].

The rate of CB has more than tripled over the past 50 years in the UK, to around 35% of all births [4]. This is a trend that is reflected across the world and seen in both an elective and emergency setting [4–6]. Reasons for this rise are extensive and beyond the scope of this textbook, but are thought partly to be related to the increased medical complexity of pregnant women, and changes in guidelines (including guidance around "maternal request" CB) [7].

CB has some significant risks in both the short- and long-term to both mother and baby, when compared to vaginal birth (VB) and instrumental birth (IB), including complicating any future pregnancies. It also, however, has benefits. The risks and benefits of CB must be considered

© The Author(s), under exclusive license to Springer Nature Switzerland AG 2024
A. H. Sultan et al. (eds.), *Pelvic Floor, Perineal, and Anal Sphincter Trauma During Childbirth*,
https://doi.org/10.1007/978-3-031-43095-4_6

individually by each woman to make a fully informed decision about her mode of birth and will be discussed in this chapter.

It is also important to note that a woman's planned mode of birth may deviate from the actual mode of birth. Newer research is attempting to review the implications of *planned* (rather than actual) mode of birth. However, in this chapter, outcomes will be presented by *actual* mode of birth, as this is what the majority of published research examines.

6.2 Short-term Implications of CB

There is no mode of birth which is free of risk, but the risk of severe maternal complications is higher in CB when compared to VB [8] (Table 6.1). Newer research has begun to evaluate the difference in short-term risks in planned versus unplanned CB and VB, as there is a significantly higher risk of complications, particularly at advanced dilation. The risk of an unplanned CB in a primigravida is around 25%. However, as noted earlier, this chapter remains focused on *actual* mode of birth.

It is important to note that there are some occasions where the risks of labour and VB may be too high to mother or baby (e.g. significant fetal compromise, morbidly adherent placenta,

and decompensated cardiac failure) and CB offers a safer, more predictable mode of birth, eliminating the stress of labour.

6.2.1 Bleeding

A common intraoperative complication in CB is excess blood loss, with the average blood loss at planned CB of around 500 mL [37–39]. The risk of primary postpartum haemorrhage (generally considered blood loss >1000 mL) is between 2 and 6%, but higher in unplanned CB [10, 11]. Although the risk of haemorrhage may be lower in an uncomplicated VB, it still complicates up to 4% of vaginal births. IB and the use of episiotomy further increase this risk [40]. Limited evidence suggests that there is no difference in rates of major haemorrhage between planned VB and planned CB [41].

The risk of peripartum hysterectomy for haemorrhage is low in a first pregnancy, but CB increases this risk. However, other risk factors (such as abnormal placentation) appear to be a more significant risk factor for both major haemorrhage and hysterectomy [17, 42].

6.2.2 Surgical Site Infection and Wound Complications

The incidence of surgical site infection (including superficial and deep wound infection, and endometritis) after CB is 9–11% and can lead to significant morbidity and extended hospital stay [15, 16]. This risk is reduced using perioperative antibiotic prophylaxis [43], but is increased further by in CB performed in an emergency setting [44]. A rare complication of CB is severe, invasive infection, including necrotizing fasciitis. This type of infection can require multiple further surgeries and cause significant morbidity, with a mortality rate of 20–40% [45]. There are other risks of wound complications, such as persistent pain, haematoma formation, and wound dehiscence; these increase in the obese population. With a BMI above 50, the risk of any wound complication is 25% [12, 13].

Table 6.1 Complications of caesarean birth

Risk	Rate (in 1000 women)
Persistent pain [9]	60–420
Haemorrhage (blood loss >1000 mL) [10, 11]	20–60
Wound complication (pain, infection, dehiscence) [12, 13]	30–150
Fetal Injury [14]	10–20
Postoperative infection [15, 16]	90–110
Peripartum hysterectomy [17–19]	0.06–0.15
Need for further surgery [20–22]	5–20
Admission to ICU [23–26]	4–9
Venous thromboembolism [27, 28]	0.4–3
Bladder injury [29]	1
Ureteric injury [30, 31]	Rare
Bowel injury [32, 33]	0.1
Maternal death [23, 34–36]	0.12–0.5

6.2.3   Return to Theatre

The most common indications for return to the operating theatre after CB is severe, uncontrollable bleeding or invasive infection. The most common secondary procedures performed are exploratory laparotomy for haemostasis, or wound exploration. Rates vary widely depending on the literature but lie somewhere between 0.005 and 0.2% [20–22].

6.2.4   Venous Thromboembolism (VTE)

The risk of VTE, including deep vein thrombosis and pulmonary embolism, is increased in all postnatal periods, by up to 20-fold compared to non-pregnant individuals. The risk with CB is around four times higher than after VB [27, 28]. VTE is associated with a risk of severe maternal morbidity and mortality [46, 47]. It was the leading direct cause of death in women in the UK who were pregnant, or up to 6 weeks postnatal in the UK between 2017 and 2019 [48].

6.2.5   Visceral Injury

There is a small risk of visceral injury at CB, which can include injury to bladder, bowel, or ureters [49]. The risk of bladder injury is around 1 in 1000. Where the repair is performed at the time of injury the long-term outcome is generally good, but, it can lead to long-term catheterisation. The risk of incidental cystotomy is increased in the setting of a previous CB, in patients with significant adhesions, and in cases of a more complex operation (including uterine rupture) [29].

Ureteric injury is a rare complication of CB, generally occurring during the placing of blind haemostatic sutures. It is often subject to a delayed diagnosis and can result in significant morbidity including ureterouterine fistula [30, 31].

The risk of bowel injury in CB is around 1 in 10,000. This is twice the risk than that of VB and this risk increases with increasing number of CBs. It most commonly affects the colon, and may require extensive resection and stoma formation [32, 33].

6.2.6   Maternal Mortality

Although the absolute risk is low, maternal mortality rate for CB is around three times higher than VB in an elective setting, and up to nine times higher in an emergency setting [23, 34–36]. There is also a small, but slight increase in risk of intensive care admission, which is between 4 and 9 per 1000 women. This risk may be related to the reason for CB, but this has not been fully explored in research [23–26].

6.2.7   Neonatal Implications

Neonates born by CB have nearly double the risk of short-term respiratory issues, including respiratory distress, when compared to VB. This risk is reduced when birth occurs after 39 weeks, and after labour has begun, but neonates may need neonatal unit admission and further care [50, 51]. The overall risk of neonatal death is very similar with each mode of birth, but there may be a very small increase in mortality in a planned CB compared to planned VB [52, 53].

The risk of fetal injury is around 1% at CB, but the overall risk of birth trauma is up to 60% lower than VB. The risk of neonatal trauma at birth is particularly increased in IB [14].

6.2.8   Recovery Time

CB requires an increased length of hospital stay, with the average is around 2–4 days [54–56]. It also has a significant recovery time, lasting months in some cases, although anecdotally this appears to vary greatly depending on the woman, the operation itself, and any complications which may arise [57].

6.3   Long Term Implications of CB

6.3.1   Future Pregnancies

Previous CB can complicate a future pregnancy for the mother, both antenatally and intrapartum and the risk of complications increase with an

Table 6.2 The estimated risks of planned vaginal birth after caesarean, in comparison to planned vaginal birth after previous vaginal birth

Future pregnancy complication	Risk after a single CB (in 1000 women)	Risk in primigravida or after single VB (in 1000 women)
Need for unplanned CB [38, 60, 61]	250	10–63
Peripartum hysterectomy [18, 62]	0.4–1.7	0.03
Uterine rupture [63–67]	5–7	0.06–0.08
Placenta Praevia [68]	8.7	4.4
Placenta Accreta Spectrum [69]	0.9	0.03
Perinatal Mortality [70]	0.4	Similar
Maternal mortality [48, 71] (188)	0.4	0.08
Preterm labour (before 37 weeks) [72–74]	Unknown–Small increase	Around 80

increasing number of CBs. However, planned vaginal birth after CB (VBAC) has been deemed a safe option for most women after one CB [58, 59]. This risks of VBAC (Table 6.2) must be discussed when the patient is exploring her options for mode of birth.

6.3.1.1 Birth Complications

Women opting for VBAC after one previous CB have approximately a 25% risk of requiring unplanned CB, which is significantly higher than women who have not had a prior CB [60, 61]. Even a single previous CB, in an otherwise uncomplicated pregnancy, increases the risk of peripartum hysterectomy [18, 62]. However, the risk of delivery-related perinatal mortality is similar to that of a nulliparous woman [70].

6.3.1.2 Uterine Rupture

Women planning VBAC must consider the risk of uterine rupture, which can have catastrophic consequences for mother and baby. The incidence of rupture has increased significantly over the years [63]. Uterine rupture often presents with severe, constant abdominal pain, vaginal bleeding, haematuria, and signs of fetal distress [64, 75]. Perinatal mortality is estimated to be between 4 and 8% [65, 70]. There is also a significantly higher risk of birth asphyxia, major haemorrhage

and need for hysterectomy, although outcomes have improved over the years [63]. The overall risk of rupture in VBAC is 5–7 per 1000 women, but increases as the number of previous CBs increases. It most commonly occurs in labour, and the risk increases with interventions such as induction of labour [63, 66, 67, 70]. Uterine rupture can occur without a history of a previous CB at a much lower rate (0.06–0.08 in 1000 women), but is usually associated with other risk factors [63–65].

6.3.1.3 Placenta Praevia

The risk of placenta praevia (placenta covering the internal cervical os) increases from 4 in 1000 women with no previous CB, to 8 in 1000 in women with one prior CB. This is a condition that can be accompanied by a risk of major haemorrhage and usually requires a CB [68].

6.3.1.4 Placenta Accreta Spectrum (PAS)

PAS is an umbrella term describing several types of abnormal implantation of the placenta. International classification includes (1) placenta accreta (placental villi adherent to the myometrium), (2) increta (villi invade the myometrium) and (3) percreta (villi invade the full thickness of the myometrium and other pelvic structures) [76]. The pathophysiology is complex, but in the presence of the abnormal surface caused by a uterine scar, the placental villi are thought to invade inappropriately into the myometrium, and beyond [77]. Increasing number of CBs increases the risk of PAS. This risk increases exponentially as the number of CB increases [62, 78, 79]. The risk in no previous CBs is 0.3 in 10,000 women and increases to 9 in 10,000 after one CB [69]. Women with PAS are at significantly increased risk of major haemorrhage requiring hysterectomy and transfusion, as well as serious intraoperative complications [80].

6.3.1.5 Preterm Labour (PTL)

Studies are small and inconsistent, but a history of a previous CB may confer a small increase in risk of spontaneous PTL in future pregnancies, which is most commonly observed between 34 and 37 weeks [72]. A six-fold rise in risk of future PTL has been observed when the CB is performed at full dilatation [73]. It has been hypothesised that this association may be caused by cervical trauma at the time of CB. There is currently research underway to further understand this association and determine interventions to reduce the risk of PTL after full-dilatation CB [73, 81].

6.3.1.6 Spontaneous Abortion and Ectopic Pregnancy

While anecdotally it was thought that uterine scarring may increase the risk of spontaneous abortion in future pregnancies, the evidence does not support this. Although smaller studies identify a small increased risk, larger reviews found inconsistent evidence subject to confounding [78]. On the other hand, the increased association between spontaneous abortion after CB in a pregnancy conceived with reproductive technology (ART) is a little better established. This may relate to the formation of a niche (small outpouching) in the scar (discussed later in this chapter), causing issues with implantation during IVF/ICSI, thus making the pregnancy is more prone to spontaneous abortion [82, 83].

Small studies have also found a slight increase in risk of ectopic pregnancy after CB, and this risk increases with increasing number of CBs; again, the quality of this evidence is variable and unreliable. It may be related to patients who had significant postoperative infection or adhesion formation, but currently there is little evidence to support this theory [84–86].

6.3.1.7 Caesarean Scar Ectopic Pregnancy (CSEP)

A CSEP was first described 40 years ago, but is being reported with increasing frequency as the rates of CB rise [87, 88]. CSEP is a pregnancy which implants into the uterine scar and is surrounded by myometrium and recently there has been speculation that CSEP may represent an extreme end of the spectrum of invasive placental disorders [89]. The absolute risk of CSEP is about 1 per 1800 pregnancies, but is exclusively seen in women with at least one previous CB, and an accompanying scar [88, 90]. Nearly half of all women with CSEP will spontaneously abort, which is accompanied by a high risk of bleeding and need for hysterectomy [90].

In those that don't abort spontaneously, the pregnancy will either (1) grow outwards (towards the abdominal cavity) which is accompanied by a high risk of uterine rupture and bleeding, or (2) grow into the endometrial cavity, where it may be relatively safe to continue the pregnancy [91, 92]. However, continuing a CSEP has significantly increased risks of serious morbidity, including spontaneous uterine rupture in the second trimester, PAS, major haemorrhage and need for hysterectomy [92]. Unfortunately, currently there is no consensus about management of these patients, and it remains a focus of research [88].

6.3.1.8 Fetal Demise

It is thought that CB may increase the risk of antepartum fetal demise by up 20%, but it is difficult to identify reasons for this association, as the demise itself often remains unexplained. A large study suggested a there would need to be 3333 CBs to cause a single fetal demise [78, 93, 94]. Evidence is conflicting, but it appears the risk of intrauterine demise is more pronounced in women with a previous emergency CB. It has therefore been suggested that the indication for CB may confer the future risk of stillbirth [94–96].

6.3.2 Gynaecological Issues

An area of developing interest is the impact of CB on the development of gynaecological problems, including chronic pain, infertility, irregular bleeding and development of endometriosis.

6.3.2.1 Fertility

The relationship between fertility and CB has been widely debated without achieving a consensus, with most studies suggesting that women who undergo CB have a wider pregnancy interval and a reduction in the number of pregnancies [97–100]. This is also reflected across the world, even in developing countries with higher parities [101]. However, it has been observed that most often this related to maternal choice, with no robust evidence of a true reduction in fertility [102, 103]. It is also known that women with fertility issues are more likely to have a CB than those without, and this could confound results [104].

Women with a previous CB have a lower live birth rate after ART, which is most prominently seen in women with a persistent scar defect [83, 105, 106]. Tubal infertility does not seem to be related to mode of birth [107, 108]. There are some reports of CB causing vaginal atresia, significant uterine adhesions, and adherence of the anterior uterine wall, but these remain isolated cases [109, 110].

Emerging evidence has identified that some women with previous CB develop a niche (indentation of the scar of at least 2 mm) and this may have an impact on fertility, particularly in ART, either by acting as a physical barrier to implantation or a psychogenic barrier to conception (by causing dyspareunia and bleeding with intercourse) [105, 111, 112].

6.3.2.2 Chronic Pelvic or Abdominal Pain

Chronic pelvic pain affects up to 11.5% of all women after childbirth, irrespective of mode of birth, and the reasons for it are complex and wide-ranging. Although 6–42% of women will experience chronic pain after CB, evidence suggests that CB reduces the risk of perineal pain, which appears to impact women more significantly [9, 113]. The risk of long-term pain is highest in those with the most severe postoperative pain, suggesting it may be related to individual patient or operation factors [113, 114]. There is no robust evidence to link mode of birth and dyspareunia, as it is observed in all modes of birth [115]. However, although evidence remains sparse, it is thought that the presence of a uterine niche after CB may be responsible for chronic pain, dyspareunia, and irregular bleeding in some women [116].

6.3.2.3 Development of Endometriosis

Endometriosis is a condition which affects up to 10% of all women and can cause major morbidity. With caesarean scar endometriosis, endometrial deposits are found in the operative scar, and it has been postulated that on uterine entry, endometrial tissue can spread. Evidence for this remains sparse [117, 118]. This condition can present with cyclical abdominal pain and an abdominal mass, which often requires excision. The actual incidence of this condition is unclear but can also cause significant morbidity to patients [119].

6.4 Emotional and Psychological Wellbeing and Birth Satisfaction

A woman's birth choice is complex and is dictated by personal preference, as well as by social, cultural, and economic factors. See Fig. 6.1 for a flowchart describing the factors involved in decision-making around mode of birth. Whether having a CB affects a woman's emotional well-being or psychological health remains somewhat unclear [120, 121]. CB does not independently seem to have an impact in psychological well-being or birth satisfaction early in the postnatal period or in the long-term. Instead, other factors, such as a protracted labour or deviation from planned mode of birth, seem to have more of an effect [122–124]. This is also reflected in women's assessment of their birth experience. For example, a poor overall experience in labour is more likely to confer dissatisfaction than their experience of CB itself. However, it should be noted that those with an unplanned CB express the highest rates of dissatisfaction [125, 126].

Unplanned CB and other factors relating to the patient's experience in labour are risk factors for maternal psychological birth trauma and post-traumatic stress disorder. These conditions can lead to difficulties in the postnatal period and impact future pregnancies including choice of future mode of birth. This risk is lower in planned CB and highest after IB [127, 128].

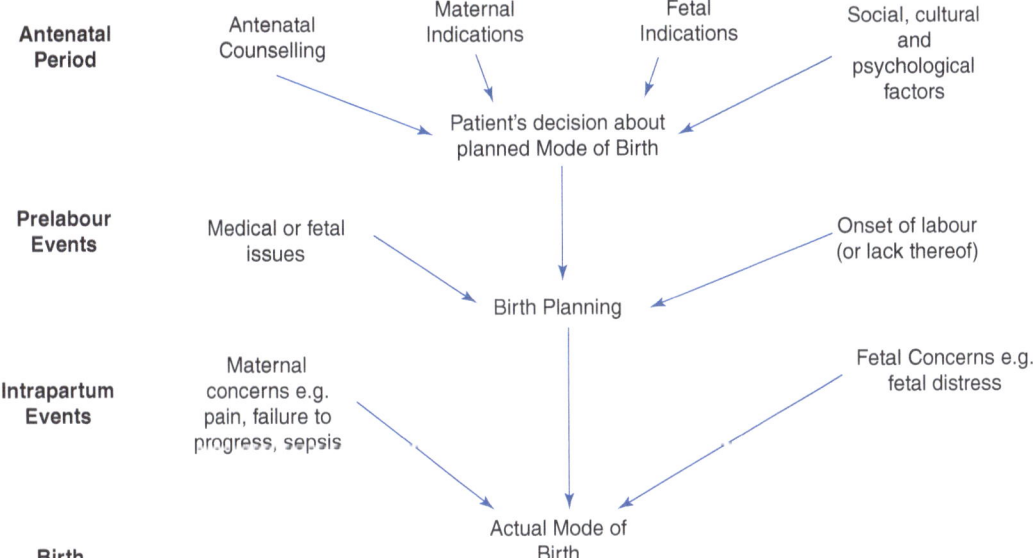

Fig. 6.1 Flowchart reviewing all the factors involved in decision-making around mode of birth planning, from antenatal period to delivery

Planned VB is often unpredictable, with a relatively high risk of intervention and complications, particularly for the nulliparous woman, depending on her choice of mode of birth. For example, a low-risk nulliparous woman has a 26% chance of IB and 12.5% chance of unplanned CB. The risk of CB doubles in high-risk nulliparous women, but is much lower in multiparous women who have not had a previous CB [38]. In view of this unpredictability and considering the psychological risks these deviations from the planned birth experience may pose, there may be some benefit to a planned CB in reducing the risk of maternal birth trauma in those who are felt to be high-risk.

6.5 Childhood Wellbeing Implications

The implications of CB on long-term childhood development and wellbeing have been debated widely. Suggestions have been made that CB may have associations with the development of neurodevelopmental and physical conditions, but evidence remains inconsistent. It has been postulated that CB causes changes in the neonatal microbiome and endocrine system which could affect the child's development in later life [129–131].

6.5.1 Cerebral Palsy and Neuropsychological Development

It is known that deprivation of oxygen at birth (birth asphyxia) is a risk factor for cerebral palsy, and there is some evidence to suggest it may have an association with the development of conditions such as autism spectrum disorder [132–134]. It is thought that the acute stress of CB could have similar effects on neuropsychiatric development [135]. However, there is currently no evidence to support the theory that delivery by CB is an independent risk factor for cerebral palsy. It is thought that the increased incidence of cerebral palsy seen in those delivered by emergency CB may be instead related to the indication for the CB [130, 136]. There are some situations in which CB is required to prevent birth asphyxia in the neonate, such as major placental abruption, where urgent CB would in fact reduce the risk of cerebral palsy (180). Despite a lack of evidence of real-world associations, studies in mice and rat models have demonstrated changes in the brain after CB, regardless of the presence of asphyxia. The relevance of this to humans is not known, but affected animals did show some cognitive impairment in early life [129, 135].

There is also no robust evidence for an association between CB and development of autism spectrum disorder, or any other neuropsychiatric disorder [130, 137].

6.5.2 Development of Physical Health Conditions

Emerging evidence suggests that CB may cause alterations in the neonatal microbiome. This change in flora has been implicated in several health conditions in later life [138, 139]. However, it is important to note that these studies are generally small and observational.

There seems to be an increased risk of obesity (5 in 1000) in children born via CB, and this is seen in children up to 5 years old [140–142]. Similarly, a 20% increased risk of type 1 diabetes mellitus in children delivered by CB has been observed, but again, evidence remains conflicting [52, 141].

Multiple studies have observed a small increase in risk of developing asthma (3 per 1000) [52, 140, 143, 144]. There may also be a small increase in risk of allergic disorders, atopy and severe respiratory infections, but evidence is less robust [145, 146].

6.6 Implications to Perineal Problems, Prolapse and Incontinence

While avoidance of VB reduces the risk of many pelvic floor disorders, it is important to note that pregnancy itself can contribute to pelvic floor dysfunction, irrespective of mode of delivery [147].

6.6.1 Perineal and Anal Sphincter Injury

The rates of perineal trauma after birth are highlighted in Table 6.3.

Only 10% of primiparous women and 31% of multiparous women will have a VB with an intact perineum [148]. The risk of this type of trauma is removed by planned CB. Although most perineal trauma heals well, there is a significant rate of infection and wound dehiscence [151, 152]. It can also be associated with dyspareunia and sexual dysfunction up to a year postpartum and can cause significant long-term morbidity (including pain, incontinence, and psychological issues). Some research suggests it may affect a woman's future pregnancy and birth planning [152, 153]. Although CB reduces this risk, there is a risk of other types of chronic pain and the risk of dyspareunia appears unrelated to mode of birth [9, 115].

Table 6.3 The risks of perineal and anal sphincter trauma after birth (first and second degree removed for instrumental birth due to RCOG recommendation that most should have prophylactic episiotomy) [38, 148–150]

	Type of perineal trauma	Risk in primigravida (in 100)	Risk in multiparous woman (if previous vaginal delivery) (in 100)
Vaginal birth	First and second degree	90	69
	Third and fourth degree	6	1–2
Instrumental birth	Third and fourth degree	Up to 12	

Table 6.4 The effect of CB on long-term risk factors (see relevant references and discussion in chapter)

Risks increased by CB	Risks similar in VB and CB	Risks decreased by CB	Conflicting or poor evidence
Lower live birth rate after IVF/ICSI	Dyspareunia	Perineal/vaginal pain	Spontaneous abortion
Development of childhood asthma	Development of cerebral palsy	Post-traumatic stress disorder (if planned CB)	Ectopic pregnancy
Development of childhood obesity	Faecal incontinence in later life	Perineal trauma	Fertility
		Obstetric anal sphincter injury	Intrauterine fetal demise
		Urinary incontinence	Endometriosis
		Pelvic organ prolapse	Birth satisfaction
		Postpartum Faecal incontinence	Childhood diabetes
			Childhood neuropsychiatric disorders

Nulliparous women have a 6% risk of obstetric anal sphincter injury (OASI) from VB, and can be as high as 12% in IB. This risk is reduced in multiparous women [38, 102, 149, 150]. This is a major obstetric complication, which is accompanied by a high risk of long-term faecal incontinence and occasionally requires further operative intervention [154, 155]. The question of whether CB should be recommended after OASI is a complex one, and discussion is likely to be different for every woman. It is known that the risk of recurrent injury is similar to that of a nulliparous woman [155]. The advice given depends on the severity of the initial injury and the significance of chronic morbidity – for example, a woman with complete faecal incontinence is unlikely to gain any benefit from CB and will risk the accompanying morbidity [155]. Refer to Chap. 5 for further information on this topic.

It should be mentioned that a major benefit of CB in cases of obstructed labour is that it has almost eliminated the development of obstetric fistulae in labour in the developed world [156].

6.6.2 Pelvic Organ Prolapse (POP) and Incontinence

POP is an umbrella term which encompasses prolapse of uterus, cervix, bladder, and rectum. It is a condition which can cause significant morbidity to women for many years. Although CB reduces the risk of POP, it is still seen in women who are nulliparous or have had only CB [147].

The risk of persistent urinary incontinence is reduced in women who only have CBs but it returns to the same as VB if combination of VB and CB occurs. The rate of persistent urinary incontinence is around 25%, again suggesting it may also be related to other factors, including the pressure caused by pregnancy itself, and woman-specific factors, including high BMI [157].

Evidence suggests that the risk of faecal incontinence is similar in CB and unassisted VB but doubled in IB, and as previously mentioned, the risk of IB as a primigravida is relatively high [158].

6.7 Conclusion

In counselling a patient about her risks with mode of birth, there are several short- and long-term morbidities for both mother and child associated with CB which must be weighed against those of VB. See Table 6.4 for a summary of the long-term risks of CB. These risks must be balanced, and the stratification of these is different for every woman. There are times when planning VB would confer such a significant risk to either mother or baby that it is contraindicated, but most women lie somewhere in the middle of the spectrum. These women must be allowed to consider every implication of CB.

Take Home Messages

- Caesarean section is a commonly performed operation
- Caesarean birth is accompanied by significant risks and some benefits to the woman and the fetus
- Risk benefit ratio should be considered when counselling women who are planning their mode of birth.

Appendix: MCQ

Mark each item TRUE or FALSE

Questions

1. What is the estimated future risk of uterine rupture in a second pregnancy after a single caesarean birth?
   (A) 1 in 1000 births.
   (B) 5–7 in 1000 births.
   (C) 1 in 100 births.
   (D) 5–7 in 10000 births.
   (E) 2–3 in 100 births.

2. Which of the below long-term outcomes are more common after caesarean birth (choose all that apply)?
   (A) Development of cerebral palsy.
   (B) Development of childhood asthma.
   (C) Type 1 diabetes.
   (D) Obesity (up to the age of 5 years old).
   (E) Obesity (beyond 5 years of age).

3. The long-term risk of which of the following gynecologic conditions is reduced after caesarean birth (in comparison to vaginal birth) (choose all that apply)?:
   (A) Pelvic organ prolapse.
   (B) Faecal incontinence.
   (C) Dyspareunia.
   (D) Urinary incontinence.
   (E) Endometriosis.

4. Which of the below risks are more common complications of caesarean birth that occur in at least 1 in 1000 patients (choose all that apply)?:
   (A) Fetal injury or laceration.
   (B) Major Haemorrhage (> 1 litre blood loss).
   (C) Need for Peripartum Hysterectomy.
   (D) Ureteric injury.
   (E) Bladder injury.

5. Which of the below conditions are more common in a future pregnancy after a first pregnancy caesarean birth?
   (A) Placenta Praevia and Placenta Accreta Spectrum.
   (B) Preterm labour (34–37 weeks).
   (C) Spontaneous miscarriage.
   (D) Ectopic Pregnancy.
   (E) Uterine rupture.

Answers

1. What is the estimated future risk of uterine rupture in a second pregnancy after a single caesarean birth?
   (A) FALSE
   (B) TRUE
   (C) FALSE
   (D) FALSE
   (E) FALSE

2. Which of the below long-term outcomes are more common after caesarean birth (choose all that apply)?
   (A) FALSE
   (B) TRUE
   (C) FALSE
   (D) TRUE
   (E) FALSE

3. The long-term risk of which of the following gynecologic conditions is reduced after caesarean birth (in comparison to vaginal birth) (choose all that apply)?:
   (A) TRUE

(B) FALSE
(C) FALSE
(D) TRUE
(E) FALSE

4. Which of the below risks are more common complications of caesarean birth that occur in at least 1 in 1000 patients (choose all that apply)?:
(A) TRUE
(B) TRUE
(C) FALSE
(D) FALSE
(E) TRUE

5. Which of the below conditions are more common in a future pregnancy after a first pregnancy caesarean birth?
(A) TRUE
(B) TRUE
(C) FALSE
(D) FALSE
(E) TRUE

References

1. Sewell JE. Cesarean section—a brief history. 1998. https://www.nlm.nih.gov/exhibition/cesarean/part1.html
2. Rosenberg KR, Trevathan WR. Evolutionary perspectives on cesarean section. Evol Med Public Health. 2018;2018(1):67–81.
3. Halperin ME, Moore DC, Hannah WJ. Classical versus low-segment transverse incision for preterm caesarean section: maternal complications and outcome of subsequent pregnancies. Br J Obstet Gynaecol. 1988;95(10):990–6.
4. The Scottish Government. The best start—caesarean section rates: review report. Scottish Government; 2021.
5. Betran AP, Ye J, Moller A, Souza JP, Zhang J. Trends and projections of caesarean section rates: global and regional estimates. BMJ Global Health. 2021;6:e005671.
6. Wilkinson C, McIllwaine G, Boulton-Jones C, Cole S. Is a rising caesarean section rate inevitable? BJOG Int J Obstet Gynaecol. 1998;105(1):45–52.
7. Parliamentary Office of Science and Technology. Caesarean sections. 2002.
8. Koroukian SM. Relative risk of postpartum complications in the Ohio Medicaid population: vaginal versus cesarean delivery. Med Care Res Rev. 2004;61(2):203–24.
9. Yimer H, Woldie H. Incidence and associated factors of chronic pain after caesarean section: a systematic review. J Obstet Gynaecol Can. 2019;41(6):840–54.
10. Kolås T, Øian P, Skjeldestad FE. Risks for peroperative excessive blood loss in cesarean delivery. Acta Obstet Gynecol Scand. 2010;89(5):658–63.
11. Magann EF, Evans S, Hutchinson M, Collins R, Lanneau G, Morrison JC. Postpartum hemorrhage after cesarean delivery: an analysis of risk factors. South Med J. 2005;98(7):681–5.
12. Słabuszewska-Jóźwiak A, Szymański JK, Jóźwiak Ł, Sarecka-Hujar B. A systematic review and meta-analysis of wound complications after a caesarean section in obese women. J Clin Med. 2021;10(4):675.
13. Conner SN, Verticchio JC, Tuuli MG, Odibo AO, Macones GA, Cahill AG. Maternal obesity and risk of post-cesarean wound complications. Am J Perinatol. 2014;31(4):299–304.
14. Baskett TF, Allen VM, O'Connell CM, Allen AC. Fetal trauma in term pregnancy. Am J Obstet Gynecol. 2007;197(5):499.e1–7.
15. Johnson A, Young D, Reilly J. Caesarean section surgical site infection surveillance. J Hosp Infect. 2006;64(1):30–5.
16. Wloch C, Wilson J, Lamagni T, Harrington P, Charlett A, Sheridan E. Risk factors for surgical site infection following caesarean section in England: results from a multicentre cohort study. BJOG. 2012;119(11):1324–33.
17. Kallianidis A, Maraschini A, Danis J, Colmorn LB, Deneux-Tharaux C, Donati S, et al. Epidemiological analysis of peripartum hysterectomy across nine European countries. Acta Obstet Gynaecol Scand. 2020;99(10):1364–73.
18. Knight M, Kurinczuk JJ, Spark P, Brocklehurst P. Cesarean delivery and peripartum hysterectomy. Obstet Gynecol. 2008;111(1):97–105.
19. Knight M. Peripartum hysterectomy in the UK: management and outcomes of the associated haemorrhage. BJOG. 2007;114(11):1380–7.
20. Ahmed M, Pandya ST, Supraneni T. Return to the operation theatre: an analysis of repeat surgeries in operative obstetrics. J Obstet Gynecol India. 2015;66(Suppl 1):117–21.
21. Levin I, Rapaport AS, Satzer L, Maslovitz S, Lessing JB, Almog B. Risk factors for relaparotomy after cesarean delivery. Int J Gynecol Obstet. 2012;119(2):163–5.
22. Gedikbasi A, Akyol A, Asar E, Bingol B, Sargin A, Ceylan Y. Re-laparotomy after cesarean section: operative complications in surgical delivery. Arch Gynecol Obstet. 2008;278:419–25.
23. Deneux-Tharaux C, Carmona E, Bouvier-Colle M, Bréart G. Postpartum maternal mortality and

cesarean delivery. Obstet Gynecol. 2006;108(3 Part 1):541–8.

24. Morris EP. Caesarean section: consent advice no. 7. Consent Group of the RCOG.

25. National Collaborating Centre for Women's and Children's health. Caesarean section; 2004.

26. Zandvakili F, Rezaie M, Shahoei R, Roshani D. Abstract. CNRS Éditions; 2022.

27. Blondon M, Casini A, Hoppe KK, Boehlen F, Righini M, Smith NL. Risks of venous thromboembolism after cesarean sections: a meta-analysis. Chest. 2016;150(3):572–96.

28. National Collaborating Centre for Women's and Children's Health. Caesarean section CG132 full guideline appendices A-K. 2011.

29. Phipps MG, Watabe B, Clemons JL, Weitzen S, Myers DL. Risk factors for bladder injury during cesarean delivery. Obstet Gynecol. 2005;105(1):156–60.

30. Lo T, Wijaya T, Lo L, Kao C, Wu P, Cortes EFM, et al. Clinical relevance and treatment selection of ureteral injury after cesarean section. Female Pelvic Med Reconstr Surg. 2016;22(5):303–6.

31. Ku JH, Kim ME, Jeon YS, Lee NK, Park YH. Minimally invasive management of ureteral injuries recognized late after obstetric and gynaecologic surgery. Injury. 2003;34(7):480–3.

32. Visconti F, Quaresima P, Rania E, Palumbo AR, Micieli M, Zullo F, et al. Difficult caesarean section: a literature review. Eur J Obstet Gynecol Reprod Biol. 2020;246:72–8.

33. Mesdaghinia E, Abedzadeh-Kalahroudi M, Hedayati M, Moussavi-Bioki N. Iatrogenic gastrointestinal injuries during obstetrical and gynecological operation. Arch Trauma Res. 2013;2(2):81–4.

34. Crowhurst JA, Plaat F. Why mothers die—report on confidential enquiries into maternal deaths in the United Kingdom 1994–96. Anaesthesia. 1999;54(3):207–9.

35. Stationary Office. Why mothers die. Report on confidential enquiries into maternal deaths in the United Kingdom 1994–96. 1998.

36. Villar J, Carroli G, Zavaleta N, et al. Maternal and neonatal individual risks and benefits associated with caesarean delivery: multicentre prospective study. BMJ. 2007;335:1025.

37. Suwal A, Shrivastava VR, Giri A. Maternal and fetal outcome in elective versus emergency cesarean section. JNMA J Nepal Med Assoc. 2013;52(192):563–6.

38. Jardine J, Blotkamp A, Gurol-Urganci I, Knight H, Harris T, Hawdon J, et al. Risk of complicated birth at term in nulliparous and multiparous women using routinely collected maternity data in England: cohort study. BMJ. 2020;371:m3377.

39. Duthie SJ, Ghosh A, Ng A, Ho PC. Intra-operative blood loss during elective lower segment caesarean section. BJOG. 1992;99(5):364–7.

40. Combs CA, Murphy EL, Laros RK. Factors associated with postpartum hemorrhage with vaginal birth. Obstet Gynecol. 1991;77(1):69–76.

41. Herstad L, Klungsøyr K, Skjærven R, Tanbo T, Forsén L, Åbyholm T, et al. Elective cesarean section or not? Maternal age and risk of adverse outcomes at term: a population-based registry study of low-risk primiparous women. BMC Pregnancy Childbirth. 2016;16:230.

42. Huque S, Roberts I, Fawole B, Chaudri R, Arulkumaran S, Shakur-Still H. Risk factors for peripartum hysterectomy among women with postpartum haemorrhage: analysis of data from the WOMAN trial. BMC Pregnancy Childbirth. 2018;18(1):186.

43. Smaill F, Hofmeyr GJ. Antibiotic prophylaxis for cesarean section. Cochrane Database Syst Rev. 2002;(3):CD000933.

44. Leth RA, Møller JK, Thomsen RW, Uldbjerg N, Nørgaard M. Risk of selected postpartum infections after cesarean section compared with vaginal birth: a five-year cohort study of 32,468 women. Acta Obstet Gynecol Scand. 2009;88(9):976–83.

45. von Glinski M, Dadras M, Wallner C, Wagner JM, Behr B, Lehnhardt M. [Necrotizing Fasciitis]. Handchir Mikrochir Plast Chir. 2021;53(3):312–319.

46. Jackson E, Curtis KM, Gaffield ME. Risk of venous thromboembolism during the postpartum period: a systematic review. Obstet Gynecol. 2011;117(3):691–703.

47. Pomp ER, Lenselink AM, Rosendaal FR, Doggen CJM. Pregnancy, the postpartum period and prothrombotic defects: risk of venous thrombosis in the MEGA study. J Thromb Haemost. 2008;6(4):632–7.

48. MBRRACE-UK. Saving lives, improving mothers' care lessons learned to inform maternity care from the UK and Ireland confidential enquiries into maternal deaths and morbidity 2017–19. Maternal, newborn and infant clinical outcome review programme 2021.

49. Zwergel C, von Kaisenberg CS. Maternal and fetal risks in higher multiple cesarean deliveries. IntechOpen; 2019.

50. Hansen AK, Wisborg K, Uldbjerg N, Henriksen TB. Risk of respiratory morbidity in term infants delivered by elective caesarean section: cohort study. BMJ. 2007;336:85–7.

51. Tefera M, Assefa N, Mengistie B, Abrham A, Teji K, Worku T. Elective cesarean section on term pregnancies has a high risk for neonatal respiratory morbidity in developed countries: a systematic review and meta-analysis. Front Pediatr. 2020;8:286.

52. National Institute for Health and Care Excellence. NG192 Caesarean birth appendix A: benefits and risks of vaginal and caesarean birth. 2021.

53. Paixao ES, Bottomley C, Pescarini JM, Wong KLM, Cardim LL, de Cássia Ribeiro Silva R, et al. Associations between cesarean delivery and child mortality: a national record linkage longitudinal study of 17.8 million births in Brazil. PLoS Med. 2021;18(10):e1003791.

54. Federspiel JJ, Suresh SC, Darwin KC, Szymanski LM. Hospitalization duration following uncompli-

cated cesarean delivery: predictors, facility variation, and outcomes. AJP Rep. 2020;10(2):e187–97.

55. Digenis C, Salter A, Cusack L, Koch A, Turnbull D. Reduced length of hospital stay after caesarean section: a systematic review examining women's experiences and psychosocial outcomes. Midwifery. 2020;91:102855.

56. Roy S, Montgomery IL. Caesarean section rate and postnatal bed occupancy: a retrospective study replacing assumptions with evidence. BMC Health Serv Res. 2018;18(1):760.

57. Kealy MA, Small RE, Liamputtong P. Recovery after caesarean birth: a qualitative study of women's accounts in Victoria, Australia. BMC Pregnancy Childbirth. 2010;10(1):47.

58. Gupta JK, Smith G, Chodankar RR. Birth after previous caesarean birth: GTG no. 45. RCOG; 2015:2.

59. Tunc SY, Agacayak E, Sak S, Basaranoglu S, Goruk NY, Turgut A, et al. Multiple repeat cae-sarean deliveries: do they increase maternal and neonatal morbidity? J Matern Fetal Neonatal Med. 2017;30(6):739–44.

60. Mozurkewich EL, Hutton EK. Elective repeat cesar-ean delivery versus trial of labor: a meta-analysis of the literature from 1989 to 1999. Am J Obstet Gynecol. 2000;183(5):1187–97.

61. Guise J, Berlin M, McDonagh M, Osterweil P, Chan B, Helfand M. Safety of vaginal birth after cesarean: a systematic review. Obstet Gynecol. 2004;103(3):420–9.

62. Marshall NE, Fu R, Guise J. Impact of multiple cesar-ean deliveries on maternal morbidity: a systematic review. Am J Obstet Gynecol. 2011;205(3):262.e1–8.

63. Al-Zirqi I, Stray-Pedersen B, Forsén L, Daltveit A, Vangen S. Uterine rupture: trends over 40 years. BJOG. 2016;123(5):780–7.

64. Yap OW, Kim ES, Laros RK. Maternal and neonatal outcomes after uterine rupture in labor. Am J Obstet Gynecol. 2001;184(7):1576–81.

65. Zwart JJ, Richters JM, Ory F, de Vries JIP, Bloemenkamp KWM, van Roosmalen J. Uterine rupture in the Netherlands: a nationwide population-based cohort study. BJOG. 2009;116(8):1069–80.

66. Chibber R, El-Saleh E, Al Fadhli R, Al Jassar W, Al Harmi J. Uterine rupture and subsequent pregnancy outcome—how safe is it? A 25-year study. J Matern Fetal Neonatal Med. 2010;23(5):421–4.

67. Al-Zirqi I, Stray-Pedersen B, Forsén L, Vangen S. Uterine rupture after previous caesarean section. BJOG. 2010;117(7):809–20.

68. Gurol-Urganci I, Cromwell DA, Edozien LC, Smith G, Onwere C, Mahmood TA, et al. Risk of placenta previa in second birth after first birth cesarean sec-tion: a population-based study and meta-analysis. BMC Pregnancy Childbirth. 2011;11:95.

69. Fitzpatrick KE, Sellers S, Spark P, Kurinczuk JJ, Brocklehurst P, Knight M. Incidence and risk fac-tors for placenta accreta/increta/percreta in the UK: a National Case-Control Study. PLoS One. 2012;7(12):e52893.

70. Landon MB, Hauth JC, Leveno KJ, Spong CY, Leindecker S, Varner MW, et al. Maternal and perina-tal outcomes associated with a trial of labor after prior cesarean delivery. N Engl J Med. 2004;351(25):2581–9.

71. Guise J, Eden K, Emeis C, Denman MA, Marshall N, Fu R, et al. Results. Agency for Healthcare Research and Quality (US); 2010.

72. Visser L, Slaager C, Kazemier BM, Rietveld AL, Oudijk MA, Groot C, et al. Risk of preterm birth after prior term cesarean. BJOG Int J Obstet Gynaecol. 2020;127(5):610–7.

73. Levine LD, Sammel MD, Hirshberg A, Elovitz MA, Srinivas SK. Does stage of labor at time of cesarean delivery affect risk of subsequent preterm birth? Am J Obstet Gynecol. 2015;212(3):360.e1–7.

74. Blencowe H, Cousens S, Oestergaard MZ, Chou D, Moller A, Narwal R, et al. National, regional, and worldwide estimates of preterm birth rates in the year 2010 with time trends since 1990 for selected countries: a systematic analysis and implications. Lancet. 2012;379(9832):2162–72.

75. Guise J, McDonagh MS, Osterweil P, Nygren P, Chan BKS, Helfand M. Systematic review of the incidence and consequences of uterine rupture in women with previous caesarean section. BMJ. 2004;329(7456):19–25.

76. Jauniaux E, Ayres-de-Campos D. FIGO consensus guidelines on placenta accreta spectrum disorders: introduction. Int J Gynecol Obstet. 2018;140(3):261–4.

77. Mitsui T, Mishima S, Tani K, Maki J, Eto E, Hayata K, et al. Clinical course of 60 cesarean scar pregnan-cies. Acta Med Okayama. 2021;75(4):439–45.

78. O'Neill SM, Kearney PM, Kenny LC, Khashan AS, Henriksen TB, Lutomski JE, et al. Caesarean delivery and subsequent stillbirth or miscarriage: systematic review and meta-analysis. PLoS One. 2013;8(1):e54588.

79. Usta IM, Hobeika EM, Musa AAA, Gabriel GE, Nassar AH. Placenta previa-accreta: risk factors and complications. Am J Obstet Gynecol. 2005;193(3 Pt 2): 1045–9.

80. Silver RM, Barbour KD. Placenta accreta spectrum: accreta, increta, and percreta. Obstet Gynecol Clin N Am. 2015;42(2):381–402.

81. Glazewska-Hallin A, Story L, Suff N, Shennan A. Late-stage cesarean section causes recurrent early preterm birth: how to tackle this problem? Ultrasound Obstet Gynaecol. 2019;54(3):293–6.

82. Zhao J, Hao J, Xu B, Wang Y, Li Y. Impact of pre-vious caesarean section on reproductive outcomes after assisted reproductive technology: systematic review and meta-analyses. Reprod Biomed Online. 2021;43(2):197–204.

83. Wang L, Yao W, Tang X, Yao H, Wei S, Huang J, et al. Fertility outcomes of IVF/ICSI after caesar-ean section: a cohort study. Reprod Biomed Online. 2020;40(5):719–28.

84. Karaer A, Avsar FA, Batioglu S. Risk factors for ectopic pregnancy: a case-control study. Aust N Z J Obstet Gynaecol. 2006;46(6):521–7.

85. O'Neill SM, Khashan AS, Kenny LC, Greene RA, Henriksen TB, Lutomski JE, et al. Caesarean section and subsequent ectopic pregnancy: a systematic review and meta-analysis. BJOG. 2013;120(6):671–80.
86. Bowman ZS, Smith KR, Silver RM. Cesarean delivery and risk for subsequent ectopic pregnancy. Am J Perinatol. 2015;32(9):815–20.
87. Larsen JV, Solomon MH. Pregnancy in a uterine scar sacculus—an unusual cause of postabortal haemorrhage. A case report. S Afr Med J. 1978;53(4):142–3.
88. Jayaram PM, Okunoye GO, Konje J. Caesarean scar ectopic pregnancy: diagnostic challenges and management options. Obstet Gynaecol. 2017;19(1):13–20.
89. Timor-Tritsch IE, Monteagudo A, Cali G, Palacios-Jaraquemada JM, Maymon R, Arslan AA, et al. Cesarean scar pregnancy and early placenta accreta share common histology. Ultrasound Obstet Gynecol. 2014;43(4):383–95.
90. Jurkovic D, Hillaby K, Woelfer B, Lawrence A, Salim R, Elson CJ. First-trimester diagnosis and management of pregnancies implanted into the lower uterine segment cesarean section scar. Ultrasound Obstet Gynecol. 2003;21(3):220–7.
91. Mohapatra I, Samantray SR. Scar ectopic pregnancy—an emerging challenge. Cureus. 2021;13(7):e16673.
92. Tamada S, Masuyama H, Maki J, Eguchi T, Mitsui T, Eto E, et al. Successful pregnancy located in a uterine cesarean scar: a case report. Case Rep Womens Health. 2017;14:8–10.
93. Smith GC, Pell JP, Bobbie R. Caesarean section and risk of unexplained stillbirth in subsequent pregnancy. Lancet. 2003;362(9398):1779–84.
94. Moraitis AA, Oliver-Williams C, Wood AM, Fleming M, Pell JP, Smith G. Previous caesarean delivery and the risk of unexplained stillbirth: retrospective cohort study and meta-analysis. BJOG. 2015;122(11):1467–74.
95. Wood S, Ross S, Sauve R. Cesarean section and subsequent stillbirth, is confounding by indication responsible for the apparent association? An updated cohort analysis of a large perinatal database. PLoS One. 2015;10(9):e0136272.
96. Wood SL, Chen S, Ross S, Sauve R. The risk of unexplained antepartum stillbirth in second pregnancies following caesarean section in the first pregnancy. BJOG Int J Obstet Gynaecol. 2008;115(6):726–31.
97. Gurol-Urganci I, Bou-Antoun S, Lim CP, Cromwell DA, Mahmood TA, Templeton A, et al. Impact of caesarean section on subsequent fertility: a systematic review and meta-analysis. Hum Reprod. 2013;28(7):1943–52.
98. Kjerulff KH, Paul IM, Weisman CS. Association between mode of first delivery and subsequent fecundity and fertility. JAMA Newt Open. 2020;3(4):e203076.
99. Kjerulff KH, Zhu J, Weisman CS, Ananth CV. First birth caesarean section and subsequent fertility: a population-based study in the USA, 2000-2008. Hum Reprod. 2013;28(12):3349–57.
100. Jacob L, Weber K, Sechet I, Macharey G, Kostev K, Ziller V. Caesarean section and its impact on fertility and time to a subsequent pregnancy in Germany: a database analysis in gynecological practices. Arch Gynecol Obstet. 2016;294(5):1005–10.
101. Collin SM, Marshall T, Filippi V. Caesarean section and subsequent fertility in sub-Saharan Africa. BJOG Int J Obstet Gynaecol. 2006;113(3):276–83.
102. Gurol-Urganci I, Cromwell DA, Mahmood TA, van der Meulen JH, Templeton A. A population-based cohort study of the effect of caesarean section on subsequent fertility. Hum Reprod. 2014;29(6):1320–6.
103. Bhattacharya S, Porter M, Harrild K, Naji A, Mollison J, van Teijlingen E, et al. Absence of conception after caesarean section: voluntary or involuntary? BJOG. 2006;113(3):268–75.
104. Lodge-Tulloch NA, Elias FTS, Pudwell J, Gaudet L, Walker M, Smith GN, et al. Caesarean section in pregnancies conceived by assisted reproductive technology: a systematic review and meta-analysis. BMC Pregnancy Childbirth. 2021;21(1):244.
105. Vissers J, Sluckin TC, van Driel-Delprat CC, Repelaer SR, Groot CJM, Lambalk CB, et al. Reduced pregnancy and live birth rates after in vitro fertilization in women with previous caesarean section: a retrospective cohort study. Hum Reprod. 2020;35(3):595–604.
106. Diao J, Gao G, Zhang Y, Wang X, Zhang Y, Han Y, et al. Caesarean section defects may affect pregnancy outcomes after in vitro fertilization-embryo transfer: a retrospective study. BMC Pregnancy Childbirth. 2021;21(1):487.
107. Saraswat L, Porter M, Bhattacharya S, Bhattacharya S. Caesarean section and tubal infertility: is there an association? Reprod Biomed Online. 2008;17(2):259–64.
108. Farhi J, Oron G, Orbach S, Levran D, Barkat J, Tzelnick S, et al. A previous caesarean section is not a risk factor for tubal abnormalities in the infertile population. J Obstet Gynaecol. 2018;38(4):466–9.
109. Sethi P, Mohanty GS, Kumari S. Secondary vaginal atresia following caesarean section: an unreported entity. BMJ Case Rep. 2021;14(2):e238427.
110. El-Shawarby SA, Salim R, Lavery S, Saridogan E. Uterine adherence to anterior abdominal wall after caesarean section. BJOG. 2011;118(9):1133–5.
111. Vissers J, Hehenkamp W, Lambalk CB, Huirne JA. Post-caesarean section niche-related impaired fertility: hypothetical mechanisms. Hum Reprod. 2020;35(7):1484–94.
112. Jordans IPM, de Leeuw RA, Stegwee SI, Amso NN, Barri-Soldevila PN, van den Bosch T, et al. Sonographic examination of uterine niche in non-pregnant women: a modified Delphi procedure. Ultrasound Obstet Gynecol. 2019;53(1):107–15.
113. Lavand'homme P. Postpartum chronic pain. Minerva Anestesiol. 2019;85(3):320–4.

114. Jin J, Peng L, Chen Q, Zhang D, Ren L, Qin P, et al. Prevalence and risk factors for chronic pain following cesarean section: a prospective study. BMC Anesthesiol. 2016;16:99.

115. Lal M, Pattison HM, Allan TF, Callender R. Does post-caesarean dyspareunia reflect sexual malfunction, pelvic floor and perineal dysfunction? J Obstet Gynaecol. 2011;31(7):617–30.

116. Kulshrestha V, Agarwal N, Kachhawa G. Post-caesarean niche (Isthmocele) in uterine scar: an update. J Obstet Gynecol India. 2020;70(6):440–6.

117. Zondervan KT, Becker CM, Koga K, Missmer SA, Taylor RN, Viganò P. Endometriosis. Nat Rev Dis Primers. 2018;4(1):1–25.

118. Andolf E, Thorsell M, Källén K. Caesarean section and risk for endometriosis: a prospective cohort study of Swedish registries. BJOG Int J Obstet Gynaecol. 2013;120(9):1061–5.

119. Zhang P, Sun Y, Zhang C, Yang Y, Zhang L, Wang N, et al. Cesarean scar endometriosis: presentation of 198 cases and literature review. BMC Womens Health. 2019;19:14.

120. McGrath P, Ray-Barruel G. The easy option? Australian findings on mothers' perception of elective caesarean as a birth choice after a prior caesarean section. Int J Nurs Pract. 2009;15(4):271–9.

121. O'Donovan C, O'Donovan J. Why do women request an elective cesarean delivery for non-medical reasons? A systematic review of the qualitative literature. Birth. 2018;45(2):109–19.

122. Fobelets M, Beeckman K, Buyl R, Healy P, Grylka-Baeschlin S, Nicoletti J, et al. Preference of birth mode and postnatal health related quality of life after one previous caesarean section in three European countries. Midwifery. 2019;79:102536.

123. Hanlon AJM, Beckmann MM. Mode of birth and early postnatal psychological morbidity. Aust N Z J Obstet Gynaecol. 2015;55(6):578–83.

124. Henderson I, Quenby S. The association between caesarean and postnatal psychological distress: effect modification by mental health history. Paediatr Perinat Epidemiol. 2021;35(6):635–44.

125. Blomquist JL, Quiroz LH, Macmillan D, McCullough A, Handa VL. Mothers' satisfaction with planned vaginal and planned cesarean birth. Am J Perinatol. 2011;28(5):383–8.

126. Fenaroli V, Molgora S, Dodaro S, Svelato A, Gesi L, Molidoro G, et al. The childbirth experience: obstetric and psychological predictors in Italian primiparous women. BMC Pregnancy Childbirth. 2019;19(1):419.

127. Taghizadeh Z, Irajpour A, Arbabi M. Mothers' response to psychological birth trauma: a qualitative study. Iran Red Crescent Med J. 2013;15(10):e10572.

128. Harrison SE, Ayers S, Quigley MA, Stein A, Alderdice F. Prevalence and factors associated with postpartum posttraumatic stress in a population-based maternity survey in England. J Affect Disord. 2021;279:749–56.

129. Huang K, Hu Y, Sun Y, Yu Z, Liu W, Zhu P, et al. Elective caesarean delivery and offspring's cognitive impairment: implications of methylation alteration in hippocampus glucocorticoid signaling genes. Brain Res Bull. 2019;144:108–21.

130. Sandall J, Tribe RM, Avery L, Mola G, Visser GH, Homer CS, et al. Short-term and long-term effects of caesarean section on the health of women and children. Lancet. 2018;392(10155):1349–57.

131. Shao Y, Forster SC, Tsaliki E, Vervier K, Strang A, Simpson N, et al. Stunted microbiota and opportunistic pathogen colonization in caesarean-section birth. Nature. 2019;574(7776):117–21.

132. Zhang S, Li B, Zhang X, Zhu C, Wang X. Birth asphyxia is associated with increased risk of cerebral palsy: a meta-analysis. Front Neurol. 2020;11:704.

133. Gardener H, Spiegelman D, Buka SL. Perinatal and neonatal risk factors for autism: a comprehensive meta-analysis. Pediatrics. 2011;128(2):344–55.

134. van Handel M, Swaab H, de Vries LS, Jongmans MJ. Long-term cognitive and behavioral consequences of neonatal encephalopathy following perinatal asphyxia: a review. Eur J Pediatr. 2007;166(7):645–54.

135. Zuena AR, Casolini P, Venerosi A, Alemà GS, Nicoletti F, Calamandrei G. Selective reduction in the expression of type-1 metabotropic glutamate receptors in the hippocampus of adult rats born by caesarean section. Int J Dev Neurosci. 2021;81(4):333–41.

136. O'Callaghan M, MacLennan A. Cesarean delivery and cerebral palsy: a systematic review and meta-analysis. Obstet Gynecol. 2013;122(6):1169–75.

137. Curran EA, Cryan JF, Kenny LC, Dinan TG, Kearney PM, Khashan AS. Obstetrical mode of delivery and childhood behavior and psychological development in a British cohort. J Autism Dev Disord. 2016;46(2):603–14.

138. Salas Garcia M, Yee A, Gilbert J, Dsouza M. Dysbiosis in children born by caesarean section. Ann Nutr Metab. 2018;73(Suppl 3):24–32.

139. Mueller NT, Bakacs E, Combellick J, Grigoryan Z, Dominguez-Bello MG. The infant microbiome development: mom matters. Trends Mol Med. 2015;21(2):109–17.

140. Keag OE, Norman JE, Stock SJ. Long-term risks and benefits associated with cesarean delivery for mother, baby, and subsequent pregnancies: systematic review and meta-analysis. PLoS Med. 2018;15(1):e1002494.

141. Cardwell CR, Stene LC, Joner G, Cinek O, Svensson J, Goldacre MJ, et al. Caesarean section is associated with an increased risk of childhood-onset type 1 diabetes mellitus: a meta-analysis of observational studies. Diabetologia. 2008;51(5):726–35.

142. Kuhle S, Tong OS, Woolcott CG. Association between caesarean section and childhood obesity: a systematic review and meta-analysis. Obes Rev. 2015;16(4):295–303.

143. Thavagnanam S, Fleming J, Bromley A, Shields MD, Cardwell CR. A meta-analysis of the association between caesarean section and childhood asthma. Clin Exp Allergy. 2008;38(4):629–33.

144. Håkansson S, Källén K. Caesarean section increases the risk of hospital care in childhood for asthma and gastroenteritis. Clin Exp Allergy. 2003;33(6):757–64.

145. Renz-Polster H, David MR, Buist AS, Vollmer WM, O'Connor EA, Frazier EA, et al. Caesarean section delivery and the risk of allergic disorders in childhood. Clin Exp Allergy. 2005;35(11):1466–72.

146. Alterman N, Kurinczuk JJ, Quigley MA. Caesarean section and severe upper and lower respiratory tract infections during infancy: evidence from two UK cohorts. PLoS One. 2021;16(2):e0246832.

147. Gyhagen M, Bullarbo M, Nielsen TF, Milsom I. Prevalence and risk factors for pelvic organ prolapse 20 years after childbirth: a national cohort study in singleton primiparae after vaginal or caesarean delivery. BJOG Int J Obstet Gynaecol. 2013;120(2):152–60.

148. Smith LA, Price N, Simonite V, Burns EE. Incidence of and risk factors for perineal trauma: a prospective observational study. BMC Pregnancy Childbirth. 2013;13:59.

149. Thiagamoorthy G, Johnson A, Thakar R, Sultan AH. National survey of perineal trauma and its subsequent management in the United Kingdom. Int Urogynecol J. 2014;25(12):1621–7.

150. Edozien LC, Gurol-Urganci I, Cromwell DA, Adams EJ, Richmond DH, Mahmood TA, et al. Impact of third- and fourth-degree perineal tears at first birth on subsequent pregnancy outcomes: a cohort study. BJOG. 2014;121(13):1695–703.

151. Jones K, Webb S, Manresa M, Hodgetts-Morton V, Morris RK. The incidence of wound infection and dehiscence following childbirth-related perineal trauma: a systematic review of the evidence. Eur J Obstet Gynecol Reprod Biol. 2019; 240:1–8.

152. Gommesen D, Nøhr E, Qvist N, Rasch V. Obstetric perineal tears, sexual function and dyspareunia among primiparous women 12 months postpartum: a prospective cohort study. BMJ Open. 2019;9(12):e032368.

153. Williams A, Herron-Marx S, Carolyn H. The prevalence of enduring postnatal perineal morbidity and its relationship to perineal trauma. Midwifery. 2007;23(4):392–403.

154. Kulkarni J, Patil AJ, Musande B, Bhamare AB. Management of fourth degree obstetric perineal tear without colostomy using non–stimulated gracilis—our experience over eleven years. Indian J Plast Surg. 2016;49(1):26–34.

155. Jha S, Parker V. Risk factors for recurrent obstetric anal sphincter injury (rOASI): a systematic review and meta-analysis. Int Urogynecol J. 2015;27(6):849–57.

156. Wall LL. Overcoming phase 1 delays: the critical component of obstetric fistula prevention programs in resource-poor countries. BMC Pregnancy Childbirth. 2012;12:68.

157. MacArthur C, Wilson D, Herbison P, Lancashire RJ, Hagen S, Toozs-Hobson P, et al. Urinary incontinence persisting after childbirth: extent, delivery history, and effects in a 12–year longitudinal cohort study. BJOG Int J Obstet Gynaecol. 2016;123(6): 1022–9.

158. MacArthur C, Wilson D, Herbison P, Lancashire RJ, Hagen S, Toozs-Hobson P, et al. Faecal incontinence persisting after childbirth: a 12 year longitudinal study. BJOG Int J Obstet Gynaecol. 2013;120(2):169–79.

Sexual Dysfunction After Childbirth

7

Lisa C. Hickman and Christina Lewicky-Gaupp

Overview
Test your learning and check your understanding of this book's contents: use the "Springer Nature Flashcards" app to access questions using ▶ https://sn.pub/wqrf89. To use the app, please follow the instructions in Chap. 1.

Learning Objectives

- To appreciate the incidence and definition of sexual dysfunction postpartum
- To understand the risk factors for postpartum sexual dysfunction
- To gain competency in the evaluation and management of sexual dysfunction in the postpartum population

L. C. Hickman (✉)
The Ohio State University Wexner Medical Center, Female Pelvic Medicine & Reconstructive Surgery, Columbus, OH, USA
e-mail: lisa.hickman@osumc.edu

C. Lewicky-Gaupp
Department of Obstetrics and Gynecology, Section of Urogynecology and Reconstructive Pelvic Medicine, University of Chicago Pritzker School of Medicine, Chicago, IL, USA
e-mail: Christina.Lewicky-Gaupp@bsd.uchicago.edu

7.1 Introduction

Pregnancy and the postpartum period are the time in a woman's reproductive life associated with the most dynamic change. This is due to a variety of factors including alterations in the hormonal milieu, bodily and body image changes, fatigue, stress, and relationship factors. One area that can be significantly affected during this time is sexual function. In pregnancy, while 90% of women continue to be sexually active, two-thirds of women refrain from sexual activity in the ninth month [1]. While numerous physical and psychological factors can be attributed to women abstaining from intercourse in the later portion of pregnancy, changes in clitoral sensation, lack of libido, and difficulty achieving orgasm in the third trimester have all been reported [2]. Altered sexual function continues postpartum, at which time the waning pregnancy hormones, disrupted sleep, stress, body image changes, anatomic sequelae from birth, mood disorders, and breastfeeding can impact desire and sexual activity. In fact, 41–83% of women report sexual dysfunction at 2–3 months postpartum, which not surprisingly has a negative impact on quality of life [3–6]. While many women attend a postpartum visit with their obstetric provider in the fourth trimester, only a minority (15%) discuss concerns about sexual dysfunction [5]. Although sexual dysfunction generally does improve with time, 64% of women continue to report sexual dys-

© The Author(s), under exclusive license to Springer Nature Switzerland AG 2024
A. H. Sultan et al. (eds.), *Pelvic Floor, Perineal, and Anal Sphincter Trauma During Childbirth*, https://doi.org/10.1007/978-3-031-43095-4_7

105

function at 6 months; some women continue to report a negative impact on sexual satisfaction at greater than 18 months postpartum [7]. In this chapter, we aim to (1) describe the incidence and definition of postpartum sexual dysfunction, (2) highlight the risk factors for postpartum sexual dysfunction and (3) describe the evaluation and management of sexual dysfunction in the postpartum population.

7.2 Sexual Function and Dysfunction in Women

Sexual function in women is a complex response process, which has evolved from the original four stage, linear description of physiological arousal (excitement, plateau, orgasm, and resolution) as description by Masters and Johnson. More recent models, such as that described by Basson, purports the important role of the interpersonal relationship on sexual function and outlines the non-linear progression through the sexual response [8, 9]. Biopsychosocial models gained

favor in the early 2000s including Bancroft's Dual Control Model (Fig. 7.1) [10]. This theory posits that the sexual response occurs due to the interplay between excitatory and inhibitory processes, and the complex relationship between these factors varies from individual to individual.

The definition of sexual dysfunction, on the other hand, is outlined in the fifth edition of the Diagnostic and Statistical Manual of Mental Disorders (DSM-5) which describes disorders as those of interest/arousal, orgasm, and pain (Table 7.1) [12]. Compared to the fourth edition, the fifth edition of the DSM places a new emphasis on characterizing both duration (presence ≥6 months) and severity of the patient's sexual symptoms. Importantly, sexual symptoms are not considered dysfunctional per the DSM-5 unless they lead to "clinically significant distress in the individual" [12]. An IUGA/ICS joint report by Rogers et al. further outlines terminology utilized to describe sexual function and dysfunction in women with pelvic floor disorders and provides over 100 separate definitions [13]. In the peripartum literature, most studies utilize the terminol-

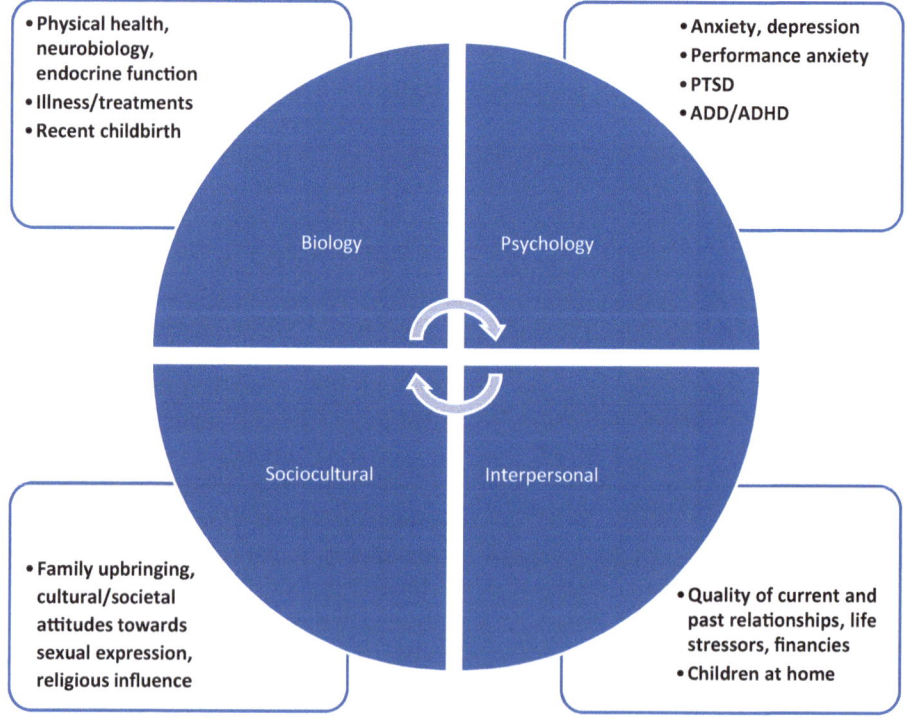

Fig. 7.1 Biopsychosocial model of female sexual response. (Adapted from Kinsberg and Reszaee [11])

Table 7.1 DSM-5 classification of sexual dysfunction

Diagnosis	Criteria
Female orgasmic disorder	Presence of either of the following on all or almost all (75–100%) occasions of sexual activity 1. Marked delay in, marked infrequency of, or absence of orgasm 2. Markedly reduced intensity of orgasmic sensations
Female sexual interest/arousal disorder	Lack of or significantly reduced, sexual interest/arousal as manifested by 3 of the following: 1. Absent/reduced interest in sexual activity 2. Absent/reduced sexual/erotic thoughts or fantasies 3. No/reduced initiation of sexual activity and unreceptive to partner's attempts to initiate 4. Absent/reduced sexual excitement/pleasure during sexual activity in almost all or all (75–100%) sexual encounters 5. Absent/reduced sexual interest/arousal in response to any internal or external sexual/erotic cues (written, verbal, visual) 6. Absent/reduced genital or nongenital sensations during sexual activity in almost all or all (75–100%) sexual encounters
Genito-pelvic pain/penetration disorder	Persistent or recurrent difficulties with 1 or more of the following: 1. Vaginal penetration during intercourse 2. Marked vulvovaginal or pelvic pain during intercourse or penetration attempts 3. Marked fear or anxiety about vulvovaginal or pelvic pain in anticipation of, during, or as a result of vaginal penetration 4. Marked tensing or tightening of the pelvic floor muscles during attempted vaginal penetration

Diagnosis requires presence of symptoms ≥6 months and after excluding co-existing conditions, significant stress or alternative etiologies

ogy of "dyspareunia" and "sexual dysfunction" without further specificity which contributed to difficulty providing personalized care to affected women.

7.3 Risk Factors

Many studies have investigated the risk factors associated with the development of sexual dysfunction, dyspareunia, and vaginal dryness postpartum, however conflicting data remains due to a relative paucity of research in this area and overall lower quality evidence of the currently available research; much data arises from case series or retrospective literature. Risk factors commonly identified as contributors to sexual dysfunction include mode of childbirth, perineal trauma especially in the form of obstetric anal sphincter injury (OASI), episiotomy, breastfeeding and postpartum depression (see Table 7.2) [14]. It is important to note that sexual dysfunction is likely multifactorial in etiology. This creates a challenge in isolating individual factors, due to the interplay between risk factors and other confounding variables such as fatigue from sleep deprivation, stress associated with new family dynamics, relationship factors, body image alterations, and the changing hormonal milieu.

7.3.1 Mode of Childbirth

Studies evaluating the impact of a spontaneous vaginal birth versus cesarean section on sexual dysfunction are inconclusive. At 2 years after childbirth, women in a retrospective cohort study who underwent a vaginal birth had lower sexual satisfaction scores than those who had an elective cesarean section, however rates of urinary incontinence, flatal incontinence, subjective depression and dyspareunia were higher in the vaginal birth group [15]. A smaller study of primiparous women compared those who underwent vaginal birth versus those who underwent cesarean section and followed Female Sexual Function Inventory (FSFI) scores upwards of 12 months [16]. In this study, there was significantly more dyspareunia at 3 months in the vaginal birth group, but this resolved by 12 months. A prospective study of Australian women found that at 12 months postpartum, those who experienced a cesarean delivery were more likely to be experiencing a sexual health issue than those who had a

Table 7.2 Risk and protective factors for postpartum sexual dysfunction and dyspareunia

Outcome	Variable	Comparator	Summary OR (95% CI)	Number of participants	Number of studies
Sexual dysfunction	Assisted vaginal delivery	Spontaneous vaginal birth	1.70 (1.05–2.76)	533	4
	OASI	No OASI	3.00 (1.28–7.03)	872	1
	Contraception	No contraception	0.41 (0.27–0.64)	864	3
Dyspareunia	Maternal age ≥ 35 years	Maternal age < 35 years	0.43 (0.23–0.81)	925	2
	Cesarean section	Spontaneous vaginal birth	0.68 (0.54–0.86)	2200	6
	OASI	No OASI	1.92 (1.47–2.52)	2982	5
	Episiotomy	No episiotomy	1.64 (1.25–2.14)	1210	5

Adapted from Cattani et al. [21]

spontaneous vaginal birth without a significant laceration [17]. Another prospective study recruited nulliparous patients during pregnancy and followed over 1500 women out to 18 months postpartum [18]. Women who experienced a cesarean section for an emergency indication had a two-fold increased odds of persistent dyspareunia at 18 months postpartum compared to women who had a spontaneous vaginal birth over an intact perineum [18]. Similar increased odds were found for with women who experienced a vacuum extraction or had pre-pregnancy dyspareunia. On the other hand, two other prospective studies found no difference in sexual function at 12 months postpartum [19, 20]. A recent systematic review of 26 studies by Cattani et al. evaluated predictors of sexual dysfunction in the first year postpartum [21]. Compared to spontaneous vaginal birth, the authors found no difference in sexual dysfunction, but a lower incidence in dyspareunia in women who underwent a cesarean section; operative vaginal birth was associated with a higher incidence of sexual dysfunction compared to spontaneous vaginal birth, but was not associated with an increase in dyspareunia [21].

Other factors associated with vaginal birth that impact sexual function are anatomic and include pudendal neuropathy and levator ani avulsion. Ischemic or stretch injury of the pudendal nerve occurs during vaginal birth, and due to its innervation of the pelvic floor and clitoris, it is likely that short- or long-term damage can affect sexual domains. Similarly, levator avulsion, which can also be a sequela of vaginal birth, affects the vagi-

nal opening width, pelvic floor muscle strength and can result in a feeling of vaginal laxity. In a study of postpartum women, over 20% had levator ani avulsion on ultrasonography [22]. Those with more severe levator ani injuries were less likely to be sexually active and reported both reduced vaginal sensation and a feeling of the vaginal opening being "too loose" [22].

7.3.2 Perineal Trauma and Episiotomy

7.3.2.1 Obstetric Anal Sphincter Injuries

OASI is associated with a significant negative impact on sexual function. A large prospective cohort study of women who experienced OASI in the UK found at 3 months postpartum, less than 60% of women had resumed intercourse, and of these nearly one-third reported dyspareunia [23]. A long-term follow up study of women who experienced OASI and their male partners evaluated FSFI and Golombok-Rust Inventory of Sexual Satisfaction scores 4 years from their index birth [24]. Nearly half of women and nearly one-third of male partners met criteria for sexual dysfunction, with infrequency of intercourse being the most problematic aspect. Women were also found to have greater problems in psychosocial and emotional domains rather than physical aspects of intercourse [24]. In the systematic review by Cattani et al., OASI was associated with an increased incidence of both sexual dysfunction and dyspareunia [21].

7.3.2.2 Episiotomy

Studies on the impact of episiotomy on sexual dysfunction have found varying results, although low data quality is likely a contributing factor. A 2017 Cochrane review reported no difference in whether or not episiotomy had been performed in women experiencing dyspareunia at 6 or greater months after birth [25]. In contrast, in a more recent systematic review, episiotomy was associated with an increased incidence of dyspareunia, but not sexual dysfunction [21].

7.3.3   Breast Feeding

Breast feeding affects sexual function multiple ways. First, increasing levels of prolactin result in suppression of the hypothalamic-pituitary-ovarian axis. This creates a menopausal state with both low estrogen and testosterone levels. Such changes in hormone levels result in vaginal atrophy and decreased desire, which can in turn affect timing of intercourse resumption in this population. During intercourse, women feel less lubrication and increased discomfort. Increasing oxytocin levels from nipple stimulation can also result in breast sensitivity and for some a troubling sense of sexual arousal or orgasm associated with breastfeeding. A longitudinal prospective cohort study found a negative impact of breastfeeding on sexuality, specifically with a negative impact on arousal and sexual satisfaction [26]. Another longitudinal cohort study utilizing FSFI questionnaires found breastfeeding was a significant risk factor for sexual dysfunction postpartum [27].

7.3.4   Postpartum Depression

One in ten women will experience postpartum depression, which has a negative impact on sexual satisfaction and desire [28]. At 8–12 weeks postpartum, women with depression have decreased frequency and interest in intercourse and continue to have decreased desire at 6 months [3]. Selective Serotonin Reuptake Inhibitors (SSRI) medications, which are commonly prescribed in the postpartum population, can further exacerbate these symptoms, as a well-known side effect is sexual dysfunction. Unfortunately, resolution of sexual dysfunction may not occur after treatment is initiated or after depressive symptoms have resolved.

7.3.5   Other Contributing Factors

7.3.5.1 Fatigue

Fatigue is a common plight of the new mother. Sleep deprivation occurs due to interruptions in the sleep cycle to address the demands of the infant. This maternal effect of fatigue can frequently last greater than 6 months postpartum, and has been associated with a negative impact on desire, frequency of coitus, and sexual satisfaction.

7.3.5.2 Body Image

Changes in body image also has a deleterious impact on sexual function. Satisfaction with body image has been found to decline throughout pregnancy and declines further after birth. This negative impact has been found to extend even out to 6 months postpartum, which was associated with lower scores on the FSFI in a study by Pauls et al. [29] Importantly, poorer body image concerns were not correlated with BMI at 6 months postpartum, indicating that factors other than weight impact postpartum body image [30].

7.3.5.3 Interpersonal Relationships

Relationship quality is also affected by the new infant, with the care required by a newborn sometimes resulting in a maternal feeling of isolation. A cross-sectional survey study of new parents found that postpartum sexual concerns were highly prevalent in both new fathers and mothers and primarily related to decreased relationship well-being [31].

7.3.5.4 Obstetric Trauma/Post-Traumatic Stress Disorder

Traumatic obstetrical events, especially those associated with maternal morbidity, can also impact sexual function and maternal well-being. Up to 16% of women experience postpartum post-traumatic stress disorder (PTSD) from a traumatic birth experience, and the inciting event for PTSD is highly variable [32]. Traumatic obstetrical events in turn can cause women to avoid intercourse due to associated sequelae, low desire, and/or fear of conceiving.

7.3.5.5 Pelvic Floor Disorders

Pelvic floor disorders are known to have a negative impact on sexual well-being in women. For example, in the postpartum population, urinary incontinence at 6 months postpartum was associated with lower FSFI scores [29]. Bowel control issues in women who have experienced OASI are also a significant risk factor for delayed return to intercourse [33]. Damage to the pudendal nerve, which innervates the pelvic floor, anorectum and the clitoris, is believed to play a role in pelvic floor disorders. Similarly, pelvic floor hypertonicity, which is associated with sexual dysfunction, can also occur after a vaginal birth.

7.4 Natural History of Sexual Dysfunction Postpartum

Sexual activity is resumed by half of women at 5–6 weeks postpartum, and this increases to nearly 90% at 12 weeks [34, 35]. In contrast, it has been shown that when women have an OASI, only 40% will have resumed intercourse by 12 weeks postpartum [33]. It is important to note that in women who have resumed intercourse, regardless of birth type, greater than 80% will report some associated sexual difficulties at 2–3 months, including sexual pain [3]. By 6 months postpartum, some women will have improvement in dyspareunia, however, 30% will still suffer from it; sexual dysfunction is reported in as many as two-thirds [35]. Fortunately, at 12 months, the majority of women have returned to their baseline sexual function, but for nearly half there continues to be a decreased interest in sex and persistent pain in just less than one-third [17]. Additionally, there remains a negative impact of the peripartum on sexual satisfaction past 18 months after childbirth [7].

As described above, while a variety of factors contribute to timing of sexual activity resumption, it is important to keep in mind that some women may choose to delay coitus due to concerns about becoming pregnant. As such, professional societies, including the American College of Obstetricians and Gynecologists (ACOG) and others, recommend discussion of family planning at both antepartum and postpartum visits. Multiparous patients are more likely to resume intercourse postpartum, likely due to lower incidence of dyspareunia and greater confidence from previous experience with the postpartum period. In a planned secondary analysis of a prospective cohort study of postpartum sexual function among primiparous women, 54% of women with OASI noted they would wait 1–2 years prior to attempting another pregnancy [36].

Another factor that contributes to timing of intercourse is cultural expectations. Specifically, some developing world countries dictate a specified amount of time postpartum before intercourse can be resumed, such as in the African subcontinent where postpartum abstinence can last out to 12 months. Lastly, predictors of lower satisfaction with intercourse at 1 year postpartum is lack of sexual activity at 12 weeks gestational age and older age at birth [19].

7.5 Screening for Sexual Dysfunction

Identifying patients with postpartum sexual dysfunction starts with initiating a conversation with the patient about sexual function postpartum. ACOG recommends contact with an obstetric provider within 3 weeks of childbirth, with ongoing care as needed, tailored to the patient's concerns, as well as a comprehensive postpartum visit before the end of the fourth trimester [37]. Despite these recommendations, approximately 40% of women do not attend a postpartum visit. As such, ACOG recommends anticipatory guidance should be initiated antenatally when engagement is high, including a discussion of planned contraception and suggestions for potential postpartum problems such vaginal lubricants for dyspareunia. ACOG also outlines components for postpartum care, which include evaluation of many of the components which affect sexual function: mood and emotional well-being; sexuality, contraception and birth spacing; sleep and fatigue; and physical recovery from birth (see Box 7.1).

In the UK, the National Institute for Health and Care Excellence (NICE) guidance recommends that the first postnatal visit by a midwife takes place within 36 hours after transfer of care from the place of birth or after a home birth. The visit should be face-to-face and usually at the woman's home, depending on her circumstances and preferences. Further it is recommended to arrange the first postnatal health visitor home visit to take place between 7 and 14 days after transfer of care from midwifery care so that the timing of postnatal contacts is evenly spread out [38].

Box 7.1: Selected Recommendations from the American College of Obstetricians and Gynecologists for the Ambulatory Evaluation of Postpartum Sexual Function

Mood and Emotional Well-Being
- Screen for postpartum depression and anxiety with a validated instrument [1, 2]
- Provide guidance regarding local resources for mentoring and support
- Follow-up on preexisting mental health disorders, refer for or confirm attendance at mental health-related appointments, and titrate medications as appropriate for the postpartum period

Infant Care and Feeding
- Assess comfort and confidence with caring for newborn
- Assess comfort and confidence with breastfeeding

Sexuality, Contraception and Birth Spacing
- Provide guidance regarding sexuality, management of dyspareunia, and resumption of intercourse
- Assess desire for future pregnancies and reproductive life plan
- Explain the rationale for avoiding an interpregnancy interval of less than 6 months and discuss the risks and benefits of repeat pregnancy sooner than 18 months

- Select a contraceptive method that reflects patient's stated needs and preferences, with same-day placement of LARC, if desired

Sleep and Fatigue
- Discuss coping options for fatigue and sleep disruption
- Engage family and friends in assisting with care responsibilities

Physical Recovery from Birth
- Assess presence of perineal or cesarean incision pain; provide guidance regarding normal versus prolonged recovery
- Assess for presence of urinary and fecal continence, with referral to physical therapy or urogynecology as indicated
- Provide actionable guidance regarding resumption of physical activity and attainment of healthy weight

Adapted from Committee Opinion No. 736: Optimizing Postpartum Care, May 2018.

Previous research suggests providers often neglect to inquire about sexual function in patients, with less than 25% of patients recalling whether or not they were asked about sexual health [17]. This may reflect insufficient provider time or expertise. Additionally, women who had a cesarean section in one study had lower odds of being asked by their provider about sexual health issues [17]. Patients often fail to disclose difficulties with sexual function due to embarrassment. Indeed, only 15% of postpartum women in one study voluntarily discussed concerns about sexual dysfunction [5]. And while nearly two-thirds of women reported that they had been told when they were permitted to resume intercourse postpartum, less than 20% had been informed about changes in sexual function after birth [5].

To combat this paucity in postpartum healthcare, providers should start implementing a simple screening questionnaire. The three-question tool described by Plouffe et al. is one option, asking

Table 7.3 Selected questionnaires to evaluate sexual function

	Instrument	Number of questions	Areas assessed	Reference
Validated in postpartum population	Intimate Relationship Scale	12	Changes in intimacy and sexuality in heterosexual couples: personal, physical, and cognitive domains	Fischman et al. [43]
	McCoy Female Sexuality Questionnaire	19	Arousal, desire, orgasm, pain	McCoy and Davidson [47]
	Pelvic Floor Birth Questionnaire	23	Arousal, desire, orgasm, pain; prolapse and pelvic floor muscle function	Thibault-Gagnon et al. [44]
Not validated in postpartum population	Brief Sexual Symptom Checklist for Women	4	Arousal, desire, orgasm, pain	Hatzichristou et al. [41]
	Female Sexual Distress Scale	13	Distress due to sexual dysfunction	Derogatis et al. [48]
	Female Sexual Function Index (FSFI)	19	Arousal, desire, orgasm, pain	Rosen et al. [45]
	FSFI-6 Item	6	Arousal, desire, orgasm, pain	Isidori et al. [46]
	Golombok Rust Inventory of Sexual Satisfaction (GRISS)	28	Sexual satisfaction in heterosexual couples	Rust and Glombok [49]
	Pelvic Organ Prolapse/ Urinary Incontinence Sexual Questionnaire (PISQ-12)	12	Sexual function in women with prolapse or urinary incontinence	Rogers and Espuña Pons [50]
	Plouffe Simple Questionnaire	3	Sexual dysfunction, pain	Plouffe [39]

whether or not the patient is sexually active, followed by if active, do any problems exist and whether or not sexual pain is experienced (see Table 7.3) [39]. A study utilizing this questionnaire found that while 37% of women in the study had a sexual complaint, yet only 20% volunteered this information upon provider questioning [40]. Another screening tool is the Brief Sexual Symptom Checklist. This is four questions in length, and inquires whether or not the respondent is satisfied with their sexual function, and if not, how long she has been dissatisfied, what problems are present with her sexual function/what is most bothersome, and whether or not she would like to discuss the concerns with her doctor (see Table 7.3) [41].

7.6 Clinical Evaluation of Sexual Dysfunction

When sexual difficulties or dysfunction are identified, the provider should obtain a thorough medical, surgical, obstetric, psychosocial, and sexual history to better understand the current

condition. It is also important to appreciate the duration of the symptoms, as sexual dysfunction that preexisted the pregnancy will likely require a different management approach than that which developed in the postpartum period. Postpartum depression occurs in approximately 10% of women [28]. Being mindful of the use of medications to treat this condition is important, as some may have a deleterious effect on sexual function. It is also important that the provider inquire whether or not the patient is breast feeding and/or pumping, as the hormonal changes associated with these activities often result in vaginal atrophy. The provider should also evaluate for other comorbid conditions or medications that may impact sexual function.

7.7 Screening and Diagnostic Questionnaires

As previously discussed, providers may find it easier to administer a questionnaire to screen and explore patient concerns with sexual function postpartum (Table 7.3). Indeed, previous research suggests patients may be more forthcoming regarding sexual concerns when provided with a survey as compared to direct inquiry [40, 42]. The Intimate Relationship Scale is one tool that can be utilized to evaluate postpartum sexual function. It is a 12-item questionnaire that was validated in postpartum couples [43]. Yet another tool is the Pelvic Floor Birth Questionnaire, which is a 23-question survey with 5 domains, 3 of which focus on sexual function and utilizes a Likert-type scale for responses [44]. The FSFI is a 19 question survey (an abbreviated 6 item questionnaire was subsequently validated), however neither of these surveys have been validated in a postpartum population despite their common use in research studies [45, 46]. Other sexual function tools include the McCoy Female Sexuality Questionnaire, the Female Sexual Distress Scale, and the Pelvic Organ Prolapse/Urinary Incontinence Sexual Questionnaire [47–51].

7.8   Physical Exam

In the postpartum population, a thorough physical exam should be performed as part of the sexual dysfunction evaluation. From a gynecologist's perspective, the provider should start with inspection of the vulva. Evaluation of vulvar healing should be noted, as well as the presence of any granulation tissue, atrophy, or evidence of either urinary or fecal incontinence. Additionally, on inspection of the anal opening, one should note whether or not the anus appears patulous or if the dovetail sign is present, which typically represents decreased anal tone and anal sphincter separation. These findings are often associated with the clinical symptoms of anal and/or fecal incontinence. Next, palpation of the vulva should be performed, evaluating sensory function as well as the presence of any provoked pain. If there is concern for pain in the vestibule, a moistened

Q-tip examination can be performed to further discern the location and extent of pain. Next a speculum exam should be performed evaluating for healing, tissue quality/atrophy, and granulation tissue. A bimanual exam can evaluate motor function of the pelvic floor muscles by having the patient perform a pelvic floor muscle contraction. Additionally, the presence of myofascial pain should be evaluated. A cough stress test can be performed to assess for stress urinary incontinence.

7.9   Clinical Counseling and Addressing Patient Goals

When sexual dysfunction or bothersome dyspareunia is reported by a new mother, taking a patient-centered approach to address her symptoms is essential. Allowing the patient to discuss her concerns and providing validation is the first step. Permitting the patient to outline her goals is also important. This discussion can be nuanced and take time, which a provider may not have when a busy clinical schedule is present. If this is the case, having an abbreviated discussion and recommending the patient reschedule so that adequate time can be provided is appropriate. Even with a brief discussion, the provider may be able to offer a few interventions, such as placing a referral to physical therapy, suggesting the use of vaginal lubricants and moisturizers for the breastfeeding and/or pumping patient, or recommending trial of alternative sexual positions to begin to improve her symptoms. Referral to a sex counselor or therapist can be done as well. Lastly, the provider can offer educational resources for the patient to review, such as those available through ACOG, the Royal College of Obstetrician Gynaecologists, the International Urogynecological Association and the American Urogynecologic Society (see Table 7.4).

Table 7.4 Resources for patients with sexual dysfunction/dyspareunia

Organization	Patient resource	Website
American College of Obstetricians and Gynecologists	When Sex is Painful	https://www.acog.org/womens-health/faqs/when-sex-is-painful
	Your Sexual Health	https://www.acog.org/womens-health/faqs/your-sexual-health
American Urogynecologic Society	Vaginal Estrogen Therapy (focus on genitourinary syndrome of menopause)	https://www.voicesforpfd.org/assets/2/6/Vaginal_Estrogen_Therapy.pdf
International Urogynecological Association	Painful Sex (Dyspareunia)	https://www.yourpelvicfloor.org/conditions/dyspareunia
	Low Dose Vaginal Estrogen Therapy	https://www.yourpelvicfloor.org/conditions/low-dose-vaginal-estrogen-therapy//
	Maternal Pelvic Floor Trauma	https://www.yourpelvicfloor.org/conditions/maternal-pelvic-floor-trauma/
Royal College of Obstetrician Gynaecologists	Care of a third- or fourth-degree tear that occurred during childbirth (OASI)	https://www.rcog.org.uk/en/patients/patient-leaflets/third%2D%2Dor-fourth-degree-tear-during-childbirth/
	This hub aims to inform about the types of tears that can occur during childbirth, how to minimize risk of deeper tearing, and what can be done to help recovery if a tear	https://www.rcog.org.uk/for-the-public/perineal-tears-and-episiotomies-in-childbirth/

7.10 Therapeutic Strategies

Therapeutic strategies for treatment of sexual dysfunction and dyspareunia should be tailored to the patient's clinical concerns, her detailed history and physical exam findings. The most basic interventions include oral and topical analgesics if the patient has perineal pain and a history of an obstetric laceration or episiotomy. If a patient complains of vaginal dryness, over the counter lubricants for intercourse and vaginal moisturizers are simple interventions that can provide relief. If the patient is breastfeeding and/or pumping and vaginal atrophy is present on exam, a prescription for vaginal estrogen may be beneficial. Breastfeeding and/or pumping patients should be counseled that with proper use, vaginal estrogen will not diminish her milk supply. If granulation tissue is identified on exam, this can be excised sharply or cauterized using silver nitrate, depending on the size of the lesion. If a vulvovaginal trigger point is present, offering a trigger point injection may be efficacious.

Referral to pelvic floor physical therapy is also a critical strategy that has been shown to be beneficial for a variety of postpartum concerns. A systematic review on pelvic floor muscle training found that most studies demonstrate improvement in sexual function in women with pelvic floor dysfunction, including in a postpartum population [52]. Furthermore, in a systematic review and meta-analysis of postpartum women, those undergoing physical therapy were less likely to report symptoms of prolapse, sexual dysfunction, urinary incontinence [53]. Sobhgol et al. found that physical therapy positively affects sexual desire, arousal, orgasm and satisfaction postpartum [54]. In women who have levator ani defects, a secondary analysis of a randomized control trial found those who underwent pelvic floor physical therapy had improvement in the sensation of the vagina feeling "loose or lax" [55]. While the authors found no difference in sexual dysfunction at 6 months postpartum between the physical therapy group and controls, this is likely a result of insufficient power to assess this outcome. Physical therapy also has a well-established role for treatment of vulvovaginal pain, bowel or bladder control issues, prolapse, and pelvic muscle weakness, all of which can negatively affect sexual function. The long-term effect of physical therapy on sexual function, however, is less clear [56].

For patients experiencing postpartum depression, treatment of their condition may improve sexual dysfunction. Referral to psychotherapy should be the initial step for mild to moderate symptoms and avoids the initiation of pharmacotherapy. Initiation of anti-depressants can be considered for patients with more severe symptoms or who have an insufficient response to psychotherapy alone. SSRI's, which are the preferred medication for lactating women, can negatively affect sexual function through reduced libido and impaired ability to achieve orgasm. If these medications are selected, the patient should be counseled accordingly. When appropriate, prescribing a medication that does not have side effects on sexual function should be prioritized.

For women with persistent sexual dysfunction, referral to a sex counselor or therapist may be warranted. Depending upon the patient's concerns, this can be attended by the patient alone or in combination with her partner. Other considerations include addressing stress and fatigue through lifestyle changes and working to improve body image concerns.

Lastly, the provider should address other underlying conditions that may be contributing to symptoms. Regardless of the contributing factor and treatment plan, maintaining an open, non-judgmental dialog with the patient, and scheduling follow up appointments to revisit their symptoms is an essential component in the care of women with postpartum sexual dysfunction.

7.11 Conclusions

Postpartum sexual dysfunction is highly prevalent and multifactorial in etiology. A discussion of changes in postpartum sexual function should begin antenatally and revisited at the first encounter postpartum. A variety of interventions, which are mostly conservative in nature, are available. The selected treatment strategy should be tailored to the patient's clinical concerns, exam findings, and personal goals. Follow up should be continued until the patient's sexual symptoms have satisfactorily improved or resolved.

Take Home Messages

- Sexual dysfunction is very common postpartum, with up to 83% experiencing symptoms at 2–3 months after childbirth.
- While sexual dysfunction improves with time, some women continue to experience reduced sexual satisfaction at greater than 18 months postpartum.
- Sexual dysfunction is likely multifactorial in the postpartum population, with common risk factors including operative vaginal birth, higher order perineal lacerations, breastfeeding and depression.
- Providers should inquire whether or not women are experiencing sexual difficulties as the majority of women will not disclose issues voluntarily.
- When sexual dysfunction or bothersome dyspareunia is reported by a patient, a patient-centered approach should be taken to managing her symptoms and outpatient follow up continued until symptoms sufficiently improve or resolve.
- While there remains a paucity of data, the benefits and risks of cesarean section should be discussed with the patient, and shared-decision making should be individualized to take into account the woman's personal experience, goals, and choice.

Appendix: MCQ

Questions

1. Which of the following is true regarding sexual function in the postpartum period?
   - (A) Most women discuss sexual dysfunction during this time with their provider.
   - (B) 41–83% of women report sexual dysfunction at 2–3 months postpartum.
   - (C) At 6 months postpartum, less that 50% of women continue to report sexual dysfunction.
   - (D) Sexual symptoms are considered dysfunctional, regardless of the degree of bother they pose to the patient.

2. All of the following are risk factors for post-partum sexual dysfunction/dyspareunia *except*:
   (A) Mode of delivery.
   (B) Perineal trauma.
   (C) Episiotomy.
   (D) Maternal age < 35 years old.

3. All of the following statements are true *except*:
   (A) Postpartum sexual dysfunction is highly prevalent and multifactorial in etiology.
   (B) While sexual dysfunction improves with time, some women continue to experience reduced sexual satisfaction at greater than 18 months postpartum.
   (C) Referral to pelvic floor physical therapy is also a critical strategy that has been shown to be beneficial for a variety of postpartum concerns.
   (D) SSRIs, which are the preferred medication for lactating women, should not negatively affect sexual function.

4. Which of the following statements is true?
   (A) ACOG recommends contact with an obstetric provider within 2 weeks of childbirth.
   (B) In the UK, the National Institute for Health and Care Excellence (NICE) guidance recommends that the first post-natal visit by a midwife takes place within 72 hours after transfer of care from the place of birth or after a home birth.
   (C) Research suggests patients may be more forthcoming regarding sexual concerns when provided with a survey as compared to direct inquiry.
   (D) Breastfeeding and/or pumping patients should be counseled that vaginal estrogen will diminish her milk supply.

5. All of the following statements are true *except*:
   (A) The female sexual response is not linear.
   (B) The 5th edition of the DSM places a new emphasis on characterizing both dura-

tion (presence ≥ 6 months) and severity of the patient's sexual symptoms.
   (C) In a more recent systematic review, episiotomy was associated with an increased incidence of dyspareunia, but not sexual dysfunction.
   (D) One in seven women will experience postpartum depression, which has a negative impact on sexual satisfaction and desire.

Answers

1. Which of the following is true regarding sexual function in the postpartum period?
   (A) FALSE
   (B) TRUE
   (C) FALSE
   (D) FALSE

2. All of the following are risk factors for postpartum sexual dysfunction/dyspareunia *except*:
   (A) FALSE
   (B) FALSE
   (C) FALSE
   (D) TRUE

3. All of the following statements are true *except*:
   (A) FALSE
   (B) FALSE
   (C) FALSE
   (D) TRUE

4. Which of the following statements is true?
   (A) FALSE
   (B) FALSE
   (C) TRUE
   (D) FALSE

5. All of the following statements are true *except*:
   (A) FALSE
   (B) FALSE
   (C) FALSE
   (D) TRUE

References

1. Von Sydow K. Sexuality during pregnancy and after childbirth: a metacontent analysis of 59 studies. J Psychosom Res. 1999;47(1):27–49.
2. Erol B, Sanli O, Korkmaz D, Seyhan A, Akman T, Kadioglu A. A cross-sectional study of female sexual function and dysfunction during pregnancy. J Sex Med. 2007;4(5):1381–7.
3. Glazener CMA. Sexual function after childbirth: women's experiences, persistent morbidity and lack of professional recognition. Br J Obstet Gynaecol. 1997;104(3):330–5.
4. Signorello LB, Harlow BL, Chekos AK, Repke JT. Postpartum sexual functioning and its relationship to perineal trauma: a retrospective cohort study of primiparous women. Am J Obstet Gynecol. 2001;184(5):881–90.
5. Barrett G, Pendry E, Peacock J, Victor C, Thakar R, Manyonda I. Women's sexual health after childbirth. BJOG. 2000;107(2):186–95.
6. Lagaert L, Weyers S, Van Kerrebroeck H, Elaut E. Postpartum dyspareunia and sexual functioning: a prospective cohort study. Eur J Contracept Reprod Health Care. 2017;22(3):200–6.
7. McDonald E, Woolhouse H, Brown SJ. Sexual pleasure and emotional satisfaction in the first 18 months after childbirth. Midwifery. 2017;55:60–6.
8. Masters W, Johnson V. Human Sexual Response. Bantam Books; 1966.
9. Basson R. The female sexual response: a different model. J Sex Marital Ther. 2000;26(1):51–65.
10. Bancroft J, Graham CA, Janssen E, Sanders SA. The dual control model: current status and future directions. J Sex Res. 2009;46(2–3):121–42.
11. Kinsburg SA, Rezaee RL. Hypoactive sexual desire in women. Menopause. 2013;20(12):1284–300.
12. American Psychiatric Association. Diagnostic and statistical manual of mental disorders. 5th ed; 2013.
13. Rogers RG, Pauls RN, Thakar R, et al. An International Urogynecological Association (IUGA)/International Continence Society (ICS) joint report on the terminology for the assessment of sexual health of women with pelvic floor dysfunction. Neurourol Urodyn. 2018;37(4):1220–40.
14. Gutzeit O, Levy G, Lowenstein L. Postpartum female sexual function: risk factors for postpartum sexual dysfunction. Sex Med. 2020;8(1):8–13.
15. Griffiths A, Watermeyer S, Sidhu K, Amso NN, Nix B. Female genital tract morbidity and sexual function following vaginal delivery or lower segment caesarean section. J Obstet Gynaecol. 2006;26(7):645–9.
16. Klein K, Worda C, Leipold H, Gruber C, Husslein P, Wenzl R. Does the mode of delivery influence sexual function after childbirth? J Womens Health (Larchmt). 2009;18(8):1227–31.
17. Mcdonald E, Woolhouse H, Brown SJ. Consultation about sexual health issues in the year after childbirth: a cohort study. Birth. 2015;42(4):354–61. https://doi.org/10.1111/BIRT.12193.
18. McDonald EA, Gartland D, Small R, Brown SJ. Dyspareunia and childbirth: a prospective cohort study. BJOG. 2015;122(5):672–9.
19. Van Brummen HJ, Bruinse HW, Van De Pol G, Heintz APM, Van Der Vaart CH. Which factors determine the sexual function 1 year after childbirth? BJOG. 2006;113(8):914–8.
20. De Souza A, Dwyer PL, Charity M, Thomas E, Ferreira CHJ, Schierlitz L. The effects of mode delivery on postpartum sexual function: a prospective study. BJOG An Int J Obstet Gynaecol. 2015;122(10):1410–8.
21. Cattani L, De Maeyer L, Verbakel JY, Bosteels J, Deprest J. Predictors for sexual dysfunction in the first year postpartum: a systematic review and meta-analysis. BJOG. Published online 2021.
22. Van Delft K, Sultan AH, Thakar R, Schwertner-Tiepelmann N, Kluivers K. The relationship between postpartum levator ani muscle avulsion and signs and symptoms of pelvic floor dysfunction. BJOG. 2014;121(9):1164–72.
23. Marsh F, Lynne R, Christine L, Alison W. Obstetric anal sphincter injury in the UK and its effect on bowel, bladder and sexual function. Eur J Obstet Gynecol Reprod Biol. 2011;154(2):223–7.
24. O'Shea MS, Lewicky-Gaupp C, Gossett DR. Long-term sexual function after obstetric anal sphincter injuries. Female Pelvic Med Reconstr Surg. 2018;24(2):82–6.
25. Jiang H, Qian X, Carroli G, Garner P. Selective versus routine use of episiotomy for vaginal birth. Cochrane Database Syst Rev. 2017;2017(2).
26. Avery MD, Duckett L, Frantzich CR. The experience of sexuality during breastfeeding among primiparous women. J Midwifery Women's Heal. 2000;45(3):227–37.
27. Wallwiener S, Müller M, Doster A, et al. Sexual activity and sexual dysfunction of women in the perinatal period: a longitudinal study. Arch Gynecol Obstet. 2017;295(4):873–83.
28. ACOG Committee Opinion No. 757: screening for perinatal depression. Obstet Gynecol. 2018;132(5):E208–12.
29. Pauls RN, Occhino JA, Dryfhout VL. Effects of pregnancy on female sexual function and body image: a prospective study. J Sex Med. 2008;5(8):1915–22.
30. Pauls RN, Occhino JA, Dryfhout V, Karram MM. Effects of pregnancy on pelvic floor dysfunction and body image; a prospective study. Int Urogynecol J Pelvic Floor Dysfunct. 2008;19(11):1495–501.
31. Schlagintweit HE, Bailey K, Rosen NO. A new baby in the bedroom: frequency and severity of postpartum sexual concerns and their associations with relation-

ship satisfaction in new parent couples. J Sex Med. 2016;13(10):1455–65.

32. Grekin R, O'Hara MW. Prevalence and risk factors of postpartum posttraumatic stress disorder: a meta-analysis. Clin Psychol Rev. 2014;34(5):389–401.

33. Leader-Cramer A, Kenton K, Davé B, Gossett DR, Mueller M, Lewicky-Gaupp C. Factors associated with timing of return to intercourse after obstetric anal sphincter injuries. J Sex Med. 2016;13(10):1523–9.

34. Rogers RG, Borders N, Leeman LM, Albers LL. Does spontaneous genital tract trauma impact postpartum sexual function? J Midwifery Womens Health. 2009;54(2):98–103.

35. Brubaker L, Handa VL, Bradley CS, et al. Sexual function 6 months after first delivery. Obstet Gynecol. 2008;111(5):1040–4.

36. O'Shea M, Zandi R, Kamat N, et al. Postpartum contraceptive uptake and fertility desires following obstetric anal sphincter injury. Int Urogynecol J. 2021;32(7):1833–8.

37. McKinney J, Keyser L, Clinton S, et al. ACOG Committee Opinion No. 736: optimizing postpartum care. Obstet Gynecol. 2018;132(3):784–5.

38. Postnatal care. Postnatal care. Published online 2021. https://pubmed.ncbi.nlm.nih.gov/34197057/. Accessed 24 July 2022.

39. Plouffe L. Screening for sexual problems through a simple questionnaire. Am J Obstet Gynecol. 1985;151(2):166–9.

40. Roos AM, Sultan AH, Thakar R. Sexual problems in the gynecology clinic: are we making a mountain out of a molehill? Int Urogynecol J. 2012;23(2):145–52.

41. Hatzichristou D, Rosen RC, Derogatis LR, et al. Recommendations for the clinical evaluation of men and women with sexual dysfunction. J Sex Med. 2010;7(1 Pt 2):337–48.

42. Rosen RC. Assessment of female sexual dysfunction: review of validated methods. Fertil Steril. 2002;77 Suppl 4(SUPPL. 4):89–93.

43. Fischman SH, Rankin EA, Soeken EL, Lenz ER. Changes in sexual relationships in postpartum couples. J Obstet Gynecol Neonatal Nurs JOGNN. 1986;15(1):58–63.

44. Thibault-Gagnon S, Yusuf S, Langer S, et al. Do women notice the impact of childbirth-related levator trauma on pelvic floor and sexual function? Results of an observational ultrasound study. Int Urogynecol J. 2014;25(10):1389–98.

45. Rosen R, Brown C, Heiman J, et al. The female sexual function index (FSFI): a multidimensional self-report instrument for the assessment of female sexual function. J Sex Marital Ther. 2000;26(2):191–205.

46. Isidori AM, Pozza C, Esposito K, et al. Development and validation of a 6-item version of the female sexual function index (FSFI) as a diagnostic tool for female sexual dysfunction. J Sex Med. 2010;7(3):1139–46.

47. McCoy NL, Davidson JM. A longitudinal study of the effects of menopause on sexuality. Maturitas. 1985;7(3):203–10.

48. Derogatis L, Clayton A, Lewis-D'agostino D, Wunderlich G, Fu Y. Validation of the female sexual distress scale-revised for assessing distress in women with hypoactive sexual desire disorder. J Sex Med. 2008;5(2):357–64.

49. Rust J, Golombok S. The golombok rust inventory of sexual satisfaction (GRISS). Br J Clin Psychol. 1985;24(1):63–64.

50. Rogers RG, Espuña Pons ME. The pelvic organ prolapse incontinence sexual questionnaire, IUGA-revised (PISQ-IR). Int Urogynecol J. 2013;24(7):1063–4.

51. Rogers RG, Coates KW, Kammerer-Doak D, Khalsa S, Qualls C. A short form of the pelvic organ prolapse/urinary incontinence sexual questionnaire (PISQ-12). Int Urogynecol J Pelvic Floor Dysfunct. 2003;14(3):164–8; discussion 168.

52. Ferreira CHJ, Dwyer PL, Davidson M, De Souza A, Ugarte JA, Frawley HC. Does pelvic floor muscle training improve female sexual function? A systematic review. Int Urogynecol J. 2015;26(12):1735–50.

53. Wu YM, McInnes N, Leong Y. Pelvic floor muscle training versus watchful waiting and pelvic floor disorders in postpartum women: a systematic review and meta-analysis. Female Pelvic Med Reconstr Surg. 2018;24(2):142–9.

54. Sobhgol SS, Priddis H, Smith CA, Dahlen HG. The effect of pelvic floor muscle exercise on female sexual function during pregnancy and postpartum: a systematic review. Sex Med Rev. 2019;7(1):13–28.

55. Kolberg Tennfjord M, Hilde G, Stær-Jensen J, Siafarikas F, Engh ME, Bø K. Effect of postpartum pelvic floor muscle training on vaginal symptoms and sexual dysfunction-secondary analysis of a randomised trial. BJOG. 2016;123(4):634–42.

56. Battut A, Nizard J. Impact of pelvic floor muscle training on prevention of perineal pain and dyspareunia in postpartum. Prog Urol. 2016;26(4):237–44.

Impact of Pregnancy and Childbirth on Pre-existing Bowel Conditions

8

Peter Rimmer and Rachel Cooney

Overview

Test your learning and check your understanding of this book's contents: use the "Springer Nature Flashcards" app to access questions using ► https://sn.pub/wqrf89. To use the app, please follow the instructions in Chap. 1.

Learning Objectives

- To understand the impact of pregnancy on the gastrointestinal tract
- To learn about the management of inflammatory bowel disease (IBD) before and during pregnancy
- To explore the management of stomas in pregnancy
- To understand the treatment of irritable bowel syndrome (IBS) and constipation in pregnancy
- To learn about acid reflux disease, haemorrhoids, coeliac disease and gallstones in pregnancy

P. Rimmer · R. Cooney (✉)
University Hospitals Birmingham, Birmingham, UK
e-mail: peter.rimmer@uhb.nhs.uk;
Rachel.Cooney@uhb.nhs.uk

8.1 Introduction

8.1.1 The Changing Physiology of Pregnancy and the Consequences for the Gastrointestinal Tract

The gastrointestinal tract, like multiple organ systems, is impacted by the major physiological changes of pregnancy. The influences of pregnancy on gastrointestinal function can be split into those attributable to (1) direct hormonal effects, (2) physiological circulatory changes and (3) mechanical origins.

- Hormonal changes
  - Increased *progesterone* production from the corpus luteum (weeks 8–12), followed by the placenta thereafter is associated with:
    Delayed gastric emptying
    Increased small intestinal transit times [1]
    Reduced lower oesophageal sphincter tone
  - Placental production of *gastrin* is associated with increased gastric acidity [2]
  - Whilst its role is still debated, it is worth noting that when given to health subjects intravenously, oxytocin:
    Increases colonic peristalsis
    Accelerate gastric emptying [3]

- Circulatory changes in pregnancy include the following:
  - 30–50% increase in plasma volume
  - Total body water content increase by up to 8 litres [4]
  - Oestrogen-mediated upregulation of endothelial nitric oxide synthase, alongside the role of the placenta as a type of arteriovenous fistula, causes peripheral vasodilatation [5]
  - Activation of the renin-angiotensin aldosterone system (RAAS) with consequent sodium and water retention and haemodilution [5]. Activation of RAAS increases water reabsorption from the gastrointestinal tract, with consequent reduced stool volume and increased transit time
- Mechanical changes
  - As pregnancy progresses, enlargement of the uterus displaces abdominal structures and increases intra-abdominal pressure, further slowing gastrointestinal transit

Common gastrointestinal complaints during pregnancy include nausea, vomiting, constipation and gastro-oesophageal reflux. When involved in the assessment of pregnant patients, it is important to be aware of these factors, as well as other pregnancy changes. During clinical examinations, mechanical changes (for example, peritoneal stretch) can result in desensitisation and a softening of clinical signs associated with abdominal pathology [1]. A classic example of this is appendicitis, where the typical history of migratory abdominal pain, starting centrally and moving to the right iliac fossa, may not be present. Whilst interpreting blood results, the overall haemodilutional state will have consequent reductions in 'normal' haemoglobin and albumin concentrations as the pregnancy progresses. Alkaline phosphatase (ALP) is an enzyme which in humans is largely concentrated in liver, renal, intestinal and biliary mucosa, as well as bone. During pregnancy, an isoenzyme is produced by the placenta resulting in increased levels and a higher reference range. Where clinical uncertainty is present regarding the significance of an elevated ALP, this can be confirmed by measuring isoenzymes. The potential causes of elevation in ALP are outlined below:

ALP origin	Possible underlying process
Hepatic	Alcohol related liver disease, primary sclerosing cholangitis, primary biliary cholangitis, malignancy (primary or secondary), cholestasis e.g. drug induced
Biliary	Gallstones, malignancy, cholangitis
Renal	Renal osteodystrophy
Bone	Recent fracture, primary bone malignancy, bone metastases, Paget's disease of bone, hyperparathyroidism, osteomalacia
Physiological	Pregnancy, adolescence

It is important to note that conversely, alanine aminotransferase (ALT) should fall during pregnancy and values considered normal in the general population can represent pathology [6].

Please note management of pre-existing liver disease will not be discussed in this chapter.

8.2 The Gastrointestinal Microbiome and Pregnancy

The microbiota consists of up to 100 trillion microbial cells harboured by an individual, which when catalogued can be referred to as the *human microbiome* [7]. There is increasing interest in the role of the microbiome in the pathogenesis of multiple disease processes. This is particularly true of the gastrointestinal tract. There has been interest in the changes seen in during pregnancy and how these may impact the development of new pathologies and the behaviour of existing conditions.

It is recognised that as pregnancy progresses, the abundance of gut bacteria associated with inflammatory states increases in nearly 70% of women [8]. In the third trimester, alpha diversity (the overall diversity of bacterial species within the colon) is seen to be reduced, though the significance of this is not yet established [9]. These changes are in part felt to be due to the influence of oestrogen and progesterone on bacterial metabolism. Some of these changes seen in the microbiome through pregnancy mimic those of metabolic syndrome, and it is postulated that these changes may be necessary to increase the amount of energy stored as fat for subsequent utilisation for foetal growth and lactation [9]. Consequently, there is interest in the risk these changes pose to obese patients in whom there is usually an existing deviation from what would be considered a normal microbiome (term 'dysbiosis'). For example, one study has demonstrated that further loss of short-chain fatty acid producing bacteria in obese individuals during pregnancy was associated with higher maternal blood pressure [10]. At present, how to translate this into clinical practice is not clear but it is a growing field of interest.

8.3 Inflammatory Bowel Disease (IBD)

IBD refers to a group of multifactorial diseases characterised by chronic inflammation of the gastrointestinal tract. The principal forms are ulcerative colitis (UC) and Crohn's disease.

The causes of IBD are an area of great research interest. Currently, the disease is viewed as a combination of environmental triggers which result in a dysbiosis within the human intestinal microbiome. In the genetically susceptible host, this can trigger immune activation and consequent inflammation and ulceration of the digestive tract. This is summarised in Fig. 8.1.

Ulcerative colitis is limited to the large intestine and classically involves inflammation beginning in the rectum and extended proximally. The disease may be limited to the rectum (proctitis) but can extend, typically in a continuous manner, to involve the more proximal large intestine. Inflammation of the entire large intestine is referred to as *pancolitis*. Crohn's disease, on the other hand, can involve any section of the digestive tract and is characterised by patchy inflammation with areas of deeper ulceration. Crohn's can be associated with the formation of strictures and fistulae, the latter of which can involve the peri-anal area. Presentations with perianal disease are usually associated with a more aggressive disease course. Both diseases can be characterised by periods of active inflammation and by periods of relative remission. The goal of treatment is to maintain remission and allow

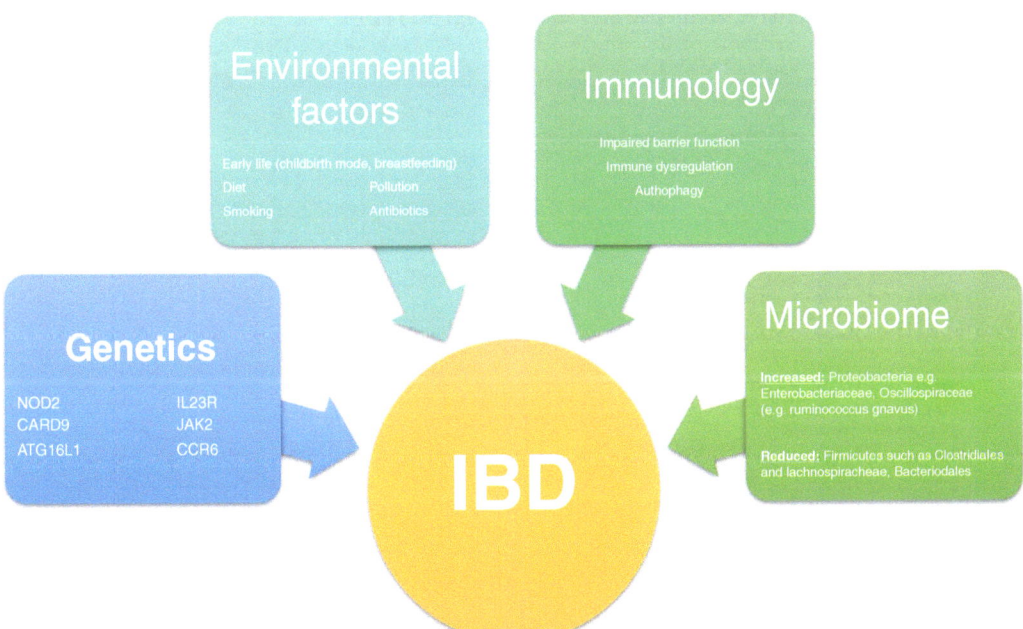

Fig. 8.1 The multifactorial aetiology of IBD. (Adapted from Oliveira and Monteiro [11])

healing of the previously inflamed intestinal mucosa. Mesalasine-based therapies are used in UC, but are not effective in Crohn's disease. Older treatments that are still used include azathioprine medications and steroids (topical, oral, intravenous). Biologic therapies which include anti-tumor necrosis factor (TNF) drugs and the newer small molecules (for example, Janus kinase (JAK) inhibitors) have recently become the mainstay of IBD treatment. Again, the goal of treatment is to promote healing of the gut mucosa, thus preventing disease flares and gut damage. How these therapies can be utilised during pregnancy is explored subsequently.

8.4   IBD and Pregnancy

It has long been recognised that though pregnancy outcomes are similar between those with IBD in sustained remission and the general population, the same is not true of those with active disease [12]. Pregnancy itself does not significant increase the risk of IBD relapse, however, inappropriate withdrawal of therapy has contributed to worse disease control. More recent meta-analyses have demonstrated that active disease remains associated with worse outcomes even in the 'post biologic era'. A large meta-analysis from 2015 revealed that those with active disease have the following outcomes [13]:

Domain	Rate in all births	Rate in IBD	Odds ratio
Pre term birth	13 per 100 births	22 per 100 births	1.85 (95% CI 1.67–2.05; $I^2 = 31\%$)
Small for gestational age birth weight	10 per 100 births	13 per 100 births	1.36 (95% CI 1.16–1.69; I^2 56%)
Stillbirth	6 per 1000 births	9 per 100 births	1.57 (95% CI 1.03–2.38; I^2 30%)
Congenital abnormality	4 per 100 births	5 per 100 births	1.29 (95% CI 1.05–1.58; I^2 46%)

Preconceptual planning for a mother with IBD should focus on ensuring disease remission at time of conception and maintenance of remission during the pregnancy. The American Gastroenterology Association break these considerations down as follows in their guidelines (Fig. 8.2) [14].

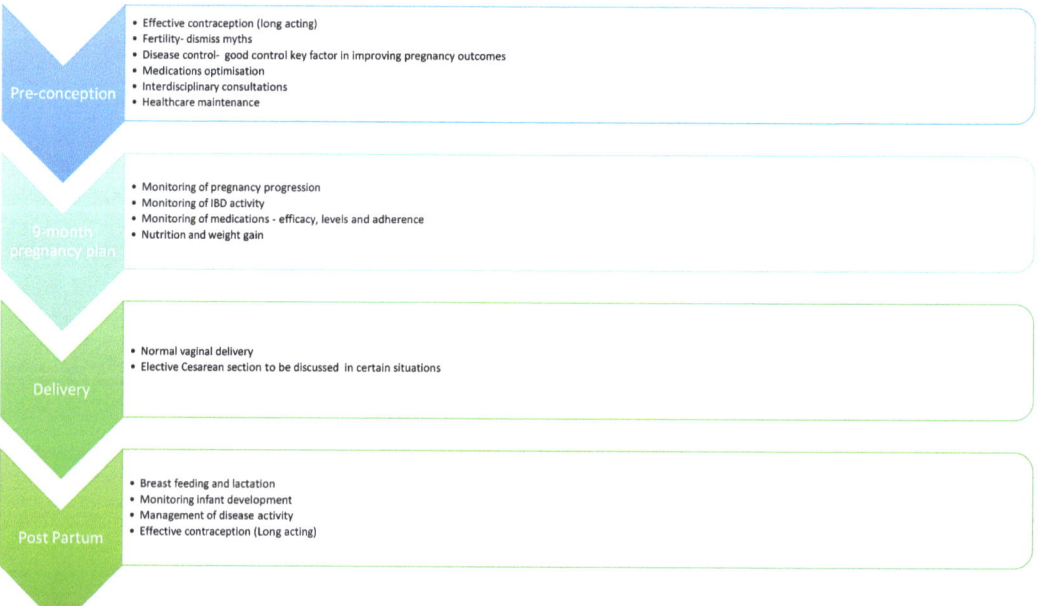

Fig. 8.2 Inflammatory bowel disease in pregnancy clinical decision support tool. (Adapted from the AGA guidelines [14])

8.4.1 Pre-conception Planning (and Fertility)

Fertility rates in IBD are equivalent to those in the general population, provided the disease is in remission and surgery has not previously been required. Reduced fertility however, can be seen in women with active inflammation and in those who have undergone surgical procedures including open ileal pouch-anal anastomoses, proctectomy and permanent stoma [14].

There is no association between the medications used for IBD control and reduced fertility. However, there is an increase in voluntary childlessness associated with IBD (17% of women with IBD vs 6% in the general population) [15]. Good pre-pregnancy counselling can help allay patients fears and dismiss any misbelieves regarding the risks of pregnancy or heritability of disease. Indeed pre-pregnancy counselling has been shown to reduce disease activity during pregnancy [16].

Recommended Pre-pregnancy Counselling Checklist

1. Ensure PAP smear tests are up to date, folic acid is being taken, iron stores are optimised, and general steps are undertaken to ensure adequate nutrition
2. Advise regarding smoking and alcohol cessation
3. Discuss mode of birth when an absolute indication of caesarean birth is present (e.g. active perianal disease)
4. Assess disease activity to ensure patient is aware of the importance of conception in remission.
   - Assessment of clinical remission on symptoms alone may not be enough, as it is well recognised that subclinical inflammation can also predict disease relapse [17].
     – Faecal calprotectin is a non-invasive method of determining mucosal healing and should be utilised to confirm remission
     – Elevated C-reactive protein (CRP) and platelets as well as low albumin can all be markers of active disease
     – The gold standard method of confirming deep remission remains flexible sigmoidoscopy or colonoscopy
5. Evaluate current medications
   - The general approach should be to continue the current medication; exceptions to this rule are detailed in the table below.
   - The previous mantra to stop anti-TNF in all patients in the third trimester no longer holds true and emphasis must be placed upon getting disease into remission thus preventing flares.

Medication	Suggested dosing	Breast feeding
Aminosalicylates Mesalazine Sulfasalazine	Continue usual maintenance. There is a preference of mesalazine over sulfasalazine, both in terms of efficacy and safety. If sulfasalazine is maintained, pre-conception folic acid should be high dose (sulfasalazine can impair folic acid absorption and metabolism)	Continue
Azathioprine	Continue if monotherapy In combination therapy, consider cessation (increased risk of infection in the neonate) If given with allopurinol, caution re potential embryo toxic effects (allopurinol mechanism of action inhibits purine synthesis. Limited data, isolated case reports of congenital malformations) Therapeutic drug monitoring (TDM) recommended. Should not be started in pregnancy if treatment naive (risk of complications e.g. pancreatitis, extended period to maximum efficacy)	Continue
Methotrexate	Must be stopped at least 3 months prior to conception	Discontinue – present in milk

Medication	Suggested dosing	Breast feeding
Ciclosporin	Relatively limited data and established as an acceptable rescue therapy in pregnancy Some associations with low birth weight, pre-term birth and maternal complications including hypertension and gestational diabetes	Minimal infant exposure, compatible with breast feeding

Anti-TNF
  Infliximab
  Adalimumab
	Current practice would generally suggest continuing through all three trimesters
	  Infliximab – if 8 weekly IV dosing, plan final dose 6–10 weeks before planned delivery
	  Adalimumab – if fortnightly dosing, place final dose 2–3 weeks before planned delivery
	This is to aim to minimise fetal transfer
		Continue

Anti IL12/23
  Ustekinumab
	Continue
	  Data is limited but no issues identified where it is available
	  Final dosing again should be timed to minimise transfer (i.e. delivery planned around time next dose due)
		Continue

Anti-integrin
(alpha4, beta7)
  Vedolizumab
	Continue
	  Similarly limited data and dosing practice as above
		Continue

Small molecules
  Tofacitinib
	Avoid if possible
	  Human data too limited
	  Known to cross the placenta
	  Higher doses teratogenic in mice
		Limited human data, not advised

Antibiotics	Not indicated for a 'flare' but may be indicated for perianal disease, pouchitis or infective complications such as Clostridium difficile. Amoxicillin or Metronidazole preferred over Ciprofloxacin	Amoxicillin (+/− clavulanic acid) considered safe Ciprofloxacin preferred over metronidazole

Optimising IBD medications for pregnancy. Adapted from AGA guidelines [14] and European Crohn's and Colitis Guidelines [18]

8.4.2 Biologic Medications

'Biologic' drugs are still relatively new in the scheme of IBD therapies. When anti-TNF drugs were first utilised, the typical practice was to stop the medication in the third trimester. This owed to their ability to cross the placenta and remain active in the foetus. There is now, however, a growing field of evidence in this area. A large prospective multi-centre study in the United States, running from 2007 to 2019, supported the continued use of biologics throughout pregnancy [19]. The key findings of the PIANO (Pregnancy in Inflammatory bowel disease And Neonatal Outcomes) study included that biologics were *not* associated with:

- Congenital malformations, pre-term birth, low birthweight or spontaneous abortion
- A negative impact on the foetus, as the drug cleared in most by 6 months and all by 9 months

Not surprisingly, increased disease activity was associated with lower birth weight and increased spontaneous abortion. Though the outcome data above is reassuring, the presence of detectable drug in the infant for 6 months mandates that live vaccinations (the only routine recommended one being rotavirus) should be delayed until after 6 months of age when the drug has cleared. This advice followed reports of death in neonates who were exposed to an Anti-TNF in utero receiving a live attenuated vaccine as per routine schedules (i.e. before 6 months).

8.4.3 Managing IBD Flares During Pregnancy

Pre-pregnancy counselling, conception while in remission and continuation of medications where possible all give the patient the best chance of maintaining remission. Nonetheless, not all pregnancies are planned, and disease can still flare unpredictably. Historic data from the pre-biologic era placed the risk of relapse in pregnant patients at 34% per year vs 32% in the non-pregnant IBD population [20]. Interestingly, the PIANO registry demonstrated lower rates of remission per trimester in patients with UC over those with Crohn's disease [19].

Consideration must also be given to physiological and biochemical changes already described when confirming a flare. Constipation and reduced transit time can increase abdominal pain. Modest elevations in CRP can occur in normal pregnancy, as can reductions in albumin. As mentioned above, faecal calprotectin, however, remains a reliable marker of disease activity. Where necessary and there is a clear potential for a consequent change in management, endoscopic assessment can be undertaken. Wherever possible, flexible sigmoidoscopy with enema preparation only is preferred. The risk of endoscopy to the patient increases after 24 weeks, particularly where bowel preparation, sedation or a full colonoscopy are required. However, endoscopy can be performed at any stage of pregnancy if required. Wherever MRI (without gadolinium) or ultrasound can be utilised, this is preferred to CT scanning.

If active disease is confirmed, medications can be utilised in a similar fashion to those that would be employed in the absence of pregnancy. Corticosteroids can be used where indicated, though this should prompt close monitoring of blood glucose levels. Prednisolone is the drug of choice due to foetal levels only reaching 10% of maternal levels via conversion to less active metabolites in the placenta [21].

8.4.4 The Post-surgical Abdomen and Pregnancy in IBD

Despite the advent of novel medical therapies, surgical approaches in IBD still form a cornerstone of treatment. The impact upon fertility and pregnancy across all these approaches is not equal, whilst different surgical procedures will have differing consequences for delivery.

In those with UC, most patients undergoing surgery will have active inflammation that is refractory to medical therapy. In that setting, patients often undergo a subtotal colectomy, whereby the diseased colon is removed with a rectal stump left in situ and a covering ileostomy left in situ. Restorative surgical options are then considered in the appropriate setting. The current operation of choice is a completion proctectomy with formation of an ileal pouch-anal anastomosis (IPAA), a schematic of which is shown in Fig. 8.3:

Other approaches which still may be encountered in clinical practice include an ileorectal anastomosis, but the risk of malignancy in the residual rectal mucosa has left this approach less common.

In Crohn's disease, on the other hand, surgical approaches vary according to the distribution of the disease and whether treatment is for perianal or luminal activity. In isolated ileal disease, an ileocaecal resection with primary anastomosis is typical, whilst transmural complications such as fistula formation can necessitate surgery elsewhere, with or without the need for an ileostomy. In those with perianal disease, initial approaches include incision and drainage of abscess, with seton placement to aid fistula drainage and consequent healing. In patients with refractory disease, again a defunctioning stoma may be necessary for bowel rest and healing.

Unfortunately, the formation of an IPAA (see Fig. 8.3) is associated with a reduction in fertility across multiple patient cohorts. Infertility is estimated to be 12% in patients prior to their restorative procedure, and up to 26% post [23]. This may owe to the risk of pelvic sepsis, whilst pouchitis may also contribute. However, completion proctectomy instead of IPAA is also associated with reduced fertility. Laparoscopic approaches to IPAA have been demonstrated to have less of an impact on fertility in comparison to open surgery [24]. For other types of surgery, particularly in the Crohn's disease cohort, the procedure of choice is often not straightforward and depends on the nature of the disease phenotype, nature of the surgery, and presence or absence of perianal disease. One large systematic review found that before age of 25, patients who had undergone surgery for Crohn's had higher rates of fertility than those who had not. This may be due to

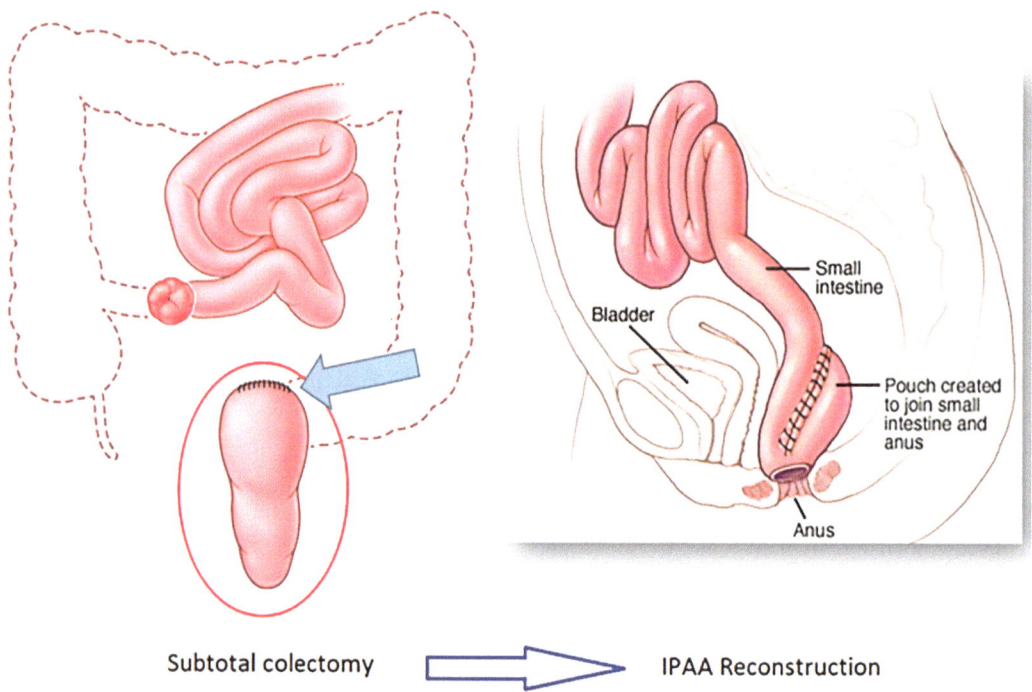

Fig. 8.3 Surgical approaches in Ulcerative colitis. (Adapted from Ordás et al. [22])

shorter duration of disease, earlier reduction in inflammatory burden/establishment of disease control and general age related rates of fertility. Overall, however, fertility rates were higher in those not requiring surgery [25].

8.4.5 Managing Stomas in Pregnancy

There has until recently been a paucity of evidence, often limited to case reports, regarding the management of patients with an 'ostomy' during pregnancy; a recent study investigated this [26]. The PAPooSE (Pregnancy outcomes & experiences in patients with ileostomies) study evaluated the outcomes of 82 pregnancies from 77 patients with an 'ostomy' (ileostomy or colostomy) as a consequence of IBD. 73% of patients required a caesarean birth, including 16% as an emergency procedure. 24% of patients suffered significant stoma related complications; 2 required surgery for stomal prolapse, 2 for parastomal hernia and 3 for bowel obstruction. In the

cohort, there was 1 miscarriage, 1 still-birth and 80 live births. Overall, the mean gestation at birth was 37 weeks (range 29–41). Delivery before week 37 occurred in 14 of 74 documented (19%) cases. Mean birth weight was 3030 g (standard deviation 720 g) with weight < 2500 g at birth in 13 of 75 documented cases (17%) [26]. This demonstrates that though pregnancy is cleared very possible in those with a stoma, it is associated with a high risk of requiring caesarean birth, as well as a significant risk of serious complications relating to the stoma. Patients in this cohort should be counselled accordingly.

8.4.6 Birth Modality

Overall, in patients with IBD, the indications for mode of delivery should be the same as for those without IBD. Nonetheless, there are some circumstances where the IBD must be factored into the decision. In those with an IPAA, there is a relative indication for an medically-indicated caesarean birth. Continence will deteriorate in the third trimester and any sphincter injury during vaginal delivery may carry a significant adverse impact on quality of life. These same considerations apply to patients who are considered likely to require a pouch (or ileorectal anastomosis) in the future. The data however is conflicting, and this is not an absolute indication, rather one that needs to be discussed with the patient and an individualised decision made [27]. Though the PAPoose data demonstrates that caesarean birth is not mandatory for patients with a stoma, the rate of caesarean is high and rates of stoma related complication can precipitate the need for an emergency procedure.

In the Crohn's patient who has not had previous surgery, the most important consideration is the presence or absence of perianal disease. Active perianal disease is associated with a 10-fold increase in perianal damage with vaginal birth [28]. With that in mind, caesarean birth is usually the preferred approach.

Another consideration is how to handle patients with one or multiple previous abdominal surgeries. In an emergency, the time from decision to perform the caesarean and birth should be <30 min [29, 30]. Shared decision making between the patient, obstetrician and even a Colorectal surgeon is recommended if there is concern that emergency c-section could be delayed due to adhesions making access to uterus difficult.

Finally, IBD is a pro-inflammatory condition and the risk of venous thromboembolism is a very relevant consideration in the post operative period, often extending up to 6 weeks post-partum.

8.5   Other Gastrointestinal Disorders and Pregnancy

8.5.1   Irritable Bowel Syndrome

Irritable bowel syndrome (IBS) is the most common GI diagnosis and is characterised by functional abdominal pain and altered bowel habits; there is an absence of organic pathology [31]. There are different subtypes such as IBS-D (diar-

rhoea predominant), IBS-C (constipation predominant) and IBS- M (mixed) as defined by Rome IV criteria. IBS is more common in woman and the population prevalence is approximately 12% [32]. IBS symptoms, most notably constipation, may worsen in pregnancy, especially in the last trimester. There is limited data, but IBS does not appear to impact fertility. There is a large retrospective study suggesting that women with IBS have a higher rate of miscarriage and ectopic pregnancy than the general population [33], however, the study has not been replicated. When compared with mothers without IBS, maternal IBS was associated with increased risk of miscarriage (odds ratio [OR] 1.21; 95% confidence interval [CI], 1.13–1.30) and ectopic pregnancy (OR 1.28; 95% CI 1.06–1.55), but not with preeclampsia (OR 1.09; 95% CI 0.85–1.39) or stillbirth (OR 1.00; 95% CI 0.69–1.44).

Dietary modification is the mainstay of treatment of IBS. The National Institute for Clinical Excellence (NICE) in the UK, recommendations outside of pregnancy include eating regular meals, avoiding caffeine. These as well as others detailed below can also be applicable during pregnancy [34]. Avoidance of food triggers which vary from individual to individual can be helpful. Some common triggers include gluten, lactose, onions, tomatoes, highly processed foods and carbonated drinks. A common recommendation is a diet low in fermentable oli-, di-, and monosaccharides and polyols (FODMAPs), as this has been shown to reduce IBS symptoms [35]. However, restrictive diets can result in deficiencies in vitamins such as folic acid and Vitamin D; this is detrimental in pregnancy and should only be undertaken with the close supervision of a dietician. Unlike insoluble fibers, soluble fibers (e.g., psyllium and ispaghula husk), can improve IBS symptoms especially in those with IBS-C; use should be encouraged in pregnancy due to the excellent safety profile [36]. Pharmacological options in the management of IBS-D are very limited due to a paucity of safety data. Drugs commonly used outside of pregnancy for IBS-D do not have adequate data available to recommend their use in pregnancy. These include loperamide, serotonin receptor uptake inhibitors and tricyclic antidepressants. However, if symptoms are debilitating their use can be discussed with the patient on a case-by-case basis. Use of cognitive behavioural therapy and acupuncture have both been shown to be effective in small studies outside pregnancy and there is no contraindication to their use in pregnancy [37].

8.5.2 Constipation

In the case of functional constipation, pregnancy can worsen this condition considerably. Initial simple, but often overlooked considerations, include ensuring adequate hydration and increasing dietary fibre. The preferred pharmacological option is a Polyethylene Glycol (PEG) containing laxative, the commonest of which in the United Kingdom is Movicol/Laxido™. Lactulose is also commonly used but can cause abdominal bloating. Stimulant laxatives are generally not recommended, as they can cause pain and there is concern about them triggering uterine contractions [38]. Newer drugs such as linaclotide and prucalopride are also not recommended in pregnancy due to reports of miscarriage in early pregnancy and the negative impact on animal models [39, 40].

8.5.3 Haemorrhoids

Haemorrhoids are exceptionally common during pregnancy and for those with pre-existing haemorrhoids, these can significantly worsen in pregnancy. They are present at some stage during 25–35% of pregnancies and are most common during the third trimester [41]. As with those occurring outside of pregnancy, conservative methods are preferred first line therapy. This involves prevention of constipation using the same approaches as described above in order to reduce straining. Stool softeners may also help. Other measures include bathing in a warm sitz bath to reduce anorectal pain. Topical anaesthetic and/or steroids agents utilised outside of pregnancy can be used, although the evidence supporting their efficacy is poor [42]. Anal fissures can be managed in a similar manner, as botulinum toxin (which can be used to treat this outside pregnancy) should be avoided in pregnancy. Fortunately, the majority of these will rapidly resolve in the post-partum period.

8.5.4 Acid Reflux and Peptic Ulcer Disease

Acid reflux is common in pregnancy for the physiological reasons highlighted earlier. For those with pre-existing conditions such as a hiatal hernia, this can be particularly problematic. In general, the diagnosis of reflux is made based on symptoms only. If there is a clinical need (e.g. haematemesis or severe pain/weight loss), an upper endoscopy can be performed during pregnancy in any trimester.

Conservative measures for these upper GI disorders include frequent and small meals, adequate fluid intake, avoiding caffeine and high fat foods; these are the first line measures for managing heartburn in pregnancy. Over-the-counter alginate-based therapies are the first line pharmacological measures, followed by histamine 2 (H2) antagonists (ranitidine/cimetidine/famotidine) [43, 44]. Proton pump inhibitors (PPI) may be required to control symptoms and can be used to treat peptic ulcer disease, erosive oesophagitis and Zollinger Ellison syndrome. It is recommended that these are taken 20–30 min before meals to maximise the benefit [45].

If Helicobacter pylori is diagnosed in pregnancy, it is reasonable to treat with a PPI only to prevent complications of infection and prescribe eradication therapy post-partum. This will avoid the risk of using combinations of antibiotics in pregnancy and their side effects.

8.5.5 Coeliac Disease

In those with a diagnosis of Coeliac disease who are well-controlled on a gluten free diet, there is little evidence of suggest any specific impacts the disease may have upon pregnancy outcomes. Note must be taken, however, of those presenting with symptoms suggestive of coeliac disease. In this setting, it is recognised that undiagnosed/untreated coeliac disease is associated with a reduced mean birth weight and premature birth [46]. Impact on fertility is debated in the literature, but there is also some suggestion that it is reduced in the two years preceding a Coeliac diagnosis and, fortunately, rapidly normalises after commencement of treatment. Finally, links have been made between undiagnosed Coeliac disease and recurrent miscarriage [47]. Though these findings can't be condensed into one single recommendation, they do highlight the importance of early screening for Coeliac disease in patients with gastrointestinal symptoms, particularly those with sub-fertility or intra-uterine growth restriction.

8.5.6 Gallstone Disease

Gallstone disease is common in developed countries. In a person's lifetime, it can be present in up to 15% of the population. After appendicitis, gallstones are the second most common non-obstetric emergency in pregnancy [48]. Gallstone disease can affect up to 12% of pregnant women; Despite this there are no UK guidelines on the management of gallstones in pregnancy. If gallstones are symptomatic prior to pregnancy, surgical management is appropriate. For these that become symptomatic in pregnancy, management varies according to presentation. Acute cholecystitis can be managed conservatively with fluids and antibiotics. Gallstone pancreatitis is an indication for Endoscopic Retrograde Cholangiopancreatogram (ERCP), although the British Society of Gastroenterology (BSG) does not mention pregnancy in it's guidelines [49]. Choledocholithiasis with associated obstructive jaundice is an indication for ERCP and stone retrieval in pregnancy. The risk of ERCP is outweighed by the risk of sepsis and liver failure from bile duct obstruction. Again, once the bile duct is cleared, cholecystectomy can be carried out post-partum – indeed up to 3% of pregnant women in the US require cholecystectomy in the first year post-partum.

8.6 Conclusions

The physiological changes of pregnancy can lead to a variety of gastrointestinal symptoms. The main bowel condition requiring careful management during pregnancy is IBD. Though pregnancy itself does not worsen the disease, there is a complex interplay between with health of the mother and that of the foetus. Careful planning pre-pregnancy, maintenance of remission and individualised care both during the pregnancy and at the time of birth are the cornerstones of management.

Take Home Messages

- Pregnancy has an impact on existing GI issues as a result of the hormonal, circulatory and mechanical changes
- In patients with IBD (Ulcerative colitis and Crohn's disease), conception during disease remission is recommended
- Most IBD medications are safe in pregnancy and should be continued to reduce the risk of disease flare up
- Active disease increases the risk of miscarriage, pre-term labour and small for gestational age infants.
- Birth mode should be discussed with patients with IBD; Caesarean birth is recommended for those with active perianal Crohn's disease
- IBD flares can have a negative impact on pregnancy and should be treated quickly with steroids and escalation of treatment as in a non-pregnant state
- Infants exposed to biologic medications in pregnancy should not receive live vaccines in the first year of life
- IBS symptoms, namely constipation, often worsen in pregnancy; there is a paucity of research on the impact of IBS on pregnancy and IBS treatments in pregnancy.
- Gallstone disease is the second most common non obstetric emergency in pregnancy

Appendix: MCQ

Mark each item TRUE or FALSE

Questions

1. In terms of the physiological changes associated with pregnancy:
   (A) Pregnancy is generally associated with increase stool transit time and reduced stool volume, manifesting as constipation.
   (B) Progesterone production from the corpus luteum increases the rate of gastric emptying.
   (C) Pregnancy is associated with an increase in plasma volume of between 60-80%.
   (D) Pregnancy is typically associated with activation of the renin-angiotensin aldosterone system.
   (E) The placenta is involved with maternal increases in gastric acidity, via the production of gastrin.

2. With respect to the impact of pregnancy on blood results (haematology and clinical biochemistry):
   (A) Haemoglobin levels increase as normal pregnancy progresses.
   (B) Albumin levels fall as normal pregnancy progress.
   (C) Alkaline phosphatase falls during normal pregnancy.
   (D) Measurement of alkaline phosphatase isoenzymes can help identify to clinically relevant elevations.
   (E) Alanine aminotransferase increases during normal pregnancy.

3. With regard to the impact of IBD on fertility and pregnancy outcomes:
   (A) IBD is typically associated with reduced fertility rates.
   (B) Pregnancy increases risk of an IBD flare.
   (C) IBD has a negative impact on pregnancy outcomes regardless of disease state.

   (D) Active IBD is associated with an increased risk of stillbirth.
   (E) Active IBD is associated with an increased risk of preterm birth.

4. In IBD, the presence of active disease has the greatest negative impact on pregnancy relative to the drugs used to control it. However, there are exceptions. Which of the following medications can be continued in pregnancy?
   (A) Mesalazine
   (B) Azathioprine
   (C) Methotrexate
   (D) Anti-TNF
   (E) Small molecules

5. With regard to mode of delivery in patients with IBD:
   (A) The presence of isolated ileal Crohn's disease is an indication for caesarean birth.
   (B) The presence of active perianal Crohn's disease is an indication for caesarean birth.
   (C) Any previous surgery for IBD is an absolute indication for caesarean birth.
   (D) The presence of, or likely future need for, an Ileal-pouch anal anastomosis (IPAA) is a relative indication for caesarean birth.
   (E) Ulcerative colitis is associated with a higher rate of anal sphincter injury during spontaneous vaginal delivery.

Answers

1. In terms of the physiological changes associated with pregnancy:
   (A) TRUE
   (B) FALSE
   (C) FALSE
   (D) TRUE
   (E) TRUE

2. With respect to the impact of pregnancy on blood results (haematology and clinical biochemistry):
   (A) FALSE
   (B) TRUE
   (C) FALSE
   (D) TRUE
   (E) FALSE

3. With regard to the impact of IBD on fertility and pregnancy outcomes:
   (A) FALSE
   (B) FALSE, though the inappropriate withdrawal of treatment during pregnancy may do.
   (C) FALSE
   (D) TRUE
   (E) TRUE

4. In IBD, the presence of active disease has the greatest negative impact on pregnancy relative to the drugs used to control it. However, there are exceptions. Which of the following medications can be continued in pregnancy?
   (A) TRUE
   (B) TRUE
   (C) FALSE
   (D) TRUE
   (E) FALSE

5. With regard to mode of delivery in patients with IBD:
   (A) FALSE
   (B) TRUE
   (C) FALSE
   (D) TRUE
   (E) FALSE

References

1. Tan EK, Tank EL. Alterations in physiology and anatomy during pregnancy. Best Pract Res Clin Obstet Gynaecol. 2013;27(6):791–802.

2. Conklin KA. Maternal physiology adaptations during gestation, labour and the puerperium. Semin Anaesth. 1991;X(4):221–34.

3. Ohlsson B, et al. Oxytocin is expressed throughout the human gastrointestinal tract. Regul Pept. 2006;135(1–2):7–11.

4. Bernstein IM, et al. Plasma volume expansion in early pregnancy. Obstet Gynecol. 2001;97(5 Pt 1):669–7.

5. Bekheirnia MR, Schrier RW. Pathophysiology of water and sodium retention: edematous states with normal kidney function. Curr Opin Pharmacol. 2006;6(2):202–7.

6. Abbassi-Ghanavati M, Greer L, Cunningham GF. Pregnancy and laboratory studies: a reference table for clinicians. Obstet Gynecol. 2009;114(6): 1326–31.

7. Mullish BH, Quraishi MN, Segal JP, Ianiro G, Iqbal TH. The gut microbiome: what every gastroenterologist needs to know. Frontline Gastroenterol. 2021;12(2):118–27. https://doi.org/10.1136/flgastro-2019-101376.

8. Edwards SM, Cunningham SA, Dunlop AL, Corwin EJ. The maternal gut microbiome during pregnancy. MCN Am J Matern Child Nurs. 2017;42(6):310–7.

9. Zakaria ZZ, Al-Rumaihi S, Al-Absi RS, Farah H, Elamin M, Nader R, Bouabidi S, Suleiman SE, Nasr S, Al-Asmakh M. Physiological changes and interactions between microbiome and the host during pregnancy. Front Cell Infect Microbiol. 2022;12:824925.

10. Gomez-Arango LF, Barrett HL, McIntyre HD, Callaway LK, Morrison M, Dekker Nitert M. Connections between the gut microbiome and metabolic hormones in early pregnancy in overweight and obese women. Diabetes. 2016;65(8):2214–23. https://doi.org/10.2337/db16-0278.

11. Oliveira SB, Monteiro IM. Diagnosis and management of inflammatory bowel disease in children. BMJ. 2017;357. https://doi.org/10.1136/bmj.j2083.

12. Miller JP. Inflammatory bowel disease in pregnancy: a review. J R Soc Med. 1986;79:221–5.

13. O'Toole A, Nwanne O, Tomlinson T. Inflammatory bowel disease increases risk of adverse pregnancy outcomes: a meta-analysis. Dig Dis Sci. 2015;60:2750–61.

14. Mahadevan U, et al. Inflammatory bowel disease in pregnancy clinical care pathway: a report from the American Gastroenterological Association IBD Parenthood Project Working Group. Gastroenterology. 2019;156(5):1508–24.

15. Selinger CP, Ghorayeb J, Madill A. What factors might drive voluntary childlessness (VC) in women with IBD? Does IBD-specific pregnancy-related knowledge matter? J Crohns Colitis. 2016;10(10): 1151–8.

16. De Lima A, et al. Preconception care reduces relapse of inflammatory bowel disease during pregnancy. Clin Gastroenterol Hepatol. 2016;14(9):1285–92.

17. STRIDE-II: An Update on the Selecting Therapeutic Targets in Inflammatory Bowel Disease (STRIDE) Initiative of the International Organization for the Study of IBD (IOIBD): determining therapeutic goals for treat-to-target strategies in IBD. Gastroenterology, 2021;160(5);1570–83.

18. Torres J, Chaparro M, Julsgaard M, Katsanos K, Zelinkova Z, Agrawal M, Ardizzone S, Campmans-Kuijpers M, Dragoni G, Ferrante M, Fiorino G, Flanagan E, Gomes CF, Hart A, Hedin CR, Juillerat P, Mulders A, Myrelid P, O'Toole A, Rivière P, Scharl M, Selinger CP, Sonnenberg E, Toruner M, Jantien Wieringa C, Van der Woude J. European Crohn's and Colitis guidelines on sexuality, fertility, pregnancy, and lactation. J Crohn's Colitis. 2022;17:jjac115.

19. Mahadevan U, et al. Pregnancy and neonatal outcomes after fetal exposure to biologics and thiopurines among women with inflammatory bowel disease. Gastroenterology. 2021;160(4):1131–9.

20. Nielsen OH, Andreasson B, Bondesen S, Jarnum S. Pregnancy in ulcerative colitis. Scand J Gastroenterol. 1983;18(6):735–42.

21. Murphy VE, Fittock RJ, Zarzycki PK, Delahunty MM, Smith R, Clifton VL. Metabolism of synthetic steroids by the human placenta. Placenta. 2007;28:39–46. https://doi.org/10.1016/j.placenta.2005.12.010.

22. Ordás I, et al. Ulcerative colitis. Lancet. 2012;380(9853):1606–19.

23. Cornish JA, et al. The effect of restorative proctocolectomy on sexual function, urinary function, fertility, pregnancy and delivery: a systematic review. Dis Colon Rectum. 2007 Aug;50(8):1128–38.

24. Beyer-Berjot L, et al. A total laparoscopic approach reduces the infertility rate after ileal pouch-anal anastomosis: a 2-center study. Ann Surg. 2013;258:275–82.

25. Ban L, Tata LJ, Humes DJ, Fiaschi L, Card T. Decreased fertility rates in 9639 women diagnosed with inflammatory bowel disease: a United Kingdom population-based cohort study. Aliment Pharmacol Ther. 2015;42(7):855–66.

26. Blackwell S, Selinger C, Brookes M, et al. PMO-32 Pregnancy outcomes after stoma surgery for IBD: the results of a multi-centre retrospective audit. Gut. 2021;70:A93.

27. Selinger CP, Nelson-Piercy C, Fraser A, Hall V, Limdi J, Smith L, Smith M, Nasur R, Gunn M, King A, Mohan A, Mulgabal K, Kent A, Kok KB, Glanville T. IBD in pregnancy: recent advances, practical management. Frontline Gastroenterol. 2020;12(3):214–24.

28. Nguyen et al. Outcomes of obstetric hospitalizations among women with inflammatory bowel disease in the United States. Clin Gastroenterol Hepatol 2009;7(3):329–334.

29. NICE guideline [NG192] Published: 31 March 2021.

30. American Academy of Pediatrics. Guidelines for perinatal care. Elk Grove Village, IL: American Academy of Pediatrics; 2017.

31. Lacy BE, Patel NK. Rome criteria and a diagnostic approach to irritable bowel syndrome. J Clin Med. 2017;6(11):99.

32. Canavan C, West J, Card T. The epidemiology of irritable bowel syndrome. Clin Epidemiol. 2014;6:71–80.

33. Khashan AS, Quigley EM, McNamee R, McCarthy FP, Shanahan F, Kenny LC. Increased risk of miscarriage and ectopic pregnancy among women with irritable bowel syndrome. Clin Gastroenterol Hepatol. 2012 Aug;10(8):902–9.

34. Irritable bowel syndrome in adults: diagnosis and management. NICE clinical guideline CG61.

35. McKenzie YA, Bowyer RK, Leach H, Gulia P, Horobin J, O'Sullivan NA, Pettitt C, Reeves LB, Seamark L, Williams M, Thompson J, Lomer MC; (IBS Dietetic Guideline Review Group on behalf of Gastroenterology Specialist Group of the British Dietetic Association). British Dietetic Association systematic review and evidence-based practice guidelines for the dietary management of irritable bowel syndrome in adults (2016 update). J Hum Nutr Diet. 2016;29(5):549–75.

36. Moayyedi P, Quigley EM, Lacy BE, et al. The effect of fiber supplementation on irritable bowel syndrome: a systematic review and meta-analysis. Am J Gastroenterol. 2014;109:1367–74.

37. Sarvee M, Pimentel M, Wong MS, Rezaie A. Irritable bowel syndrome in pregnancy. Am J Gastroenterol. 2021;116(3):480–90.

38. Gomes CF, Sousa M, Lourenço I, Martins D, Torres J. Gastrointestinal diseases during pregnancy: what does the gastroenterologist need to know? Ann Gastroenterol. 2018;31(4):385–94.

39. Constella (Linaclotide) [product monograph]. Allergan, Markham, ON, 2018. https://pdf.hres.ca/dpd_pm/00047072.PDF. Accessed 20 Oct 2020.

40. Prucalopride. In chronic constipation: poorly documented risks. Prescrire Int. 2011;20:117–20.

41. Staroselsky A, Nava-Ocampo AA, Vohra S, Koren G. Hemorrhoids in pregnancy. Can Fam Physician. 2008;54(2):189–90. PMID: 18272631; PMCID: PMC2278306

42. Vazquez JC. Constipation, haemorrhoids, and heartburn in pregnancy. BMJ Clin Evid. 2010 Aug;3(2010):1411.

43. Leiman DA, Riff BP, Morgan S, Metz DC, Falk GW, French B, Umscheid CA, Lewis JD. Alginate therapy is effective treatment for GERD symptoms: a systematic review and meta-analysis. Dis Esophagus. 2017;30(5):1–9.

44. Gill SK, O'Brien L, Koren G. The safety of histamine 2 (H2) blockers in pregnancy: a meta-analysis. Dig Dis Sci. 2009;54(9):1835–8.

45. Gill SK, O'Brien L, Einarson TR, Koren G. The safety of proton pump inhibitors (PPIs) in pregnancy: a meta-analysis. Am J Gastroenterol. 2009;104(6):1541–5.

46. Butler MM, Kenny LC, McCarthy FP. Coeliac disease and pregnancy outcomes. Obstet Med. 2011;4(3):95–8.

47. Casella G, Orfanotti G, Giacomantonio L, Bella CD, Crisafulli V, Villanacci V, Baldini V, Bassotti G. Celiac disease and obstetrical-gynecological contribution. Gastroenterol Hepatol Bed Bench. 2016;9(4):241–9.

48. Hess E, Thumbadoo RP, Thorne E, McNamee K. Gallstones in pregnancy. Br J Hosp Med (Lond). 2021;82(2):1–8.

49. Williams E, Beckingham I, El Sayed G, Gurusamy K, Sturgess R, Webster G, Young T. Updated guideline on the management of common bile duct stones (CBDS). Gut. 2017;66:765–82.

Perineal and Anal Sphincter Wound Healing Complications

9

Nicola Adanna Okeahialam, Ranee Thakar, and Abdul H. Sultan

Overview

Test your learning and check your understanding of this book's contents: use the "Springer Nature Flashcards" app to access questions using ▶ https://sn.pub/wqrf89. To use the app, please follow the instructions in Chap. 1.

Learning Objectives

- Understand the progression of healing of perineal wounds complicated by wound infection or dehiscence
- Identify causes of delayed wound healing in perineal wounds complicated by wound infection or dehiscence
- Learn how to assess perineal wound complications
- Learn the conservative and surgical management of perineal wound complications
- Understand the preventative methods that can be utilised to reduce the occurrence of perineal wound complications

N. A. Okeahialam (✉)
Croydon University Hospital, Thornton Heath, UK
e-mail: nicola.okeahialam@nhs.net

R. Thakar · A. H. Sultan
Croydon University Hospital, London, UK
e-mail: ranee.thakar@nhs.net; abdulsultan@nhs.net

9.1 Introduction

Perineal trauma following vaginal birth is very common, with 9 out of 10 women being affected [1]. Women who require an episiotomy or sustain an obstetric anal sphincter injury (OASI) are more likely to report a negative birth experience in the immediate post-partum period [2]. It is well documented that maternal morbidity is common after childbirth, as 87% of mothers report complications within 8 weeks and 76% up to 18 months after delivery [3]. This is particularly with regards to perineal wound healing and its potential complications, including wound infection and dehiscence, which are a major source of anxiety reported by mothers within in the first month following perineal trauma [4, 5]. Furthermore, these complications can be severe and lead to perinatal mortality. The Mothers and Babies: Reducing Risk through Audit and Confidential Enquiries (MMBRACE) report found that between 2006 and 2008, seven women had died from perinatal sepsis following vaginal birth, one of whom was following wound infection of a second-degree perineal tear [6]. However, despite this, postnatal maternity services give little priority to perineal health concerns, subsequently leading women to feel unsupported by health care professionals [7, 8]. This is probably due to the poor understanding by clinicians of normal and disrupted perineal wound healing process following childbirth. Moreover, many women will not seek help from a health care professional as perineal morbidity is often considered an embarrassing and taboo subject, causing women to feel isolated further [8]. To address this, since the early 2000s, there has been an increase in specialised perineal services, which allow the provision of evidence based, standardised care by experienced clinicians, to mothers with perineal complications following vaginal delivery [9–11]. The dedicated perineal clinic at Croydon University Hospital has been established since 2002 and is run by a consultant urogynaecologist and a specialist perineal midwife. Women can self-refer themselves to this clinic or be referred by their midwife or general practitioner. There were 765 new referrals with perineal complications to the clinic from January 2006 to December 2016. In 31% this was due to perineal wound infection and 27% due to perineal wound dehiscence [9]. Other postpartum problems and the role of the perineal clinic is described in Chap. 10.

In this chapter, the management of wound healing complications including wound infection and dehiscence following perineal and anal sphincter trauma will be discussed.

9.2 Normal Wound Healing

Wounds, due to acute tissue injury are stimulated to heal in four overlapping phases; this includes bleeding and haemostasis, inflammation, proliferation and remodelling (Fig. 9.1) [13, 14]. At the time of injury, vasoconstriction occurs to stem the blood loss from injured blood vessels and platelets aggregate to fill the wound with a fibrin clot [14–16]. Once the bleeding has stopped, blood vessels dilate to allows the entry of blood, fluid and inflammatory cells [14, 16]. During the inflammatory phase, neutrophils monocytes and macrophages degrade necrotic tissue, debris and local bacteria from the wound [15, 16]. Once the wound is cleaned, fibroblasts begin the proliferative stage and the fibrin clot matures into collagen-based granulation tissue and new blood vessels are formed [15, 16]. The final phase of the wound healing cascade is remodelling, where collagen maturation occurs [15, 16]. The wound then becomes avascular and a scar is formed [17, 18].

However, complications of wound healing can occur including, wound infection and dehiscence. In perineal wounds specifically, this can lead to further complications including pain, persistent granulation tissue, scar tissue and fistula. This not only affects women physically but can also significantly impact women psychologically [19].

Fig. 9.1 Mechanism of wound healing. (Reproduced with permission [12])

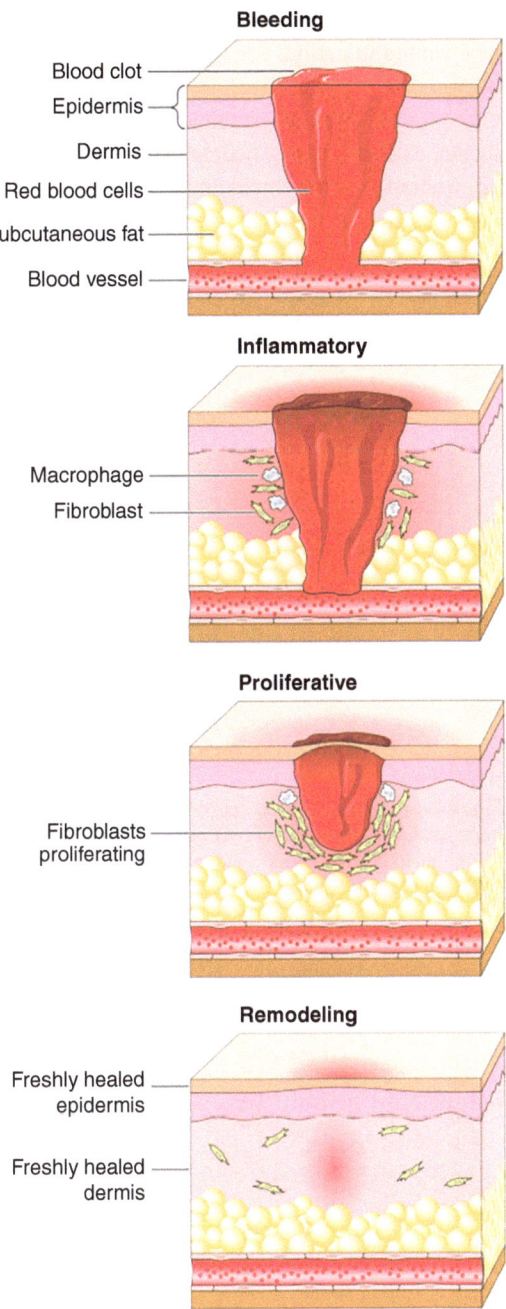

Bleeding

Blood clot
Epidermis
Dermis
Red blood cells
Subcutaneous fat
Blood vessel

Inflammatory

Macrophage
Fibroblast

Proliferative

Fibroblasts proliferating

Remodeling

Freshly healed epidermis

Freshly healed dermis

9.3 Perineal Wound Infection

9.3.1 Definition

There is a wide variation in the definition of perineal wound infection in the literature.

Wound infection can occur at a superficial level which can extend and cause deep (fascial/muscle layer) or organ space infection. Deep wound infection may be diagnosed by the presence of an abscess, wound dehiscence of the deep fascial layers and systemic signs such as fever. Organ space infection occurs when wound infection has seeded to the surrounding anatomy that was not involved in the initial primary infection and can be detected on anatomical, histopathological or radiological examination [20]. In perineal wound infection, 8% will be superficial, 5% deep and <1% organ space [21]. Features of perineal wound infection include local pain, erythema, exudate, odour, oedema and pyrexia with or without wound breakdown. As shown in Fig. 9.2 and 9.3, signs and symptoms of wound

infection may include the presence of markers such as perineal pain, purulent discharge and wound dehiscence of the surgical repair [23]. Outcome reporting in childbirth trauma research is heterogeneous. Developing, disseminating, and implementing a core outcome set in future childbirth trauma research could help address these issues [24].

9.3.2 Pathophysiology

Under normal conditions, bacteria, viruses and fungi colonise the outermost layer of the skin: the epidermis, and protect the host from overgrowth of potential pathogenic bacteria [25]. This stable ecosystem of microorganisms has an intricate relationship with the skin and its protective function [26]. However, all microorganisms have the potential to cause disease. Factors that can increase the risk of disease include the concentration of microorganisms, their virulence and the host resistance to infection [27, 28].

Normally, the epidermis is shed to remove the bacteria colonising its surface, meaning bacterial loads are higher in areas of increased moisture and hence less skin shedding [29]. In addition,

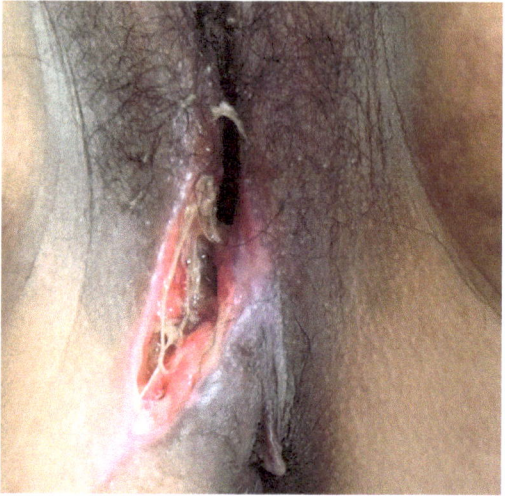

Fig. 9.2 A perineal wound (episiotomy) with a wound infection and dehiscence. Purulent discharge and loose suture material are noted within the wound. Patient informed consent obtained

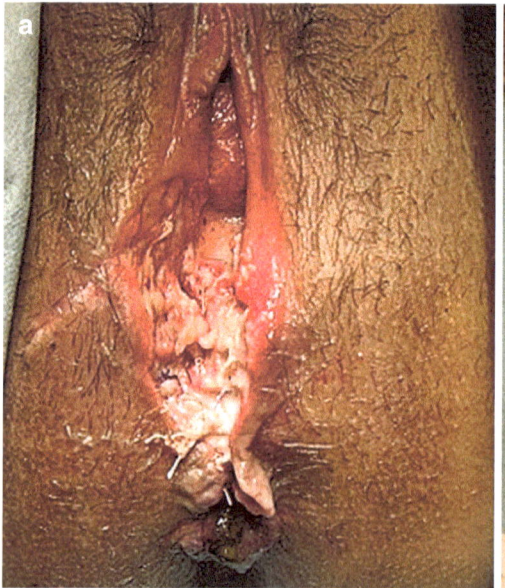
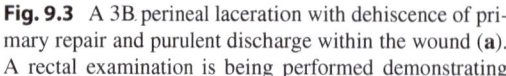
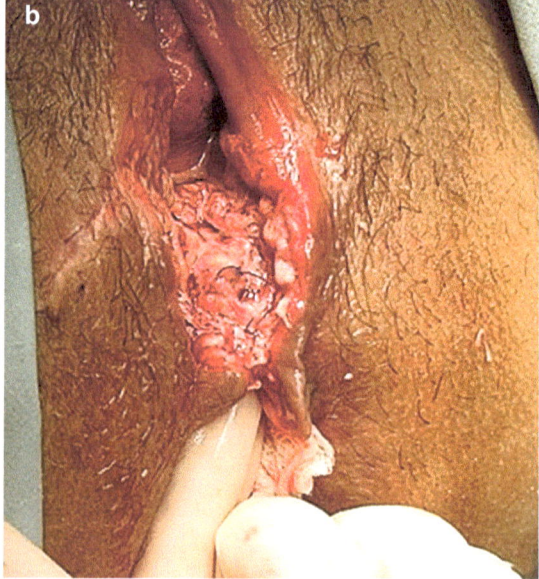

Fig. 9.3 A 3B perineal laceration with dehiscence of primary repair and purulent discharge within the wound (**a**). A rectal examination is being performed demonstrating dehiscence of the anal sphincter repair (**b**). (Reproduced with permission [22])

microorganism proliferate in warm environments [30]. As the perineum is an area of significant moisture and high surface temperature, in the presence of injury, it is a favourable environment for bacteria. Furthermore, due to its anatomical location, wound contamination can occur from the surrounding skin, genitourinary tract, gastrointestinal tract or the external environment leading to infection [31]. Examples of bacteria colonising the body surface of areas with high moisture, such as the perineum include *Staphylococcus aureus, Enterococcus, Corynebacterium, Acinetobacter and Proteus.*

If wound bacteria multiply above a critical level, this stimulates a prolonged immune response at a local and systemic level [26, 30]. In infected perineal wounds, the prolonged host response can result in signs as symptoms such as perineal pain, oedema, purulent discharge, wound dehiscence and fever. However, it is important to note that erythema, heat and oedema of a wound can also be a normal response to wound healing in the absence of infection [15].

9.3.3 Microbiology

Table 9.1 highlights the pathogens most commonly identified in perineal wound infection from the literature. The most commonly isolated pathogens in infected perineal wounds include *Escherichia spp., Staphylococcus spp., Streptococcus spp.* and both aerobic and anaerobic bacteria. However, perineal wound infections are often polymicrobial due to the complex microflora of the surrounding genitourinary and gastrointestinal tract [46]. The surface of any open wound will often be colonised with bacteria, and wound healing can occur even in the presence of bacteria [47]. This means that any microbial swab taken from the perineum, even in the absence of infection will likely isolate a number of microorganisms. Therefore, diagnosis of wound infection should be made on assessment of clinical signs and symptoms, and the results of microbiological analysis results used to guide management [48]. The critical level at which bacteria stimulate a host immune response, leading

Table 9.1 Microorganisms causing perineal wound infection following childbirth

Organisms	Author
Gram positive cocci	
Staphylococcus spp.	Ajibade et al. [32]
	Arendsen et al. [33]
	Fox [34]
	Rotas et al. [35]
	Sule and Shittu [36]
	Zhang and Han [37]
Streptococcus spp.	Ajibade et al. [32]
	Almarzouqi et al. [38]
	Arendsen et al. [33]
	Chua et al. [39]
	Fox [34]
	Shy and Eschenbach [40]
	Wiseman et al. [41],
Enterococcus spp.	Ajibade et al. [32]
	Häusler et al. [42]
	Tsenov et al. [43]
Gram positive rods	
Escherichia spp.	Almarzouqi et al. [38]
	Fox [34]
	Häusler et al. [42]
	Shy and Eschenbach [40]
	Sule and Shittu [36]
	Tsenov et al. [43]
	Zhang and Han [37]
Gram negative aerobic	
Acinetobacter spp.	Zhang and Han [37]
Pseudomonas spp.	Ajibade et al. [32]
	Zhang and Han [37]
Enterobacter spp.	Zhang and Han [37]
Proteus spp.	Rai et al. [44]
Mixed anaerobes	Arendsen et al. [33]
	Fox [34]
Gram negative rods	
Bacteroides spp.	Almarzouqi et al. [38]
	Fox [34]
	Shy and Eschenbach [40]
Gardnerella spp.	Fox [34]
Coliforms	Ajibade et al. [32]
	Arendsen et al. [33]
Anaerobic	
Klebsiella spp.	Fox [34]
	Rai et al. [44]
	Shy and Eschenbach [40]
Clostridium spp.	Shy and Eschenbach [40]
Fungi	
Candida spp.	Ajibade et al. [32]
	Fox [34]
	Zhang and Han [37]
Saccharomyces spp.	Zhang and Han [37]

Reproduced with permission [45]

to infection has been reported to be >10⁴ CFU/g on quantitative microbiological analysis. However, in the presence of sutures, the bacterial count required to cause wound infection may decrease to >10² CFU/g [49]. Semi-quantitative analysis is another technique in microbiological analysis where results are reported as none (0), light (1+) moderate (2+ to 3+) or heavy (4+) growth [50]. It is important to identify wounds with signs of infection to avoid unnecessary antibiotic provision in the presence of normal wound bacterial colonisation alone. Antimicrobial stewardship is a significant health priority and the overuse of antimicrobials is associated with antimicrobial resistance [51].

9.3.4 Incidence

There is a huge variation in the reported incidence of perineal wound infection following childbirth. In a systematic review of 17 observational studies (40,182 women), Jones et al. [52] found that the reported incidence of perineal wound infection in all degrees of perineal tears including OASI ranged from 0.1% to 23.6%. An explanation for this wide range is the lack of a standardised definition of infection. Table 9.2 lists the studies reporting the incidence of perineal wound infection identified from this review. Of the 17 observational studies, only 5 reported the incidence of perineal wound infection in

Table 9.2 The incidence of perineal wound infection and dehiscence with childbirth-related perineal trauma

Author	Date	Country	Outcome	Time point	No. of participants	No. of cases	%
Allen et al. [53]	2006	Canada	Infection	Unclear	24,609	188	0.76%
Calvia et al. [54]	2016	UK	Infection	Up to 28 days	36	5	14%
Clement and Reed [55]	1999	UK	Infection	Unclear	106	2	2%
Edwards et al. [56]	1978	USA	Infection	Unclear	416	10	2.40%
Fodstad et al. [57]	2014	Norway	Infection	Unclear	179	17	9.40%
Goldaber et al. [58]	1992	USA	Infection	Unclear	390	14	3.58%
Harris [59]	1970	USA	Infection	Unclear	870	1	0.10%
Johnson et al. [23]	2012	UK	Infection	Up to 21 days	341	39	11%
Lam et al. [60]	2006	Hong Kong	Infection	Unclear	6167	13	0.20%
Lewicky-Gaupp et al. [61]	2015	USA	Infection	Day 7	268	53	19.77%
O'Leary and O'Leary [62]	1965	USA	Infection	Unclear	1224	9	0.73%
Ridley [63]	2015	UK	Infection	Within 28 days	262	31	11.83%
Stock et al. [64]	2013	USA	Infection	Unclear	909	39	4.20%
Sule and Shittu [36]	2003	Nigeria	Infection	Day 7	76	18	23.68%
Wiseman et al. [41]	2018	UK	Infection	Unclear	828	14	1.7%
Yokoe et al. [65]	2001	USA	Infection	Unclear	2301	7	0.30%
Zhang and Han [37]	2017	China	Infection	Unclear	1200	30	2.50%
Ajibade et al. [32]	2013	UK	Dehiscence	Unclear	3218	19	0.59%
Glazener et al. [66]	1995	UK	Dehiscence	0–13 days	1068	18	1.68%
Goldaber et al. [58]	1992	USA	Dehiscence	Unclear	390	18	4.61%
Jallad et al. [67]	2016	USA	Dehiscence	Unclear	68,839	144	0.21%
Johnson et al. [23]	2012	UK	Dehiscence	Up to 21 days	341	35	10%
Lewicky-Gaupp et al. [61]	2015	USA	Dehiscence	Unclear	268	66	24.60%
Otoide et al. [68]	1999	Nigeria	Dehiscence	Unclear	627	36	5.70%
Stock et al. 2013 [64]	2013	USA	Dehiscence	Unclear	909	36	3.96%
Sule and Shittu [36]	2003	Nigeria	Dehiscence	Day 7	76	11	14.40%
Wilkie et al. [69]	2018	USA	Dehiscence	Unclear	334	7	2.10%
Wiseman et al. [41]	2018	UK	Dehiscence	Unclear	828	2	0.24%
Stock et al. [70]	2013	UK	Combined	Unclear	848	12	1.40%

Reproduced with permission [52]

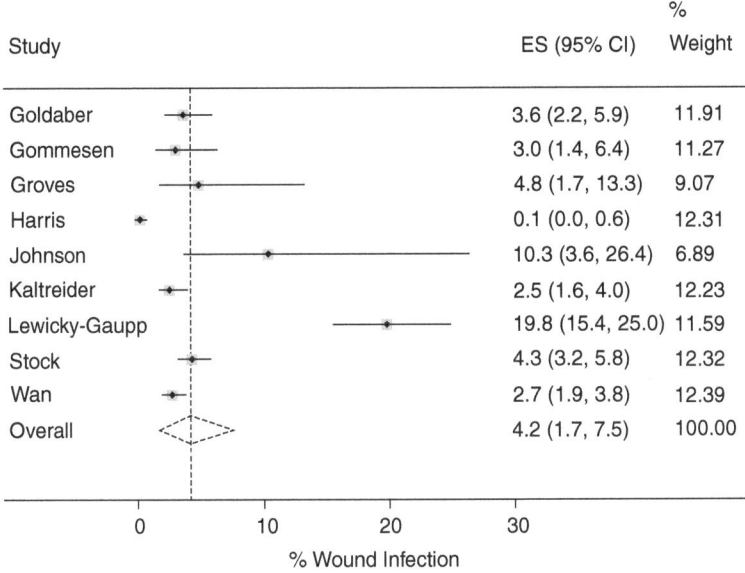

Study		ES (95% CI)	% Weight
Goldaber		3.6 (2.2, 5.9)	11.91
Gommesen		3.0 (1.4, 6.4)	11.27
Groves		4.8 (1.7, 13.3)	9.07
Harris		0.1 (0.0, 0.6)	12.31
Johnson		10.3 (3.6, 26.4)	6.89
Kaltreider		2.5 (1.6, 4.0)	12.23
Lewicky-Gaupp		19.8 (15.4, 25.0)	11.59
Stock		4.3 (3.2, 5.8)	12.32
Wan		2.7 (1.9, 3.8)	12.39
Overall		4.2 (1.7, 7.5)	100.00

% Wound Infection

Patient group	Number studies	Heterogeneity p-value I^2	Pooled Incidence (%) (95% CI)
Wound infection	9	<0.001 95%	4.2% (1.7%, 7.5%)

Fig. 9.4 The pooled incidence of wound infection (no dehiscence) following primary OASI repair. (Reproduced with permission [74])

women with an intact anal sphincter [37, 41, 55, 57, 65]. The range of perineal wound infection in these studies ranged between 0.3% and 9.4%. Nine cohort studies have reported the incidence of wound infection following primary surgical repair of OASIs ranging between 0.1% and 19.8% [9, 23, 58, 59, 61, 64, 71–73]. The overall incidence of wound infection following primary OASI repair, obtained by combining the results of these studies (4593 women) is 4.2% (95% CI 1.7–7.5%) (Fig. 9.4) [74].

9.3.5 Risk Factors

Factors in pregnancy and delivery associated with perineal wound infection identified from observational studies in the literature are summarised in Table 9.3. In a retrospective cohort study of 1200 women, Zhang and Han found that after controlling for confounding factors, raised BMI, repeated vaginal examinations, increased postoperative stay, premature rupture of mem-

branes and puerperal genital tract infection were associated with perineal wound infection [37]. Additionally, OASI has also been identified to be a risk factor for perineal wound infection in two studies, increasing its incidence approximately four-fold [67, 76]. Lewicky-Gaupp et al. [61] prospectively studied 268 women with OASI and demonstrated that operative vaginal birth was associated with wound complications such as infection, dehiscence or both (OR 2.54 [95%CI 1.32–4.87]), whilst intrapartum antibiotic use for obstetric indication decreased the risk of complications (OR 0.50 [9%CI 0.27–0.94]).

The effect of administering prophylactic antibiotics after operative vaginal birth to reduce the risk of maternal infection, has been evaluated in the ANODE trial (a randomised controlled trial [RCT] of prophylactic ANtibiotics to investigate the prevention of infection following Operative vaginal DElivery) [21]. This RCT of 3427 women from 27 maternity units in the United Kingdom found that the provision of

Table 9.3 Literature review of studies investigating risk factors for perineal wound infection following childbirth

Authors	Type of study Number in study Proportion with wound infection	Independent risk factors	Odds ratio (95% CI)
Edwards et al. [56]	Retrospective case control 416 2.40%	Obesity	9.36 (1.17–74.57)
Gommeson et al. [71]	Prospective cohort 400 5.75%	BMI >35 kg/m^2 BMI (1-unit increase) Episiotomy	7.66 (2.13–27.5) 1.12 (1.04–1.22) 2.97 (1.05–8.41)
Jallad et al. [67]	Retrospective case control 288 0.21%	Smoking Previous vaginal delivery OASI Episiotomy Instrumental delivery Midwife vs doctor repairing Chromic vs polyglactin	6.5 (1.20–38.5) 0.14 (0.05–0.30) 4.0 (1.10–15.70) 11.1 (2.9–48.8) 3.4 (1.20–10.30) 4.7 (1.50–15.80) 3.9 (1.60–9.80)
Johnson et al. [23]	Prospective audit 341 11.00%	Prolonged rupture of membranes Instrumental delivery Episiotomy	4.11 (1.48–11.37) 3.33 (1.21–9.18) 2.82 (1.21–6.58)
Lewicky-Gaupp et al.[a] [61]	Prospective cohort 268 19.8%	Instrumental delivery Antibiotic use	2.54 (1.32–4.87) 0.50 (0.27–0.94)
Macleod et al. [75]	Prospective cohort 1360 4.26%	Operative vaginal delivery and mediolateral episiotomy	4.04 (1.44–11.37)
Stock et al.[a] [64]	Retrospective cohort 909 3.96%	Instrumental delivery BMI (1-unit increase) Smoking Intrapartum antibiotics Postpartum antibiotics	1.76 (1.15–2.68) 1.06 (1.01–1.12) 4.04 (1.40–12.2) 0.29 (0.14–0.59) 2.46 (1.11–5.63)
Wilkie [69]	Retrospective cohort 529 2.10%	Opiod use post-partum Forceps Episiotomy	21.29 (5.43–83.47) 6.73 (1.99–22.78) 3.74 (1.08–12.95)
Williams and Chames [76]	Retrospective case control 117 40.70%	OASI Meconium Prolonged second stage Operative vaginal delivery and mediolateral episiotomy	3.70 (1.51–9.08) 3.22 (1.32–7.88) 3.07 (1.38–6.81) 6.36 (2.18–18.57)
Zhang and Han [37]	Retrospective Cohort 1200 2.50%	BMI >28 kg/m^2 Number of vaginal examinations >3 Postoperative hospitalisation >5 days Premature rupture of membranes Puerperal reproductive tract infection Comorbidities e.g. diabetes	2.14 (1.12–4.09) 1.85 (1.16–2.95) 2.62 (1.36–5.03) 1.62 (1.06–2.50) 1.87 (1.05–3.30) 2.02 (1.22–3.35)

[a]Women with OASI only included in this study

Amoxicillin and Clavulanic acid in comparison to placebo significantly reduced the risk of superficial perineal wound infection by 47% (OR 0.53 [95%CI 0.37–0.75]) and deep wound infection by 53% (OR 0.46 [95%CI 0.28–0.77]) [21]. As a result, in 2020 the Royal College of Obstetricians and Gynaecologists recommended the routine administration of a single prophylactic dose of intravenous Amoxicillin and Clavulanic acid following operative vaginal birth [77]. However, with episiotomy following spontaneous vaginal birth there is insufficient evidence to support the use of routine antibiotic provision [78].

9.4 Perineal Wound Dehiscence

9.4.1 Definition

Perineal wound dehiscence occurs when there is partial or complete separation of previously approximated wound edges. Following surgical repair of the perineum or anal sphincter this may involve separation of all layers of the repair, including the vaginal mucosa and perineal muscles (Superficial Transverse Perineal and Bulbospongiosus muscles). Following repair of OASIs, the external anal sphincter (EAS), internal anal sphincter (IAS) or anal epithelium can dehisce.

9.4.2 Pathophysiology

Perineal wound dehiscence often occurs concurrently with perineal wound infection [79]. However, wound dehiscence can occur in the absence of infection due to other factors which increase the stress placed on the suture line. This includes excessive tension or poor alignment of sutures, wound oedema (a normal healing response) and any local bleeding or haematoma. Additionally, other contributory factors can affect normal wound healing such as smoking, diabetes and immunocompromised states [80]. Traumatic disruption of repair of OASIs can also occur, and therefore stool softeners following surgical repair are recommended, as passage of hard stool may physically disrupt the sphincter repair [81, 82]. However, wound dehiscence may also be the initial presenting symptom in women with undiagnosed OASIs (therefore not repaired at delivery).

Taithongchai et al. [83] demonstrated in their cohort study of 40 women with missed OASIs that two women were referred to the dedicated perineal clinic with perineal wound dehiscence. Other reasons for referral included anorectal symptoms such as faecal incontinence, faecal urgency or flatal incontinence in 78%, perineal pain in 5% and a deficient perineum in 5%. Okeahialam et al. [84] found that that in their cohort of 56 dehisced perineal wounds, five (9%) women had an undiagnosed OASI. The presence of OASI (diagnosed and undiagnosed), was found to be a significant predictor of delayed perineal wound healing (>4 weeks) and reduced the odds of healing within 4 weeks by 89% (OR 0.11 (95% CI 0.02–0.77)) [85]. Of the undiagnosed OASIs in the study cohort, all had an operative vaginal birth and four women had a mediolateral episiotomy. Therefore, clinicians should consider the possibility of an undiagnosed OASI in dehisced perineal wounds with evidence of delayed healing particularly in women with risk factors for OASI such as operative vaginal birth [86].

9.4.3 Incidence

Similar to perineal wound infection, the incidence of wound dehiscence varies greatly in the literature. In the systematic review by Jones et al. [52], from 10 observational studies (73,680 women), the incidence of perineal wound dehiscence in all degrees of perineal tears including OASI ranged between 0.6% to 24.6% (Table 9.2). Of the 10 observational studies, only 1 reported the incidence of perineal wound infection in women with an intact anal sphincter (0.24%) [41]. With respect of OASI specifically, nine cohort studies (3866 women) have described the rate of dehiscence following primary OASI repair. Figure 9.5 demonstrates the pooled incidence of the studies: 6.9% (95% CI 1.6%–12.2%) [74].

Fig. 9.5 The pooled incidence of wound dehiscence following primary OASI repair. (Reproduced with permission [74])

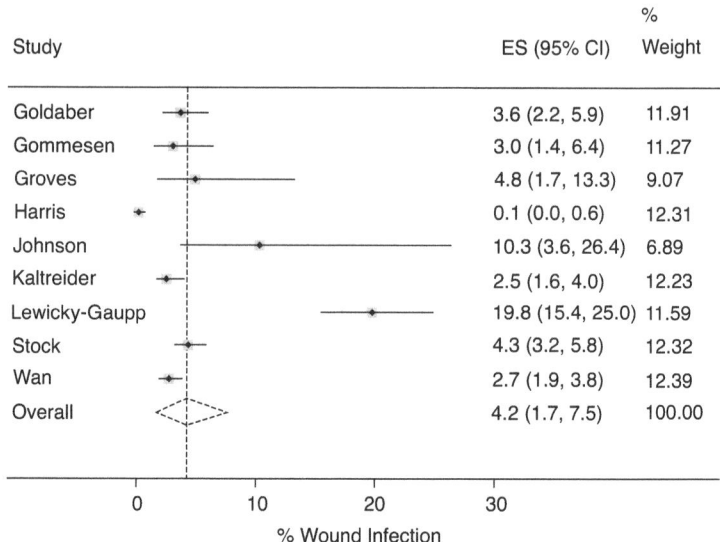

Study	ES (95% CI)	% Weight
Goldaber	3.6 (2.2, 5.9)	11.91
Gommesen	3.0 (1.4, 6.4)	11.27
Groves	4.8 (1.7, 13.3)	9.07
Harris	0.1 (0.0, 0.6)	12.31
Johnson	10.3 (3.6, 26.4)	6.89
Kaltreider	2.5 (1.6, 4.0)	12.23
Lewicky-Gaupp	19.8 (15.4, 25.0)	11.59
Stock	4.3 (3.2, 5.8)	12.32
Wan	2.7 (1.9, 3.8)	12.39
Overall	4.2 (1.7, 7.5)	100.00

% Wound Infection

Patient group	Number studies	Heterogeneity p-value	I²	Pooled Incidence (%) (95% CI)
Wound infection	9	<0.001	95%	4.2% (1.7%, 7.5%)

9.4.4 Risk Factors

Factors in pregnancy and delivery associated with perineal wound dehiscence are similar to those associated with wound infection. Suture material can act as a nidus for bacterial biofilm formation [87]. The PERINEAL study (A *Prospective observational study evaluating the sonographic appearance of the anal sphincter in women with wound infection following vaginal delivery*) performed by Okeahialam et al. [85] demonstrated that in their cohort of 80 infected perineal wounds, the use of a subcuticular repair reduced the odds of significant bacterial colonisation by 80% (OR 0.20 [95%CI 0.50–0.90]). Therefore, a continuous subcuticular technique in comparison to interrupted sutures should be considered for repair of perineal injuries, as less suture material is exposed, thereby reducing the risk of contamination from the surrounding environment. A Cochrane review of 16 studies, involving 8184 women, found that a continuous suture technique compared with interrupted for perineal closure (for all layers or perineal skin only) was also associated with a 44% reduction

in need for suture removal up to 3 months postpartum (RR 0.56 [95% CI 0.32–0.98]) [88].

9.5 Objective Assessment of Wound Healing Complications

Initial assessment should first include a detailed history, followed by examination:

1. Informed consent should be obtained for assessment of the perineum and combined vaginal and rectal examination.
2. Assist the woman into a comfortable position for the examination.
3. Ensure there is good exposure of the perineum with good lighting.
4. Offer inhalation analgesia if required, to allow unrestricted examination.
5. A systematic examination of the perineal wound should be completed including the assessment of:
   (a) Pain
   (b) Discharge

(c) Redness

(d) Oedema

(e) Presence of dehiscence (vagina or perineum)
   (i) Length, depth and width measurements
   (ii) Dehiscence close to the anus

(f) Any other abnormality

6. A rectal examination should also be performed to check for any suspected undiagnosed injury to the anal sphincter.

7. A wound swab should be taken to for microbiological confirmation.

Tools can be used to provide clinicians with a framework to systematically assess perineal wound complications. The REEDA (*Redness*, o*E*dema, *Ecchymosis*, *Discharge*, and *Approximation*) tool, which was first described by Davidson in 1974 is an example, and has a maximum score of 15, indicating the worst healing outcome (Table 9.4) [90]. The agreement of this scoring system between clinicians has been assessed by Alvarenga et al. [91] at 7–10 days post-partum and was found to be good to excellent. However, it is important to note that in their cohort of 54 women, 89% described their skin colour as white or mixed. In darker pigmented skin tones it should be considered that as well as redness, inflammation may cause other colour changes such as purple, grey, brown, dark brown or black [92].

9.5.1 Advanced Wound Assessment

Advances have been made in wound care to aid clinicians to accurately perineal wound complications. This includes imaging devices which allow real-time diagnosis of wound infection and accurate three-dimensional measurement of wound size. The MolecuLight i:X imaging device (MolecuLight, Toronto, Canada) uses bacterial fluorescence imaging technology to evaluate wounds with significant bacterial loads, at levels that are agreed to cause wound infection on traditional microbiological analysis [93, 94]. In the PERINEAL study, Okeahialam et al. [95] found that bacterial fluorescence imaging had excellent accuracy in the diagnosis of infected perineal wounds, with a positive predictive value of 92% (95% CI 0.74–0.98) and a negative predictive value of 80% (95% CI 0.58–0.92). In addition, the presence of exposed suture material increased the odds of bacterial fluorescence three-fold (OR 2.95 (95% CI 1.03–8.45)) [95]. Figure 9.6 shows images of infected perineal wounds with bacterial fluorescence present within exposed suture material. With dehisced perineal wounds, the presence of bacterial fluorescence is a significant predictor of delayed wound healing, and has been shown to reduce the odds of wound healing within 4 weeks by 76% (OR 0.24 (95%CI 0.07–0.81)) [85]. As bacterial fluorescence is associated with delayed perineal wound healing, and exposed suture material is a nidus for bacterial

Table 9.4 The REEDA wound assessment tool

Score	Redness	Oedema	Ecchymosis	Discharge	Approximation
0	None	None	None	None	Closed
1	Within 0.25 cm of incision bilaterally	<1 cm from incision	Within 0.25 cm of incision bilaterally or 0.5 cm unilaterally	Serum	Skin separation ≤3 mm
2	Within 0.5 cm of incision bilaterally	1–2 cm from incision	0.25 cm–1 cm bilaterally or between 0.5–2 cm unilaterally	Serosanguineous	Skin and subcutaneous fat separation
3	Beyond 0.5 cm of incision bilaterally	>2 cm from incision	>1 cm bilaterally or 2 cm unilaterally	Bloody, Purulent	Skin and subcutaneous fat and fascial layer separation
				Total	

Reproduced with permission [89]

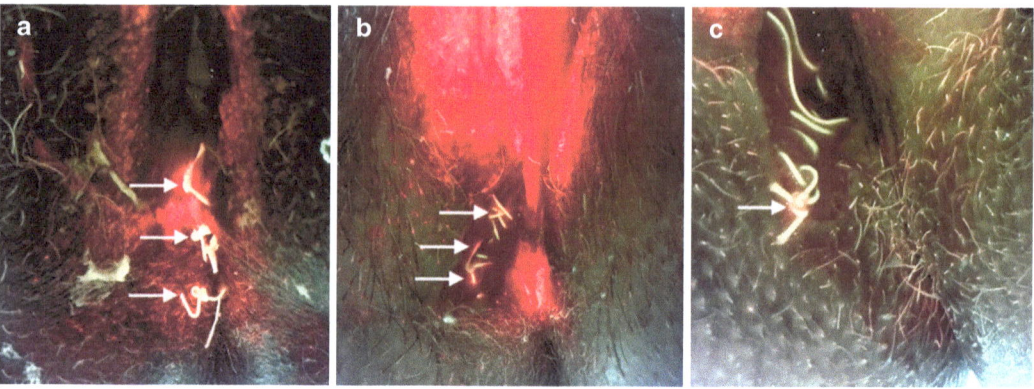

Fig. 9.6 Bacterial fluorescence images of infected perineal wounds taken using the MolecuLight i:X imaging device. Wounds showing red fluorescence (arrowed) within exposed suture material. (Reproduced with permission [85])

colonisation, it is important that loose suture material within an infected perineal wound is removed to improve wound healing outcomes.

Okeahialam et al. [85] also demonstrated wound measurements of dehisced perineal wounds, taken using the Silhouette® camera (Aranz, Christchurch, New Zealand), can predict wound healing outcomes. The Silhouette® camera uses laser assisted scanning technology in order to obtain accurate three-dimensional measurements of wounds [96]. The rate of wound edge contracture (horizontal healing) was found to be significantly slower in wounds with delayed healing in comparison to those with a normal healing rate (≤4 weeks) (0.21 cm/week vs 0.12 cm/week). In addition, a wound area of less than 1.60 cm^2 had a 70% probability of wound healing and a wound perimeter of less than 5.57 cm had a 70% probability of wound healing within 4 weeks. These threshold measurements can be used by clinicians to guide management. However, RCTs are required to evaluate the true clinical benefit of these advanced wound imaging modalities with regards to anti-microbial stewardship and wound healing outcomes before they are used routinely in clinical practice.

9.6 Management

The care of affected women should be transferred to the obstetrician, or to a multidisciplinary specialist perineal clinic which is described in Chap. 6. With perineal wound infection, broad-spectrum antibiotics are recommended until microbiological analysis results can be reviewed to guide further management [97]. However, wounds that have dehisced can be managed conservatively (healing by secondary intention with antibiotic cover) (Fig. 9.7) or surgically. With secondary intention healing, new tissue proliferates from the base of the wound to fill the space between the unopposed wound edges [98]. Figure 9.8 demonstrates that in dehisced perineal wounds, the vertical healing of wounds (depth/volume) is much faster than the horizontal healing (wound area/perimeter). In comparison to horizontal healing, vertical would healing may be a more important indicator of appropriate wound healing, as it corresponds with the rate of wound re-epithelialisation [99].

Traditionally, it was recommended that re-suturing of dehisced perineal and anal sphincter repairs should be delayed for 3–6 months, ensuring tissue viability from wound revascularisation and resolution of inflammation [100, 101]. However, this delay is associated with significant maternal morbidity due to symptoms such as pain, persistent faecal incontinence and sexual dysfunction, meaning early re-suturing has been advocated. Early re-suturing can be offered within 14 days after vaginal birth and there is a growing body of evidence from cohort studies, demonstrating its good post-operative outcomes (Fig. 9.9) [22, 100–105]. However, although a RCT by Dudley et al. [106] demonstrated that in

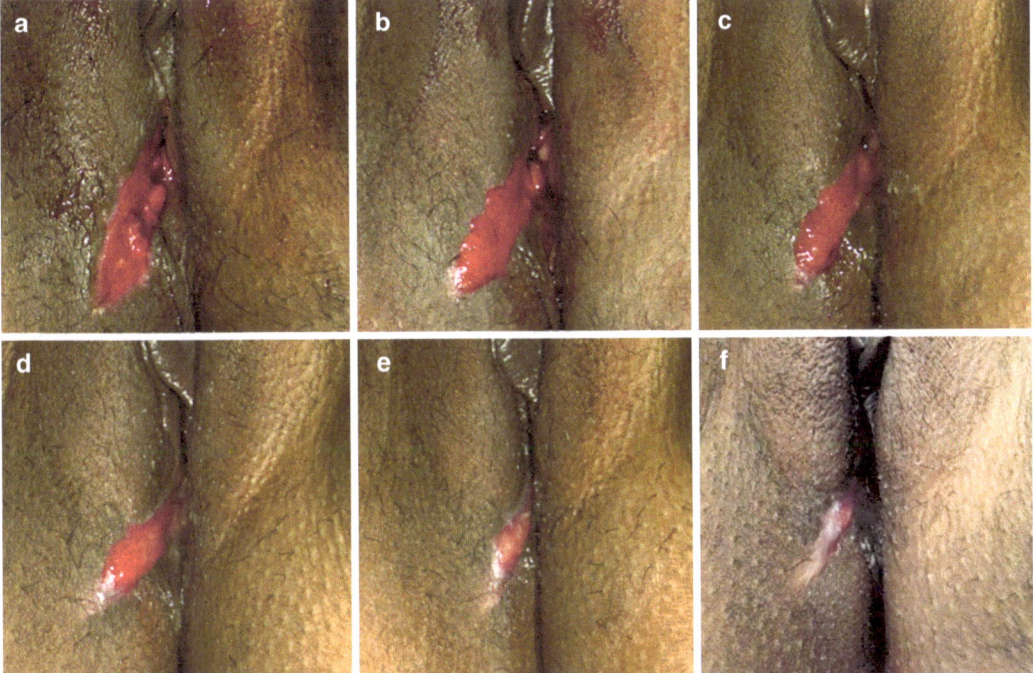

Fig. 9.7 Secondary intention wound healing of a dehisced episiotomy, 2 weeks (**a**), 3 weeks (**b**), 4 weeks (**c**), 5 weeks (**d**), 6 weeks (**e**), and 7 weeks (**f**) where the wound has healed with a wide-based scar. (Reproduced with permission [45])

comparison to conservative management, perineal re-suturing was favourable with regards to healing times and maternal satisfaction, only 26% (34 women) of potentially eligible participants were recruited, as most women opted for re-suturing rather than participating in the RCT.

When third- or fourth-degree tears breakdown, historically, the practice was to defer a second attempt at repair for 3–4 months. The delay was considered necessary to ensure adequate blood supply to the margins of the defect and restoration of tissue viability [101]. However, this delay is largely undesirable (persistent faecal incontinence, effect on sexual intercourse, muscle atrophy etc); early repair after outpatient wound debridement and preparation has been advocated more recently. In a case series of 22 patients who developed wound breakdown within a week of repair of a fourth-degree tear, all had a subsequent repair within an average of a further week. None experienced subsequent wound breakdown. One patient developed a small rectoperineal fistula that closed spontaneously after irrigation [101]. In another series of 23 patients (2 third and 21 fourth degree tears), a second repair was performed within a mean of 7 days of outpatient debridement and all repairs were successful apart from one rectoperineal fistula that healed spontaneously after 3 months [100]. The authors concluded that forcing women to wait the traditional 3–4 months before repairing such defects may be both cruel and unnecessary and perhaps should be obsolete. In a more recent case series of 18 women who underwent early repair (within 2 months) of OASIs breakdown, all repairs were successful, and the authors concluded that in women with OASIs breakdown, early secondary repair is both feasible and successful with meticulous surgical technique [107].

With regards to early secondary repair of the anal sphincter, in our literature review of 96 patients, Okeahialam et al. [22] found that although the majority of women had an uneventful post-operative recovery, complications such

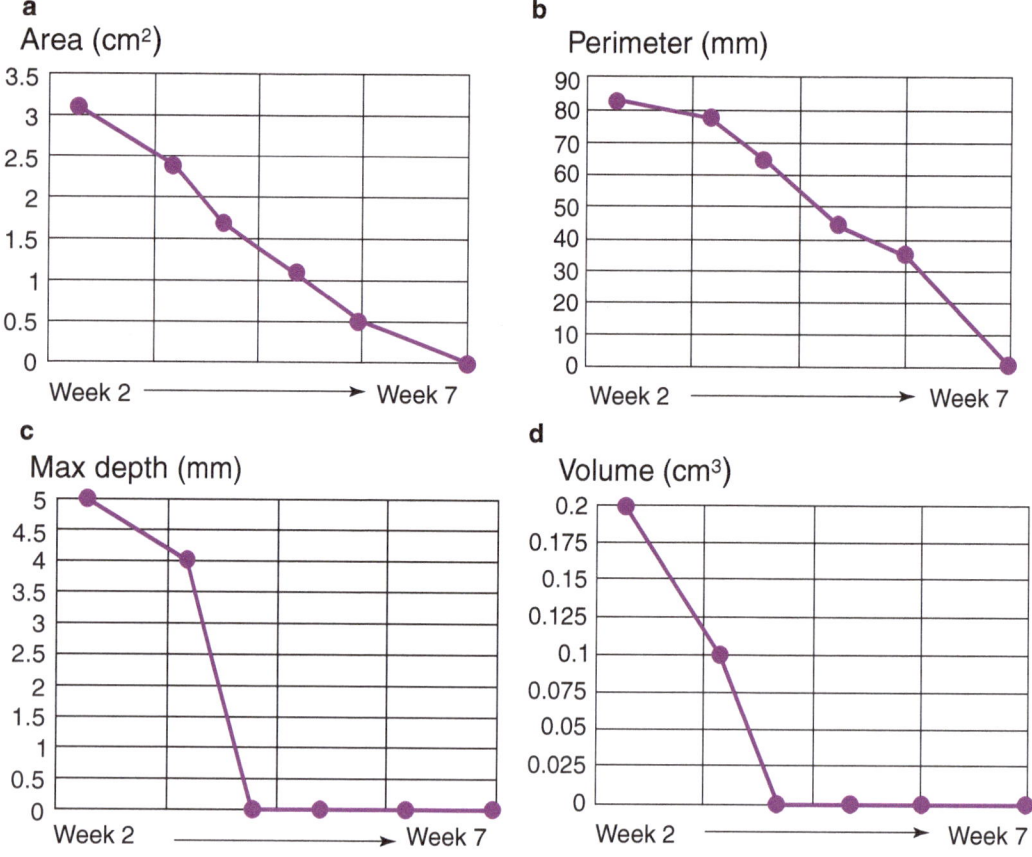

Fig. 9.8 The wound measurements of a dehisced episiotomy healing by secondary intention. Area (**a**), Perimeter (**b**), Depth (**c**), Volume (**d**). (Reproduced with permission [45])

as skin dehiscence occurred in 10%, infection in 5% and fistula formation in 8%. Therefore, at present there is no agreed recommendation for the management of perineal wound or anal sphincter dehiscence, due to a lack of robust evidence comparing the two management options [108]. It is important that women are counselled appropriately regarding both options and made aware of the lack of evidence of one method of management being superior to the other.

9.6.1 Principles and Technique of Repair

To reduce the risk of further wound complications following re-suturing, it is important that if there is any evidence of deep wound infec-

tion, women are admitted for intravenous broad-spectrum antibiotic administration and regular wound irrigation with sterile water, until the wound appears clean. Deep wound infection can be defined as wound infection that involves the deep soft tissues of the dehisced incision (muscle/fascia) and/or associated with systemic symptoms such as fever [109]. In the presence of superficial infection, oral broad-spectrum antibiotics should be given, and wound irrigation can be done by the woman with a shower-head attachment at home.

Re-suturing should only be conducted by a doctor who has been formally trained (or under direct supervision). The repair should be conducted in the operating theatre where there is access to good lighting and using an aseptic

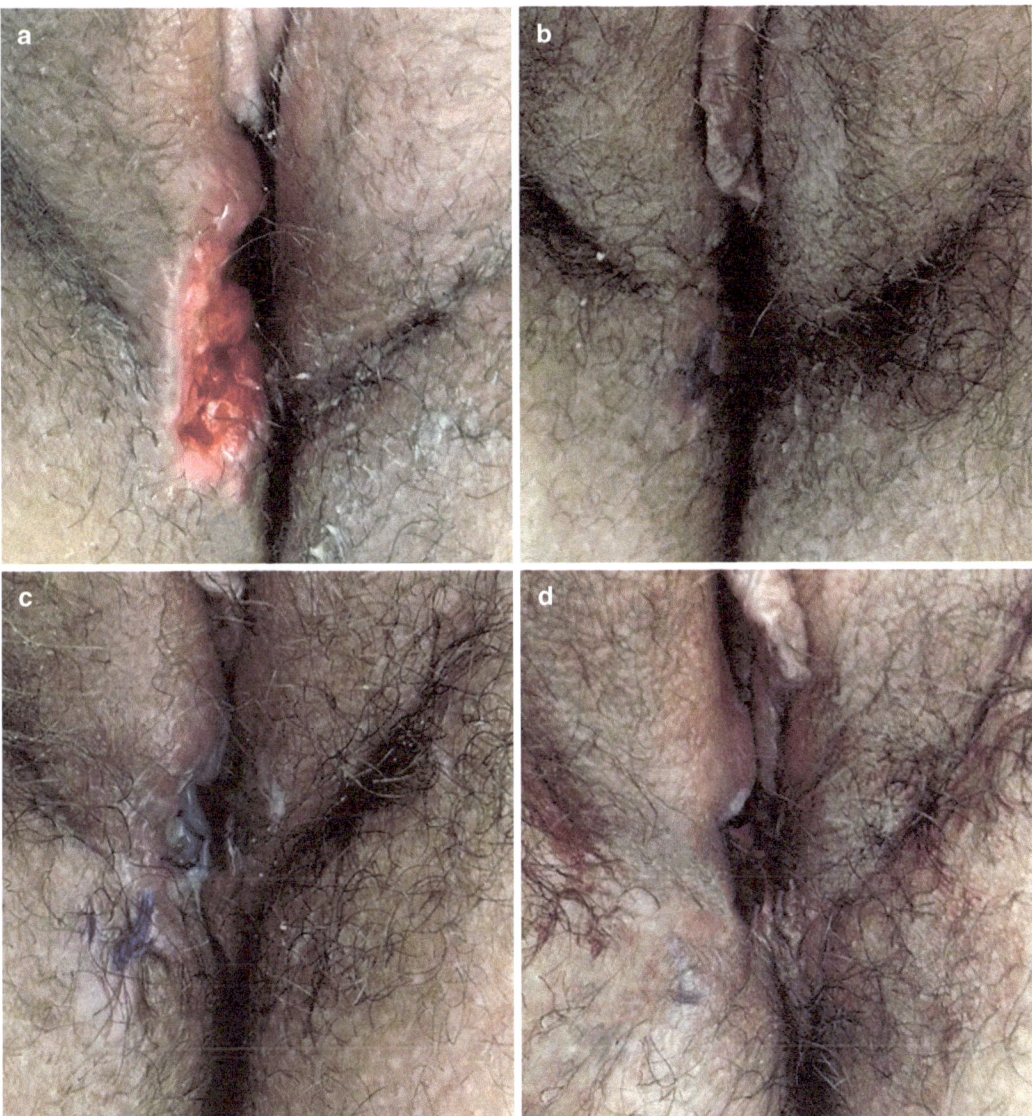

Fig. 9.9 A dehisced episiotomy diagnosed in week 1 (**a**) following a ventouse and forceps delivery. The patient opted for surgical re-suturing which was performed 2 weeks following delivery. The images show the uncom- plicated healing of the wound 2 weeks (**b**), 3 weeks (**c**) and 4 weeks (**d**) following delivery. (Reproduced with permission [45])

technique. Repairs are performed in the lithotomy position with the patient under general/ regional anaesthetic. Intravenous broad-spectrum antibiotics should be given intra-operatively. Following perineal/vaginal cleansing and application of sterile drapes, the wound should be irrigated with a 50:50 dilution of 3% Hydrogen Peroxide and 0.9% Sodium Chloride. Wound debridement should then be performed using a brush and curette. Old suture material should be removed, and devitalised vaginal or perineal tissue also be excised. It is important the full extent of the dehiscence is evaluated with careful vaginal and rectal examination. The repair techniques for re-suturing of the perineum and anal sphincter have been described previously [22, 102]. After the repair a vaginal and rectal examination should always be repeated to ensure the introitus admits two fingerbreadths, and in cases of an intact rectal mucosa, that no sutures have penetrated the mucosa. A video demonstrating these surgical steps has be published by Okeahialam et al. [102].

9.6.1.1 Perineal Repair

Perineal repair should be completed in three layers.

1. The vaginal mucosa is repaired from the apex to the hymenal remnants with a 2−0 Vicryl (Polydiaxone) suture using a continuous, non-locking technique.
2. To reduce tension on the suture line, the perineal muscles are dissected away from the overlying skin. The perineal muscles are then repaired continuously in one or two layers with 1−0 Vicryl, ensuring closure of all the dead space.
3. The perineal skin is repaired with interrupted 2−0 Vicryl mattress sutures (Fig. 9.10)

9.6.1.2 Anal Sphincter Repair

1. In the presence of a broken-down anal epithelium, this is repaired with a continuous, non-locking 3–0 Vicryl (Polyglactin) suture.
2. The sphincter muscles are repaired with a 3–0 Vicryl (Polyglactin) suture. If the IAS is broken down, it should be repaired separately with end-to-end approximation using horizontal mattress sutures. Suturing the IAS separately from the EAS during secondary sphincter repair has been shown to be associated with improved outcomes. In a prospective study of 94 women with anal incontinence following primary OASI repair undergoing sphincteroplasty, with separate suturing of the IAS, 64% experienced an improvement in anal incontinence at 2 years follow up [110].
3. The torn ends of the EAS should be identified and grasped with Allis tissue forceps. To release tension and to ensure adequate mobilisation of the torn ends, the EAS should be dissected gently away from the ischioanal fat laterally. If the full length of the EAS is identified, an overlap repair is performed. However, if the full length of the EAS cannot be identified, an end-to end repair technique can be used (Fig. 9.11).
4. Perineal repair should then be performed as described above (Sect. 9.6.1.1) to reconstruct the perineal body

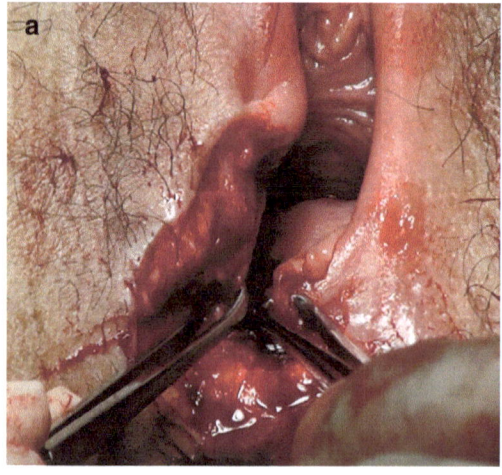
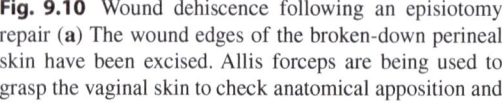
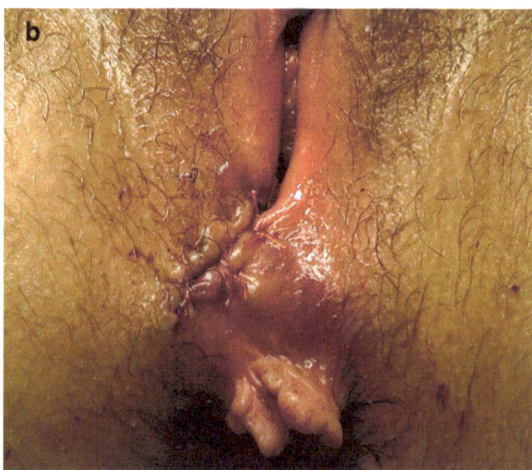

Fig. 9.10 Wound dehiscence following an episiotomy repair (**a**) The wound edges of the broken-down perineal skin have been excised. Allis forceps are being used to grasp the vaginal skin to check anatomical apposition and alignment. (**b**) The perineum after interrupted mattress sutures were inserted for skin closure, ensuring the wound is not under tension as swelling may occur post-operatively. (Reproduced with permission [102])

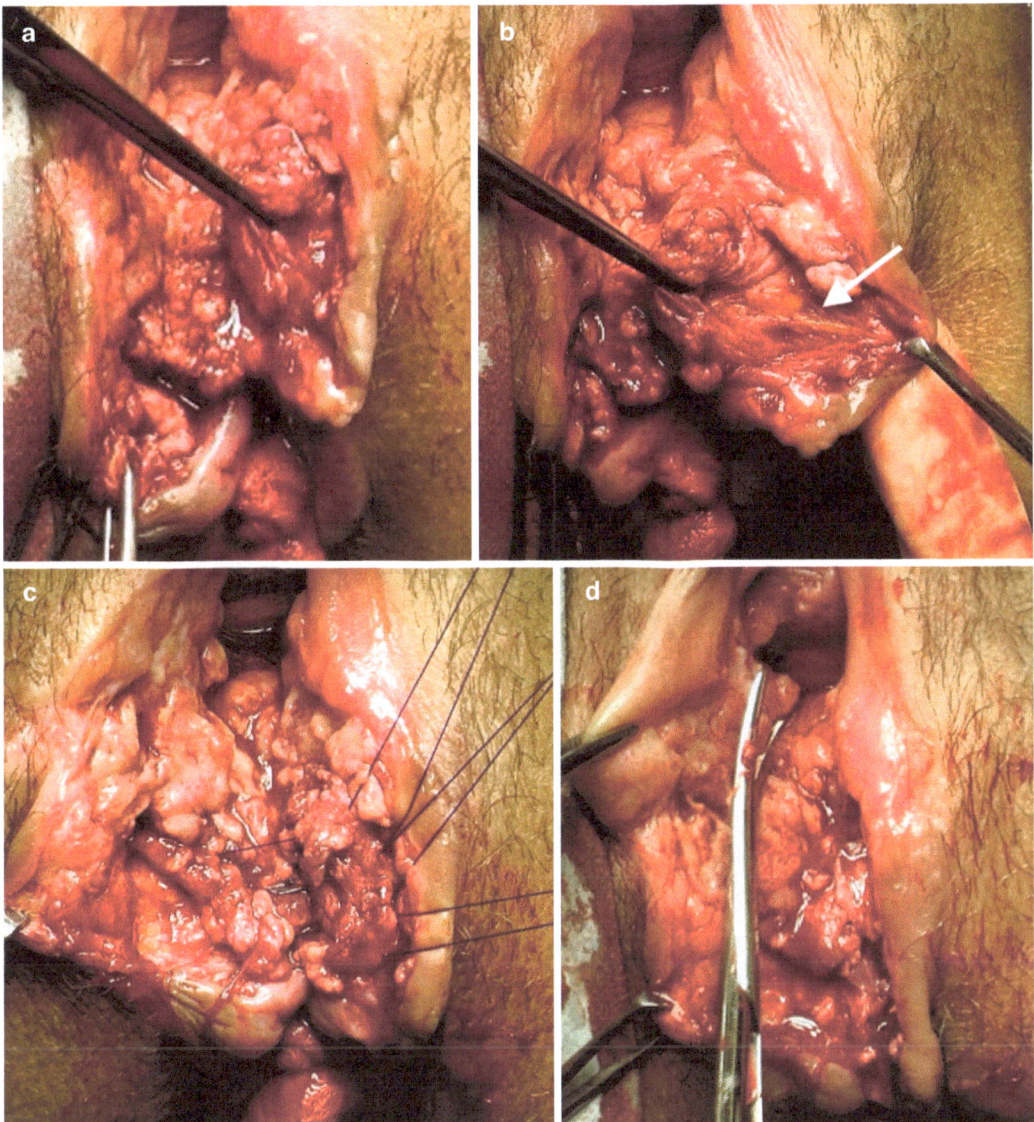

Fig. 9.11 The torn ends of the external anal sphincter (EAS) are identified and grasped with Allis forceps (**a**). The EAS is dissected laterally away from the ischioanal fat (arrow) (**b**). Reconstruction of the EAS with overlap repair using 3–0 PDS (Polydioxanone) dyed sutures (**c**). Completed overlap repair of the EAS: the edges of the vaginal skin are freshened by excision of devitalized tissue before re-suturing (**d**). (Reproduced with permission [22])

9.7   Common Complications of Disrupted Perineal Healing

9.7.1   Granulation Tissue

During the wound healing process, the transition between the inflammatory stage to the proliferative stage in critical [17]. When this phase is prolonged due to infection, hypergranulation of the wound can occur. Wounds prone to hypergranu-lation also include wounds that have dehisced, and those in areas of high moisture or friction (for example from maternity pads) [111, 112]. Symptoms women may report include bleeding, excessive discharge and pain.

Although there have been no RCTs investigating the effectiveness of treatments for over-granulated perineal wounds, cautery in the out-patient setting using silver nitrate has been described previously in the literature [9]. Figure 9.12 demonstrates the effect of silver

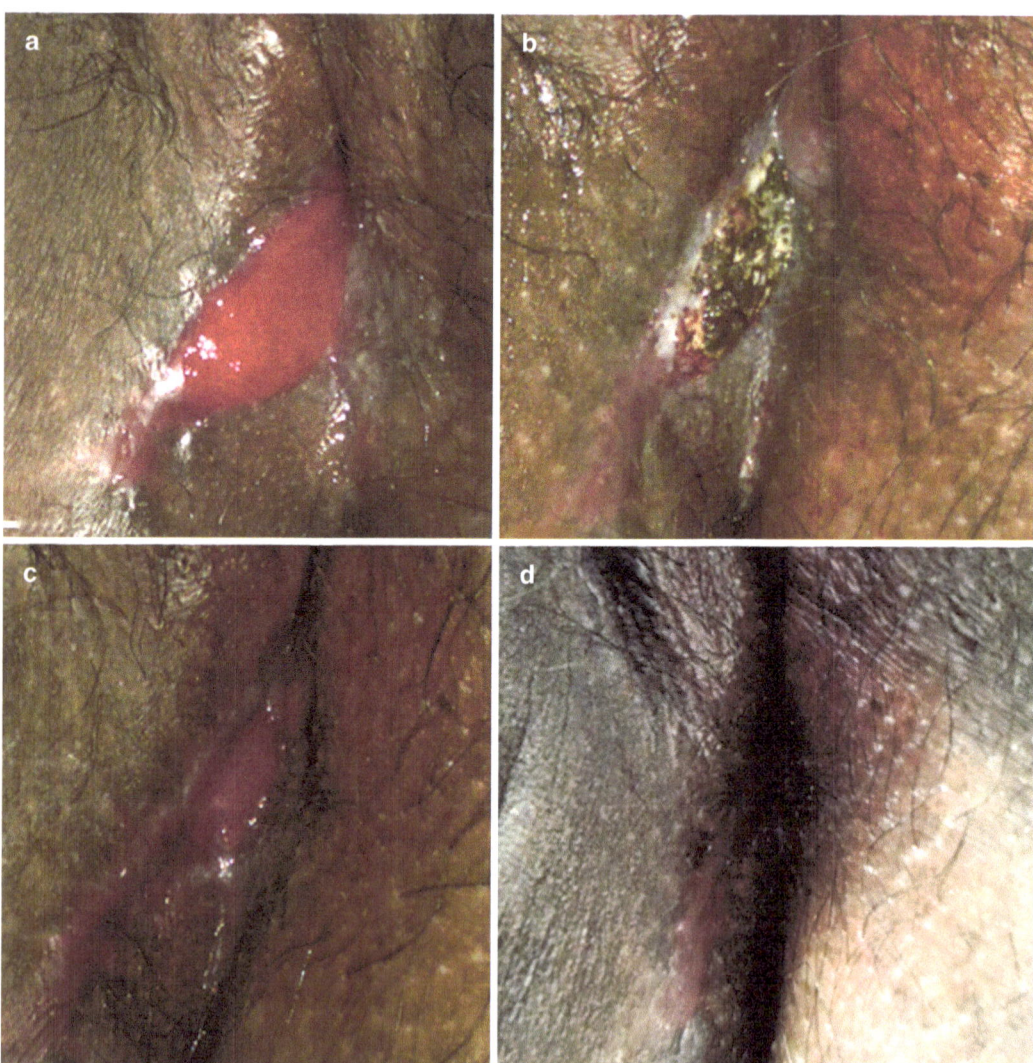

Fig. 9.12 Hypergranulation at 7 weeks postnatal following healing of a dehisced perineal wound healing by secondary intention (**a**). The area was treated with silver nitrate (**b**). The area of granulation tissue 2 weeks after treatment (**c**). The area of granulation tissue had resolved, and the wound had healed completely with a broad-based scar 4 weeks after treatment (**d**). (Reproduced with permission [45])

nitrate application on granulation tissue within a dehisced perineal wound. However, it should be applied to the wound with care, as it can be painful and potentially aggravate surrounding healthy skin [113]. Analgesics such 5% lidocaine ointment or *Instillagel®* can be applied directly to the perineal wound and surrounding skin prior to silver nitrate application. In a small number of cases resistant to treatment, surgical management with diathermy or excision may be required [97].

9.7.2 Perineal Pain/Dyspareunia

When normal wound healing is disrupted due to infection or dehiscence, excess collagen deposition occurs, leading to the formation of a hypertrophic scar [114]. In the perineum this causes scar tissue formation or a web of skin at the posterior fourchette. This can cause fissuring, bleeding and pain during sexual intercourse [115].

Perineal pain due to scar tissue formation can be managed with perineal massage and/or vaginal dilators with topical 5% lidocaine ointment [9]. However, there is limited evidence supporting the use of topical anaesthetics for perineal pain [116]. A combination of 10 ml 0.5% bupivacaine, 1500 IU hyaluronidase and 40 mg methylprednisolone acetate can be infiltrated into the perineum at the site of maximal tenderness in cases of persistent pain. In addition, perineo-

plasty may be required to surgically divide scar tissue at the introitus [9].

9.7.3 Fistula

Fistulae can occur as a result of disrupted perineal healing, leading to an abnormal connection between two epithelialized surfaces [117]. Obstetric fistula usually occur either immediately following vaginal delivery and perineal repair, or 1–2 weeks following delivery as a result of wound infection and subsequent inflammation [118]. For example, multi-resistant bacteria such as *Methicillin-resistant Staphylococcus Aureus* (MRSA) (rates of which are increasing in the obstetric population) have been shown to cause aggressive local infection at site of perineal trauma (Fig. 9.13) [119]. Fistulae can develop at number of sites between the genitourinary tract and the gastrointestinal tract. This includes, but is not limited to rectovaginal (between the rectum and vagina), vesicovaginal (between the bladder and vagina), urethrovaginal (between the urethra and vagina) and perineovaginal (between the perineum and vagina) fistulae [117]. Risk factors for fistulae development include obstetric anal sphincter injuries, episiotomy, operative vaginal delivery and perineal wound infection [118]. Women with suspected fistulae should have a complete vaginal and rectal examination, endoanal ultrasound or perineal ultrasound. However,

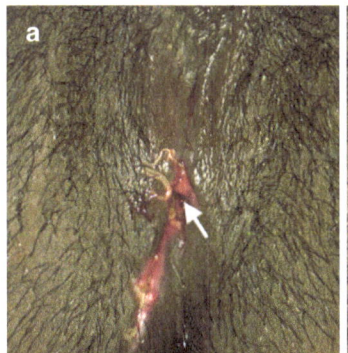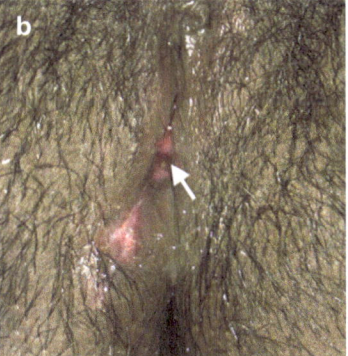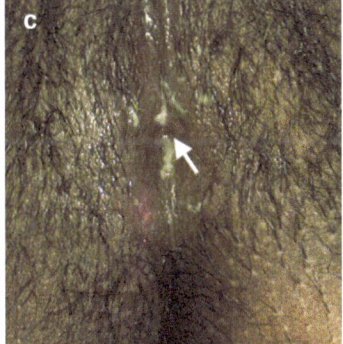

Fig. 9.13 A dehisced episiotomy which led to the formation of a perineovaginal fistula (arrows) at 1 (**a**), 3 (**b**) and 4 weeks (**c**) following delivery. Wound swabs grew Methicillin-resistant Staphylococcus aureus on microbiological analysis. Patient informed consent obtained

examination under anaesthesia may be needed to confirm fistula and investigate its full extent [9]. Not all fistulae will require surgical intervention as 50% of all small fistulae will heal spontaneously [120].

9.7.4 Psychological Impact

Perineal wound infection and dehiscence can affect women psychologically. In the nested qualitative study by Dudley et al. [19], perineal wound infection and dehiscence were found to have a significant psychosocial effect, with women experiencing denial, feelings of failure, fear, body image concerns leading to isolation.

9.8 Prevention of Wound Complications

An optimal primary repair is important in the prevention of wound complications. In a case series of six women undergoing early secondary sphincter repair, in comparison to 504 women who had a primary repair alone, residual anal sphincter defect size on endoanal ultrasound was significantly larger [22]. Not only can the risk of wound complications following perineal and anal sphincter repair in the immediate puerperium be minimised with sound surgical principles, but also by emphasising the importance of good perineal hygiene. This includes hand hygiene, regular changing of maternity pads and daily washing of the perineum with water, followed by gentle drying [121]. RCTs have been performed to assess the efficacy of perineal management practices. Barclay and Martin [122] randomised 120 women to one of five protocols including, basic perineal hygiene, warm sitz bathing, ice sitz bathing, ray lamp and witch hazel solution, and found there was no significant difference in healing times or infection rates. In Sleep and Grants [123] RCT of 1800 women, no differ-

ence in wound infection or dehiscence rates were found with adding Cetrimide and Chlorhexidine digluconate (Savlon antiseptic cream) or salt to tap water for perineal bathing in comparison to water alone. In addition, 1% of women reported that salt caused skin irritation. The benefit of antiseptics solutions such as Chloroxylenol (similar in properties to Chlorhexidine) has also been evaluated. In an RCT comparing its use to tap water, Martin et al. [124] found that there was no significant difference in the bacterial flora of the perineal skin, and no difference in healing rates or the incidence of wound breakdown. Therefore, women can be assured that tap water can be used safely in the care of perineal wounds, without additional cost and the risk of potentially affecting the barrier function of the skin with irritation.

There only one randomised trial addressing the efficacy of peripartum antibiotics in preventing perineal wound infections. In a study of 147 women who sustained an obstetric anal sphincter injury, women were randomized to receive placebo (n = 84) or single intravenous dose (n = 64) of a second-generation cephalosporin (cefotetan or cefoxitin) at the time of repair. Primary end points for the study were gross disruption or purulent discharge at site of perineal repair at 2 weeks postpartum. The authors found significantly lower rates of wound complications in those who had received antibiotics [125]. Further study in the efficacy and/or need for postpartum antibiotics after severe tears is needed.

It is however, important that clinicians acknowledge that due to an increasingly diverse population, cultural competency is imperative. This means that differences in cultural hygiene practices with regards to perineal care, such as restriction of bathing, sitz bathing or steam bathing with medicinal herbs should be recognised. This will allow the risks and benefits of the practices to be addressed, taking into account the wishes of the woman, thereby improving her healthcare experience [126].

Table 9.5 Perineal Outcomes from the ECHO Study

	Total N = 442*	Study group N = 220*	Control group N = 222*	OR 95% (CI)	p value	ARR (95% CI)	NNT (95% CI)
All infection	102 (23.1%)	19 (8.6%)	83 (37.4%)	0.16 (0.09, 0.27)	<0.001	28.8 (21.4, 36.1)	3.5 (2.8, 4.7)
Superficial /deep infection	84 (19.0%)	17 (7.7%)	67 (30.2%)	0.19 (0.11, 0.34)	<0.001	22.5 (15.4, 29.4)	4.5 (3.4, 6.5)
Organ/Space infection	80 (18.1%)	10 (4.6%)	70 (31.5%)	0.10 (0.05, 0.21)	<0.001	27.0 (20.3, 33.7)	3.7 (3.0, 4.9)

Reproduced with permission [33]
*8 patients excluded from the analysis (5 study group, 3 control group) due to loss to follow-up / missing data.
OR odds ratio, ARR absolute risk reduction, NNT number needed to treat

9.8.1 Other Treatments

Antimicrobial alternatives
The ECHO study (*E*ffect of *C*opper on the *H*ealing of *O*bstetric wounds) performed at Croydon University Hospital, investigated the effect of copper impregnated maternity pads for 2 weeks on wound infection rates. Table 9.5 shows the results from the 450 women's responses to the Health Protection Agency's Post Discharge Questionnaire (PDQ) for national Surgical Site Infection (SSI) within 30 days of vaginal birth [127] Significant differences in the incidence of wound infection (superficial, deep and organ space) were found and the number needed to treat was four, meaning four women would need to be given a copper impregnated maternity pad to prevent one additional woman developing wound infection within 30 days. There is a need for the impact of copper impregnated materials to be evaluated with more RCTs, including its costs benefit to wound management.

9.9 Conclusions

Complications of perineal and anal sphincter wound healing have a major impact on a women's short- and long-term physical and psychosocial health. Wound healing complications are an essential aspect of postnatal care, which needs to be prioritised. As outcomes reporting in childbirth trauma research are heterogeneous, developing, disseminating, and implementing a core outcome set in future childbirth trauma research could help address some of these issues. Health care professionals need to understand the clinical progression of perineal wounds and the potential wound healing complications, so women can be counselled appropriately. Knowledge of how these complications can present and their management options will improve the quality of postnatal care. These complications will continue to occur, even when preventative strategies are applied, and it is important clinicians are aware of the best management options available. The evidence base of these options needs to be reviewed and discussed openly with women, so an informed decision can be made.

Take Home Messages

- Knowledge of the clinical progression of perineal wound healing is essential for all clinicians assessing perineal wound healing complications.
- The appreciation of risk factors associated with perineal wound complications will allow for a modification of obstetric practice, which can minimise their occurrence. For example, the use of a continuous sub-cuticular repair of perineal injuries and the provision of broad-spectrum antibiotics following operative vaginal birth
- There is a lack of robust evidence comparing the outcomes of perineal re-suturing to conservative management. Therefore, women should be counselled appropriately regarding both options and made aware of the lack of

evidence of one method of management being superior to the other.

- Women should be informed about perineal hygiene techniques as it can prevent the risk of wound complications following perineal and anal sphincter repair.

Appendix: MCQ

Questions

1. With regards to the pathophysiology and microbiology of wound healing, which of the following statements is true?
   (A) There are five wound healing stages.
   (B) Wound erythema, heat and/or oedema are always indicative of a wound infection.
   (C) The critical level of bacterial colonisation at which wound infection occurs is $>10^3$ CFU/g.
   (D) One bacterial species alone is usually isolated from wound swabs in perineal wound infection.
   (E) The vertical rate of wound healing is faster than the horizontal rate.

2. In perineal wound infection/dehiscence, which of the following is true?
   (A) Up to 25% of women are affected by wound infection/dehiscence following childbirth.
   (B) OASI is not a significant risk factor for wound infection/dehiscence.
   (C) Wound dehiscence only occurs in the presence of infection.
   (D) When assessing, a rectal examination is only required if the woman has a history of OASI.
   (E) Any evidence of granulation tissue should be treated.

3. Which of the following is true concerning the prevention of perineal wound healing complications?
   (A) At the time of primary wound, perineal skin closure should be performed with interrupted sutures.
   (B) Prophylactic antibiotics should be given in all cases of perineal trauma to reduce the risk of wound complications.
   (C) Women should be instructed to ensure proper hand hygiene, regular changing of maternity pads and daily washing of the perineum.
   (D) Cleansing the wound with antiseptic solutions is better than tap water alone.

Answers

1. With regards to the pathophysiology and microbiology of wound healing, which of the following statements is true?
   (A) FALSE
   (B) FALSE
   (C) FALSE
   (D) FALSE
   (E) TRUE

2. In perineal wound infection/dehiscence, which of the following is true?
   (A) TRUE
   (B) FALSE
   (C) FALSE
   (D) FALSE
   (E) FALSE

3. Which of the following is true concerning the prevention of perineal wound healing complications?
   (A) FALSE
   (B) FALSE
   (C) TRUE
   (D) FALSE

References

1. Smith LA, Price N, Simonite V, Burns EE. Incidence of and risk factors for perineal trauma: a prospective observational study. BMC Pregnancy Childbirth. 2013;13:59.

2. Molyneux R, Fowler G, Slade P. The effects of perineal trauma on immediate self-reported birth experience in first-time mothers. Null. J Psychosom Obstet Gynaecol. 2022;43(2):228–234.

3. Glazener C, Abdalla M, Russell I, Templeton A. Postnatal care: a survey of patients' experiences. Br J Midwifery. 1993;1:67–74.

4. Li W-Y, Liabsuetrakul T, Stray-Pedersen B. Effect of mode of delivery on perceived risks of maternal health outcomes among expectant parents: a cohort study in Beijing, China. BMC Pregnancy Childbirth. 2014;14:12.

5. Perkins E, Tohill S, Kettle C, Bick D, Ismail K. Women's views of important outcomes following perineal repair. BJOG Int J Obstet Gynaecol. 2008;115(Suppl 1):67–253.

6. Knight M, Kenyon S, Brocklehurst P, editors. On behalf of MBRRACE UK. Saving lives, improving mothers' care—lessons learned to inform future maternity care from the United Kingdom and Ireland, confidential enquiries into maternal deaths and morbidity 2009–12; 2014.

7. Bick D. Postpartum management of the perineum. Br J Midwifery. 2009;17:571–7.

8. Herron-Marx S, Williams A, Hicks C. A Q methodology study of women's experience of enduring postnatal perineal and pelvic floor morbidity. Midwifery. 2007;23:322–34.

9. Wan OYK, Taithongchai A, Veiga SI, Sultan AH, Thakar R. A one-stop perineal clinic: our eleven-year experience. Int Urogynecol J. 2020;31:2317–26.

10. Fitzpatrick M, Cassidy M, O'Connell PR, O'Herlihy C. Experience with an obstetric perineal clinic. Eur J Obstet Gynecol Reprod Biol. 2002;100:199–203.

11. Brincat C, Crosby E, McLeod A, Fenner DE. Experiences during the first four years of a post-partum perineal clinic in the USA. Int J Gynecol Obstet. 2015;128:68–71.

12. Arendsen LP, Thakar R, Sultan AH. The use of copper as an antimicrobial agent in health care, including obstetrics and gynecology. Clin Microbiol Rev. 2019;32:e00125–18, /cmr/32/4/CMR.00125-18. atom.

13. Singer AJ, Clark RAF. Cutaneous wound healing. N Engl J Med. 1999;341:738–46.

14. Li J, Chen J, Kirsner R. Pathophysiology of acute wound healing. Clin Dermatol. 2007;25:9–18.

15. Reinke JM, Sorg H. Wound repair and regeneration. Eur Surg Res. 2012;49:35–43.

16. Robson MC, Steed DL, Franz MG. Wound healing: biologic features and approaches to maximize healing trajectories. Curr Probl Surg. 2001;38:A1–140.

17. Landén NX, Li D, Ståhle M. Transition from inflammation to proliferation: a critical step during wound healing. Cell Mol Life Sci. 2016;73:3861–85.

18. Gonzalez AC de O, Costa TF, Andrade Z de A, Medrado ARAP. Wound healing – a literature review. An Bras Dermatol. 2016; 91:614–20.

19. Dudley L, Kettle C, Waterfield J, Ismail KMK. Perineal resuturing versus expectant management following vaginal delivery complicated by a dehisced wound (PREVIEW): a nested qualitative study. BMJ Open. 2017;7:e013008.

20. European Centre for Disease Prevention and Control. Stockholm. Healthcare-associated infections: surgical site infections Annual Epidemiological Report for 2017; 2019.

21. Knight M, Chiocchia V, Partlett C, et al. Prophylactic antibiotics in the prevention of infection after operative vaginal delivery (ANODE): a multicentre randomised controlled trial. Lancet. 2019;393:2395–403.

22. Okeahialam NA, Thakar R, Sultan AH. Early secondary repair of obstetric anal sphincter injuries (OASIs): experience and a review of the literature. Int Urogynecol J. 2021; https://doi.org/10.1007/s00192-021-04822-x.

23. Johnson A, Thakar R, Sultan AH. Obstetric perineal wound infection: is there underreporting? Br J Nurs. 2012;21:S28–35.

24. Pergialiotis V, Durnea C, Elfituri A, Duffy J, Doumouchtsis S, International Collaboration for Harmonising Outcomes, Research, and Standards in Urogynaecology and Women's Health (CHORUS). Do we need a core outcome set for childbirth perineal trauma research? A systematic review of outcome reporting in randomised trials evaluating the management of childbirth trauma. BJOG: Int J Obstet Gy. 2018;125:1522–31.

25. Rashid M-U, Weintraub A, Nord CE. Effect of new antimicrobial agents on the ecological balance of human microflora. Anaerobe. 2012;18:249–53.

26. Bowler PG. Wound pathophysiology, infection and therapeutic options. Ann Med. 2002;34:419–27.

27. Peterson J. Bacterial pathogenesis. In: Medical microbiology. Galveston: University of Texas Medical Branch at Galveston; 1996.

28. Landis SJ. Chronic wound infection and antimicrobial use. Adv Skin Wound Care. 2008;21:531–40.

29. Tortora GJ, Funke BR, Case CL. Nonspecific defenses of the host. In: Microbiology an introduction. Pearson. 2004.

30. Bowler PG, Duerden BI, Armstrong DG. Wound microbiology and associated approaches to wound management. Clin Microbiol Rev. 2001;14:244–69.

31. Karsnitz DB. Puerperal infections of the genital tract: a clinical review. J Midwifery Womens Health. 2013;58:632–42.

32. Ajibade F, De la Horra A, Street P, Motara K. Surveillance of perineal breakdown during childbirth : essential audit. BJOG Int J Obst Gynaecol Confer RCOG World Congr. 2013;2013:476–7.

33. Arendsen LP, Thakar R, Bassett P, Sultan AH. A double blind randomized controlled trial using copper impregnated maternity sanitary towels to reduce perineal wound infection. Midwifery. 2020;92:102858.

34. Fox A. Challenges: perineal wound care in the community. World Ir Nurs Midwifery. 2011;19:48–50.
35. Rotas M, McCalla S, Liu C, Minkoff H. Methicillin-resistant Staphylococcus aureus necrotizing pneumonia arising from an infected episiotomy site. Obstet Gynecol. 2007;109:533–6.
36. Sule S, Shittu S. Puerperal complications of episiotomies at Ahmadu Bello University Teaching Hospital, Zaria, Nigeria. East Afr Med J. 2004;80:351–6.
37. Zhang H, Han S. Risk factors and preventive measures for postoperative infection in episiotomy of puerperal. Biomed Res. 2017;28:8857–61.
38. Almarzouqi F, Grieb G, Klink C, Bauerschlag D, Fuchs PC, Alharbi Z, Vasku M, Pallua N. Fatal necrotizing fasciitis following episiotomy. Case Rep Surg. 2015;2015:1–4.
39. Chua WC, Mazlan MZ, Ali S, et al. Post-partum streptococcal toxic shock syndrome associated with necrotizing fasciitis. IDCases. 2017;9:91–4.
40. Shy KK, Eschenbach DA. Fatal perineal cellulitis from an episiotomy site. Obstet Gynecol. 1979;54:292.
41. Wiseman O, Rafferty AM, Stockley J, Murrells T, Bick D. Infection and wound breakdown in spontaneous second-degree perineal tears: an exploratory mixed methods study. Birth. 2019;46:80–9.
42. Häusler G, Hanzal E, Dadak C, Gruber W. Necrotizing fasciitis arising from episiotomy. Arch Gynecol Obstet. 1994;255:153–5.
43. Tsenov D, Shopova E, Chamova M, Garnizov T, Ganeva G, Diakova D. [Microbiology of open surgical wounds after delivery--episiotomy and cesarean section]. Akush Ginekol (Sofiia). 2001;40(Suppl 5):19–21.
44. Rai S, Medhi R, Das A, Ahmed M, Das B. Necrotizing fasciitis – a rare complication following common obstetric operative procedures: report of two cases. IJWH. 2015;7:357.
45. Okeahialam NA, Thakar R, Sultan AH. Healing of disrupted perineal wounds after vaginal delivery: a poorly understood condition. Br J Nurs. 2021;30:S8–S16.
46. Childs C, Sandy-Hodgetts K, Broad C, Cooper R, Manresa M, Verdú-Soriano J. Risk, prevention and management of complications after vaginal and caesarean section birth. J Wound Care. 2020;29:S1–S48.
47. Angel DE, Lloyd P, Carville K, Santamaria N. The clinical efficacy of two semi-quantitative wound-swabbing techniques in identifying the causative organism(s) in infected cutaneous wounds. Int Wound J. 2011;8:176–85.
48. Healy B, Freedman A. ABC of wound healing: infections. BMJ. 2006;332:838–41.
49. Edmiston CE Jr, Krepel CJ, Marks RM, Rossi PJ, Sanger J, Goldblatt M, Graham MB, Rothenburger S, Collier J, Seabrook GR. Microbiology of explanted suture segments from infected and noninfected surgical patients. J Clin Microbiol. 2013;51:417–21.
50. Mahon CR, Lehman DC, Manuselis G. Specimen collection and processing. In: Textbook of diagnostic microbiology. Elsevier Health Sciences; 2018. p. 106–20.
51. National Institute for Health and Care Excellence. Antimicrobial stewardship: systems and processes for effective antimicrobial medicine use. NICE guideline [NG15]; 2015.
52. Jones K, Webb S, Manresa M, Hodgetts-Morton V, Morris RK. The incidence of wound infection and dehiscence following childbirth-related perineal trauma: a systematic review of the evidence. Eur J Obstet Gynecol Reprod Biol. 2019;240:1–8.
53. Allen VM, O'Connell CM, Baskett TF. Maternal morbidity associated with cesarean delivery without labor compared with induction of labor at term. Obstet Gynecol. 2006;108:286.
54. Calvia A, Natarajan D, Denman K, Kaur K. Surgical site infection surveillance-perineal wounds 2015. BJOG Int J Obstet Gynaecol. 2016;123:168.
55. Clement S, Reed B. To stitch or not to stitch? A long-term follow-up study of women with unsutured perineal tears. Pract Midwife. 1999;2:20–8.
56. Edwards LE, Dickes WF, Alton IR, Hakanson EY. Pregnancy in the massively obese: course, outcome, and obesity prognosis of the infant. Am J Obstet Gynecol. 1978;131:479–83.
57. Fodstad K, Staff AC, Laine K. Effect of different episiotomy techniques on perineal pain and sexual activity 3 months after delivery. Int Urogynecol J Pelvic Floor Dysfunct. 2014;25:1629–37.
58. Goldaber KG, Wendel PJ, McIntire DD, Wendel GD. Postpartum perineal morbidity after fourth-degree perineal repair. Am J Obstet Gynecol. 1993;168:489–93.
59. Harris RE. An evaluation of the median episiotomy. Am J Obstet Gynecol. 1970;106:660–5.
60. Lam KW, Wong HS, Pun TC. The practice of episiotomy in public hospitals in Hong Kong. Hong Kong Med J. 2006;12:94–8.
61. Lewicky-Gaupp C, Leader-Cramer A, Johnson LL, Kenton K, Gossett DR. Wound complications after obstetric anal sphincter injuries. Obstet Gynecol. 2015;125:1088–93.
62. O'Leary J, O'Leary J. The complete episiotomy analysis of 1224 complete lacerations, sphincterotomies, and episiproctotomies. Obstet Gynecol. 1965;25:235.
63. Ridley N. Perineal wound infections: an audit. Pract Midwife. 2015;18:28–32.
64. Stock L, Basham E, Gossett DR, Lewicky-Gaupp C. Factors associated with wound complications in women with obstetric anal sphincter injuries (OASIS). Am J Obstet Gynecol. 2013;208:327.e1–6.
65. Yokoe DS, Christiansen CL, Johnson R, Sands K, Livingston J, Shtatland ES, Platt R. Epidemiology of and surveillance for postpartum infections. Emerg Infect Dis. 2001;7:837–41.
66. Glazener CMA, Abdalla M, Stroud P, Templeton A, Russell IT, Naji S. Postnatal maternal morbidity: extent, causes, prevention and treatment. BJOG Int J O&G. 1995;102:282–7.

67. Jallad K, Steele SE, Barber MD. Breakdown of perineal laceration repair after vaginal delivery: a case-control study. Female Pelvic Med Reconstr Surg. 2016;22:276–9.

68. Otoide VO, Ogbonmwan SM, Okonofua FE. Episiotomy in Nigeria. Int J Gynecol Obstet. 2000;68:13–7.

69. Wilkie GL, Saadeh M, Robinson JN, Little SE. Risk factors for poor perineal outcome after operative vaginal delivery. J Perinatol. 2018;38:1625–30.

70. Stock SJ, Josephs K, Farquharson S, Love C, Cooper SE, Kissack C, Akolekar R, Norman JE, Denison FC. Maternal and neonatal outcomes of successful Kielland's rotational forceps delivery. Obstet Gynecol. 2013;121:1032–9.

71. Gommesen D, Nohr EA, Drue HC, Qvist N, Rasch V. Obstetric perineal tears: risk factors, wound infection and dehiscence: a prospective cohort study. Arch Gynecol Obstet. 2019;300:67–77.

72. Groves JW Jr, Foster RT, Kuehl TJ, Yandell PM. Risk and outcome of obstetrical anal sphincter injury. J Pelvic Med Surg. 2007;13:171–6.

73. Kaltreider DF, Dixon DM. A study of 710 complete lacerations following central episiotomy. South Med J. 1948;41:814–20.

74. Okeahialam NA, Wong KW, Thakar R, Sultan AH. The incidence of wound complications following primary repair of Obstetric Anal Sphincter Injuries (OASIS): a systematic review and meta-analysis. Am J Obstet Gynecol. 2022;S0002937822003568.

75. Macleod M, Strachan B, Bahl R, Howarth L, Goyder K, Van de Venne M, Murphy D. A prospective cohort study of maternal and neonatal morbidity in relation to use of episiotomy at operative vaginal delivery. BJOG Int J Obstet Gynaecol. 2008;115:1688–94.

76. Williams MK, Chames MC. Risk factors for the breakdown of perineal laceration repair after vaginal delivery. Am J Obstet Gynecol. 2006;195:755–9.

77. Murphy D, Strachan B, Bahl R. The Royal College of Obstetricians and Gynaecologists, Assisted vaginal birth: green-top guideline no. 26. BJOG: Int J Obstet Gy. 2020; https://doi.org/10.1111/1471-0528.16092.

78. Bonet M, Ota E, Chibueze CE, Oladapo OT. Antibiotic prophylaxis for episiotomy repair following vaginal birth. Cochrane Database Syst Rev. 2017; https://doi.org/10.1002/14651858.CD012136.pub2.

79. Dudley L, Kettle C, Ismail K. Prevalence, pathophysiology and current management of dehisced perineal wounds following childbirth. Br J Midwifery. 2013;21:160–71.

80. Wound International. World Union of Wound Healing Societies (WUWHS). Consensus Document Surgical wound dehiscence: improving prevention and outcomes; 2018.

81. Sultan AH, Monga AK, Kumar D, Stanton SL. Primary repair of obstetric anal sphincter rupture using the overlap technique. BJOG Int J O&G. 1999;106:318–23.

82. Royal College of Obstetrics and Gynaecology. Management of third and fourth degree perineal tears. Greentop guideline number 29; 2015.

83. Taithongchai A, Veiga SI, Sultan AH, Thakar R. The consequences of undiagnosed obstetric anal sphincter injuries (OASIS) following vaginal delivery. Int Urogynecol J. 2020;31:635–41.

84. Okeahialam NA, Thakar R, Sultan AH. Perineal wound infection and its effect on anal sphincter integrity following vaginal delivery. The Herbert Reiss Prize and Dame Josephine Barnes Prize webinar; 2022

85. Okeahialam NA, Thakar R, Sultan AH. The clinical progression and wound healing rate of dehisced perineal tears healing by secondary intention: a prospective observational study. Eur J Obstet Gynecol Reprod Biol. 2022;274:191–6.

86. McPherson KC, Beggs AD, Sultan AH, Thakar R. Can the risk of obstetric anal sphincter injuries (OASIs) be predicted using a risk-scoring system? BMC Res Notes. 2014;7:471.

87. Ercan UK, İbiş F, Dikyol C, Horzum N, Karaman O, Yıldırım Ç, Çukur E, Demirci EA. Prevention of bacterial colonization on non-thermal atmospheric plasma treated surgical sutures for control and prevention of surgical site infections. PLoS One. 2018;13:e0202703.

88. Kettle C, Dowswell T, Ismail K. Continuous and interrupted suturing techniques for repair of episiotomy or second-degree tears. Cochrane Database Syst Rev. 2012; https://doi.org/10.1002/14651858.CD000947.pub3.

89. Hill P. Psychometric properties of the REEDA. J Nurse Midwifery. 1990;35:162–5.

90. Davidson N. REEDA: evaluating postpartum healing. J Nurse Midwifery. 1974;19:6–8.

91. Alvarenga MB, Francisco AA, Oliveira SMJV de, Silva FMB da, Shimoda GT, Damiani LP. Episiotomy healing assessment: Redness, Oedema, Ecchymosis, Discharge, Approximation (REEDA) scale reliability. Rev Latino-Am Enfermagem. 2015;23:162–8.

92. Finlay AY, Griffiths TW, Belmo S, Chowdhury MMU. Why we should abandon the misused descriptor 'erythema'. Br J Dermatol. 2021;185:1240–1.

93. Rennie M, Dunham D, Lindvere-Teene L, Raizman R, Hill R, Linden R. Understanding real-time fluorescence signals from bacteria and wound tissues observed with the MoleculLight i:XTM. Diagnostics. 2019;9:22.

94. Ottolino-Perry K, Chamma E, Blackmore KM, et al. Improved detection of clinically relevant wound bacteria using autofluorescence image-guided sampling in diabetic foot ulcers: autofluorescence image-guided wound sampling. Int Wound J. 2017;14:833–41.

95. Okeahialam NA, Thakar R, Sultan AH. Visualising bacteria from infected perineal wounds using a bacterial autofluorescence device. The Herbert Reiss Prize and Dame Josephine Barnes Prize webinar; 2022.

96. Jørgensen LB, Sørensen JA, Jemec GB, Yderstraede KB. Methods to assess area and volume of wounds – a systematic review: review of methods to assess wound size. Int Wound J. 2016;13:540–53.

97. Webb S, Sherburn M, Ismail KMK. Managing perineal trauma after childbirth. BMJ. 2014;349:–g6829.

98. Norman G, Dumville JC, Mohapatra DP, Owens GL, Crosbie EJ. Antibiotics and antiseptics for surgical wounds healing by secondary intention. Cochrane Database Syst Rev. 2016; https://doi.org/10.1002/14651858.CD011712.pub2.

99. Sangwine SJ, Sangwine SJ, Horne REN. Wound metrics- the background and motivation. In: The colour image processing handbook. Boston: Springer US: imprint: Springer; 1998. p. 359–60.

100. Arona AJ, al-Marayati L, Grimes DA, Ballard CA. Early secondary repair of third- and fourth-degree perineal lacerations after outpatient wound preparation. Obstet Gynecol. 1995;86:294–6.

101. Hankins GD, Hauth JC, Gilstrap LC, Hammond TL, Yeomans ER, Snyder RR. Early repair of episiotomy dehiscence. Obstet Gynecol. 1990;75:48–51.

102. Okeahialam N, Thakar R, Kleprlikova H, Taithongchai A, Sultan A. Early re-suturing of dehisced obstetric perineal wounds: a 13-year experience. Eur J Obstet Gynecol Reprod Biol. 2020;254:69–73.

103. Uygur D, Yesildaglar N, Kis S, Sipahi T. Early repair of episiotomy dehiscence. Aust N Z J Obstet Gynaecol. 2004;44:244–6.

104. Ramin SM, Ramus RM, Little BB, Gilstrap LC. Early repair of episiotomy dehiscence associated with infection. Am J Obstet Gynecol. 1992;167:1104–7.

105. Soerensen MM, Bek KM, Buntzen S, Højberg K-E, Laurberg S. Long-term outcome of delayed primary or early secondary reconstruction of the anal sphincter after obstetrical injury. Dis Colon Rectum. 2008;51:312–7.

106. Dudley L, Kettle C, Thomas PW, Ismail KMK. Perineal resuturing versus expectant management following vaginal delivery complicated by a dehisced wound (PREVIEW): a pilot and feasibility randomised controlled trial. BMJ Open. 2017;7:e012766.

107. Lewicky-Gaupp C, Mueller MG, Collins SA, Tavathia M, Geynisman-Tan J, Kenton KS. Early secondary repair of obstetric anal sphincter injury breakdown: contemporary surgical techniques and experiences from a peripartum subspecialty clinic. Female Pelvic Med Reconstr Surg. 2021;27:e333–5.

108. Dudley LM, Kettle C, Ismail KMK. Secondary suturing compared to non-suturing for broken down perineal wounds following childbirth. Cochrane Database Syst Rev. 2013;2013:CD008977.

109. Horan TC, Andrus M, Dudeck MA. CDC/NHSN surveillance definition of health care-associated infection and criteria for specific types of infections in the acute care setting. Am J Infect Control. 2008;36:309–32.

110. Berg MR, Gregussen H, Sahlin Y. Long-term outcome of sphincteroplasty with separate suturing of the internal and the external anal sphincter. Tech Coloproctol. 2019;23:1163–72.

111. Vuolo J. Hypergranulation: exploring possible management options. Br J Nurs. 2010;19:S4–8.

112. Kornhaber R, Jaeger M, Harats M, Aviv U, Zerach A, Haik J. Treatment of hypergranulation tissue in burn wounds with topical steroid dressings: a case series. IMCRJ. 2016;9:241–5.

113. Hampton S. Understanding overgranulation in tissue viability practice. Br J Community Nurs. 2007;12:S24–30.

114. Martin P, Nunan R. Cellular and molecular mechanisms of repair in acute and chronic wound healing. Br J Dermatol. 2015;173:370–8.

115. Kettle C, Ismail KM, O'Mahony F. Dyspareunia following childbirth. The Obstet Gynaecol. 2005;7:245–9.

116. Hedayati H, Parsons J, Crowther C. Topically applied anaesthetics for treating perineal pain after childbirth. Cochrane Database Syst Rev. 2005; https://doi.org/10.1002/14651858.CD004223.pub2.

117. Brown HW, Wang L, Bunker CH, Lowder JL. Lower reproductive tract fistula repairs in inpatient US women, 1979–2006. Int Urogynecol J. 2012;23:403–10.

118. Abulafi AM, Sultan AH. Rectovaginal Fistulae. In: Santoro GA, Wieczorek AP, Sultan AH, editors. Pelvic floor disorders: a multidisciplinary textbook. Cham: Springer International Publishing; 2021. p. 975–94.

119. Beigi RH. Clinical implications of methicillin-resistant Staphylococcus aureus in pregnancy. Curr Opin Obstet Gynecol. 2011;23:82–6.

120. Homsi R, Daikoku NH, Littlejohn J, Wheeless CR. Episiotomy: risks of dehiscence and rectovaginal fistula. Obstet Gynecol Surv. 1994;49:803–8.

121. National Institute for Health and Care Excellence. Postnatal care up to 8 weeks after birth (CG37). 2006.

122. Barclay L, Martin N. A sensitive area (care of the episiotomy in the post-partum period). Aust J Adv Nurs. 1983;1:12–9.

123. Sleep J, Grant A. Effects of salt and Savlon bath concentrate post-partum. Nurs Times. 1988;84:55–7.

124. Martin RT, Reiss HE, Milne SE. Vulval and perineal toilet in the puerperium. Br Med J. 1957;2:670–2.

125. Duggal N, Mercado C, Daniels K, Bujor A, Caughey AB, El-Sayed YY. Antibiotic prophylaxis for prevention of postpartum perineal wound complications: a randomized controlled trial. Obstet Gynecol. 2008;111:1268–73.

126. Dennis C-L, Fung K, Grigoriadis S, Robinson GE, Romans S, Ross L. Traditional postpartum practices and rituals: a qualitative systematic review. Women's Health (Lond Engl). 2007;3:487–502.

127. Health Protection Agency. Protocol for the surveillance of surgical site infection, surgical site infection surveillance service; 2013.

Post-partum Problems and the Perineal Clinic

10

Ranee Thakar, Abdul H. Sultan,
and Christina Lewicky-Gaupp

Overview

Test your learning and check your understanding of this book's contents: use the "Springer Nature Flashcards" app to access questions using ▶ https://sn.pub/wqrf89. To use the app, please follow the instructions in Chap. 1.

Learning Objectives

- To help providers familiarise themselves with common postpartum problems to be able to identify and treat them
- To understand that postpartum issues include those related to the perineum, the bladder and bowel, as well as pelvic floor disorders
- To appreciate that maternal recovery clinics/ perineal clinics are an important resource for women in the postpartum time

R. Thakar · A. H. Sultan
Croydon University Hospital, London, UK

C. Lewicky-Gaupp (✉)
Department of Obstetrics and Gynecology, Section of Urogynecology and Reconstructive Pelvic Surgery, University of Chicago Pritzker School of Medicine, Chicago, IL, USA
e-mail: Christina.Lewicky-Gaupp@bsd.uchicago.edu

10.1 Introduction

Over the last century there has been a dramatic decrease in maternal morbidity and mortality especially in developed countries. Women, therefore, have high expectations of pregnancy and childbirth and consequently feel disillusioned when complications occur in the postpartum period. Up to 87% of mothers experience at least one health problem in the first 8 weeks postpartum, with 76% reporting health issues up to 18 months after delivery [1]. MacArthur et al. [2] found that majority of symptoms that persisted for more than a year after birth were still present 1–8 years later, clearly suggesting that problems arising after childbirth can have long-term consequences. Common postnatal health problems include fatigue [1, 3, 4], headache [1, 3], haemorrhoids [1, 3, 4], perineal pain [1, 5], breast conditions [1], constipation [1], dyspareunia [4, 6], backache [7], and urinary [8–10] and anal incontinence [11–14]. In the United States, 1 in 6 women has urinary incontinence, 1 in 30 has symptomatic pelvic organ prolapse, and 1 in 10 has faecal incontinence [15]. These unexpected symptoms can often leave a woman lonely, isolated, and ashamed [16]. However, majority of women do not consult a health professional even if they feel that they need help [3]. These conditions are more prevalent in primiparas and more likely to occur following instrumental rather than spontaneous vaginal or caesarean birth [2].

In this chapter, management of problems pertaining to the perineum or pelvic floor during pregnancy and the early postpartum period will be discussed.

10.2 Perineal Concerns

10.2.1 Perineal Pain

Perineal pain is a common symptom following vaginal birth, regardless of the presence of perineal trauma. However, the severity of perineal pain is directly proportional to the severity of perineal trauma [5, 17]. Perineal pain occurs in 42% of women immediately after delivery, but significantly reduces to 22% and 10% at 8 and 12 weeks respectively. Compared to a spontaneous vaginal birth, perineal pain occurs more frequently and persists for a longer period after assisted vaginal birth (forceps, vacuum delivery, vaginal breech delivery) [18]. Risk factors for persistent pain include having perineal stitches, episiotomy, primiparity, assisted vaginal birth and using Entonox for analgesia in labour [18].

Perineal pain may be due to soft tissue trauma with or without suturing. The pain becomes exaggerated if there is an associated inflammatory process which can range from mild inflammation to cellulitis and even to florid inflammation with wound breakdown and/or abscess formation. Precipitating factors for wound complications can include lack of aseptic techniques, poor surgical techniques which can result in poor apposition and/or granulation tissue or a stitch placed inadvertently in the rectal mucosa.

10.2.1.1 Treatment of Perineal Pain

In addition to treating the underlying condition, treatment options used to relieve perineal pain may be divided into local and systemic. Perineal pain is often accompanied with dyspareunia. Figure 10.1 shows a pathway that can be followed to manage both perineal pain and dyspareunia. Further details on management of perineal wound infections and its sequelae are in Chap. 9.

Local Treatment

Local application of cooling treatments such as ice or cold gel pad, are often included in contemporary maternity practice to obtain relief from pain from perineal trauma. There is very low-certainty evidence that may support the use of cooling treatments, in the form or ice packs or cold gel pads, for the relief of perineal pain in the first 2 days following childbirth. The concurrent use of several treatments is required to adequately address this issue, including prescription and non-prescription analgesia [19].

Bathing in water with or without salt additives (Sitz baths) has been traditionally used to relieve perineal wound pain and promote healing. A three-arm randomised controlled trial (n = 1800) examined the effectiveness of adding (1) salt, (2) a 25 ml sachet of 'Savlon' or (3) nothing to the bath water each day for the first 10 days following delivery [20]. At 10 days and at 3 months, the prevalence of pain and pattern of wound healing was similar in all groups. Although bath additives did not enhance healing or reduce pain or dyspareunia, most of the women reported that bathing did provide some relief of the discomfort. Similarly, lavender oil added to bath water has been evaluated in a randomised trial and found to be ineffective [21]. Therapeutic ultrasound has been suggested as a means to alleviate perineal pain, but data are inconclusive [22].

Local anaesthetics that can be applied directly to the perineum include lidocaine which can be administered as a spray, gel, cream or Epifoam (anti-inflammatory steroid-based foam containing 1% hydrocortisone acetate and 1% pramoxine hydrochloride). However, the evidence for the effectiveness of topically applied anaesthetics is not compelling. Furthermore, there has been no evaluation regarding any long-term effects of topically applied anaesthetics [23].

Systemic Treatment

Oral Analgesics

Paracetamol (acetaminophen) is one of the most used analgesics to relieve mild postnatal perineal pain. A recent Cochrane review suggested that a single dose of paracetamol (either 650 mg or

Fig. 10.1 Suggested regimen for management of perineal pain and dyspareunia

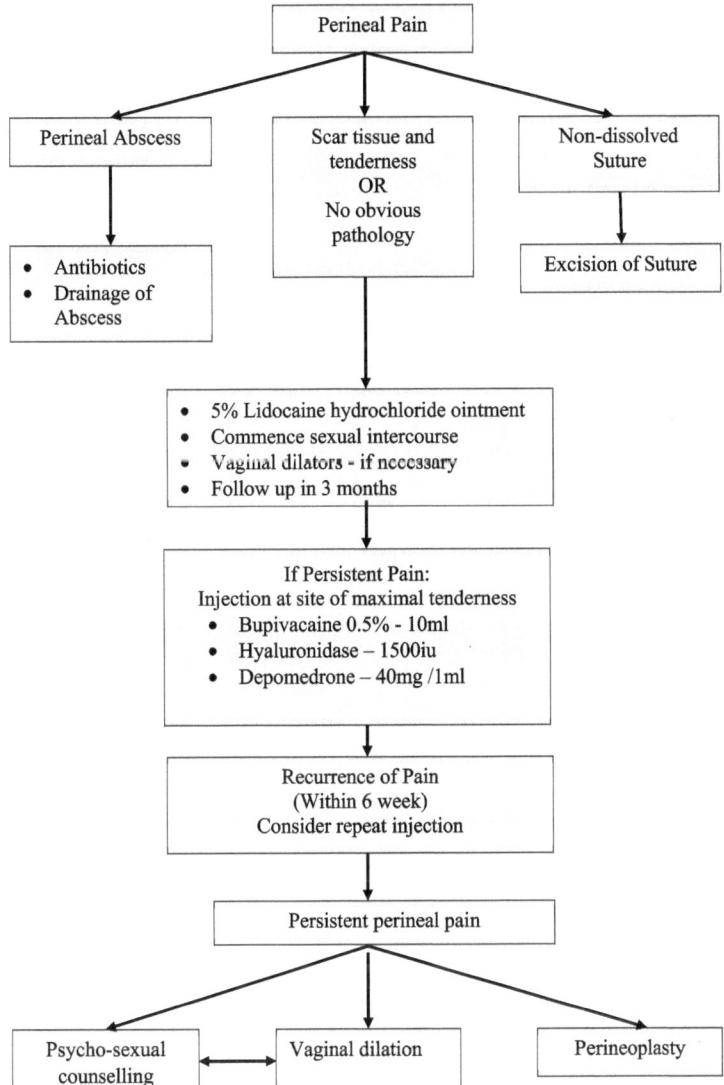

1000 mg) may be effective for reducing the incidence of perineal pain after childbirth. All ten studies included looked at perineal pain relief associated with trauma, and no studies where the pain was associated with intact perineum were found. Overall, the evidence was of low quality due to the unclear methodology reported and the variation of findings. However, it is relatively inexpensive, does not carry a risk of dependence, and is effective and free of side effects to the mother and child [24]. If pain is at moderate and severe levels, stronger analgesics such as opioid analgesics and non-opioid analgesics including non-steroidal anti-inflammatory drugs (NSAIDS) can be considered. However, one must be aware that opioids can cause constipation (and in extreme cases, addiction) and NSAIDS can cause gastric irritation, renal failure, and haematological problems. In addition, these drugs can be secreted in breast milk. In women who sustain perineal trauma, NSAIDs (compared to placebo or paracetamol) may provide greater pain relief for acute perineal pain [24, 25]. In the presence of pain after episiotomy a single dose of aspirin may increase adequate pain relief compared with placebo [26]. Of note, all trials included in these reviews excluded women with intact perineums and those who were breastfeeding.

Suppositories

Rectal analgesia may be preferred in certain situations e.g. nausea and vomiting and/or gastric irritation. The mother should be informed about the route of administration and verbal consent obtained. About 50% of the drug administered via the rectum will bypass the liver resulting in faster pain relief and more local action [27]. In a systematic review set out to assess the effectiveness of analgesic rectal suppositories for perineal pain after childbirth, Hedayati et al. [27] found that compared to placebo, women were less likely to experience pain at or close to 24 hours after birth if they received NSAIDs in the form of suppositories such as Diclofenac. In addition, they required less additional analgesia in the first 24 hours after birth and this effect was still evident at 48 hours. The effect, if any, on longer-term pain relief and analgesia is not known. At the time of birth, proven strategies to reduce perineal pain include use of continuous absorbable synthetic sutures [28].

10.2.2 Perineal Haematoma

A haematoma may be infralevator (vulval, perineal, vaginal) or supralevator (in the broad ligament or paravaginal area). Fortunately, haematomas occur infrequently, with an incidence of between 1:500 and 1:900 vaginal deliveries. Although frequently related to an unrecognised incomplete episiotomy repair (due to suboptimal visualisation of the entire tear) and lack of obliteration of the "dead space" between tissues of the laceration, about 20% of cases occur even with an apparently intact perineum due to a concealed ruptured vessel [29, 30]. A supralevator haematoma forms in the broad ligament and could be due to an extension of a tear of the cervix, vaginal fornix, or uterus. As the haematoma distends, it displaces the uterus contralaterally and bulges into the upper vagina.

With both infralevator and supralevator haematomas, the patient often presents with pain and swelling in the perineal area immediately after delivery or in the postpartum period. However, with a supralevator haematoma, shock may ensue without any obvious swelling. The classical presentation is pain, restlessness, an inability to pass urine and rectal tenesmus within a few hours after delivery. On examination, there is usually an obvious tender swelling of the perineal area with purple and glistening overlying skin.

Management of these haematomas includes immediate treatment of shock, if present. Analgesics, ice-packs and pressure dressings can be used if the haematoma is small (less than 5 cm) and not expanding. Surgical evacuation of the infralevator haematoma by incision and drainage should be carried out only if the haematoma is large and expanding. The incision should preferably be made in the vagina to avoid scar formation, and deep sutures will need to be placed at the base of the haematoma. It is advisable to leave a drain or pack for at least 24 hours.

In contrast to an infralevator haematoma, the management of the supralevator haematoma is largely conservative and a blood transfusion may be necessary. Surgical exploration by laparotomy is usually very frustrating, as the bleeding point almost always cannot be identified; the ureter can be injured with the insertion of deep sutures. In this situation, options include evacuation of the clot and packing the cavity for 24 hours or performing an internal iliac artery ligation. The ideal approach when conservative management fails is to involve an intervention radiologist to perform angiographic embolisation of the bleeding vessel in order to avoid operating [30].

10.2.3 Perineal Wound Healing Complications

Perineal wound healing complications are discussed in Chap. 9.

10.3 Bowel Concerns

10.3.1 Anal Fissures

An anal fissure is an ulcer in the squamous epithelium of the anus located just distal to the mucocutaneous junction; fissures usually occur in the posterior midline [31]. The mucosa in this area has a robust somatic nerve supply (see Chap. 1), and therefore can be extremely painful. Anal fissures are believed to be caused by trauma to the anal mucosa, usually after passage of hard, bulky stools. Constipation is the most common predisposing factor, although diarrhoea may also be a cause [32, 33]. Atypical fissures (large, irregular, multiple and non-midline) may be caused by inflammatory bowel disease, local or systemic malignancy, venereal infection, trauma, tuberculosis, or chemotherapy [31].

In a prospective study before and after delivery of 163 consecutive women (84 primiparous), Abramowitz et al. [34] reported anal fissures in 15% during the first 2 months postpartum. Others have reported an incidence of 9% during a 6 week follow-up period of primiparous women [32]. Risk factors associated with the development of anal fissure include dyschezia (painful defaecation), heavier babies, long second stage of labour, anal incontinence after delivery [34], primiparity, forceps deliveries and perineal damage [35]. Caesarean section did not appear to be protective against anal fissure [24, 32].

Anal fissures typically cause episodic pain that occurs during defaecation and for 1–2 h afterwards. The diagnosis is suspected from the patient's history and frequently confirmed by visual examination of the anal margin. The most consistent finding in typical fissures is spasm of the internal anal sphincter, which is so severe that the pain caused by the fissure is thought to be due to ischaemia of the sphincter [36]. Relief of the spasm has been associated with relief of pain and healing of the fissure without recurrence.

Treatment of fissures is aimed at relieving constipation using a high fibre diet with along with fibre supplements such as Psyllium seed supplement (Fybogel). Iron preparations should be avoided. Local application of Lidocaine in the anal canal can provide effective analgesia as well. After defaecation, water (preferably a hand-held shower) should be used to clean the anus rather than wiping with toilet paper to avoid abrasions. Medical treatment is aimed at relaxing the internal anal sphincter. Nitroglycerin ointment, calcium channel blockers (either given as tablets or applied topically) and/or injection of botulinum toxin [31] have proven efficacy. In a systematic review, nitroglycerin ointment was found to have a healing rate of about 55%. Combining all analyses in which a placebo was used as the comparison group, the healing rate in the placebo group was found to be 35%, which was significantly lower. In comparisons of nitroglycerin ointment to botulinum toxin injection or calcium channel blockers, no significant difference in efficacy of healing was found. However nitroglycerin ointment was associated with headache in almost 40% of subjects, which was often severe enough to stop treatment [37]. Conservative treatment (stool softeners, laxatives and local anaesthetic cream) has been shown to be successful in 97% of postpartum women [32, 33, 38]. There is no data regarding the use of medical treatments for anal fissure during pregnancy. A suggested pathway for the management of anal fissures in postpartum women is shown in Fig. 10.2.

Non-pregnant or postpartum women who fail to respond to these conservative measures are candidates for surgical procedures. However, in a prospective sonographic study it has been shown that division of the internal anal sphincter in most females tends to be more extensive than intended, likely due to a shorter anal canal [31].

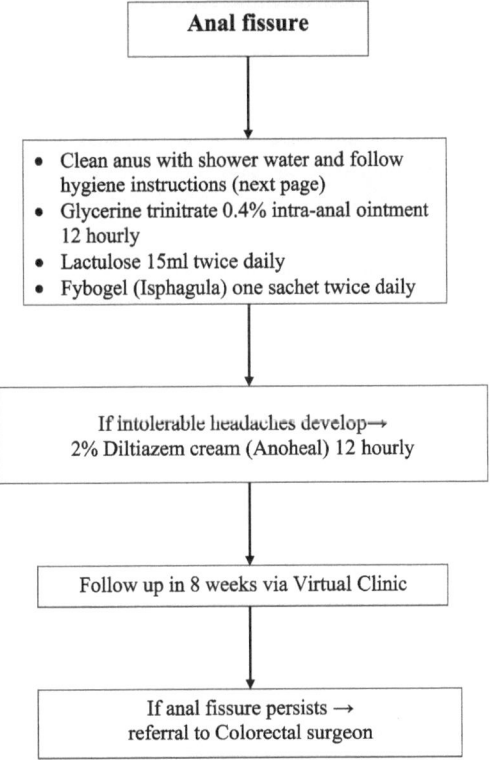

Fig. 10.2 Management of anal fissures (legend)

Furthermore, postpartum anal fissures are associated with low anal canal pressures and surgical interference with the anal sphincter mechanism. Therefore sphincterotomy should only be used a last resort, so as not to put the patient at risk for anal incontinence [32]. For those patients requiring surgery for anal fissure, open and closed partial lateral internal sphincterotomy appear to be equally efficacious. It is less clear whether posterior sphincterotomy should be performed as the primary treatment of anal fissure [39].

10.3.2 Haemorrhoids

Haemorrhoids (piles) are swollen veins at or near the anus. During bowel evacuation, normal haemorrhoids are compressed and drained, facilitating the emptying of the rectum. Haemorrhoids can become symptomatic if there is damage to their structure and/or alteration in function. Associated factors for development of painful haemorrhoids include straining at defaecation, constipation, vascular enlargement secondary to increased intra-abdominal pressure, erect posture and heredity.

Several physiological changes during pregnancy may lead to development of haemorrhoids. Firstly, constipation is likely to be due to smooth muscle inhibition by high levels of circulating progesterone or by mechanical obstruction by the gravid uterus. Secondly, venous engorgement and dilatation may occur during pregnancy as the circulating blood volume is increased by 25–40%. Furthermore, hormonal changes result in increased laxity of connective tissue, especially in the pelvis [34]. In the postnatal period, haemorrhoids are possibly a consequence of pushing in the second stage of labour. Risk factors include instrumental vaginal delivery [1–3] a longer second stage of labour [2] and vaginal birth of a heavier baby [2].

From an anatomic standpoint, haemorrhoids are either internal or external. Internal haemorrhoids originate from the internal haemorrhoidal plexus above the dentate line, while external haemorrhoids originate from the external plexus below the dentate line. Internal haemorrhoids

may be classified according to the degree of prolapse, although this may not necessarily reflect the severity of the woman's symptoms. Haemorrhoids are classified as follows [40]: (1) first degree: bleed but do not prolapse, (2) second degree: prolapse on straining but reduce spontaneously, (3) third degree: prolapse on straining and require manual reduction and (4) fourth degree: prolapsed and incarcerated.

In an observational study of 11,701 women, MacArthur et al. [2] found that 8% of women reported haemorrhoids of more than 6 weeks duration for the first time within 3 months of birth; an additional 10% reported haemorrhoids as "ongoing" or "recurrent" symptoms. Two thirds of women reported the presence of haemorrhoids 1–9 years after delivery. Glazener et al. [1] found that 17% of postnatal women reported haemorrhoids (new and recurrent) when questioned in hospital, 22% between delivery and 8 weeks postpartum and 15% after 2 months.

Symptomatically, haemorrhoids can manifest in a wide range of ways such as a burning sensation, itching, intermittent bleeding of the anus, varying degrees of leakage of mucus, faeces or flatus, sensation of fullness or a lump, perianal hygienic problems, discomfort and/or pain. The most common symptoms during pregnancy and the puerperium are intermittent bleeding from the anus and pain. Depending on the degree of pain, women's quality of life could be compromised, as pain can affect the activities of everyday life, such as walking, sitting down, emptying bowels, sleeping, caring for the family or a new baby. Assessment should include anoscopy and a digital examination in the left lateral position.

The treatment for haemorrhoids during pregnancy and the postpartum period should be tailored to the severity of the disease and duration of symptoms. Treatment is mainly directed at the relief of symptoms, especially pain control. For many women, symptoms will resolve spontaneously soon after birth, and so any corrective treatment is usually deferred to sometime after birth. However, complications of haemorrhoids (acute thrombosis, incarceration of a prolapsed internal haemorrhoid, unremitting pain) may require more aggressive treatment such as a closed excisional haemorrhoidectomy under local anaesthetic [41].

External haemorrhoids require treatment only for acute thrombosis. Internal haemorrhoids are best managed conservatively. Management can be broadly classified as (i) conservative, (ii) alternative, and (iii) surgical [42, 43]. Conservative treatment is based on (a) dietary modifications (high fibre intake, high liquid intake, stool softeners); (b) stimulants or depressants of the bowel transit (depending if the woman has constipation or diarrhoea); (c) local treatments (sitz baths, creams, ointments or suppositories containing anaesthetics, anti-inflammatory drugs, steroids, etc., alone or in combination); (d) drugs of the flavonoids family such as rutosides that cause decreased capillary fragility, improving the microcirculation in venous insufficiency. Most minor haemorrhoidal symptoms can be treated this way.

Alternative treatment is required if the haemorrhoids are severe and non-responsive to conservative treatment. This can include a number of ambulatory interventions that usually do not need anaesthetics, such as injection sclerotherapy, rubber band ligation, cryotherapy, infrared photocoagulation, laser therapy, etc. Injection sclerotherapy has been effectively used during pregnancy.

Surgical treatment includes excision surgery and stapled anopexy. These methods are usually a third line therapy after other treatments have failed. There are no known trials that have specifically evaluated treatments for severe haemorrhoids during pregnancy and the postpartum period. However, it is important to enquire about anal incontinence symptoms in antenatal women who have previously undergone haemorrhoidectomy as there could be inadvertent sphincter damage [44].

10.3.3 Anal Incontinence

The diagnosis and management of anal incontinence are discussed in Chaps. 18, 19 and 20.

10.3.4 Constipation

About 80% of people suffer from constipation at some time during their lives, and brief periods of constipation are normal. Some of the most used definitions of constipation include infrequent bowel movements typically less than 2 bowel actions per week, difficulty in defacation (straining at passing stools for more than 25% of bowel movements or a subjective sensation of hard stools), or the sensation of incomplete bowel emptying.

The percent of women who suffer symptoms of constipation in pregnancy is reported to be anywhere from 11% to 38% [45]. The pathogenesis is not fully understood, however, it appears to be related to the effect of progesterone on gastrointestinal motility, as there is an increase in gut transit time in the second and third trimester compared with both the first trimester and the postpartum period. Fibre supplements are effective in managing constipation, and raise no serious concerns about side effects to mother or fetus. Stimulant laxatives can be more effective than bulk-forming laxatives but are more likely to cause side-effects that reduce their acceptability to patients. Therefore, it is recommended that women endorsing constipation in pregnancy be treated with daily dietary supplements of fibre in the form of bran or wheat fibre. If these are ineffective, stimulant laxatives may be used. The management of constipation is discussed in Chap. 8.

10.4   Bladder Concerns

10.4.1 Postpartum Urinary Retention

There is no standardised definition for postpartum urinary retention. A commonly used symptom-based definition is the absence of spontaneous voiding of urine within 6 hours of delivery. After caesarean delivery, if a catheter is used, retention is defined as "no spontaneous voiding within 6 hours after removal of the indwelling catheter" [46]. Another commonly used definition is based on the post void residual bladder volume as estimated by ultrasound or catheterisation. Although most experts agree that residual volumes of less than 50 ml are normal and more than 200 ml are abnormal, little agreement exists on the intervening grey zone [47].

Postpartum urinary retention can be classified into covert and overt forms. The covert form is asymptomatic and recognised by demonstrating an elevated post void residual measurement of more than or equal to 150 ml, either with ultrasound scanning or with catheterisation. Clinically overt post-partum urinary retention refers to the inability to void spontaneously after delivery [48]. Risk factors for urinary retention in the postpartum period include nulliparity [49, 50], instrumental delivery [48, 49, 51], prolonged first and second stage of labour [50, 52] and severe perineal trauma [50, 52]. Although there is a lack of consensus in the literature regarding the effect of epidural analgesia on postpartum retention [47], the bladder appears to be the last to regain sensation and the Royal College of Obstetricians and Gynaecologists (RCOG) guidelines recommend catheterisation for at least 12 hours following regional anaesthesia [53].

The incidence of postpartum urinary retention ranges between 0.5% and 14% and varies depending on the definition used [47]. Often, the mother will present with an inability to pass urine that is associated with acute lower abdominal pain. Occasionally she may complain of continuous leakage of urine in the presence of a large palpable bladder. Other presenting symptoms may be hesitancy, slow or intermittent stream, straining to void and a sense of incomplete emptying. On examination, a suprapubic mass will often be palpable. However, the diagnosis is confirmed after catheterisation or ultrasound imaging. There is no consensus on the minimal urine volume that constitutes postpartum urinary retention as measured on ultrasound [52]. It should be noted that ultrasound estimation of post-void residual urine in postpartum women can be measured accurately and is not confounded by the enlarged postpartum uterus.

There is also no consensus of opinion on the management of postpartum urinary retention [54, 55] and various treatment regimens have been described [47, 48, 50, 51, 56]. Initial treatment includes administration of oral analgesia, helping the woman to mobilise, ensuring privacy during voiding and having a warm bath. If these conservative measures fail, it is advisable to insert a Foley catheter. A voiding trial can then be attempted after 24–48 h. If the voiding trial is failed, the catheter should again be replaced. However, the duration of catheterisation is empirical, and no standard has been agreed. Burkhart et al. [57] found that no postpartum women with a residual urine volume of less than 700 ml required repeat catheterisation, but repeat catheterisation was required in 14% of patients with 700–999 ml of residual urine. If the voiding trial fails again, the woman can be taught intermittent self-catheterisation every 4–6 hourly until she is able to void and her residual is less than 150 ml. If this is not feasible, she should be sent home with an indwelling catheter for 2–3 days and the voiding trial repeated. A suggested regime for management of postpartum urinary retention is shown in Fig. 10.3.

There are very few studies on the sequelae of postpartum urinary retention but published data suggests that this condition usually resolves within a short period of time and specific treatment is not necessary [48, 49]. Yip et al., in a case controlled study, found that women with postpartum urinary retention did not have a higher incidence of urinary incontinence, frequency nocturia or urgency [58]. In a more recent study of over 60 women, Mohr et al. reported long-term voiding disorders in 8.2%, 6.7%, and 4.9% after 1, 2, and 3 years respectively. The authors emphasized that 89% of the patients with urinary retention had operative vaginal births, clearly identifying this as a risk factor [59].

10.4.2 Urinary Incontinence

Childbirth is an established risk factor for urinary incontinence [60, 61]. Although vaginal birth has been implicated as the main contributory factor, the exact mechanism is not known. Pregnancy itself may cause mechanical and/or hormonal changes that can lead to urinary incontinence.

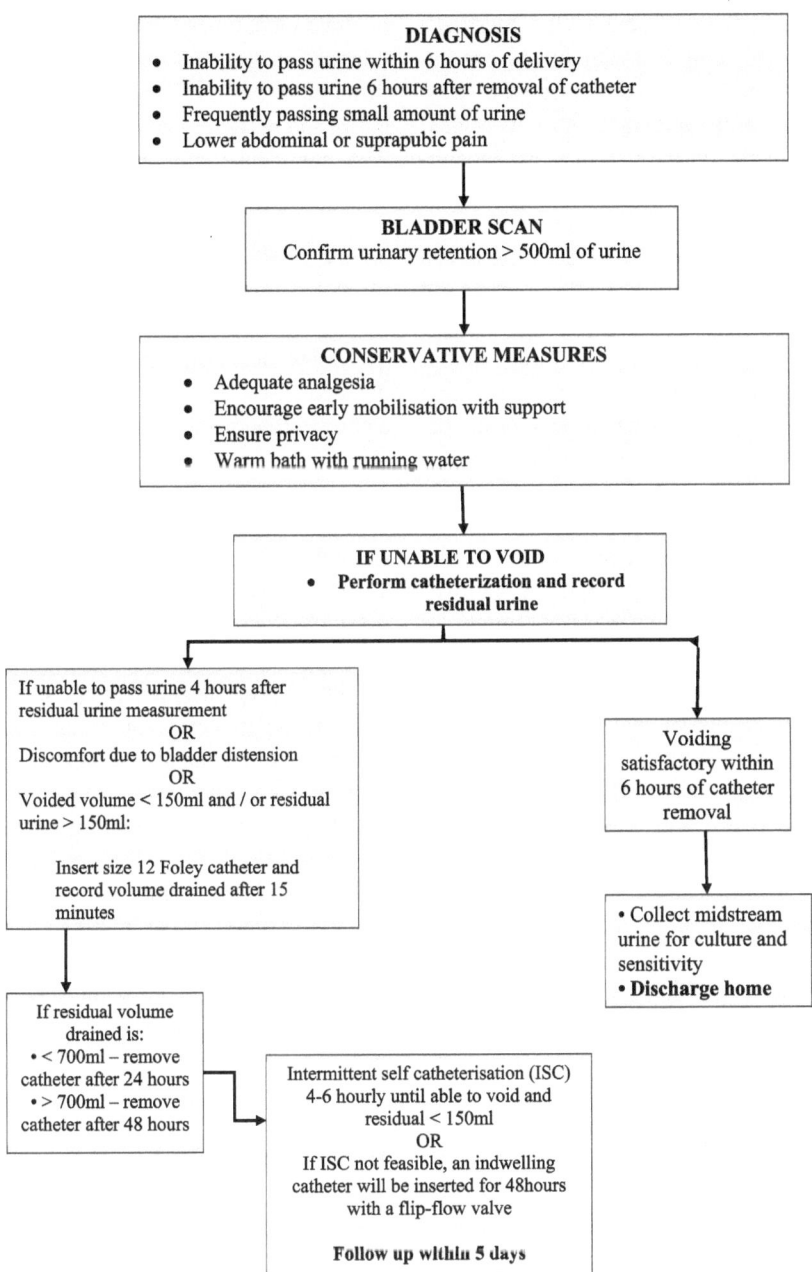

Fig. 10.3 Management of postpartum urinary retention

There is evidence that the prevalence of urinary incontinence is highest during pregnancy and decreases in the puerperium [62, 63]. Interestingly, stress or urge incontinence during the first pregnancy and puerperium predicts an increased risk of having the symptom 5 years later [64]. In a large community based epidemiological study, Rortveit et al. [65] found that compared to nulliparous women, those delivered by caesarean section were at higher risk for any incontinence and those who delivered vaginally were at an even greater increase in risk of developing urinary incontinence. The risk of moderate or severe incontinence was also higher in the vaginal-birth group compared to the caesarean section group. As compared with nulliparous status, caesarean section was associated with stress and mixed type of incontinence, whereas vaginal birth further increased the risk of stress incontinence only. Interestingly, there was no difference in the prevalence of incontinence in women who underwent elective versus emergency caesarean section. The authors suggest that this data should therefore not be used as an argument for increased use of caesarean section, as a very large number of women would have to have a caesarean section to prevent urinary incontinence. Moreover, the decrease in incontinence after caesarean section would apply until 50 years of age, since there was no association of incontinence with mode of delivery in the older age groups.

More recent studies have supported the association of urinary incontinence and mode of delivery. In 2011, Handa et al. found that in a cohort of over 1100 women five to 10 years after delivery, spontaneous vaginal birth was associated with a significantly greater odds of stress incontinence (odds ratio [OR] 2.9, 95% confidence interval [CI] 1.5–5.5) when compared to women who underwent scheduled cesarean section [66]. Similarly, in a study from 2018 of more than 1500 women looking at mode of delivery and the development of pelvic floor disorders, Blomquist et al. found that compared with spontaneous vaginal birth, caesarean birth was associated with significantly lower hazard for stress urinary incontinence as well as overactive bladder [67].

Current evidence suggests that intensive supervised pelvic floor muscle training should be offered to antenatal women [68] and/or to postnatal high risk women i.e. instrumental delivery, obstetric anal sphincter injury, delivery of a large baby, pre-pregnancy and antenatal stress incontinence, persistent postnatal urinary incontinence, family history of incontinence, pre-pregnancy obesity, increased bladder neck mobility [68, 69]. For example, Blomquist showed that in women with at least one vaginal delivery, a pelvic floor muscle strength of <20 cm H_2O was associated with a shorter time to event for the development

of stress incontinence (time ratio, 0.67; 95% confidence interval, 0.50–0.90), overactive bladder (time ratio, 0.67; 95% confidence interval, 0.51–0.86), and pelvic organ prolapse (time ratio, 0.76; 95% confidence interval, 0.65–0.88); in women who had only delivered via caesarean sections, these associations were not found [70]. In a randomised control study evaluating effects of pelvic floor muscle training by a physical therapist within 9 weeks of delivery on the rate of urinary and/or anal leakage, the authors found that training decreased the rate of urinary incontinence and related bother at 6 months postpartum, while also increasing pelvic floor and anal sphincter muscle strength and endurance [71]. Interestingly, in another study of 175 postpartum, primiparous women, pelvic floor muscle training within 8 weeks of delivery did not impact the development of pelvic organ prolapse [72]. A systematic review of the effect of pelvic floor muscle training during pregnancy and after childbirth on prevention and treatment of urinary incontinence, the authors concluded that pelvic floor muscle training is effective if done in a supervised fashion; they recommended that further, high-quality studies are needed in the immediate postpartum period [73]. While some studies suggest that the benefits of pelvic floor muscle training persist beyond 1 year postpartum [74] others found that the early benefits do not seem to persist on long term follow-up probably due to reduced compliance [75].

10.5 Sexual Problems

Sexual dysfunction is discussed in Chap. 7.

10.6 Pelvic Organ Prolapse

Injury to the pelvic floor during childbirth is incriminated in the development of pelvic organ prolapse. Other risk factors include defective collagen, race, advancing age, hysterectomy, certain medical illnesses, and states of chronically raised intra-abdominal pressure. In a large study in the

United States, Swift et al. [76] found an association between gravidity, parity, number of vaginal deliveries, vaginal delivery of a macrosomic infant, and an increased pelvic organ prolapse quantification system stage. In a prospective study conducted to document pelvic organ prolapse throughout the pregnancy, O'Boyle et al. [77] found that the POPQ-stage was significantly higher in the third rather than in the first trimester. They concluded that these findings probably represent normal physiological changes of the pelvic floor during pregnancy but suggested that significant changes may be objectively demonstrated prior to delivery.

The effect of mode of delivery on pelvic organ prolapse has been investigated by numerous groups. In one of the first studies to look at this association, Sze et al. [78] found pelvic organ prolapse to be present in 46% of women (26% had POPQ-stage II) at the 36-week antepartum visit. At 6 weeks postpartum, 83% met the definition of prolapse, however, out of these 52% had only stage II prolapse. In the 2011 study of Handa et al., the authors found that operative vaginal birth significantly increased the odds for all pelvic floor disorders, especially prolapse (OR 7.5, 95% CI 2.7–20.9) [66]. More recently in 2018, Blomquist et al. published a cohort study of over 1500 women recruited 5–10 years after their first delivery and followed up annually for up to 9 years. They found that the cumulative incidence of pelvic organ prolapse after first birth was 30% (95% CI, 25.1–34.9%) and operative vaginal birth was associated with significantly higher hazard of pelvic organ prolapse (aHR, 1.88 [95% CI, 1.28–2.78]) [67].

If a patient develops a bothersome vaginal bulge, a pessary can be placed as the first option to relieve the symptom of prolapse in the antenatal and postnatal woman with prolapse. To date, there is a paucity of data on recommendation for mode of delivery in a pregnant woman who presents with prolapse and there is no data regarding the utility of pelvic floor physical therapy in this specific population. See Chap. 11 for the management of subsequent pregnancy after incontinence and prolapse surgery.

10.7   Maternal Recovery Clinics

In a survey of 1249 women in the postnatal period, Glazener et al. found that 85% of women who reported at least one health problem in the hospital received help or treatment for it. Although just as many had problems upon discharge (87%), only a small proportion (69%) were treated; of the 75% who had a health problem after the first 2 months, only about half received treatment. Reasons for the apparent lack of treatment included a perceived notion that it is inappropriate to ask for help or that professional help was not available, unsatisfactory or ineffective [1]. Perhaps it was perceived that health professionals might only treat women with more severe problems, or that women felt that their doctors may not be able to treat their condition or that they should cope with the problem themselves [79]. This pattern of care-seeking waning over time might be due to the natural resolution of the problem or its decrease in severity with time. However, this trend might also reflect a lack of recognition of the impact of continuing maternal morbidity in the postpartum period by health professionals and even mothers themselves.

The RCOG have recommended that where possible all women sustaining OASIs should have an assessment around 6–12 weeks postpartum by clinicians with a special interest in OASI [80]. A survey of clinical leads of hospitals in the UK demonstrated that only 32% offered a dedicated outpatient clinic follow-up for women after OASI [83]. The American College of Obstetricians and Gynecologists (ACOG), on the other hand, recommends an initial assessment, either in person or by phone, within the first 3 weeks postpartum to address acute postpartum issues; specialty care is not specified. Furthermore, postpartum women with perineal complications not related to OASIs (for example those with prolapse, perineal wound infections, urinary incontinence) should also be expected to have an opportunity for a similar assessment.

Women with female genital mutilation (FGM) have been reported to have poorer obstetric outcomes in both low-resource and resource-rich countries [79] with a contributing factor being lack of knowledge and experience of healthcare professionals. However, when appropriate antenatal counselling and management are available via a dedicated perineal clinic, obstetric outcomes showed no difference from those without FGM [81, 82]. See Chap. 13 for further details of management of women with FGM.

There is a wide variation in the follow-up of women after they sustain an OASI [83, 84] and various different models of perineal clinics have been reported. These include clinics led by consultant urogynaecologists [83] consultant obstetrician and gynaecologists [86, 87], with some triaged or assisted by specialised midwives/nurses [85, 87–89], and clinics led by a specialist midwife [89]. Formats of clinics include: one-stop clinics offering all necessary investigations and referrals [91, 92] a standard outpatient set-up where investigations are performed either at a later date or prior to initial assessment, [86–89], and those where only limited investigations are available, or telephone follow-up is utilised [89, 90]. Different management protocols have also been used for the management of OASI patients [93–95].

A survey of healthcare providers (obstetrics and gynaecology trainees, attending physicians, certified nurse midwives, and advanced practice providers) from an academic tertiary level service found that introduction of a peripartum pelvic floor disorder clinic resulted in high obstetric provider satisfaction which positively impacts on patient care through increased provider knowledge and awareness on the management of OASI [96]. Service evaluation of the first 36-month experience of this clinic demonstrated both sustainability and feasibility, with consistent clinical growth over time: 483 new consultations, 2/3 of which were for OASI and the other 1/3 for a variety of peripartum pelvic floor indications [97]. It should be noted that this is the experiences of an academic medical centre primarily serving white, primiparous, obese women and may not have external validity or be reproducible for smaller volume medical centres or those with differing patient populations.

The establishment of a dedicated multidisciplinary, subspecialty clinic has numerous benefits, as it enables provision of evidence-based quality care by experienced professionals. A dedicated perineal or maternal recovery clinic also provides women an opportunity to be explained the circumstances under which the perineal injury occurred, and counsel them appropriately regarding mode of subsequent delivery. Due to time constraints and inappropriate expertise, explanation and counseling are often suboptimal in a busy postnatal or gynaecology clinic. These clinics may allocate resources more effectively by avoiding visits to an obstetrical provider for specific pelvic floor concerns. Furthermore, subspecialty clinics can fulfill a niche of quality improvement. In addition, these clinics offer an exceptional opportunity for trainee involvement and education, because trainees often are not exposed to the aftermath of birth and the sequelae of, for example, operative vaginal birth.

Although perineal clinics are now becoming very popular, there appear to be a variety of models of care. Ki Wan et al. describe the 11-year experiences of the original perineal clinic in the Croydon UK [98], with 3254 new consultations during that time period. This one -stop clinic is run by a consultant urogynaecologist (trained in anal manometry and ultrasound) and a trained nurse/midwife. There is easy access to a physiotherapist, a continence nurse specialist, colorectal nurse specialist, colorectal surgeon and psychosexual counsellor. Integration of multidisciplinary professionals promotes a holistic approach to pelvic floor and perineal problems. This clinic is restricted to childbirth related problems including conditions such as dyspareunia, perineal pain, wound breakdown, infection, prolapse, anal and urinary incontinence that occur during pregnancy and up to 16 weeks after childbirth. Women who sustain obstetric anal sphincter injuries (OASIs) are seen within 3 months postpartum. In addition, pregnant women with a history of OASI are evaluated and counselled regarding subsequent mode of delivery (See Chap. 5). The clinic is equipped with facilities for endoanal and pelvic floor ultrasound, as well as anal manometry to facilitate a one-stop approach. The most common reason for referral was OASIs, with the second being perineal wound complications, with a high proportion requiring further management.

The establishment of a dedicated one-stop clinic enables provision of evidence-based standardised care by experienced professionals. The model of the one-stop provision offers multiple benefits: the opportunity to explore the circumstances under which their perineal injury occurred, understand the extent of trauma and in many cases provide simple reassurance. A duty of candour and giving consistent advice to women is important from a medicolegal perspective particularly as this is an area of obstetrics where there is increasing litigation. It is also an arena where taboo topics such as FGM could be openly discussed and managed by experienced professionals with little to no barriers (See Chap. 13). This is particularly important for antenatal patients as it is a crucial time to identify these women and arrange appropriate treatment options. The one-stop model avoids multiple visits to the hospital, an important consideration in postpartum women. The combined anal manometry and endoanal ultrasound performed by the same physician at one visit optimizes the management plan by correlating with symptoms enabling a holistic approach to women with clinically recognised and unrecognised OASIs.

Following the original Croydon model as described above, numerous clinics have mushroomed in the United States. In a more recent clinical commentary, Hickman et al. not only highlighted the experiences of 3 tertiary care perineal clinics (University of Michigan, Cleveland Clinic and Northwestern University), but also shared an algorithm for the successful creation of a subspecialty clinic [99]. In this paper, the combined experiences of over 4000 peri- and postpartum women are described. The authors conclude that these clinics, which can be established with careful planning, create an opportunity to improve patient satisfaction and outcomes, educate patients and providers alike, and contribute to the growing body of evidence-based practice in this area.

There are different choices to consider when developing a perineal clinic [100] and these are dependent on local resources. Thus, a substantial variation in the organization and availability of equipment in perineal clinics and the protocol used to advise the mode of delivery for subsequent pregnancies is present.

There are many reasons to advocate for establishment of perineal services. Dedicated perineal clinics could help women suffering from postpartum problems to find multidisciplinary support such as physiotherapy, psychology and psychosexual counselling. It is also an opportunity to review and debrief women regarding the previous delivery events. They provide an opportunity for systematic, evidence-based evaluation and provide personalised care.

10.8 Conclusion

Postpartum problems are clearly an integral part of care of childbearing women. Ideally, a team of health care providers with the knowledge and expertise to care for these women in a single clinic setting should be available to mothers. More research is needed in the management of perineal problems including perineal wounds, OASIs in subsequent pregnancies and perineal pain. As perineal clinics become the standard of care, they will continue to serve as an ideal setting to advance our knowledge, develop local experts and provide comprehensive care. More importantly, these clinics will continue to serve as resources to unravel this under-studied patient population and to develop sound, evidence-based practices for new mothers. Furthermore, these clinics will serve as a foundation for peripartum intervention, preventative work and rehabilitation, helping to reduce the risk of future pelvic floor disorders in this at-risk patient population.

Take Home Messages

- Postpartum problems are clearly an integral part of care of childbearing women
- A team of health care providers with the knowledge and expertise to care for these women should be available to new mothers
- As perineal/maternal recovery clinics become the standard of care, they will continue to serve as an ideal setting to advance our knowl-

edge and develop our resources to study this under-studied patient population and ultimately, to develop sound, evidence-based practices for new mothers.

Appendix: MCQ

Questions

1. Which of the following statements is true?
   (A) Up to 87% of mothers experience at least one health problem in the first 8 weeks postpartum.
   (B) Rectal analgesia should not be used in the postpartum period.
   (C) At the time of delivery, proven strategies to reduce perineal pain include use of continuous delayed absorbable synthetic sutures.
   (D) Narcotics should always be given for perineal pain.

2. Regarding treatment of supralevator hematomas, all of the following statements are true *except*:
   (A) It is mainly conservative.
   (B) Surgical intervention is helpful.
   (C) Radiologic embolization can be used.
   (D) Blood transfusion may be necessary.

3. Anal fissures:
   (A) Typically cause episodic pain that occurs during defaecation and for 1–2 hours afterwards.
   (B) Cause pain secondary to spasm of the external anal sphincter.
   (C) Are always healed with nitroglycerine ointment.
   (D) Can rarely be treated with conservative measures in the postpartum period.

4. Which of the following is a true statement?
   (A) Constipation is likely to be due to smooth muscle inhibition by high levels of circulating estrogen.
   (B) Internal haemorrhoids originate from the internal haemorrhoidal plexus above the dentate line, while external haemorrhoids originate from the external plexus below the dentate line.
   (C) Three quarters of women reported the presence of haemorrhoids 1–9 years after delivery.
   (D) Assessment of hemorrhoids should include colonoscopy.

Answers

1. Which of the following statements is true?
   (A) TRUE
   (B) FALSE
   (C) FALSE
   (D) FALSE

2. Regarding treatment of supralevator hematomas, all of the following statements are true *except*:
   (A) FALSE
   (B) TRUE
   (C) FALSE
   (D) FALSE

3. Anal fissures:
   (A) TRUE
   (B) FALSE
   (C) FALSE
   (D) FALSE

4. Which of the following is a true statement?
   (A) FALSE
   (B) TRUE
   (C) FALSE
   (D) FALSE

References

1. Glazener CM, Abdalla M, Stroud P, Naji S, Templeton A, Russell IT. Postnatal maternal moridity: extent, causes, prevention and treatment. Br J Obstet Gynaecol. 1995;102:282–7.
2. MacArthur C, Lewis M, Knox EG. Health after childbirth. Br J Obstet Gynaecol. 1991;98(12):1193–5.

3. Brown S, Lumley J. Maternal health after childbirth: results of an Australian population based survey. Br J Obstet Gynaecol. 1998;105(2):156–61.

4. Schytt E, Lindmark G, Waldenstrom U. Physical symptoms after childbirth: prevalence and associations with self-rated health. BJOG. 2005;112(2):210–7.

5. Albers L, Garcia J, Renfrew M, McCandlish R, Elbourne D. Distribution of genital tract trauma in childbirth and related postnatal pain. Birth. 1999;26(1):11–7.

6. Barrett G, Pendry E, Peacock J, Victor C, Thakar R, Manyonda I. Women's sexual health after childbirth. BJOG. 2000;107(2):186–95.

7. Thompson JF, Roberts CL, Currie M, Ellwood DA. Prevalence and persistence of health problems after childbirth: associations with parity and method of birth. Birth. 2002;29(2):83–94.

8. Hojberg KE, Salvig JD, Winslow NA, Lose G, Secher NJ. Urinary incontinence: prevalence and risk factors at 16 weeks of gestation. Br J Obstet Gynaecol. 1999;106(8):842–50.

9. Foldspang A, Mommsen S, Djurhuus JC. Prevalent urinary incontinence as a correlate of pregnancy, vaginal childbirth, and obstetric techniques. Am J Public Health. 1999;89(2):209–12.

10. Wilson PD, Herbison RM, Herbison GP. Obstetric practice and the prevalence of urinary incontinence three months after delivery. Br J Obstet Gynaecol. 1996;103:154–61.

11. Sultan AH, Kamm MA, Hudson CN, Thomas JM, Bartram CI. Anal sphincter disruption during vaginal delivery. N Engl J Med. 1993;329:1905–11.

12. Abramowitz L, Sobhani I, Ganansia R, Vuagnat A, Benifla JL, Darai E, et al. Are sphincter defects the cause of anal incontinence after vaginal delivery? Results of a prospective study. Dis Colon Rectum. 2000;43(5):590–6.

13. MacArthur C, Bick DE, Keighley MRB. Faecal incontinence after childbirth. Br J Obstet Gynaecol. 1997;104:46–50.

14. Chaliha C, Sultan AH, Bland JM, Monga AK, Stanton SL. Anal function: effect of pregnancy and delivery. Am J Obstet Gynecol. 2001;185(2):427–32.

15. Nygaard IE, Barber MD, Burgio KL, Kenton K, Meikle S, Schaffer J, et al. Prevalence of symptomatic pelvic floor disorders in US women. JAMA. 2008;300(11):1311–6.

16. Pipitone F, DeLancey JO. The postpartum silence. BJOG. 2022;129(8):1231–3.

17. Macarthur AJ, MacArthur C. Incidence, severity, and determinants of perineal pain after vaginal delivery: a prospective cohort study. Am J Obstet Gynecol. 2004;191(4):1199–204.

18. Glazener CM. Women's health after delivery. In: Henderson C, Bick D, editors. Perineal care: an international issue. 1st ed. Salisbury: Quay Books Division, MA Healthcare Ltd; 2005. p. 11–7.

19. East CE, Dorward ED, Whale RE, Liu J. Local cooling for relieving pain from perineal trauma sustained during childbirth. Cochrane Database Syst Rev. 2020;10(10):CD006304.

20. Sleep J, Grant A. Relief of perineal pain following childbirth: a survey of midwifery practice. Midwifery. 1988;4(3):118–22.

21. Dale A, Cornwell S. The role of lavender oil in relieving perineal discomfort following childbirth: a blind randomized clinical trial. J Adv Nurs. 1994;19(1):89–96.

22. Hay-Smith J, Herbison P, Mørkved S. Physical therapies for prevention of urinary and faecal incontinence in adults. Cochrane Database Syst Rev. 2002;(2):CD003191.

23. Hedayatl H, Parsons J, Crowther CA. Topically applied anaesthetics for treating perineal pain after childbirth. Cochrane Database Syst Rev. 2005;(2):CD004223.

24. Abalos E, Sguassero Y, Gyte GM. Paracetamol/acetaminophen (single administration) for perineal pain in the early postpartum period. Cochrane Database Syst Rev. 2021;1(1):CD008407.

25. Wuytack F, Smith V, Cleary BJ. Oral non-steroidal anti-inflammatory drugs (single dose) for perineal pain in the early postpartum period. Cochrane Database Syst Rev. 2021;1(1):CD011352.

26. Shepherd E, Grivell RM. Aspirin (single dose) for perineal pain in the early postpartum period. Cochrane Database Syst Rev. 2020;7(7):CD012129.

27. Hedayati H, Parsons J, Crowther CA. Rectal analgesia for pain from perineal trauma following childbirth. Cochrane Database Syst Rev. 2003;(3):CD003931.

28. Frohlich J, Kettle C. Perineal care. BMJ Clin Evid. 2015;2015:1401.

29. Ridgway LE. Puerperal emergency. Vaginal and vulvar hematomas. Obstet Gynecol Clin N Am. 1995;22(2):275–82.

30. Villella J, Garry D, Levine G, Glanz S, Figueroa R, Maulik D. Postpartum angiographic embolization for vulvovaginal hematoma. A report of two cases. J Reprod Med. 2001;46(1):65–7.

31. Sultan AH, Kamm MA, Nicholls RJ, Bartram CI. Internal anal sphincter division during lateral sphincterotomy. Prospective ultrasound study. Dis Colon Rectum. 1994;37:1031–3.

32. Nelson RL. Treatment of anal fissure. BMJ. 2003;327(7411):354–5.

33. Corby H, Donnelly VS, O'Herlihy C, O'Connell PR. Anal canal pressures are low in women with postpartum anal fissure. Br J Surg. 1997;84(1):86–8.

34. Medich DS, Fazio VW. Hemorrhoids, anal fissure, and carcinoma of the colon, rectum, and anus during pregnancy. Surg Clin North Am. 1995;75(1):77–88.

35. Abramowitz L, Sobhani I, Benifla JL, Vuagnat A, Darai E, Mignon M, et al. Anal fissure and thrombosed external hemorrhoids before and after delivery. Dis Colon Rectum. 2002;45(5):650–5.
36. Martin JD. Postpartum anal fissure. Lancet. 1953;1(6):271–3.
37. Schouten WR, Briel JW, Auwerda JJ, Boerma MO. Anal fissure: new concepts in pathogenesis and treatment. Scand J Gastroenterol Suppl. 1996;218:78–81.
38. Nelson R. Non-surgical therapy for anal fissure. Cochrane Database Syst Rev. 2003;(4):CD003431.
39. Nelson R. Operative procedures for fissure in ano. Cochrane Database Syst Rev. 2005;(2):CD002199.
40. Nisar PJ, Scholefield JH. Managing haemorrhoids. BMJ. 2003;327(7419):847–51.
41. Saleeby RG Jr, Rosen L, Stasik JJ, Riether RD, Sheets J, Khubchandani IT. Hemorrhoidectomy during pregnancy: risk or relief? Dis Colon Rectum. 1991;34(3):260–1.
42. Quijano C, Abalos E. Conservative management of symptomatic and/or complicated haemorrhoids in pregnancy and the puerperium. Cochrane Database Syst Rev. 2005;(3):CD004077.
43. Vazquez JC. Constipation, haemorrhoids, and heartburn in pregnancy. BMJ Clin Evid. 2010;2010:1411.
44. Read MG, Read NW, Haynes WG, Donnelly TC, Johnson AG. A prospective study of the effect of haemorrhoidectomy on sphincter function and faecal continence. Br J Surg. 1982;69(7):396–8.
45. Jewell DJ, Young G. Interventions for treating constipation in pregnancy. Cochrane Database Syst Rev. 2001;(2):CD001142.
46. Kermans G, Wyndaele JJ, Thiery M, De SW. Puerperal urinary retention. Acta Urol Belg. 1986;54(4):376–85.
47. Yip SK, Sahota D, Pang MW, Day L. Postpartum urinary retention. Obstet Gynecol. 2005;106(3):602–6.
48. Carley ME, Carley JM, Vasdev G, Lesnick TG, Webb MJ, Ramin KD, et al. Factors that are associated with clinically overt postpartum urinary retention after vaginal delivery. Am J Obstet Gynecol. 2002;187(2):430–3.
49. Andolf E, Iosif CS, Jorgensen C, Rydhstrom H. Insidious urinary retention after vaginal delivery: prevalence and symptoms at follow-up in a population-based study. Gynecol Obstet Investig. 1994;38(1):51–3.
50. Ching-Chung L, Shuenn-Dhy C, Ling-Hong T, Ching-Chang H, Chao-Lun C, Po-Jen C. Postpartum urinary retention: assessment of contributing factors and long-term clinical impact. Aust N Z J Obstet Gynaecol. 2002;42(4):365–8.
51. Glavind K, Bjork J. Incidence and treatment of urinary retention postpartum. Int Urogynecol J Pelvic Floor Dysfunct. 2003;14(2):119–21.
52. Yip SK, Brieger G, Hin LY, Chung T. Urinary retention in the post-partum period. The relationship between obstetric factors and the post-partum post-
void residual bladder volume. Acta Obstet Gynecol Scand. 1997;76(7):667–72.
53. Royal College of Obstetricians and Gynaecologists. Operative vaginal delivery Guideline NO 26 2020.
54. Yip SK, Sahota D, Chang AM. Determining the reliability of ultrasound measurements and the validity of the formulae for ultrasound estimation of postvoid residual bladder volume in postpartum women. Neurourol Urodyn. 2003;22(3):255–60.
55. Zaki MM, Pandit M, Jackson S. National survey for intrapartum and postpartum bladder care: assessing the need for guidelines. BJOG. 2004;111(8):874–6.
56. Yang DL. Acupuncture therapy in 49 cases of postpartum urinary retention. J Tradit Chin Med. 1985;5(1):26.
57. Burkhart FL, Porges RF, Gibbs CE. Bladder capacity postpartum and catheterization. Obstet Gynecol. 1965;26:176–9.
58. Yip SK, Sahota D, Chang AM, Chung TK. Four-year follow-up of women who were diagnosed to have postpartum urinary retention. Am J Obstet Gynecol. 2002;187(3):648–52.
59. Mohr S, Raio L, Gobrecht-Keller U, Imboden S, Mueller MD, Kuhn A. Postpartum urinary retention: what are the sequelae? A long-term study and review of the literature. Int Urogynecol J. 2022;33(6):1601–8.
60. Rortveit G, Hannestad YS, Daltveit AK, Hunskaar S. Age- and type-dependent effects of parity on urinary incontinence: the Norwegian EPINCONT study. Obstet Gynecol. 2001;98(6):1004–10.
61. Chiarelli P, Brown W, McElduff P. Leaking urine: prevalence and associated factors in Australian women. Neurourol Urodyn. 1999;18(6):567–77.
62. Viktrup L, Lose G, Rolff M, Barfoed K. The symptom of stress incontinence caused by pregnancy or delivery in primiparas. Obstet Gynecol. 1992;79(6):945–9.
63. Thorp JM Jr, Norton PA, Wall LL, Kuller JA, Eucker B, Wells E. Urinary incontinence in pregnancy and the puerperium: a prospective study. Am J Obstet Gynecol. 1999;181(2):266–73.
64. Viktrup L, Lose G. Lower urinary tract symptoms 5 years after the first delivery. Int Urogynecol J. 2000;11:336–40.
65. Rortveit G, Daltveit AK, Hannestad YS, Hunskaar S. Urinary incontinence after vaginal delivery or cesarean section. N Engl J Med. 2003;348(10):900–7.
66. Handa VL, Blomquist JL, Knoepp LR, Hoskey KA, McDermott KC, Muñoz A. Pelvic floor disorders 5-10 years after vaginal or cesarean childbirth. Obstet Gynecol. 2011;118(4):777–84.
67. Blomquist JL, Muñoz A, Carroll M, Handa VL. Association of delivery mode with pelvic floor disorders after childbirth. JAMA. 2018;320(23):2438–47.
68. Adult conservative management [computer program]. Paris: Health Publications Ltd; 2005.

69. Freeman RM. The role of pelvic floor muscle training in urinary incontinence. BJOG. 2004;111(Suppl 1):37–40.

70. Blomquist JL, Carroll M, Muñoz A, Handa VL. Pelvic floor muscle strength and the incidence of pelvic floor disorders after vaginal and cesarean delivery. Am J Obstet Gynecol. 2020;222(1):62. e1–8.

71. Sigurdardottir T, Steingrimsdottir T, Geirsson RT, Halldorsson TI, Aspelund T, Bø K. Can postpartum pelvic floor muscle training reduce urinary and anal incontinence?: an assessor-blinded randomized controlled trial. Am J Obstet Gynecol. 2020;222(3):247. e1–8.

72. Bø K, Hilde G, Stær-Jensen J, Siafarikas F, Tennfjord MK, Engh ME. Postpartum pelvic floor muscle training and pelvic organ prolapse--a randomized trial of primiparous women. Am J Obstet Gynecol. 2015;212(1):38.e1–7.

73. Mørkved S, Bø K. Effect of pelvic floor muscle training during pregnancy and after childbirth on prevention and treatment of urinary incontinence: a systematic review. Br J Sports Med. 2014;48(4):299–310.

74. Mørkved S, Bø K. Effect of postpartum pelvic floor muscle training in prevention and treatment of urinary incontinence: a one-year follow up. BJOG. 2000;107(8):1022–8.

75. Glazener CM, Herbison GP, MacArthur C, Grant A, Wilson PD. Randomised controlled trial of conservative management of postnatal urinary and faecal incontinence: six year follow up. BMJ. 2005;330(7487):337.

76. Swift SE. The distribution of pelvic organ support in a population of female subjects seen for routine gynecologic health care. Am J Obstet Gynecol. 2000;183(2):277–85.

77. O'Boyle ALO, O'Boyle JD, Ricks RE, Patience TH, Calhoun B, Davis G. The natural history of pelvic organ support in pregnancy. Int Urogynecol J Pelvic Floor Dysfunct. 2003;14:46–9.

78. Sze EH, Sherard GB III, Dolezal JM. Pregnancy, labor, delivery, and pelvic organ prolapse. Obstet Gynecol. 2002;100(5 Pt 1):981–6.

79. Bick DE, MacArthur C. Attendance, content and relevance of the six week postnatal examination. Midwifery. 1995;11(2):69–73.

80. Royal College of Obstetricians and Gynaecologists. Management of third and fourth degree perineal tears. Guideline NO 29 2021.

81. Wuest S, Raio L, Wyssmueller D, Mueller MD, Stadlmayr W, Surbek DV, et al. Effects of female genital mutilation on birth outcomes in Switzerland. BJOG. 2009;116:1204–9.

82. Balachandran AA, Duvalla S, Sultan AH, Thakar R. Are obstetric outcomes affected by female genital mutilation? Int Urogynecol J. 2018;29:339–44.

83. Ismail SI. The management of obstetric anal sphincter injuries (OASIS): a national postal questionnaire survey in hospitals in the U.K. J Obstet Gynaecol. 2015;35(3):229–34.

84. Roper JC, Amber N, Wan OYK, Sultan AH, Thakar R. Review of available national guidelines for obstetric anal sphincter injury. Int Urogynecol J. 2020;31(11):2247–59.

85. Brincat C, Crosby E, McLeod A, Fenner DE. Experiences during the first four years of a postpartum perineal clinic in the USA. Int J Gynecol Obstet. 2015;128:68–71.

86. Pretlove SJ, Thompson PJ, Toozs-Hobson PM, Radley S. The first 18 months of a new perineal trauma clinic. J Obstet Gynaecol. 2004;24:399–402.

87. Fitzpatrick M, Cassidy M, O'Connell PR, O'Herlihy C. Experience with an obstetric perineal clinic. Eur J Obstet Gynecol Reprod Biol. 2002;100: 199–203.

88. Fowler G, Williams A, Murphy G, Taylor K, Wood C, Adams E. How to set up a perineal clinic. Obstet Gynaecol. 2009;11:129–32.

89. Corry E, O'Connor E, Eogan M, Fitzpatrick M, O'Sullivan S, Imcha M. A dedicated perineal clinic – an audit in support. Ir Med J. 2019;112:913.

90. Shawer S, Innayat S, Hutchinson H, Ballard P, Khunda A. Introducing a new service of a midwife-led telephone follow-up clinic for 3a & 3b Obstetric Anal Sphincter Injury: retrospective service evaluation and patients' satisfaction survey. Pelviperineology. 2019;38(2):49–52.

91. Scheer I, Andrews V, Thakar R, Sultan AH. Urinary incontinence after obstetric anal sphincter injuries (OASIS)—is there a relationship? Int Urogynecol J Pelvic Floor Dysfunct. 2008;19:179–83.

92. Taithongchai A, Veiga SI, Sultan AH, Thakar R. The consequences of undiagnosed obstetric anal sphincter injuries (OASIS) following vaginal delivery. Int Urogynecol J. 2020;31:635–41.

93. Jordan PA, Naidu M, Thakar R, Sultan AH. Effect of subsequent vaginal delivery on bowel symptoms and anorectal function in women who sustained a previous obstetric anal sphincter injury. Int Urogynecol J. 2018;29(11):1579–88.

94. Karmarkar R, Bhide A, Digesu A, Khullar V, Fernando R. Mode of delivery after obstetric anal sphincter injury. Eur J Obstet Gynecol Reprod Biol. 2015;194:7–10.

95. Cassis C, Giarenis I, Mukhopadhyay S, Morris E. Mode of delivery following an OASIS and caesarean section rates. Eur J Obstet Gynecol Reprod Biol. 2018;230:28–31.

96. Propst K, Hickman LC. Peripartum pelvic floor disorder clinics inform obstetric provider practices. Int Urogynecol J. 2021;32(7):1793–9.

97. Hickman LC, Yao M, Propst K. Starting a peripartum pelvic floor disorder clinic: what to expect in the first thirty-six months. Int Urogynecol J. 2022. https://doi.org/10.1007/s00192-022-05246-x. Epub ahead of print.

98. Wan OYK, Taithongchai A, Veiga SI, Sultan AH, Thakar RA. One stop perineal clinic: our eleven year experience. Int Urogynecol J. 2020;31:2317–26.

99. Hickman LC, Propst K, Swenson CW, Lewicky-Gaupp C. Subspecialty care for peripartum pelvic floor disorders. Am J Obstet Gynecol. 2020;223(5):709–14.

100. Fehlmann A, Reichetzer B, Ouellet S, Tremblay C, Clermont ME. Establishing a peripartum perineal trauma clinic: a narrative review. Int Urogynecol J. 2021;32(7):1653–62.

Management of Subsequent Pregnancy After Incontinence and Prolapse Surgery

11

Sarah A. Collins and Victoria Handa

Overview

Test your learning and check your understanding of this book's contents: use the "Springer Nature Flashcards" app to access questions using ▶ https://sn.pub/wqrf89. To use the app, please follow the instructions in Chap. 1.

Learning Objectives

After reading this chapter, readers should

- Be able to identify risks specific to pregnant women who have undergone midurethral sling surgery, sacral neuromodulation, and uterine-sparing surgery for pelvic organ prolapse.
- Recognize the paucity of evidence-based guidance to support the management of pregnancy and birth after surgery for urinary incontinence and/or pelvic organ prolapse.
- Have confidence to counsel women about what is known about the outcomes of specific urogynecologic surgeries after subsequent pregnancy.

S. A. Collins (✉)
Northwestern Medical Group, Chicago, IL, USA
e-mail: scollins2@bsd.uchicago.edu

V. Handa
Johns Hopkins University School of Medicine, Baltimore, MD, USA
e-mail: vhanda1@jhmi.edu

11.1 Introduction

In the United States, the peak incidence of surgical treatment of stress urinary incontinence (SUI) and pelvic organ prolapse (POP) occurs between the ages of 60 and 79 [1–3]. However, younger women also experience surgery for pelvic floor disorders. For example, among US women aged 25–34 years, almost 5% undergo surgical treatment for stress incontinence, and approximately 1% in this age group undergo surgery for pelvic organ prolapse [2, 3].

Thus, women may undergo surgery for pelvic floor disorders at the same stage in life that they are experiencing childbirth. This is especially true as childbirth becomes more common at older ages. At present, the peak birth rate in the US and most European countries is between 30 and 34 years of age [4–6]. Among US women over 40 years of age, childbirth is experienced by almost 12 per 1000 [4].

Traditionally, women have been discouraged from seeking surgery for pelvic floor disorders until childbearing is completed [7]. Nevertheless, as younger women seek treatment for pelvic floor disorders, and as childbirth becomes increasingly common among older women, it is inevitable that some women will become pregnant after surgical treatment for urinary incontinence (UI) or prolapse. This is especially true as more prolapse surgeries are performed with uterine conservation [8–10], thus leading to potential pregnancies after surgical treatment of POP. In this chapter, we discuss specific considerations for these pregnancies.

11.2 Safety Concerns During Pregnancy

Safety for the mother and fetus is a primary concern for women and their obstetricians during all pregnancies, but after surgery for UI and POP, limited data suggests that there may be specific risks to consider. Below, these risks are reviewed according to prior procedure type.

11.2.1 Previous Surgery for SUI

There are few data available on pregnancy risks in women who have undergone surgery for SUI, but what has been published is reassuring. The authors of a 2012 systematic review analyzing the safety of pregnancy after surgery for stress incontinence concluded that there is likely minimal risk to women during these pregnancies [11]. In addition, the authors of a 2021 retrospective cohort study estimated the prevalence during pregnancy of symptoms among women who became pregnant after midurethral sling (MUS; see Fig. 11.1). They found a 2% risk of urinary tract infection, a 4% risk of UI symptoms, and a 9% risk of pelvic, perineal, or abdominal pain. These may not differ from risks

of these problems in pregnant women without prior anti-incontinence surgery [12].

Obstructive urinary symptoms have been reported in pregnant women with history of anti-incontinence surgery. A case report from 2001 describes a 26 year old who developed progressively worsening urethral pain and voiding dysfunction beginning at 18 weeks gestation, with complete urinary retention at 25 weeks. Prior to her pregnancy, she had undergone a needle suspension for SUI, as well as a subsequent bone anchor pubovaginal sling using a bovine collagen injected woven polyester mesh. She required a Foley catheter until her voiding dysfunction resolved later in the pregnancy. After cesarean delivery, she developed recurrent stress incontinence [13]. A more recent case report describes a 35 year old with a history of a transobturator MUS who developed mixed urinary incontinence and nocturnal enuresis at 17 weeks' gestation. She was found to have a post-void residual volume of 750 mL, which was managed with clean intermittent self-catheterization until symptoms worsened; she ultimately required sling lysis under local anesthesia in the second trimester. Intraoperatively, her sling was found to be under significant tension, obstructing the urethra. She had recurrent SUI during her pregnancy which persisted until 1 year postpartum [14]. In summary, the incidence of de novo voiding obstruction during pregnancy after SUI surgery is uncertain but appears to be low.

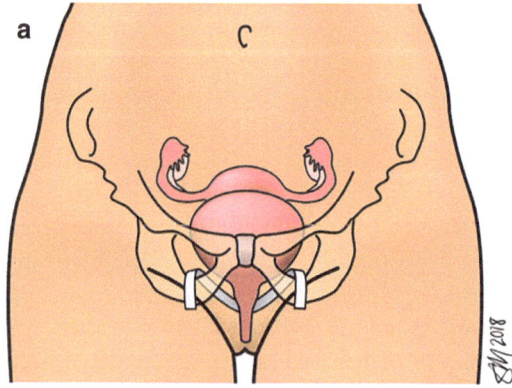
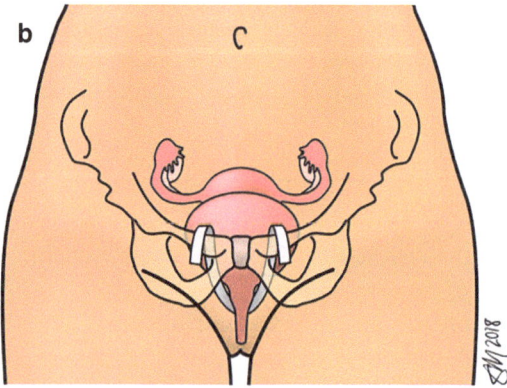
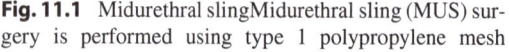

Fig. 11.1 Midurethral slingMidurethral sling (MUS) surgery is performed using type 1 polypropylene mesh passed either through a transobturator (**a**) or a retropubic (**b**) approach

11.2.2 Previous Sacral Neuromodulation

Animal studies suggest that electrical stimulation of the sacrum is safe in pregnant rats, with no fetal anomalies or pregnancy losses noted [15]. Human studies of sacral nerve stimulation on uterine activity in nonpregnant women showed that sacral neuromodulation (SNM; see Fig. 11.2) had an inhibitory effect on uterine activity. However, the effect on the pregnant uterus is unknown [16].

As the effects of electrical stimulation during pregnancy are unknown, both the device manufacturer and the International Urogynecological Association (IUGA) recommend turning off the device when planning pregnancy or during pregnancy [17, 18]. However, a survey of sacral neuromodulation in pregnant women showed that only 2/3 of those who became pregnant switched off the device [19].

Maternal and fetal risks attributable to SNM during pregnancy are difficult to identify due to the paucity of data available. However, there have been several case series and case reports documenting pregnancies and maternal and fetal outcomes in women with implanted SNM systems. Case series including pregnant women using SNM for different indications (some of whom deactivated their SNM systems during pregnancy and some who did not) are reassuring about the safety of SNM for fetal development [20–23] Two adverse outcomes were described in a single patient who kept her system on during both pregnancies to control chronic bladder pain. It is unclear if these outcomes were attributable to

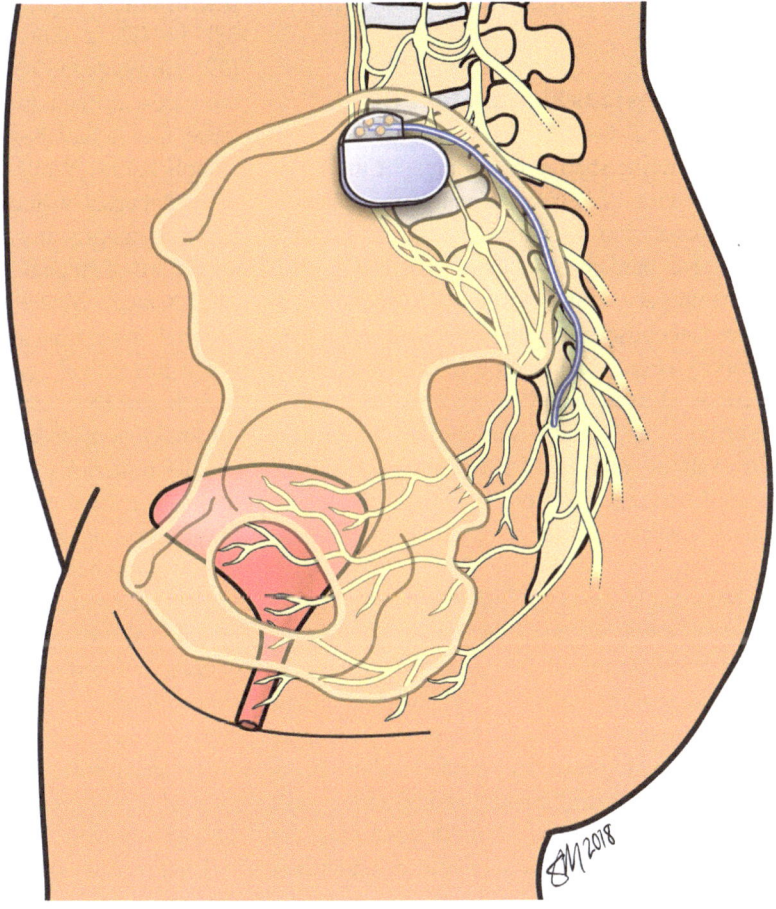

Fig. 11.2 Sacral neuromodulationSacral neuromodulation (SNM) systems, used for the treatment of urinary retention, urgency urinary incontinence, and fecal incontinence, include a flexible electrical lead implanted along the third sacral nerve root on one or both sides of the body. An implantable pulse generator (IPG) connects to the lead to provide the neuromodulation therapy

SNM. Her first baby developed a chronic motor tic at age 2, and her second child had a pilonidal cyst [21].

Obstetric complications reported in these case series include urinary tract infection (especially in women with chronic urinary retention who turned their devices off during pregnancy) and pre-term delivery [20–23]. Lead revision, replacement, and explantation have been described as well. In one patient, pain associated with an abdominally implanted neurostimulator led to explantation of the device during pregnancy [24]. Another patient with two successful pregnancies after initial SNM device implantation required surgery during both pregnancies for SNM lead replacement/revision. She experienced lead migration during the first pregnancy and surgical site infection requiring lead revision during the second pregnancy. There were no obstetric complications or adverse fetal outcomes [25].

11.2.3 Previous Surgery for POP

Several uterine sparing procedures for the surgical correction of POP exist, and there is increasingly reassuring data about the anatomic and subjective outcomes of these procedures [26]. Contemporary options for apical support procedures that conserve the uterus include sacral hysteropexy (Fig. 11.3), sacrospinous hysteropexy, uterosacral hysteropexy, transvaginal mesh hysteropexy, and the Manchester procedure. Pregnancies after all of these approaches have been described, but there is limited data about safety concerns during pregnancies after these surgeries.

Most case series of pregnancies following sacral hysteropexy describe women whose prolapse repair involved using only a posteriorly attached vaginal mesh [27, 28]. In these cases, the selection of this surgical approach was presumably due to theoretical concerns about pregnancy after the use of anterior and posterior mesh for sacral hysteropexy, as mesh encircling the lower uterine segment could restrict pregnancy related uterine changes required to support the growing fetus [26]. Yet, successful pregnancies

after sacral hysteropexy including anterior *and* posterior vaginal mesh attachments have been described, resulting in normal weight, full-term infants [29, 30]. Pelvic pain during pregnancy attributed to prior sacral hysteropexy using isolated posterior vaginal mesh also has been described [31, 32]. One case of complete (180 °) uterine torsion, incidentally discovered at the time of cesarean section in a woman who had previously undergone sacral hysteropexy, has been described. There were no adverse fetal outcomes, and the uterus was easily returned to its normal orientation after the full-term baby was delivered. Intraoperative de-torsion before the delivery was attempted but failed, and the hysterotomy was created in the anteriorly facing posterior lower uterine segment [33].

Very few pregnancy complications have been attributed to previous transvaginal native-tissue (sacrospinous or uterosacral) hysteropexy [27, 32, 34–36] or transvaginal mesh hysteropexy [37]. However, the Manchester procedure, one of the oldest techniques to treat uterovaginal prolapse, has, in fact, been associated with obstetric complications. While it is rarely performed in premenopausal women due to the high risk of cervical stenosis and menstrual disorders, there are reports of pregnancy after this procedure [38]. The "Classic Manchester Procedure" involves cervical amputation and reattachment of the cervix to the cardinal ligaments, while the "Modified Manchester Procedure" includes plication of the cardinal ligaments anteriorly and uterosacral ligaments posteriorly *without* cervical amputation to improve the support of the apex [38, 39]. The Manchester operation is performed less commonly today, but an historic case series published in 1951 of women who underwent this procedure included 14 post-procedural pregnancies. Seven of these resulted in spontaneous abortion. There also were four premature births, three of which delivered vaginally and one of which delivered by cesarean section with neonatal death. Only three of the 14 pregnancies were carried to term and delivered via cesarean section [40].

Until recently, there were not enough reports in the literature of pregnancies after uterine-sparing prolapse surgery to compare obstetrical outcomes

Fig. 11.3 Sacral hysteropexySacral hysteropexy (SH) involves the placement of type 1 polypropylene mesh to the vagina, sometimes including the cervix and lower uterine segment, and suspension of these structures to the anterior longitudinal ligament of the sacrum distal to the promontory. This figure depicts an anterior and a posterior mesh attachment, but many surgeons use only the posterior attachment to avoid theoretical risks in case of subsequent pregnancy

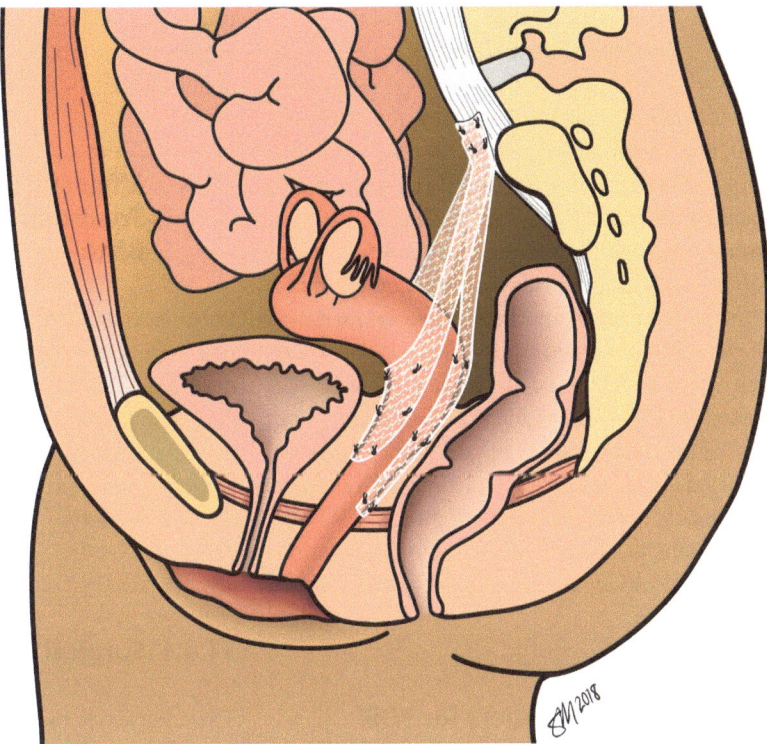

by specific procedure performed for POP. However, a systematic review and meta-analysis of obstetric outcomes after uterine-sparing prolapse surgery was published in September 2021 [41]. This analysis revealed that the Manchester procedure is associated with the highest risk of adverse outcomes including preterm premature rupture of membranes. Sacral hysteropexy was lower in risk than the Manchester procedure but associated with more adverse outcomes than native tissue hysteropexy. The authors suggested that native tissue hysteropexy may be the most prudent choice for women who desire surgery for POP but are considering future pregnancy [41].

11.3 Mode of Delivery

When pregnancies occur after surgery for pelvic floor disorders, decisions around mode of birth can be challenging. Considerations to be weighed include risk of recurrent pelvic floor symptoms, maternal and fetal outcomes, and obstetrical concerns.

11.3.1 Previous Surgery for SUI

Literature guiding decisions about vaginal versus cesarean birth in pregnancies after anti-incontinence surgery is equivocal and includes case reports, case series, and surveys of healthcare providers.

Several case reports have described outcomes for women who had births after midurethral sling procedures, including transobturator and retropubic approaches. These have suggested low rates of recurrent SUI after both vaginal and cesarean births [42–44]. Given the small number of cases and the absence of any randomized trials, evidence based recommendations for route of birth after midurethral sling surgery are not possible. Most authors agree that mode of birth for women with a history of surgery for stress incontinence should be chosen according to individual, case-specific factors but that a vaginal route is reasonable [45–47]. Some have gone so far as to express that women of childbearing age who desire future pregnancies should be offered surgical treatment for stress incontinence if conservative therapies have failed [48].

11.3.2 Previous Sacral Neuromodulation

Device malfunction has been reported after vaginal and cesarean birth [21]. A displaced and broken IPG lead has also been reported after a vacuum-assisted vaginal birth in a full-term infant [49]. Similarly, a case series of 20 births reported reduction in device efficacy after system reactivation postpartum in four women, two of whom had vaginal births and two had cesarean section [22]. The decreased efficacy was linked to lead displacement in two women, but no cause was found in the other women. Neuraxial anesthesia (spinal or epidural) does not appear to cause lead migration [24, 50]. More data is needed before recommendations regarding mode of subsequent birth can be made.

11.3.3 Previous Surgery for POP

There were no cases of vaginal birth after mesh sacrohysteropexy (SH) identified in the literature during the preparation of this chapter. This may be due to theoretical concerns about the rigidity of the mesh over the anterior and/or posterior vaginal walls and how this may impact the mechanics of the birthing process.

Births after vaginal approach uterine-sparing prolapse procedures are have been reported in the literature, but due to very limited data, it is not possible to make recommendations regarding the mode of subsequent birth after these procedures. Sacrospinous ligament hysteropexy (SSLH) is a vaginal procedure in which the cervix and upper vagina are affixed with sutures to one (usually the right) or both sacrospinous ligaments. Both vaginal and cesarean births have been described after sacrospinous ligament hysteropexy [34, 35]. Women with a history of a Modified Manchester procedure can have a vaginal birth [38], while women who have had a traditional Manchester operation with cervical amputation might have preterm labor and labor abnormalities [40].

11.4 Efficacy of Prior Surgical Treatment After Subsequent Birth

Pregnancy and the birthing process are known risk factors for the development of pelvic floor disorders. Therefore, pregnant women who have undergone prior treatments for pelvic floor disorders may be apprehensive about recurrence after pregnancy and birth. At present, there are limited data to inform women about their likely prognosis.

11.4.1 Surgical Treatment for SUI

Two case series by Adams-Piper, et al., report on pregnancies after midurethral sling in a large managed-care organization in California. Both series included women who had vaginal and cesarean births, and they suggest a rate of recurrent stress incontinence of 2–25% of women with a history of a successful midurethral sling [51, 52]. Smaller case series and case reports corroborate these findings and include examples of outcomes after both vaginal birth [53–55] and cesarean birth [56, 57]. One case series demonstrates normal positioning of the sling mesh beneath the urethra on ultrasound postpartum [54]. Additionally, there are reports describing maintenance of continence following vaginal birth after full-length and single-incision transobturator midurethral slings [58, 59]. There also are cases in which SUI recurs. One such case is described in a report of a primiparous woman who underwent a successful retropubic midurethral sling at the age 29. She became unexpectedly pregnant 10 months later, and her SUI recurred after a vaginal birth. After a second, less successful sling, she became pregnant again and underwent a cesarean birth 2 years later. Unfortunately, her SUI symptoms worsened, and she underwent an unsuccessful retropubic colposuspension [60].

There is limited evidence of the efficacy of retropubic colpususpension surgeries after subsequent births. There are two case series of Marchetti procedures from the 1950s and 1970s, one published by Dr. Marchetti himself, that describe over 400 patients. After the eight pregnancies described, all women apparently were continent postpartum, though no outcome measures or follow-up duration were documented [61, 62]. Case reports and case series suggest similar outcomes after Burch retropubic colposuspension [63, 64].

A case series of nine women who completed pregnancies after autologous pubovaginal sling reported persistent efficacy after birth in all but one woman, and seven of the nine delivered vaginally. Eight of the women who had good outcome from the sling reported unchanged continence postpartum [65].

11.4.2 Previous Sacral Neuromodulation

As previously noted, it is recommended that women with an SNM implant turn off the device during pregnancy [17, 18]. When the device is reactivated, efficacy may be reduced in some cases. Several case reports and series have addressed the efficacy of neuromodulation and the need for device revision or replacement after childbirth [22, 24, 49, 66–71]. Two larger studies describe recurrent urinary symptoms in women who turned off their devices during pregnancy and maintenance of good symptom control in those who kept theirs activated. Several cases of decreased device efficacy postpartum after reactivating the systems which had been turned off were reported [21, 22].

11.4.3 Previous Treatment for POP

There are several case series [27–30, 72–74] and case reports [32, 37, 75] in the literature describing women have become pregnant after open or laparoscopic sacrohysteropexy (SH). While the procedures described vary by approach and graft material, the majority involved placement of a posterior vaginal mesh only. Data from these studies is heterogenous, though most describe pregnancies delivered by cesarean and suggest continued pelvic organ support postpartum. In one case series [27], Pelvic Organ Prolapse Quantification System (POP-Q) measurements from three time points (before SH, after SH and before subsequent pregnancy, and at postpartum follow up) were reported upon. All five women completed pregnancies after posterior mesh SH by a single surgeon, three abdominally and three robotically. All five women underwent cesarean section. Comparing uterovaginal support before and after delivery, mean differences in POPQ measurements Aa, Ba, and C were 0.2, 0.2, and 0.4, respectively, with no statistically significant changes from before pregnancy [27].

We are aware of only one reported case of pregnancy after transvaginal mesh for prolapse [37]. In this case report, a Turkish woman with recurrent stage III anterior vaginal prolapse underwent placement of an anterior polypropylene transvaginal mesh with prepubic and transobturator arms. She became pregnant 8 weeks postoperatively and underwent an elective cesarean section at term. She did not have any subjective or objective POPQ evidence of prolapse at 2 years follow-up.

Two case series describe four women who became pregnant after laparoscopic uterosacral ligament hysteropexy [76, 77]. All four women underwent cesarean section, and three remained without prolapse recurrence at a mean follow-up of 12 months. One of the patients experienced recurrent prolapse at 11 months postpartum and underwent a repeat prolapse repair.

Several case series describe pregnancies after sacrospinous ligament hysteropexy (SSLH) [34–36, 78]. One of these series reports on nine pregnancies. All patients had vaginal births, and the authors report only one prolapse recurrence [35]. There are more series describing cesarean section after SSLH, and these describe prolapse recurrence rates of 0–50% [34, 78, 79]. Prolapse outcomes are reported using heterogenous measures in these series, and most are subjective.

A recent meta-analysis by Gutman and Maher describes twelve pregnancies after the Manchester procedure with mostly full-term vaginal births and one documented prolapse recurrence [38].

11.5   Conclusions

In summary, pregnancies in women who have undergone surgical treatment for UI or POP are occurring with increasing frequency. While most guidance about the prenatal, obstetric, and post-partum care of these women is based on case reports, case series, and expert opinion, patients can be reassured that pregnancy after MUS, SNM, SSLH, and sacral hysteropexy is likely to be uncomplicated and that they may continue to experience relief from pelvic floor symptoms if their index surgeries were successful. There is limited evidence-based guidance on mode of birth for these women, and the rate of recurrence of POP and UI postpartum is difficult to determine. Because, with few exceptions, best practice recommendations suggest performing surgery for pelvic floor disorders only in women who have completed childbearing, prospective studies on the management and outcomes of these pregnancies is unlikely. As more cases occur, however, we can look forward to larger case series that may help guide practice in the future.

Take Home Messages

Surgical history:	Surgery for stress urinary incontinence (SUI)	Sacral neuromodulation (SNM)	Surgery for pelvic organ prolapse (POP)
Safety concerns during pregnancy	Urinary obstruction during pregnancy has been described after midurethral sling surgery	Conservative recommendations have been to turn the device off during pregnancy because minimal data on risks are available Reports in a small number of women who have kept devices active during pregnancy do not reveal any adverse fetal effects attributable to SNM	Obstetric complications during pregnancy after sacral hysteropexy and vaginal native tissue hysteropexy appear to be unlikely Obstetric complications during pregnancy after Manchester operations include preterm delivery and spontaneous abortion
Mode of future birth	Vaginal and cesarean births have been described after anti-incontinence surgery There is inadequate data available to guide evidence-based decisions about mode of birth	Vaginal and cesarean births have been described after SNM There is inadequate data available to guide evidence-based decisions about mode of birth	Vaginal and cesarean births have been described after surgery for POP There is inadequate data available to guide evidence-based decisions about mode of birth
Durability of surgical treatment postpartum	There is likely a high probability of continued efficacy of MUS surgery after vaginal and cesarean births, though recurrent SUI postpartum has been described	There may be a clinically significant risk of decreased SNM efficacy postpartum, sometimes due to lead disruption	After apical prolapse surgery, including sacral hysteropexy and sacrospinous hysteropexy, POP recurrence has been documented despite cesarean section, but the incidence of recurrence is difficult to estimate as data are limited

Appendix: MCQ

Questions

1. According to a 2012 systematic review, which of the following is true regarding the safety of pregnancy after surgery for stress incontinence?
   - (A) The risk to women during these pregnancies is minimal
   - (B) After delivery, the risk of recurrent stress incontinence is >25%
   - (C) 10–15% of these women develop symptoms of voiding obstruction during the third trimester
   - (D) The risk of voiding obstruction during pregnancy is significantly higher after retropubic versus transobturator sling
   - (E) De novo vaginal mesh exposure has been documented in 3–5% during pregnancy

2. Which of the following uterine-sparing prolapse surgeries is associated with the highest risk of adverse pregnancy outcomes:
   - (A) Sacral hysteropexy
   - (B) Sacrospinous hysteropexy
   - (C) Uterosacral hysteropexy
   - (D) Transvaginal mesh hysteropexy
   - (E) Manchester procedure

3. Which of the following is true about recurrent stress incontinence among women who become pregnant after midurethral sling for stress incontinence:
   - (A) Women should be counseled they are more likely to experience recurrent stress incontinence after operative delivery versus spontaneous vaginal delivery
   - (B) The risk of recurrent stress incontinence is higher if the original procedure was a retropubic versus transobturator sling
   - (C) They are likely to continue to experience relief from stress incontinence but only if their index surgery was successful
   - (D) Cesarean birth is preferred to avoid the risk of sling displacement associated with vaginal birth
   - (E) Case series of retropubic urethropexy suggest that very few women remain continent postpartum

Answers

1. According to a 2012 systematic review, which of the following is true regarding the safety of pregnancy after surgery for stress incontinence?
   - (A) TRUE
   - (B) FALSE
   - (C) FALSE
   - (D) FALSE
   - (E) FALSE

2. Which of the following uterine-sparing prolapse surgeries is associated with the highest risk of adverse pregnancy outcomes:
   - (A) FALSE
   - (B) FALSE
   - (C) FALSE
   - (D) FALSE
   - (E) TRUE

3. Which of the following is true about recurrent stress incontinence among women who become pregnant after midurethral sling for stress incontinence:
   - (A) FALSE
   - (B) FALSE
   - (C) TRUE
   - (D) FALSE
   - (E) FALSE

References

1. Urologic Diseases in America (US Government Printing Office); 2018.
2. Shah AD, Kohli N, Rajan SS, Hoyte L. The age distribution, rates, and types of surgery for stress urinary incontinence in the USA. Int Urogynecol J Pelvic Floor Dysfunct. 2008;19(1):89–96. https://doi.org/10.1007/s00192-007-0392-y.
3. Shah AD, Kohli N, Rajan SS, Hoyte L. The age distribution, rates, and types of surgery for pelvic organ prolapse in the USA. Int Urogynecol J Pelvic Floor Dysfunct. 2008;19(3):421–8. https://doi.org/10.1007/s00192-007-0457-y.

4. Martin JA, Hamilton BE, Osterman M. Births in the United States, 2020. NCHS Data Brief. 2021;418:1–8.

5. Age of mothers at childbirth and age-specific fertility. SF 2.3. August, 2021. https://www.oecd.org/els/family/database.htm. Accessed 20 Feb 2022.

6. Clark D. Average age of mothers in Europe 1955-2020. Statista. July 26, 2019. https://www.statista.com/statistics/1251578/average-age-of-mothers-europe/. Accessed 20 Feb 2022.

7. Wieslander CK, Weinstein MM, Handa VL, Collins SA. Pregnancy in women with prior treatments for pelvic floor disorders. Female Pelvic Med Reconstr Surg. 2020;26(5):299–305. https://doi.org/10.1097/SPV.0000000000000822.

8. Enklaar RA, van IJsselmuiden MN, IntHout J, et al. Practice pattern variation: treatment of pelvic organ prolapse in The Netherlands. Int Urogynecol J. 2021; https://doi.org/10.1007/s00192-021-04968-8.

9. Hickman LC, Tran MC, Paraiso MFR, Walters MD, Ferrando CA. Intermediate term outcomes after transvaginal uterine-preserving surgery in women with uterovaginal prolapse. Int Urogynecol J. 2021; https://doi.org/10.1007/s00192-021-04987-5.

10. Zacche MM, Mukhopadhyay S, Giarenis I. Trends in prolapse surgery in England. Int Urogynecol J. 2018;29(11):1689–95. https://doi.org/10.1007/s00192-018-3731-2.

11. Pollard ME, Morrisroe S, Anger JT. Outcomes of pregnancy following surgery for stress urinary incontinence: a systematic review. J Urol. 2012;187(6):1966–70. https://doi.org/10.1016/j.juro.2012.01.068.

12. Tulokas SA, Rahkola-Soisalo P, Gissler M, Mikkola TS, Mentula MJ. Pregnancy and delivery after mid-urethral sling operation. Int Urogynecol J. 2021;32(1):179–86. https://doi.org/10.1007/s00192-020-04497-w.

13. Lynch CM, Powers AK, Keating AB. Pregnancy complicated by a suburethral sling: a case report. Int Urogynecol J Pelvic Floor Dysfunct. 2001;12(3):218–9.

14. Shveiky D, Sokol AI, Iglesia CB. A case report of antepartum bladder outlet obstruction following transobturator sling placement. Int Urogynecol J. 2010;21(3):379–81.

15. Wang Y, Hassouna MM. Electrical stimulation has no adverse effect on pregnant rats and fetuses. J Urol. 1999;162(5):1785–7.

16. Govaert B, Pares D, Delgado-Aros S, La Torre F, Van Gemert WG, Baeten CG. A prospective multicentre study to investigate percutaneous tibial nerve stimulation for the treatment of faecal incontinence. Colorectal Dis. 2010;12(12):1236–41.

17. Medtronic. Indications insert medtronic InterStim therapy. Retrieved December, 14, 2018. https://www.medtronic.com/content/dam/emanuals/neuro/MA12896A_a_004_view.pdf

18. (IUGA) IUA. Sacral neuromodulation: a guide for women. Washington, DC: IUGA Office; 2018.

19. Siegel S. Use and management of InterStim sacral neuromodulation in pregnant patients: a survey of active implanters – sessions highlights. In: Urodynamics & Female Urology (SUFU) 2009 Winter meeting. 2009; February 25–28, 2009, Las Vegas, NV, USA.

20. Khunda A, Karmarkar R, Abtahi B, Gonzales G, Elneil S. Pregnancy in women with Fowler'syndrome treated with sacral neuromodulation. Int Urogynecol J. 2013;24(7):1201–4. https://doi.org/10.1007/s00192-012-1999-1.

21. Mahran A, Soriano A, Safwat AS, et al. The effect of sacral neuromodulation on pregnancy: a systematic review. Int Urogynecol J. 2017;28(9):1357–65. https://doi.org/10.1007/s00192-017-3272-0.

22. Roulette P, Castel-Lacanal E, Sanson S, et al. Sacral neuromodulation and pregnancy: results of a national survey carried out for the neuro-urology committee of the French Association of Urology (AFU). Neurourol Urodyn. 2018;37(2):792–8. https://doi.org/10.1002/nau.23349.

23. Agnello M, Vottero M, Bertapelle P. Do you really want to deactivate your sacral neuromodulation device during pregnancy? A single center case series. Int Urogynecol J. 2021;32(3):709–17. https://doi.org/10.1007/s00192-020-04594-w.

24. Yaiesh SM, Al-Terki AE, Al-Shaiji TF. Safety of sacral nerve stimulation in pregnancy: a literature review. Neuromodulation. 2016;19(7):770–9. https://doi.org/10.1111/ner.12450.

25. Alghazwani Y, Alghafees MA, Alfraidi O, Aldarrab R. Sacral neuromodulation in a pregnant patient with Fowler's syndrome: A case report. Cureus. 2020;12(11):e11796. https://doi.org/10.7759/cureus.11796.

26. Ridgeway BM. Does prolapse equal hysterectomy? The role of uterine conservation in women with uterovaginal prolapse. Am J Obstet Gynecol. 2015;213(6):802–9. https://doi.org/10.1016/j.ajog.2015.07.035.

27. Adegoke TM, Vragovic O, Yarrington CD, Larrieux JR. Effect of pregnancy on uterine-sparing pelvic organ prolapse repair. Int Urogynecol J. 2020;31(3):657–62. https://doi.org/10.1007/s00192-019-04179-2.

28. Banu LF. Synthetic sling for genital prolapse in young women. Int J Gynaecol Obstet. 1997;57(1):57–64. https://doi.org/10.1016/s0020-7292(97)02847-6.

29. Jefferis H, Price N, Jackson S. Pregnancy following laparoscopic hysteropexy-a case series. Gynecol Surg. 2017;14(1):16. https://doi.org/10.1186/s10397-017-1017-1.

30. Rahmanou P, Price N, Black RS, Jackson SR. Pregnancy post-laparoscopic hysteropexy. J Obstet Gynaecol. 2015;35(3):303–4. https://doi.org/10.3109/01443615.2014.948406.

31. Busby C, Hamdan M, Ariabi E. Cancer, infant mortality and birth sex-ratio in Fallujah, Iraq 2005-2009. Int J Environ Res Public Health. 2010;7(7):2828–37.

32. Lewis CM, Culligan P. Sacrohysteropexy followed by successful pregnancy and eventual reoperation for prolapse. Int Urogynecol J. 2012;23(7):957–9.

33. Bagli I, Erdem S. Uterine torsion at term pregnancy associated with a previous pelvic organ prolapse (POP) surgery. J Obstet Gynaecol. 2020;40(4):569–70. https://doi.org/10.1080/01443615.2019.1615042.

34. Cavkaytar S, Kokanali MK, Tasdemir U, Doganay M, Aksakal O. Pregnancy outcomes after transvaginal sacrospinous hysteropexy. Eur J Obstet Gynecol Reprod Biol. 2017;216:204–7. https://doi.org/10.1016/j.ejogrb.2017.08.003.

35. Kovac SR, Cruikshank SH. Successful pregnancies and vaginal deliveries after sacrospinous uterosacral fixation in five of nineteen patients. Am J Obstet Gynecol. 1993;168(6 Pt 1):1778–83.; discussion 1783-6. https://doi.org/10.1016/0002-9378(93)90689-g.

36. Maher CF, Cary MP, Slack MC, Murray CJ, Milligan M, Schluter P. Uterine preservation or hysterectomy at sacrospinous colpopexy for uterovaginal prolapse? Int Urogynecol J Pelvic Floor Dysfunct. 2001;12(6):381–4; discussion 384-5. https://doi.org/10.1007/s001920170017.

37. Kumtepe Y, Cetinkaya K, Karasu Y. Pregnancy and delivery after anterior vaginal mesh replacement: a case presentation. Int Urogynecol J. 2013;24(2):345–7. https://doi.org/10.1007/s00192-012-1800-5.

38. Gutman R, Maher C. Uterine-preserving POP surgery. Int Urogynecol J. 2013;24(11):1803–13. https://doi.org/10.1007/s00192-013-2171-2.

39. Williams BF. Surgical treatment for uterine prolapse in young women. Am J Obstet Gynecol. 1966;95(7):967–71.

40. Fisher JJ. The effect of amputation of the cervix uteri upon subsequent parturition; a preliminary report of seven cases. Am J Obstet Gynecol. 1951;62(3):644–8.

41. Barba M, Schivardi G, Manodoro S, Frigerio M. Obstetric outcomes after uterus-sparing surgery for uterine prolapse: a systematic review and meta-analysis. Eur J Obstet Gynecol Reprod Biol. 2021;256:333–8. https://doi.org/10.1016/j.ejogrb.2020.11.054.

42. Cavkaytar S, Kokanali MK, Ozer I, Erkilinc S, Aksakal OS, Doganay M. Effect of pregnancy and delivery on urinary incontinence after the midurethral sling procedure. Int Urogynecol J. 2015;26(5):693–8. https://doi.org/10.1007/s00192-014-2568-6.

43. Demoulin G, Thubert T, Faivre E, Trichot C, Deffieux X. Pregnancy and postpartum of women with midurethral sling procedure: a review of the literature. J Gynecol Obstet Biol Reprod (Paris). 2013;42(6):518–24. https://doi.org/10.1016/j.jgyn.2012.10.004. Grossesse et post-partum des patientes porteuses de bandelette sous-uretrale: revue de la litterature

44. Huser M, Belkov IA, Janku P, Sedlakova K. Pregnancy and delivery following midurethral sling surgery for stress urinary incontinence. Int J Gynaecol Obstet. 2012;119(2):117–20. https://doi.org/10.1016/j.ijgo.2012.05.038.

45. Kohorst F, Flock F, Kreienberg R, Reich A. Pregnancy and delivery after tension-free vaginal tape (TVT) procedure: literature review and case report. Eur J Obstet Gynecol Reprod Biol. 2010;151(1):10–3.

46. Malabarey OFL, Gazzard L, et al. Results of a nationwide survey on practice patterns of Canadian obstetricians and gynaecologists regarding the mode of delivery after pelvic floor surgery. Gynecol Surg. 2016;13:159–64.

47. Panel L, Triopon G, Courtieu C, Marès P, de Tayrac R. How to advise a woman who wants to get pregnant after a sub-urethral tape placement? Int Urogynecol J Pelvic Floor Dysfunct. 2008;19(3):347–50.

48. Panel L, Mares P, de Tayrac R. Urinary incontinence, should fertile women undergo surgical procedure? Gynecol Obstet Fertil. 2009;37(2):167–71.

49. Moya P, Navarro JM, Arroyo A, López A, Ruiz-Tovar J, Calpena R. Sacral nerve stimulation during pregnancy in patients with severe fecal incontinence. Tech Coloproctol. 2013;17(2):245–6.

50. Anso M, Veiga-Gil L, De Carlos J, Hualde A, Perez-Cajaraville J. Neuraxial analgesia in a pregnant woman with Fowler's syndrome and sacral neuromodulation. Int J Obstet Anesth. 2017;30:58–61. https://doi.org/10.1016/j.ijoa.2016.11.008.

51. Adams-Piper E, Buono K, Whitcomb E, Mallipeddi P, Castillo P, Guaderrama N. A large retrospective series of pregnancy and delivery after midurethral sling for stress urinary incontinence. Female Pelvic Med Reconstr Surg. 2016;22(5):307–10. https://doi.org/10.1097/SPV.0000000000000276.

52. Adams-Piper E, Darbinian J, Postlethwaite D, Castillo PA. Pregnancy after transvaginal sling for stress urinary incontinence: a case series. Female Pelvic Med Reconstr Surg. 2014;20(4):212–5. https://doi.org/10.1097/SPV.0000000000000096.

53. Demaria F, Chanelles O, Boquet B, Bricou A, Amarenco G, Benifla J-L. Vaginal delivery after tension-free vaginal tape procedure. Int Urogynecol J Pelvic Floor Dysfunct. 2007;18(11):1363–5.

54. Seeger D, Truong ST, Kimmig R. Spontaneous delivery following tension-free vaginal tape procedure. Int Urogynecol J Pelvic Floor Dysfunct. 2006;17(6):676–8.

55. Vella M, Robinson D, Brown R, Cardozo L. Pregnancy and delivery following tension-free vaginal tape. Int Urogynecol J Pelvic Floor Dysfunct. 2007;18(3):347–8.

56. Iskander MN, Kapoor D. Pregnancy following tension-free vaginal taping. Int Urogynecol J Pelvic Floor Dysfunct. 2000;11(3):199–200.

57. Gauruder-Burmester A, Tunn R. Pregnancy and labor after TVT-plasty. Acta Obstet Gynecol Scand. 2001;80(3):283–4.

58. Hassan MSM, Yossri N, Davies A. Vaginal delivery after surgical treatment for stress incontinence using transobturator tape: a case report. BJOG. 2007;114(1):113–4.

59. Tommaselli GA, Di Carlo C, Formisano C, Fabozzi A, Nappi C. Vaginal delivery following single incision

sling (TVT-Secur) for female stress urinary incontinence. J Obstet Gynaecol Res. 2013;39(2):608–10.

60. Sergent F, Marpeau L. Recurrence of stress urinary incontinence after tension-free vaginal tape and childbirth. Gynecol Obstet Fertil. 2007;35(12):1239–41.

61. Marchetti AA. Urinary incontinence. J Am Med Assoc. 1956;162(15):1366–8.

62. Giesen JE. A review of 270 Marchetti operations. Aust NZ J Obstet Gynaecol. 1974;14:216.

63. Cutner A, Cardozo LD, Benness CJ. Assessment of urinary symptoms in early pregnancy. Br J Obstet Gynaecol. 1991;98(12):1283–6.

64. Casper FW, Linn JF, Black P. Obstetrical management following incontinence surgery. J Obstet Gynaecol Res. 1999;25(1):51–3.

65. Tan A, Cao Y, Xia N, Mo Z, Gao F. The addition of pioglitazone in type 2 diabetics poorly controlled on insulin therapy: a meta-analysis. Eur J Intern Med. 2010;21(5):398–403.

66. Wiseman OJ, van den Hombergh U, Koldewijn EL, Spinelli M, Siegel SW, Fowler CJ. Sacral neuromodulation and pregnancy. J Urol. 2002;167(1):165–8.

67. Khunda A, Karmarkar R, Abtahi B, Gonzales G, Elneil S. Pregnancy in women with Fowler's syndrome treated with sacral neuromodulation. Int Urogynecol J. 2013;24(7):1201–4.

68. Nanninga JB, Einhorn C, Deppe F. The effect of sacral nerve stimulation for bladder control during pregnancy: a case report. J Urol. 1988;139(1):121–2.

69. El-Khawand D, Montgomery OC, Wehbe SA, Whitmore KE. Sacral nerve stimulation during pregnancy: case report and review of the literature. Female Pelvic Med Reconstr Surg. 2012;18(2):127–9. https://doi.org/10.1097/SPV.0b013e3182436ae9.

70. Silva PS, Cavallerano JD, Sun JK, Soliman AZ, Aiello LM, Aiello LP. Peripheral lesions identified by mydriatic ultrawide field imaging: distribution and potential impact on diabetic retinopathy severity. Ophthalmology. 2013;120(12):2587–95.

71. Mamopoulos A, Stavrakis T, Mavromatidis G, Rousso D. Active sacral neuromodulator during pregnancy: a unique case report. Am J Obstet Gynecol. 2014;211(1):e4–5. https://doi.org/10.1016/j.ajog.2014.04.015.

72. Aboulghar MA, El-Kateb Y. Treatment of uterine prolapse in young women. Sacral cervicopexy by polyvinyl alcohol sponge. J Egypt Med Assoc. 1978;61(1-2):127–34.

73. Bagli I, Tahaoglu AE. Pregnancy outcomes after laparoscopic pectopexy surgery: a case series. J Obstet Gynaecol Res. 2020;46(8):1364–9. https://doi.org/10.1111/jog.14337.

74. Barranger E, Fritel X, Pigne A. Abdominal sacrohysteropexy in young women with uterovaginal prolapse: long-term follow-up. Am J Obstet Gynecol. 2003;189(5):1245–50. https://doi.org/10.1067/s0002-9378(03)00665-3.

75. Pilka R, Gagyor D, Huml K, Soviar P, Benicka A. Laparoscopic hysterosacropexy with subsequent pregnancy and delivery by cesarean section: case report with short term follow-up. Ceska Gynekol. 2019;84(6):430–4. Laparoskopicka hysterosakropexe s naslednym těhotenstvim ukončenym cisařskym řezem: kazuistika s kratkodobym follow-up

76. Maher CF, Carey MP, Murray CJ. Laparoscopic suture hysteropexy for uterine prolapse. Obstet Gynecol. 2001;97(6):1010–4.

77. Kow N, Goldman HB, Ridgeway B. Uterine conservation during prolapse repair: 9-year experience at a single institution. Female Pelvic Med Reconstr Surg. 2016;22(3):126–31.

78. Lin TY, Su TH, Wang YL, et al. Risk factors for failure of transvaginal sacrospinous uterine suspension in the treatment of uterovaginal prolapse. J Formos Med Assoc. 2005;104(4):249–53.

79. Maher CF, Baessler KK, Barber MD, et al. Summary: 2017 international consultation on incontinence evidence-based surgical pathway for pelvic organ prolapse. Female Pelvic Med Reconstr Surg. 2018; https://doi.org/10.1097/SPV.0000000000000591.

Prevention of Perineal Trauma

12

Nicola Adanna Okeahialam, Timothy J. Draycott, and Ranee Thakar

Overview

Test your learning and check your understanding of this book's contents: use the "Springer Nature Flashcards" app to access questions using ▶ https://sn.pub/wqrf89. To use the app, please follow the instructions in Chap. 1.

Learning Objectives

- Understand risk factors associated with intrapartum perineal and pelvic floor trauma
- Learn about antenatal and intrapartum interventions known to reduce the risk of perineal and pelvic floor trauma

N. A. Okeahialam
Croydon University Hospital, Thornton Heath, UK
e-mail: nicola.okeahialam@nhs.net

T. J. Draycott
Southmead Hospital, Bristol, UK
e-mail: tim.draycott@bristol.ac.uk

R. Thakar (✉)
Croydon University Hospital, Thornton Heath, UK

St George's University of London, London, UK
e-mail: ranee.thakar@nhs.net

12.1 Introduction

Intrapartum perineal trauma can be associated with considerable short and long-term morbidity. Perineal lacerations and episiotomies can be painful, incur blood loss, may become infected; fistulae can rarely occur. Long-term pelvic floor dysfunction associated with obstetric trauma can have a significant impact on a woman's quality of life. For example, postnatal dyspareunia may last for months or even years. Pelvic floor injury [1] and nerve damage [2, 3] are associated with urinary leakage, urgency and/or incontinence of faeces or flatus, and pelvic organ prolapse. Obstetric anal sphincter injury (OASI) is a risk factor for the development of anal incontinence, with approximately 10% of women developing symptoms within a year following vaginal birth [4]. Similarly, levator ani avulsion is strongly associated with the development of pelvic organ prolapse later in life [5].

The management of perineal trauma and its sequelae also contributes significantly to healthcare costs. In 2013/14 the economic burden of OASI in the United Kingdom (UK) ranged between £3.7 million (for assisted vaginal birth) and £9.8 million (for spontaneous vaginal birth). This is based on the length of stay attributed to the incident and additional management required to address postnatal symptoms [6]. Therefore, the prevention of obstetric perineal and pelvic floor trauma in even a modest proportion of vaginal births would reduce the requirement for postnatal repair, including sutures and suturing time [7]. More importantly, it would reduce costs and the preventable morbidity associated with sequelae such as urinary and faecal incontinence.

The case for perineal trauma prevention is compelling. In the last few decades, important progress has been made toward a robust evidence base for effective prevention strategies. However, much of the research is limited by the range of perineal outcomes studied, as well as short follow-up duration. In this chapter we will summarise and review the evidence for interventions associated with decreasing perineal and anal sphincter trauma as well as levator ani avulsion, focusing primarily on randomized controlled trials.

12.2   Risk Factors

12.2.1 Perineal Trauma Including Anal Sphincter Injury

Risk factors can broadly be divided into modifiable and non-modifiable risks and we acknowledge that these can overlap. Therefore, we will focus on *modifiable intrapartum risk factors* to prevent pelvic floor dysfunction. Modifiable risk factors associated with second-degree perineal trauma [8] include assisted vaginal birth and maternal birth positions (such as lithotomy, supine and sitting as opposed to squatting, kneeling and lateral); on the other hand, fetal macrosomia is a non-modifiable risk factor. As far as OASI is concerned, a recent meta-analysis reported [8] several non-modifiable risk factors such as fetal malposition (occiput posterior) (RR 2.73 [95% CI 2.08, 3.58]), Asian ethnicity (RR 1.87 [95% CI 1.46, 2.39]), primiparity (RR 1.59 [95% CI 1.45, 1.75]), augmentation of labour (RR 1.46 [95%CI 1.32, 1.62]), epidural (RR 1.21 [95% CI 1.08, 1.36]), induction of labour (RR 1.05 [95%CI 0.97, 1.15]), and fetal birthweight (mean difference 163.71 [95%CI 115.37, 212.06]). Modifiable risk factors included assisted vaginal birth (RR 3.38 [95%CI 2.21, 5.18]) and midline episiotomy (RR 2.88 [95%CI

1.79, 4.65]). Interestingly, nulliparous women with a perineal body length of less than 3 cm have a higher risk of anal sphincter tears [9]. In multiparous women, risk is increased if perineal body length is less than 2.5 cm [10]. However, there is no evidence to suggest that performing an episiotomy in women with a perineal body length of less than 3 cm reduces the incidence of OASI.

Previously there has been disagreement between observational studies that water immersion for labour and birth is a risk factor for OASI [11, 12]. Evidence from two RCTs suggested that waterbirth is not associated with OASI. It is important to note that these studies were underpowered with regards to OASI incidence and only included 57 women with OASI [13, 14]. But, a systematic review of theses RCTs and observational studies ($n = 15$ studies, 93, 630 women) demonstrated that waterbirth did not affect OASI incidence [15].

Caesarean birth and perineal trauma have also been identified as risk factors for OASIS. The risk of OASI has been shown to increase by 21% (RR 1.21 [95% CI 1.07–1.38]) at vaginal birth after previous caesarean birth (VBAC) [16] compared to primparous women having a vaginal birth. Some authors have proposed that this may be related to a "nulliparous perineum" and/or a possible cephalopelvic disproportion that may have been the indication for the first caesarean section [16, 17]. Also, women having a VBAC may share other risk factors for OASI such as forceps or vacuumassisted vaginal birth [16]. Perineal trauma at first birth has been associated with a threefold increased risk of spontaneous tears at subsequent birth; there is also a direct relationship with the severity of the perineal trauma at first birth [18]. This particularly marked in centres using midline episiotomy [19, 20] and not in those who employ mediolateral episiotomy [21]. Given that the average rate of first OASI is 6.1% and 1.7% in primiparous and multiparous women respectively [19], the expected rate in women who experienced a previous OASI would be expected to be the same rate as multiparous women. However, women with previous OASIs are at increased risk of a repeat OASI in a subsequent birth [22] with an average rate of repeat OASI of 6.3% (range of 2–13.4%) [23].

Interestingly, socio-cultural factors appear to play a role as well in OASI. A Swedish cohort study found that, in comparison to non-migrants, newly arrived migrants from South Asia had a fourfold increase in risk of OASI. The risk also increased two to threefold in women from Sub-Saharan Africa, Southeast Asia, East Asia, the Pacific, North Africa, and the Middle East. Interestingly, increased time of residency in a more resourced country was demonstrated to be associated with a reduced risk of OASIs [24]. It is important that clinicians receive training with regards to the diverse needs of migrant women, including methods of prevention. In addition, migrant women need to be empowered early in the antenatal period with information about maternity services and labour care [25].

12.2.2 Levator Injury

Several risk factors have been reported be associated with levator avulsion, however, by far the use of forceps is the most significant modifiable risk factor (OR 7.09 [95%CI 4.77–10.54) [26]. Significant non-modifiable risk factors include OASI (OR 2.96 [95% CI 1.47–5.97]), larger fetal head circumference (OR 1.24 [95%CI 1.06–1.44]), older maternal age (OR 1.20 [95%CI 1.03–1.22]) and ethnicity (OR 0.55 [95%CI 0.36–0.84]) [26].

12.3 Interventions to Prevent Perineal Trauma (Not Involving the Anal Sphincter)

12.3.1 Antenatal

12.3.1.1 Perineal Massage
Antenatal perineal massage prior to vaginal birth may be useful to prevent perineal tears; there is good evidence of a modest protective effect of third trimester perineal massage in nulliparous women (Fig. 12.1). Four published RCTs have evaluated the effectiveness of prenatal perineal massage with almond oil by the pregnant woman and/or her partner [27–30]. In nulliparous women, perineal massage reduced the incidence of any grade of perineal trauma requiring suturing by 9% (risk ratio (RR) 0.91 [95%CI 0.83–1.08]) [30] (Fig. 12.2).

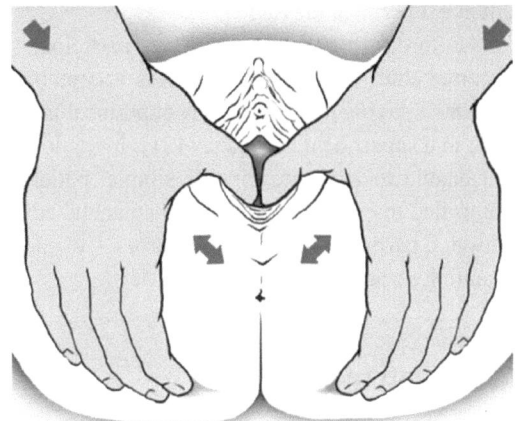

Fig. 12.1 Antenatal perineal massage technique. Massage can be performed by applying downward pressure in a U-shape (arrowed)

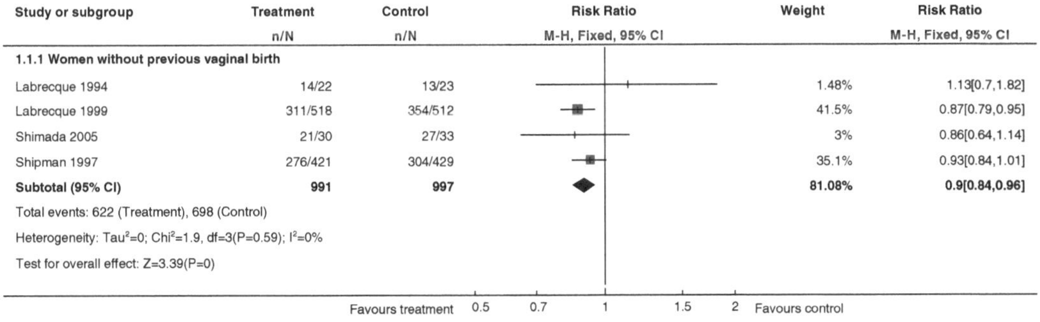

Study or subgroup	Treatment n/N	Control n/N	Risk Ratio M-H, Fixed, 95% CI	Weight	Risk Ratio M-H, Fixed, 95% CI
1.1.1 Women without previous vaginal birth					
Labrecque 1994	14/22	13/23		1.48%	1.13[0.7,1.82]
Labrecque 1999	311/518	354/512		41.5%	0.87[0.79,0.95]
Shimada 2005	21/30	27/33		3%	0.86[0.64,1.14]
Shipman 1997	276/421	304/429		35.1%	0.93[0.84,1.01]
Subtotal (95% CI)	991	997		81.08%	0.9[0.84,0.96]
Total events: 622 (Treatment), 698 (Control)					
Heterogeneity: Tau²=0; Chi²=1.9, df=3(P=0.59); I²=0%					
Test for overall effect: Z=3.39(P=0)					

Favours treatment   0.5   0.7   1   1.5   2   Favours control

Fig. 12.2 Forest plot of the risk of perineal trauma requiring suturing in RCTs of antenatal perineal massage

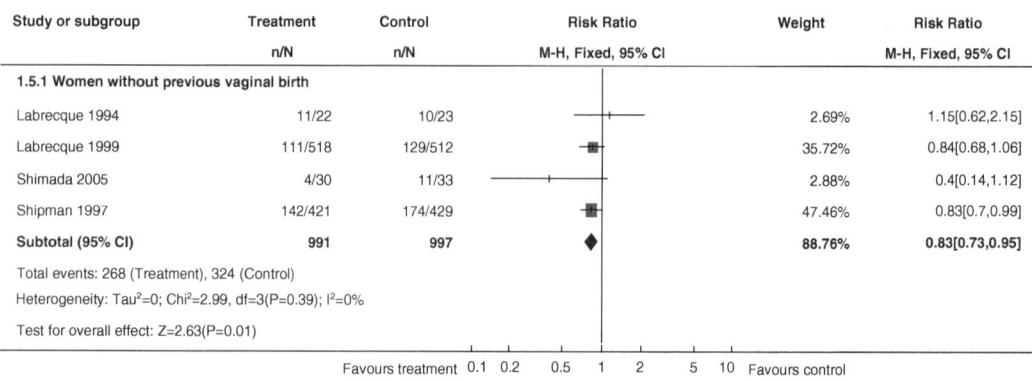

Study or subgroup	Treatment	Control	Risk Ratio	Weight	Risk Ratio
	n/N	n/N	M-H, Fixed, 95% CI		M-H, Fixed, 95% CI
1.5.1 Women without previous vaginal birth					
Labrecque 1994	11/22	10/23		2.69%	1.15[0.62,2.15]
Labrecque 1999	111/518	129/512		35.72%	0.84[0.68,1.06]
Shimada 2005	4/30	11/33		2.88%	0.4[0.14,1.12]
Shipman 1997	142/421	174/429		47.46%	0.83[0.7,0.99]
Subtotal (95% CI)	**991**	**997**		**88.76%**	**0.83[0.73,0.95]**
Total events: 268 (Treatment), 324 (Control)					
Heterogeneity: Tau²=0; Chi²=2.99, df=3(P=0.39); I²=0%					
Test for overall effect: Z=2.63(P=0.01)					

Favours treatment 0.1 0.2   0.5   1   2   5   10 Favours control

Fig. 12.3 Forest plot of the risk of episiotomy in RCTs of antenatal perineal massage

For multiparous women, there was no significant benefit [30]. There was an additional 16% (RR 0.84 [95%CI 0.74–0.95]) reduction in the rate of episiotomy in nulliparous women (Fig. 12.3); one woman would avoid an episiotomy for every 21 nulliparous women undertaking antenatal perineal massage [30].

At three months postpartum, participants reported that perineal massage was acceptable, with 80% saying they would repeat perineal massage in a subsequent pregnancy [31]. It would be reasonable to advocate for this simple, patient-controlled intervention in standard antenatal education, particularly in nulliparous women planning a vaginal birth.

12.3.2 Intrapartum

12.3.2.1 Maternal Position During Labour and Birth

There are a number of RCTs related to maternal position for the second stage of labour and birth, but the current evidence on the effectiveness of different maternal positions to prevent perineal trauma remains inconclusive. Optimal birthing positions in women without epidural anaesthesia has been assessed in one Cochrane review [32]. Thirty RCTs were included, evaluating the effect of upright position, birth or squat stool, birth cushion, and birth chair versus supine positions. An upright position was associated with a 25% reduction in episiotomies (RR 0.75 [95%CI 0.61–0.92]). No significant difference in the prevention of other grades of perineal trauma was reported. However, there was a medium to high risk of bias across the

studies, and therefore these findings should be interpreted with caution [32]. Also, there was no benefit associated with an upright birth position for women *with* an epidural with regards to perineal trauma [32]. As the causes of perineal trauma are multifactorial, maternal positions during labour may contribute to reductions in other intrapartum factors that increase the risk of perineal trauma, such as the length of the second stage of labour and rates of assisted vaginal birth.

12.4 Interventions to Prevent OASI

12.4.1 Antenatal

12.4.1.1 Perineal Massage
A recent meta-analysis reported that antenatal perineal massage was associated with a significant reduction in the incidence of OASI by 64% (RR 0.36 [95% CI 0.14–0.89]) [33]. However, subgroup analysis based on parity was not performed and there was significant study heterogeneity and publication bias.

12.4.2 Intrapartum

12.4.2.1 Second Stage Perineal Massage
Perineal massage in the second stage of labour can be performed using two gloved fingers inserted inside the vagina, moving laterally and carefully with simultaneous downward pressure towards the rectum [34]. This perineal massage

technique has been demonstrated to reduce the risk of OASI by 51% (RR 0.49 [95% CI 0.25–0.94]). However, it carries no significant effect on other grades of perineal trauma and episiotomy [35].

12.4.2.2 Second Stage Perineal Warm Compress

Applying heat to a muscle improves stretch and elasticity by increasing blood flow and promoting relaxation [36]. The use of a warm compress on the perineum during the second stage of labour has been associated with a 54% reduction in the risk of OASI (RR 0.46 [95% CI 0.27–0.79]) [35]. The reported technique involves soaking the compress in tap water boiled at a temperature of 45–59 °C. The compress is wrung out and placed on the perineum with a rewarmed pad replaced every 15 min [37].

12.4.2.3 Manual Perineal Protection

There has been a recent resurgence in the practice of manual perineal protection during the second stage of labour (Fig. 12.4).

One recent review [38] included three RCTs and three observational studies. Within the RCTs, manual perineal protection was not associated with significant clinical benefit. However, within the observational studies, manual perineal protection was associated with a 55% reduction in severe perineal trauma (RR 0.45 [95% CI 0.40–0.50]). There was a lack of technique standardisation in the RCTs, and the effect of manual perineal protection was not a primary study outcome in some of the studies [38]. For example, the large RCT of "Hands On Or Poised" ('HOOP'), allocated women to either 'hands on' (the midwife's hands put pressure on the baby's head, supported the perineum and lateral flexion used to facilitate shoulder delivery) or the 'hands poised' (the midwife's hands were poised, not touching the head or perineum except if light pressure was needed to prevent rapid expulsion, and allowing spontaneous delivery of the shoulders). The technique for perineal support was not specified in the protocol, was not reproducible, and it is unclear if all midwives in this trial used the same technique. About 30% of the 'hands poised' group were actually delivered 'hands on' because the midwife feared impending perineal

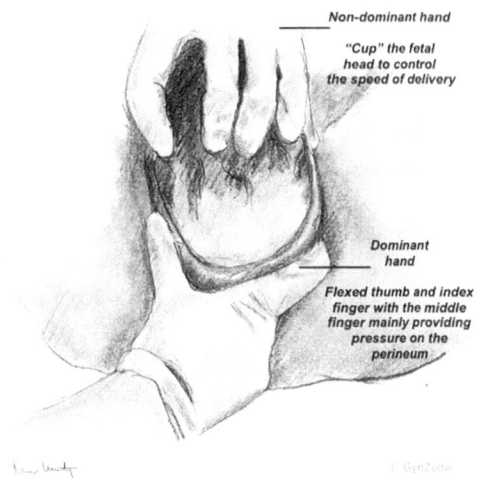

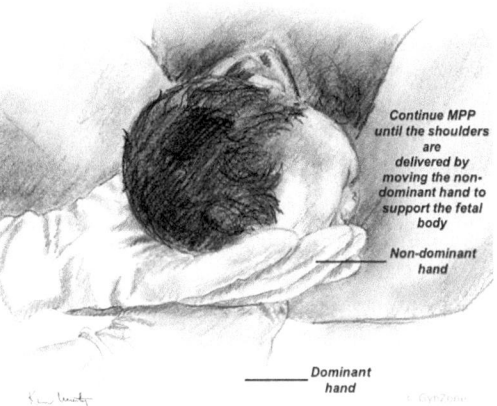

Fig. 12.4 Manual perineal protection technique. Illustrations are by courtesy of GynZone

trauma. In addition, the primary outcome measure of the study was perineal pain up to 10 days post-partum. However, the study was not powered to determine the effect of perineal support on OASI incidence [39].

A technique practiced commonly in Finland has been shown to reduce perineal muscular tension by 40%, in comparison to a hands-poised approach in bio-mechanical models [40]. The Finnish manual perineal protection involves using the technique as shown in Fig. 12.4 [41, 42]. In Norway, the application of this technique was part of a perineal protection programme. In this programme, an external midwife was employed (from a previously successful site) to educate internal trainers, who then educated staff members with practical hands-on training on a pelvic model followed by supervised hands-on training during the second stage of labour. The authors reported that the incidence of OASI fell from 4.0% to 1.9% between 2003 and 2010 [43] in an interrupted time series.

There is a growing body of evidence from several countries including the UK, Norway and Denmark, demonstrating that the implementation of perineal protection initiatives and care bundles can reduce the incidence of OASIs [44–47]. In the UK, the Royal College of Obstetricians and Gynaecologists and the Royal College of Midwives implemented an OASI Care Bundle (Fig. 12.5). The four elements of this bundle included antenatal education, manual perineal protection, use of a mediolateral episiotomy if clinically indicated, and systemic vaginal and rectal examination to assess for anal sphincter injury after birth.

Use of the OASI Care Bundle was associated with a 20% reduction in the risk of OASIs (aOR (adjusted odds ratio) 0.80, [95% CI 0.65–0.98]) with no effect on caesarean birth or episiotomy rates. Other care bundles, including the Women's Health Care Australasia Clinical Excellence Commission (WHA CEC) bundle in Australia, also include the use of warm perineal compresses in the second stage of labour [47]. Women report good experiences and feelings of support and empowerment with the implementation of these care bundles [48]. However, successful implementation of a care bundle requires clinician empowerment to change clinical practice. The STOMP (Stop OASI Morbidity Project) quality improvement project in the UK recruited clinical champions who routinely engaged with staff to empower and improve motivation. Clinicians reported feeling particularly engaged after being informed about the potential long-term morbidity associated with OASIs [49].

Controlled delivery of the fetal head by visualising the perineum throughout delivery and maternal cooperation can be protective against severe perineal trauma [50]. Having a second clinician for support can improve this further. The Oneplus multicentre RCT demonstrated that when a second midwife was present to assist with birth and perineal trauma prevention, the incidence of OASI was reduced by 31% (OR 0.69 [95%CI 0.49–0.97]) [51].

12.4.2.4 Episiotomy

The use of episiotomy has been promoted to prevent more serious tears and prevent pelvic floor relaxation [52, 53]. With unassisted vaginal

---

1. From 32 weeks in the antenatal period, the midwife or doctor will discuss OASI with the woman, including her personal risk factors and ways to minimize her risk, including the three subsequent components of the care bundle. An information leaflet (now referred to as a 'discussion guide' to highlight women's active participation) was developed with women's feedback to support this component.

2. At the time of birth and with the woman's consent, the midwife or doctor use their hands to support both the perineum and baby's head (known as manual perineal protection, or MPP) while communicating with the woman to encourage a slow and guided birth.
    - For spontaneous vaginal births, MPP should be used unless the woman's chosen birth position (i.e. water births) doesn't enable MPP to be used or she declines this technique.
    - For assisted vaginal births (i.e. forceps, ventouse), MPP should always be used unless the woman declines this technique.

3. If clinically indicated and with the woman's consent, a mediolateral episiotomy should be done at an angle of 60 degrees from the midline at crowning.

4. Following all vaginal births, a systematic examination of the vagina and a no-rectum should be offered to immediately assess whether there has been any damage to the external or internal anal sphincter and genitalia so that treatment options can be discussed and implemented as necessary. Prior discussion about the risks and benefits supports women to make an informed decision. Any tears are graded in accordance with RCOG Green-top guidelines.

Fig. 12.5 Elements of the OASI Care Bundle. From Jurczuk M, Bidwell P, Gurol-Urganci I, van der Meulen J, Sevdalis N, Silverton L, Thakar R (2021) The OASI care bundle quality improvement project: lessons learned and future direction. Int Urogynecol J 32:1989–1995 [48]

births, a policy of selective episiotomy rather than routine episiotomy has been associated with a reduction in the incidence of anal sphincter trauma by 30% (RR 0.70 [95% CI 0.52–0.94] $n = 8$ RCTs) (Fig. 12.5) [54]. Therefore, performing an episiotomy routinely to prevent a tear at spontaneous delivery has no place in modern obstetrics.

Whether midline episiotomy results in better outcomes than mediolateral episiotomy has not been definitely answered [54]. A quasi-randomised study of selective midline versus mediolateral episiotomy use [55] in 407 nulliparous women identified that OASI occurred with 24% of midline and 9% of mediolateral episiotomies. Subjects not receiving their assigned treatment were excluded from the analysis. Since the number of women in the midline episiotomy group was smaller, there may have been a clinical bias against midline episiotomy, presumably due to concern that it might extend into the anal sphincter. Pain and dyspareunia were similar in both groups, and more women resumed sexual intercourse in the first month in the midline episiotomy group. Lateral episiotomies, which are performed 2 cm away from the midline have been shown to not differ significantly from mediolateral episiotomy with respect to anal sphincter trauma incidence [56, 57]. However, for

mediolateral episiotomy, the angle from the midline seems to influence OASI rates. When the episiotomy scar angle was measured 3 months postnatally in 100 primiparous women, the incidence of OASIs was reduced by 50% for every 6° of the angle away from midline [56]. Furthermore, there is likely an underestimation of the episiotomy angle at birth due to perineal distension as a 60° mediolateral episiotomy angle at the time of birth resulted in a post-delivery angle of only 45° [56]. Similarly, when an episiotomy was performed at 45° during birth, the resultant scar was at 22.5° [56].

The effect of episiotomy at assisted vaginal birth has been most often compared to no episiotomy. A systematic review and meta-analysis which included two RCTs and an additional 29 cohort studies [58] found that with nulliparous women, in vacuum births, use of a mediolateral episiotomy significantly reduced the rate of OASIs by 49% (Fig. 12.6). This equated to a NNT to prevent one additional OASI of 28. Also, with nulliparous forceps births, there was a 68% reduction in the rate of OASIs when a mediolateral episiotomy was performed (Fig. 12.7) with a NNT of 8. There is an urgent need for an RCT, given the high rate of serious lacerations in this situation.

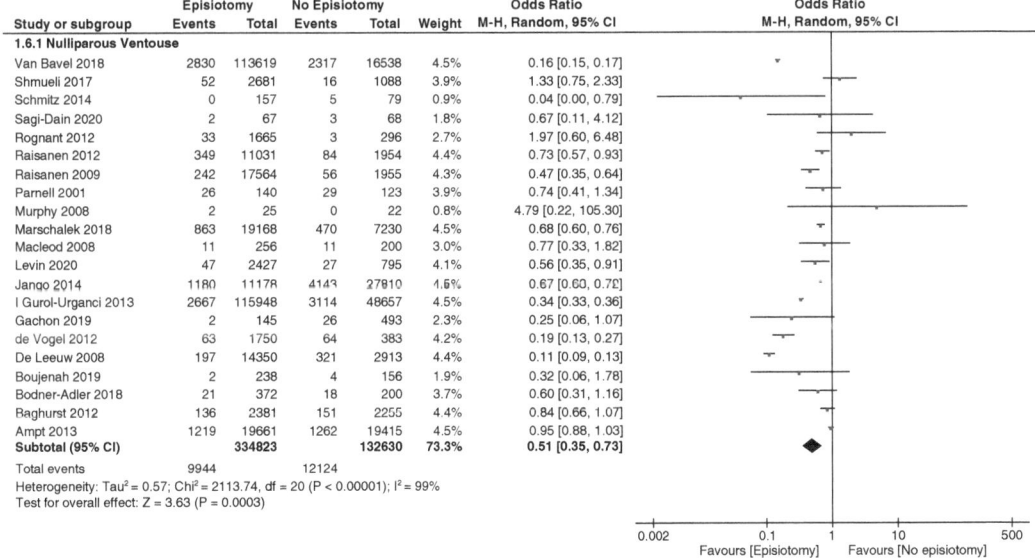

Fig. 12.6 Forest plot of the incidence of severe perineal trauma in women undergoing a vacuum assisted-birth with or without mediolateral/lateral episiotomy

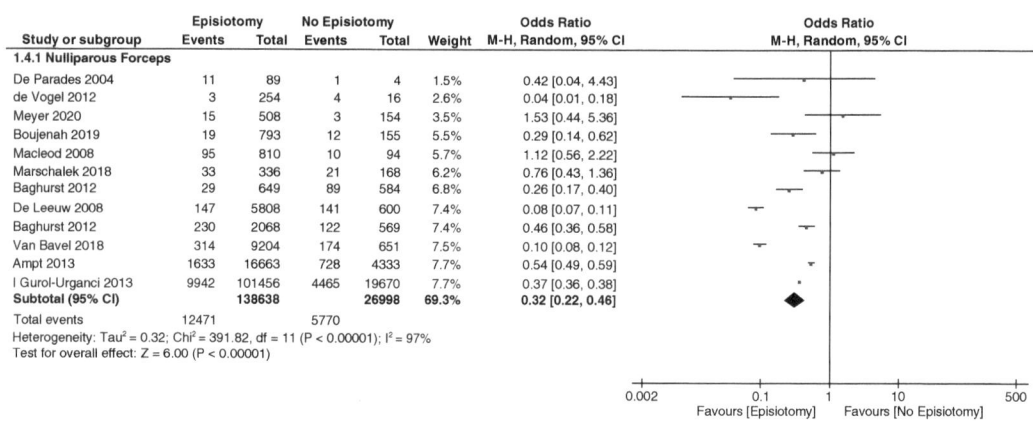

Fig. 12.7 Forest plot of the incidence of severe perineal trauma in women undergoing a forceps assisted-birth with or without mediolateral/lateral

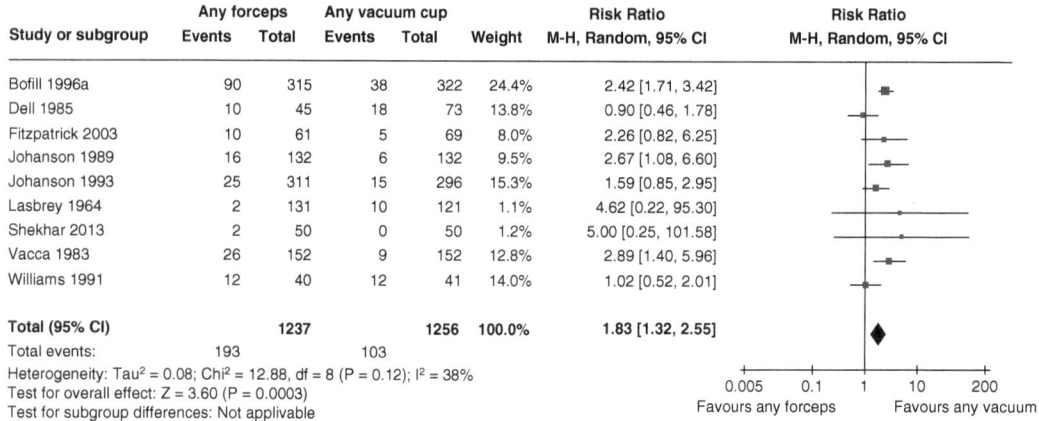

Fig. 12.8 Forest plot of the incidence of severe perineal trauma in women undergoing a vacuum or forceps assisted-birth

12.4.2.5 Assisted Vaginal Birth

In comparison to vacuum-assisted birth, forceps-assisted birth is associated with a twofold increased risk of anal sphincter trauma (RR 1.83 [95%CI 1.32–2.55]) (Fig. 12.8) [59].

Rates of anal sphincter trauma with assisted vaginal birth and episiotomy are high. A UK RCT [60] (where mediolateral episiotomy was practiced), reported severe vaginal lacerations in 17% of forceps compared to 11% of vacuum births; a Canadian RCT [61] (where midline episiotomy is practised), reported OASI in 29% of forceps compared to 12% of vacuum deliveries. Compared to vacuum extraction, forceps-assisted birth is associated with almost twice the risk of developing faecal incontinence [62].

In the UK there has been an increase in forceps use over time. One unit reported that over a

10-year period (2001–2010), the rate of forceps births had increased from 7.7% to 9.4%, whilst the rate of vacuum births decreased from 6.6% to 3.3% [63]. It is unclear why the rate of forceps has changed, however, in comparison to vacuum assisted births (particularly those with soft (silicone) cups, forceps are 42% less likely to fail in achieving a successful vaginal birth [59]. Furthermore, the failure rate of rotational forceps is 2% compared to a 25% risk of failure in rotational ventouse and/or manual rotation [64–66]. There are also significant risks associated with caesarean birth in the second stage of labour [67, 68] after failure of assisted vaginal birth.

Women recruited to a study of a new device designed to expedite birth in an emergency, expressed an aspiration for a safer, kinder alternative to forceps [69]. The BD Odon device (Fig. 12.9) uses an air chamber attached to a thin plastic sleeve, acting as the traction anchor, which reduces the traction forces applied to the fetal head and subsequent trauma to the birth canal [70, 71]. The effectiveness and safety of this device is being evaluated in the ASSIST Trial [71–74].

The choice of instrument may also be impacted by human factors. Clinicians may not only be reluctant to perform vacuum-assisted births due to fear of instrument failure, but also due to litigation [76]. This was highlighted in a retrospective cohort study [77] that demonstrated that in comparison to second stage caesarean births, more assisted vaginal births are performed during office hours when a senior obstetrician is present. However, to date no RCT has compared the risks of rotational forceps with vacuum assisted births. Al Wattar et al. [78] performed a meta-analysis of 23 non-randomised studies and demonstrated that in comparison to rotational vacuum, there was no significant difference in OASIs incidence when rotational forceps were used. It is important to note that the quality of the studies were poor with medium to high risk of bias. In addition, findings from the individual studies may not be representative of the general population, as most were performed in single centres with experienced operators [79]. There is a RCT currently funded by the NIHR to investigate the effect of different strategies for rotational birth; this study is powered for OASI as a primary outcome and we await the results [80].

12.4.2.6 Prediction Models

Prediction models have been published to improve risk reduction for OASI [81–86]. Table 12.1 describes these prediction models. The most useful prediction models are those that can be used for counselling in the antenatal period; one study attempted to address this by including variables known prior to birth. Significant predictive factors for OASIs included advanced maternal age, fetal malposition (occipito-posterior), induction/augmentation of labour and estimated infant birthweight ≥4000 g. This model had acceptable performance; 71% of the time, it would correctly assign a randomly selected patient. However, to the contrary, its low specificity could lead to a high false-positive prediction rate with potentially unnecessary interventions [84]. Further research is required to create a clinically useful prediction model which can be used to appropriately counsel women in the antenatal period.

1

The inserter is applied on the head of the baby. A soft plastic bell assures perfect adaptation to the fetal head and prevents damage.

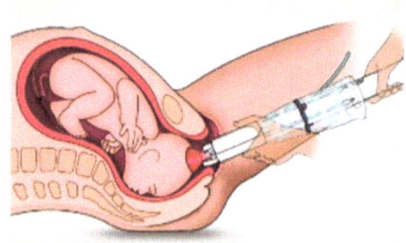

2

The inserter progressively positions the Odón device around the head of the baby. Positioning occurs as the inserter gently produces the sliding of the two surfaces of the folded sleeve along the birth canal and around the baby's head.

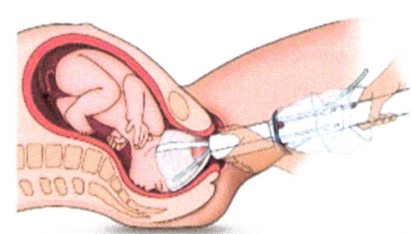

3

When the Odón device is properly positioned, a marker on the insertion handle become clearly visible in the reading window. A minimal and self-limited amount of air is pumped into an air chamber in the inner surface.

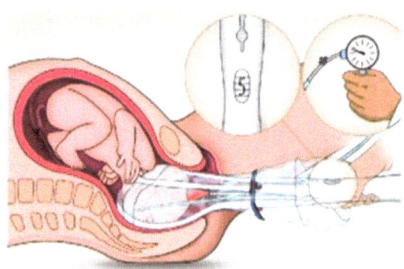

4

This produces a secure grasp around the head of the baby that fixes the inner surface and allows for traction. The inserter is removed.

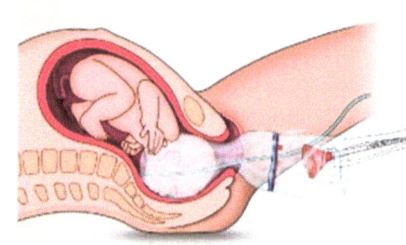

5

The head is delivered taking advantage of the sliding effect of the two surfaces of the folded sleeve. Lubrication of the surfaces further facilitates the extraction process. If needed, traction can be applied up to 19 kg (which is equivalent to the force applied with the metal vacuum extractor).

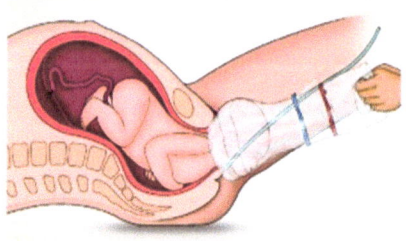

Fig. 12.9 The BD Odon device. From The World Health Organization Odon Device Research Group (2013) Feasibility and safety study of a new device (Odon device) for assisted vaginal deliveries: study protocol. Reproductive Health [75]

Table 12.1 Summary of OASI prediction models and their performance

Reference	Study design	Factors	AUC
Chill (2021) [82]	Retrospective cohort	Nulliparity Low BMI Advanced gestational age	0.76
Luchristt (2021) [86] [a]	Prospective cohort	Advanced maternal age Low BMI No previous vaginal birth Non smoker Assisted vaginal birth	0.79
McPherson (2014) [81]	Retrospective cohort	Nulliparity Ethnicity (African-Caribbean) Non-smoker Birth in hospital Water birth Assisted vaginal birth	0.64
Meister (2016) [80]	Retrospective cohort	Nulliparity Ethnicity (non-African American) Prolonged second stage Non-smoker Infant birthweight ≥3500 g Assisted vaginal birth	0.83
Webb (2017) [84]	Retrospective cohort	Nulliparity Induction/augmentation of labor Prolonged second stage Prolonged active second stage Head circumference ≥37 cm Increased birthweight (per unit (kg)) *Mediolateral episiotomy*[b]	0.77
		Pre-birth variables Advanced maternal age Fetal malposition (occipito-posterior) Induction/augmentation of labor Infant birthweight ≥4000 g	0.71
Woo (2020) [83]	Retrospective cohort	Advanced maternal age Advanced gestational age Ethnicity (Asian) Prolonged second stage Assisted vaginal birth Previous OASI	c

AUC = area under the curve (on receiver operator curve analysis), which represented the percentage of the time the prediction model would correctly assign a randomly selected patient
Study population = vaginal birth after previous cesarean section
[a] Study population = vaginal birth after previous cesarean section
[b] Mediolateral episiotomy = protective variable
[c] This study created a probability-based risk stratification tool and did not report the model AUC

12.5   Interventions to Prevent Levator Avulsion

12.5.1 Intrapartum

12.5.1.1   Mode of Birth

The incidence of levator avulsion following spontaneous vaginal, vacuum-assisted, forceps-assisted, and caesarean births has been reported in a recent systematic review (Fig. 12.10) [87]. The authors demonstrated that caesarean births resulted in a reduced incidence of levator avulsion, although its effect was not completely protective. In three studies, six primigravid women undergoing caesarean had evidence of levator avulsion [88–90]. All caesarean births were performed at full cervical dilatation with the fetal head above the ischial

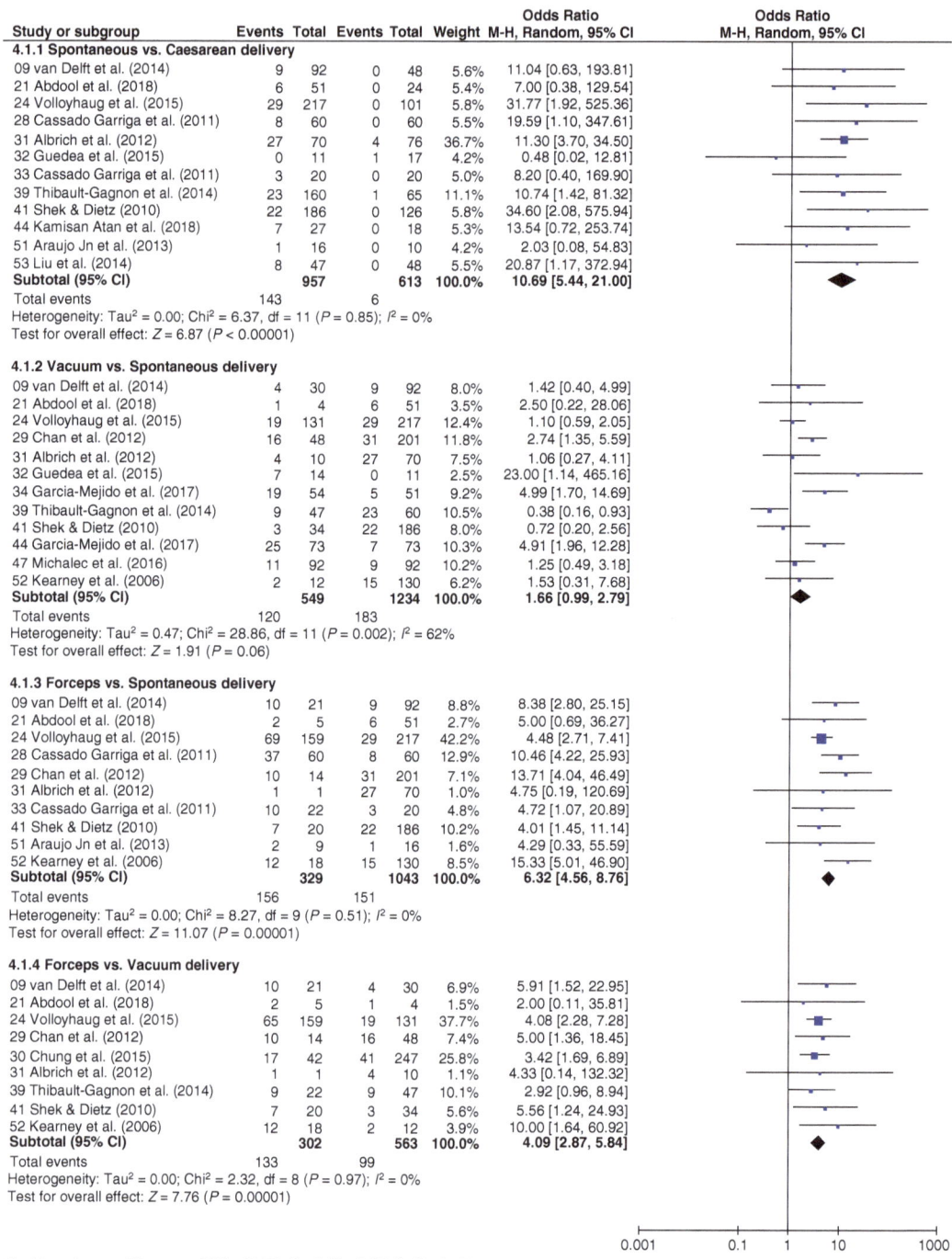

Fig. 12.10 Comparison of risk of levator avulsion between different modes of birth

spines, with no application of vacuum or forceps [88]. It is difficult to explain how levator avulsion occurred in this group, as it has been described that stretching of the levator ani does not occur until crowning of the fetal head [91].

In comparison to spontaneous vaginal births, Rusavy et al. [87] demonstrated that vacuum-assisted birth increased the odds of levator avulsion by 66%. In addition, with forceps-assisted births in comparison to spontaneous vaginal births and vacuum-assisted births, the odds of levator avulsion increased six and fourfold respectively (Fig. 12.10). The association between levator avulsion and forceps-assisted births may be due to many factors, which include an increase in pelvic outlet diameter on insertion of the blades, speed of delivery, traction force, and the subsequent quicker distension of the perineum compared to vacuum or spontaneous vaginal birth, as less maternal effort is required [92, 93].

12.5.1.2 Prediction Models

Studies have attempted to develop risk prediction models to counsel women with regards to pelvic floor trauma prevention (Table 12.2). As the majority of studies were performed in a urogynaecological population, they cannot be used to counsel pregnant women in the antenatal period. One group [94] attempted to predict levator avulsion during antepartum period in 367 women but were unsuccessful, as the only predictor identified was a lower body mass index. Subsequently, Van Delft et al. [95] identified that forceps-assisted birth, OASIs, and a prolonged second stage of labour were associated with an increased risk of levator avulsion. This risk model showed that a woman with all three risk factors would have a 75% probability of having sustained a levator avulsion. However, the results of this study should be interpreted with caution, as 80% of avulsions could not be explained by the model. This was likely due to the small number of women with levator avulsion and potential confounders not included in the model. Further research is required to create a robust risk prediction model which can be used in clinical practice.

Table 12.2 Summary of levator avulsion prediction models and their performance

Reference	Study design	Factors	R^2
Van Delft (2014) [95]	Prospective cohort	Forceps delivery OASIs Active second stage (hour)	19.2%
Lammers (2013) [96]	Retrospective cohort	Episiotomy Pelvic floor surgery Prolapse Obstructive defecation	40.0%
Dietz (2010) [97]	Retrospective cohort	Cystocele Oxford score Age Forceps/vacuum delivery History of hysterectomy Stress urinary incontinence	37.2%
Garnham (2017) [98]	Retrospective cohort	Prolapse Previous prolapse surgery Forceps delivery	[a]

[a] This study created reported the Akaike information criterion and not the model R^2

12.6 Conclusions

Every attempt should be made to prevent perineal trauma with its attendant pain, dyspareunia and longer-term sequelae such as pelvic organ prolapse and urinary and faecal incontinence. Appreciation of the modifiable and non-modifiable risk factors for pelvic floor and anal sphincter trauma is important information for clinicians and women. The implementation of care bundles to prevent perineal trauma is promising and should be explored further.

Take Home Messages

- Knowledge of the risk factors associated with perineal trauma, OASIs and levator avulsion is essential for all clinicians.
- There is a lack of robust evidence supporting the use of prediction models in clinical practice.
- The appreciation of risk factors will allow for a modification of obstetric practice.
- Forceps-assisted births are associated with worse perineal and pelvic floor outcomes than both vacuum and spontaneous births.
- Increased training in the choice and technique of assisted vaginal birth is important.

Appendix: MCQ

Questions

1. Which of the following is true regarding perineal trauma (not involving the anal sphincter):
   (A) Birthing in a lithotomy position is associated with a reduced risk of perineal trauma.
   (B) An upright birthing position can reduce the need for episiotomy.
   (C) Perineal massage in the third trimester can reduce the risk of perineal trauma in both nulliparous and multiparous women.
   (D) Perineal massage in the second stage of labour reduces the risk of perineal trauma.

   (E) Routine episiotomy can be used to prevent significant perineal trauma.

2. Which of the following statements is true regarding obstetric anal sphincter injury:
   (A) Repeat OASI affects 15% of women.
   (B) Perineal massage in the third trimester can reduce the risk of OASI in both nulliparous and multiparous women.
   (C) The use of a warm compress in the second stage of labour can prevent OASI in approximately 50% of women.
   (D) Manual perineal protection does not need to be continued once the fetal head is delivered.
   (E) A mediolateral episiotomy would need to be performed in 15 forceps births to prevent one OASI.

3. Which of the following statements regarding levator injury is false?
   (A) Levator injury can lead to the development of pelvic organ prolapse.
   (B) Forceps-assisted birth is the most significant risk factor associated with levator injury.
   (C) There is no significant difference in the incidence of levator injury between vacuum assisted birth and spontaneous vaginal birth.
   (D) There are a number of robust prediction models that can be used in the antenatal period to counsel women with regards to their risk of levator injury.

Answers

1. Which of the following is true regarding perineal trauma (not involving the anal sphincter):
   (A) FALSE
   (B) TRUE
   (C) FALSE
   (D) FALSE
   (E) FALSE

2. Which of the following statements is true regarding obstetric anal sphincter injury:
   (A) FALSE
   (B) FALSE
   (C) TRUE
   (D) FALSE
   (E) FALSE

3. Which of the following statements regarding levator injury is false?
   (A) TRUE
   (B) TRUE
   (C) TRUE
   (D) FALSE

References

1. DeLancey J. The appearance of levator ani muscle abnormalities in magnetic resonance images after vaginal delivery. Obstet Gynecol. 2003;101:46–53.
2. Allen RE, Hosker GL, Smith ARB, Warrell DW. Pelvic floor damage and childbirth: a neurophysiological study. BJOG. 1990;97:770–9.
3. Smith ARB, Hosker GL, Warrell DW. The role of partial denervation of the pelvic floor in the aetiology of genitourinary prolapse and stress incontinence of urine. A neurophysiological study. BJOG. 1989;96:24–8.
4. Sideris M, McCaughey T, Hanrahan JG, Arroyo-Manzano D, Zamora J, Jha S, Knowles CH, Thakar R, Chaliha C, Thangaratinam S. Risk of obstetric anal sphincter injuries (OASIS) and anal incontinence: a meta-analysis. Eur J Obstet Gynecol Reprod Biol. 2020;252:303–12.
5. Dietz HP. Clinical consequences of levator trauma: opinion. Ultrasound Obstet Gynecol. 2012;39:367–71.
6. Orlovic M, Carter AW, Marti J, Mossialos E. Estimating the incidence and the economic burden of third and fourth-degree obstetric tears in the English NHS: an observational study using propensity score matching. BMJ Open. 2017;7:e015463.
7. Jansson MH, Franzén K, Hiyoshi A, Tegerstedt G, Dahlgren H, Nilsson K. Risk factors for perineal and vaginal tears in primiparous women—the prospective POPRACT-cohort study. BMC Pregnancy Childbirth. 2020;20:749.
8. Pergialiotis V, Bellos I, Fanaki M, Vrachnis N, Doumouchtsis SK. Risk factors for severe perineal trauma during childbirth: an updated meta-analysis. Eur J Obstet Gynecol Reprod Biol. 2020;247:94–100.
9. Aytan H, Tapisiz OL, Tuncay G, Avsar FA. Severe perineal lacerations in nulliparous women and epi-

siotomy type. Eur J Obstet Gynecol Reprod Biol. 2005;121:46–50.
10. Deering SH, Carlson N, Stitely M, Allaire AD, Satin AJ. Perineal body length and lacerations at delivery. J Reprod Med. 2004;49:306–10.
11. Burns EE, Boulton MG, Cluett E, Cornelius VR, Smith LA. Characteristics, interventions, and outcomes of women who used a birthing pool: a prospective observational study. Birth. 2012;39:192–202.
12. Cortes E, Basra R, Kelleher CJ. Waterbirth and pelvic floor injury: a retrospective study and postal survey using ICIQ modular long form questionnaires. Eur J Obstet Gynecol Reprod Biol. 2011;155:27–30.
13. Ohlsson G, Buchhave P, Leandersson U, Nordström L, Rydhström H, Sjölin I. Warm tub bathing during labor: maternal and neonatal effects: effects of warm tub bathing during labor. Acta Obstet Gynecol Scand. 2001;80:311–4.
14. Eckert K, Turnbull D, MacLennan A. Immersion in water in the first stage of labor: a randomized controlled trial. Birth. 2001;28:84–93.
15. Burns E, Feeley C, Hall PJ, Vanderlaan J. Systematic review and meta-analysis to examine intrapartum interventions, and maternal and neonatal outcomes following immersion in water during labour and waterbirth. BMJ Open. 2022;12:e056517.
16. Uebergang J, Hiscock R, Hastie R, Middleton A, Pritchard N, Walker S, Tong S, Lindquist A. Risk of obstetric anal sphincter injury among women who birth vaginally after a prior caesarean section: a statewide cohort study. BJOG. 2022;129:1325–32.
17. Räisänen S, Vehviläinen-Julkunen K, Cartwright R, Gissler M, Heinonen S. A prior cesarean section and incidence of obstetric anal sphincter injury. Int Urogynecol J. 2013;24:1331–9.
18. Martin S, Labrecque M, Marcoux S, Bérubé S, Pinault JJ. The association between perineal trauma and spontaneous perineal tears. J Fam Pract. 2001;50:333–7.
19. Payne TN, Carey JC, Rayburn WF. Prior third- or fourth-degree perineal tears and recurrence risks. Int J Gynecol Obstet. 1999;64:55–7.
20. Peleg D. Risk of repetition of a severe perineal laceration. Obstet Gynecol. 1999;93:1021–4.
21. Harkin R, Fitzpatrick M, O'Connell PR, O'Herlihy C. Anal sphincter disruption at vaginal delivery: is recurrence predictable? Eur J Obstet Gynecol Reprod Biol. 2003;109:149–52.
22. D'Souza JC, Monga A, Tincello DG, Sultan AH, Thakar R, Hillard TC, Grigsby S, Kibria A, Jordan CF, Ashmore C. Maternal outcomes in subsequent delivery after previous obstetric anal sphincter injury (OASI): a multi-centre retrospective cohort study. Int Urogynecol J. 2019;31(3):627–33. https://doi.org/10.1007/s00192-019-03983-0.
23. Jha S, Parker V. Risk factors for recurrent obstetric anal sphincter injury (rOASI): a systematic review and meta-analysis. Int Urogynecol J. 2016;27:849–57.

24. Sørbye I, Bains S, Vangen S, Sundby J, Lindskog B, Owe K. Obstetric anal sphincter injury by maternal origin and length of residence: a nationwide cohort study. BJOG. 2022;129:423–31.

25. Higginbottom GMA, Evans C, Morgan M, Bharj KK, Eldridge J, Hussain B. Experience of and access to maternity care in the UK by immigrant women: a narrative synthesis systematic review. BMJ Open. 2019;9:e029478.

26. Subramaniam N, Eslick G, Shek K, Dietz H. P16.09: obstetric risk factors for levator avulsion: a meta-analysis and systematic review. Ultrasound Obstet Gynecol. 2019;54:208.

27. Shipman MK, Boniface DR, Tefft ME, McCloghry F. Antenatal perineal massage and subsequent perineal outcomes: a randomised controlled trial. BJOG. 1997;104:787–91.

28. Shimada M. A randomized controlled trial on evaluating effectiveness of perineal massage during pregnancy in primiparous women. J Jpn Acad Nurs Sci. 2005;25:22–9.

29. Labrecque M, Eason E, Marcoux S, Lemieux F, Pinault J-J, Feldman P, Laperrière L. Randomized controlled trial of prevention of perineal trauma by perineal massage during pregnancy. Am J Obstet Gynecol. 1999;180:593–600.

30. Beckmann MM, Stock OM. Antenatal perineal massage for reducing perineal trauma. Cochrane Database Syst Rev. 2013;(4):CD005123. https://doi.org/10.1002/14651858.CD005123.pub3.

31. Labrecque M, Eason E, Marcoux S. Women's views on the practice of prenatal perineal massage. BJOG. 2001;108:499–504.

32. Gupta JK, Sood A, Hofmeyr GJ, Vogel JP. Position in the second stage of labour for women without epidural anaesthesia. Cochrane Database Syst Rev. 2017;(5):CD002006. https://doi.org/10.1002/14651858.CD002006.pub4.

33. Abdelhakim AM, Eldesouky E, Elmagd IA, et al. Antenatal perineal massage benefits in reducing perineal trauma and postpartum morbidities: a systematic review and meta-analysis of randomized controlled trials. Int Urogynecol J. 2020;31:1735–45.

34. Albers LL, Sedler KD, Bedrick EJ, Teaf D, Peralta P. Midwifery care measures in the second stage of labor and reduction of genital tract trauma at birth: a randomized trial. J Midwifery Womens Health. 2005;50:365–72.

35. Aasheim V, Nilsen ABV, Reinar LM, Lukasse M. Perineal techniques during the second stage of labour for reducing perineal trauma. Cochrane Database Syst Rev. 2017;6(6):CD006672. https://doi.org/10.1002/14651858.CD006672.pub3.

36. Nakano J, Yamabayashi C, Scott A, Reid WD. The effect of heat applied with stretch to increase range of motion: a systematic review. Phys Ther Sport. 2012;13:180–8.

37. Dahlen HG, Homer CSE, Cooke M, Upton AM, Nunn R, Brodrick B. Perineal outcomes and maternal comfort related to the application of perineal warm packs in the second stage of labor: a randomized controlled trial. Birth. 2007;34:282–90.

38. Bulchandani S, Watts E, Sucharitha A, Yates D, Ismail K. Manual perineal support at the time of childbirth: a systematic review and meta-analysis. BJOG. 2015;122:1157–65.

39. McCandlish R, Bowler U, Asten H, Berridge G, Winter C, Sames L, Garcia J, Renfrew M, Elbourne D. A randomised controlled trial of care of the perineum during second stage of normal labour. BJOG. 1998;105:1262–72.

40. Jansova M, Kalis V, Rusavy Z, Zemcik R, Lobovsky L, Laine K. Modeling manual perineal protection during vaginal delivery. Int Urogynecol J. 2014;25:65–71.

41. Pirhonen Jouko P, Grenman Seija E, Haadem K, Gudmundsson S, Lindqvist P, Siihola S, Erkkola Risto U, Marsal K. Frequency of anal sphincter rupture at delivery in Sweden and Finland—result of difference in manual help to the baby's head. Acta Obstet Gynecol Scand. 1998;77:974–7.

42. Poulsen MØ, Madsen ML, Skriver-Møller A-C, Overgaard C. Does the Finnish intervention prevent obstetric anal sphincter injuries? A systematic review of the literature. BMJ Open. 2015;5:e008346.

43. Laine K, Skjeldestad FE, Sandvik L, Staff AC. Incidence of obstetric anal sphincter injuries after training to protect the perineum: cohort study. BMJ Open. 2012;2:e001649.

44. Hals E, Øian P, Pirhonen T, Gissler M, Hjelle S, Nilsen EB, Severinsen AM, Solsletten C, Hartgill T, Pirhonen J. A multicenter interventional program to reduce the incidence of anal sphincter tears. Obstet Gynecol. 2010;116:901–8.

45. Rasmussen OB, Yding A, Anh ØJ, Sander Andersen C, Boris J. Reducing the incidence of obstetric sphincter injuries using a hands-on technique: an interventional quality improvement project. BMJ Qual Improv Report. 2016;5:u217936.w7106.

46. Edozien L, Gurol-Urganci I, Cromwell D, Adams E, Richmond D, Mahmood T, van der Meulen J. Impact of third- and fourth-degree perineal tears at first birth on subsequent pregnancy outcomes: a cohort study. BJOG. 2014;121:1695–703.

47. Women's Healthcare Australasia. The how to guide: WHA CEC perineal protection bundle. 2019.

48. Jurczuk M, Bidwell P, Gurol-Urganci I, van der Meulen J, Sevdalis N, Silverton L, Thakar R. The OASI care bundle quality improvement project: lessons learned and future direction. Int Urogynecol J. 2021;32:1989–95.

49. Basu M, Smith D, Edwards R. Can the incidence of obstetric anal sphincter injury be reduced? The STOMP experience. Eur J Obstet Gynecol Reprod Biol. 2016;202:55–9.

50. Samuelsson E, Ladfors L, Lindblom B, Hagberg H. A prospective observational study on tears during vaginal delivery: occurrences and risk factors. Acta Obstet Gynecol Scand. 2002;81:44–9.

51. Edqvist M, Dahlen HG, Häggsgård C, Tern H, Ängeby K, Teleman P, Ajne G, Rubertsson C. The

effect of two midwives during the second stage of labour to reduce severe perineal trauma (Oneplus): a multicentre, randomised controlled trial in Sweden. Lancet. 2022;399(10331):1242–53.

52. DeLee JB. The prophylactic forceps operation. Am J Obstet Gynecol. 2002;187:254–5.

53. Pomeroy R. Shall we cut and reconstruct the perineum for every primipara? Am J Obstet Dis Women Child. 1918;78:211–20.

54. Jiang H, Qian X, Carroli G, Garner P. Selective versus routine use of episiotomy for vaginal birth. Cochrane Database Syst Rev. 2017;2(2):CD000081. https://doi.org/10.1002/14651858.CD000081.pub3.

55. Coats PM, Chan KK, Wilkins M, Beard RJ. A comparison between midline and mediolateral episiotomies. BJOG. 1980;87:408–12.

56. Kalis V, Landsmanova J, Bednarova B, Karbanova J, Laine K, Rokyta Z. Evaluation of the incision angle of mediolateral episiotomy at 60 degrees. Int J Gynaecol Obstet. 2011;112:220–4.

57. Kalis V, Laine K, de Leeuw JW, Ismail KM, Tincello DG. Classification of episiotomy: towards a standardisation of terminology. BJOG. 2012;119:522–6.

58. Okeahialam NA, Wong KW, Jha S, Sultan AH, Thakar R. Mediolateral/lateral episiotomy with operative vaginal delivery and the risk reduction of obstetric anal sphincter injury (OASI): a systematic review and meta-analysis. Int Urogynecol J. 2022;33(6):1393–405. https://doi.org/10.1007/s00192-022-05145-1.

59. Verma GL, Spalding JJ, Wilkinson MD, Hofmeyr GJ, Vannevel V, O'Mahony F. Instruments for assisted vaginal birth. Cochrane Database Syst Rev. 2021;9(9):CD005455. https://doi.org/10.1002/14651858.CD005455.pub3.

60. Johanson RB, Rice C, Doyle M, Arthur J, Anyanwu L, Ibrahim J, Warwick A, Redman CWE, O'Brien PMS. A randomised prospective study comparing the new vacuum extractor policy with forceps delivery. BJOG. 1993;100:524–30.

61. Bofill JA, Rust OA, Schorr SJ, Brown RC, Martin RW, Martin JN, Morrison JC. A randomized prospective trial of the obstetric forceps versus the M-cup vacuum extractor. Am J Obstet Gynecol. 1996;175:1325–30.

62. Fitzpatrick M, Behan M, O'Connell PR, O'Herlihy C. Randomised clinical trial to assess anal sphincter function following forceps or vacuum assisted vaginal delivery. BJOG. 2003;110:424–9.

63. Tyagi V, Perera M, Guerrero K. Trends in obstetric anal sphincter injuries over 10 years. J Obstet Gynaecol. 2013;33:844–9.

64. Tempest N, Hart A, Walkinshaw S, Hapangama D. A re-evaluation of the role of rotational forceps: retrospective comparison of maternal and perinatal outcomes following different methods of birth for malposition in the second stage of labour. BJOG. 2013;120:1277–84.

65. O'Brien S, Day F, Lenguerrand E, Cornthwaite K, Edwards S, Siassakos D. Rotational forceps versus manual rotation and direct forceps: a retrospective

cohort study. Eur J Obstet Gynecol Reprod Biol. 2017;212:119–25.

66. Stock SJ, Josephs K, Farquharson S, Love C, Cooper SE, Kissack C, Akolekar R, Norman JE, Denison FC. Maternal and neonatal outcomes of successful Kielland's rotational forceps delivery. Obstet Gynecol. 2013;121:1032–9.

67. Murphy DJ. An obstetric perspective. Lancet. 2002;360:941.

68. Cornthwaite K, Draycott T, Bahl R, Hotton E, Winter C, Lenguerrand E. Impacted fetal head: a retrospective cohort study of emergency caesarean section. Eur J Obstet Gynecol Reprod Biol. 2021;261:85–91.

69. Hotton EJ, Blencowe NS, Bale N, Lenguerrand E, Draycott TJ, Crofts JF, Wade J. Novel device for assisted vaginal birth: using integrated qualitative case study methodology to optimise Odon device use within a feasibility study in a maternity unit in the southwest of England. BMJ Open. 2022;12:e059115.

70. O'Brien S, Winter C, Burden C, Boulvain M, Draycott T, Crofts J. Fetal head position and perineal distension associated with the use of the BD Odon device™ in operative vaginal birth: a simulation study. BJOG Int J Obstet Gynaecol. 2017;124:10–8.

71. O'Brien S, Hotton EJ, Lenguerrand E, et al. The ASSIST study—the BD Odon device for assisted vaginal birth: a safety and feasibility study. Trials. 2019;20:159.

72. Schvartzman JA, Krupitzki H, Merialdi M, Betrán AP, Requejo J, Nguyen MH, Vayena E, Fiorillo AE, Gadow EC, Vizcaino FM. Odon device for instrumental vaginal deliveries: results of a medical device pilot clinical study. Reprod Health. 2018;15:1–10.

73. Schvartzman J, Krupitzki H, Merialdi M, Carroli G, von Petery F, Leberat E, Fiorillo A, Gadow E. Feasibility and safety study of a new device (Odon device) for assisted vaginal delivery: preliminary data 295| Póster perinatology. J Perinat Med. 2011;39

74. Gonçalves-Henriques M, Brandão P. The BD Odon device™: an update of its current state. J Obstet Gynaecol. 2021;41:1057–61.

75. The World Health Organization Odon Device Research Group. Feasibility and safety study of a new device (Odón device) for assisted vaginal deliveries: study protocol. Reprod Health. 2013;10:33.

76. Zwecker P, Azoulay L, Abenhaim H. Effect of fear of litigation on obstetric care: a Nationwide analysis on obstetric practice. Amer J Perinatol. 2011;28:277–84.

77. Tan P, Tan J, Tan E, Tan L. Comparison of caesarean sections and instrumental deliveries at full cervical dilatation: a retrospective review. Singapore Med J. 2019;60:75–9.

78. Al Wattar BH, Wattar BA, Gallos I, Pirie AM. Rotational vaginal delivery with Kielland's forceps: a systematic review and meta-analysis of effectiveness and safety outcomes. Curr Opin Obstet Gynecol. 2015;27:438–44.

79. Amoah A, Datta S. The Kielland's forceps: relegated to history? Obstet Gynaecol Reprod Med. 2015;25:57.

80. Siassakos D. ROTATE trial: rotation of the fetal head at full cervical dilatation. Randomised controlled trial of manual versus instrumental rotation of the fetal head in malposition at birth.

81. McPherson KC, Beggs AD, Sultan AH, Thakar R. Can the risk of obstetric anal sphincter injuries (OASIs) be predicted using a risk-scoring system? BMC Res Notes. 2014;7:471.

82. Chill HH, Guedalia J, Lipschuetz M, Shimonovitz T, Unger R, Shveiky D, Karavani G. Prediction model for obstetric anal sphincter injury using machine learning. Int Urogynecol J. 2021;32:2393–9.

83. Woo VG, Hung Y-Y, Ritterman-Weintraub ML, Painter CE, Ramm O. A clinical risk model to predict obstetric anal sphincter injuries in laboring patients. Female Pelvic Med Reconstr Surg. 2020;26:520–5.

84. Webb SS, Hemming K, Khalfaoui MY, Henriksen TB, Kindberg S, Stensgaard S, Kettle C, Ismail KMK. An obstetric sphincter injury risk identification system (OSIRIS): is this a clinically useful tool? Int Urogynecol J. 2017;28:367–74.

85. Meister MRL, Cahill AG, Conner SN, Woolfolk CL, Lowder JL. Predicting obstetric anal sphincter injuries in a modern obstetric population. Am J Obstet Gynecol. 2016;215:310.e1–7.

86. Luchristt D, Brown O, Pidaparti M, Kenton K, Lewicky-Gaupp C, Miller ES. Predicting obstetrical anal sphincter injuries in patients who undergo vaginal birth after cesarean delivery. Am J Obstet Gynecol. 2021;225:173.e1–8.

87. Rusavy Z, Paymova L, Kozerovsky M, Veverkova A, Kalis V, Kamel R, Ismail K. Levator ani avulsion: a systematic evidence review (LASER). BJOG. 2022;129:517–28.

88. Albrich S, Laterza R, Skala C, Salvatore S, Koelbl H, Naumann G. Impact of mode of delivery on levator morphology: a prospective observational study with three-dimensional ultrasound early in the postpartum period. BJOG Int J Obstet Gynaecol. 2012;119:51–61.

89. Guedea MA, Zambrano JLA, Fons JB, Viana LJ, Linaje BO, Milio JÁM. Alteration of anal sphincter function in patients with levator avulsion: observational study. Int Urogynecol J. 2015;26:985–90.

90. Thibault-Gagnon S, Yusuf S, Langer S, Wong V, Shek KL, Martin A, Dietz HP. Do women notice the impact of childbirth-related levator trauma on pelvic floor and sexual function? Results of an observational ultrasound study. Int Urogynecol J. 2014;25:1389–98.

91. Blasi I, Fuchs I, D'amico R, Vinci V, La Sala GB, Mazza V, Henrich W. Intrapartum translabial three-dimensional ultrasound visualization of levator trauma. Ultrasound Obstet Gyne. 2011;37:88–92.

92. Lurie S, Glezerman M, Baider C, Sadan O. Decision-to-delivery interval for instrumental vaginal deliveries: vacuum extraction versus forceps. Arch Gynecol Obstet. 2006;274:34–6.

93. Ashton-Miller JA, DeLancey JOL. On the biomechanics of vaginal birth and common sequelae. Annu Rev Biomed Eng. 2009;11:163–76.

94. Shek KL, Dietz HP. Can levator avulsion be predicted antenatally? Am J Obstet Gynecol. 2010;202:586.e1–6.

95. van Delft K, Thakar R, Sultan AH, Schwertner-Tiepelmann N, Kluivers K. Levator ani muscle avulsion during childbirth: a risk prediction model. BJOG. 2014;121:1155–63.

96. Lammers K, Fütterer JJ, Inthout J, Prokop M, Vierhout ME, Kluivers KB. Correlating signs and symptoms with pubovisceral muscle avulsions on magnetic resonance imaging. Am J Obstet Gynecol. 2013;208:148.e1–7.

97. Dietz HP, Kirby A. Modelling the likelihood of levator avulsion in a urogynaecological population: modelling the likelihood of levator avulsion. Aust N Z J Obstet Gynaecol. 2010;50:268–72.

98. Pattillo Garnham A, Guzman Rojas R, Shek KL, Dietz HP. Predicting levator avulsion from ICS POP-Q findings. Int Urogynecol J Pelvic Floor Dysfunct. 2017;28:907–11.

Female Genital Mutilation

13

Juliet Albert

Overview

Test your learning and check your understanding of this book's contents: use the "Springer Nature Flashcards" app to access questions using ▶ https://sn.pub/wqrf89. To use the app, please follow the instructions in Chap. 1.

Learning Objectives

- To describe classifications of female genital mutilation (FGM)
- To identify the presentation, clinical management and short term and long-term consequences of FGM
- To develop an insight into deinfibulation and how the procedure can be used in clinical care and to understand some of the concerns surrounding FGM reconstruction
- To understand the social and cultural norms around FGM, who performs it, why and when it is practiced
- To outline legal perspectives in relation to FGM
- To know how to safeguard patients and clients appropriately in the context of FGM

J. Albert (✉)
Gynaecology and Maternity, FGM Specialist Midwife and FGM Trust Lead, The Sunflower Clinic, Imperial College Healthcare NHS Trust, London, UK
e-mail: juliet.albert@nhs.net

13.1 Definition

The World Health Organisation (WHO) defines female genital mutilation (FGM) as: -.

"The *partial or total removal of, or injury to, the external female genitalia for non-medical reasons*" [1] and estimates that more than 200 million girls and women alive today have undergone FGM [1]. Female genital mutilation is recognised as a form of gender-based violence [2], and in 2015, ending FGM was made one of the United Nations Sustainable Development Goals [3]. Treatment of the health complications of FGM in 27 high prevalence countries is estimated to cost 1.4 billion USD per year [1].

13.2 Historical Perspective

Several authors have suggested that FGM has existed since the fifth century BC [4]. Gordon writes *"Herodotus (420 BC) stated that Egyptians, Phoenicians, Hittites and Ethiopians practised female genital excision. A Greek papyrus from 163 BC exists in the British Museum, and refers to circumcised girls in Egypt… However, no evidence exists of FGM in Egyptian mummies."* [5] Interestingly, the phrase "pharaonic circumcision" is commonly used by East African women to describe Type 3 FGM, suggesting an origin in ancient Egypt.

Although FGM was believed to have originated in Africa, it is now known to exist worldwide. A UNICEF report in 2020 reveals that FGM has been found in Eastern Europe, Latin America, South-Eastern Asia and the Middle East and among diaspora communities in Western Europe, North America and Australia. FGM cases have been discovered in Yemen, Syria, Northern Iraq, amongst Kurdish populations in Russia, in Dawoodi Bohra Muslim communities in Pakistan and India, in Colombia and Peru and in parts of Indonesia, Malaysia and Papa New Guinea [6]. There is clearly no one, homogenous, FGM practising community; instead, it exists in the practices of a variety of diverse people, customs, and traditions. This complexity has contributed to the endurance of the practice.

13.3   Why Is FGM practiced?

Various institutionalised social and cultural factors are cited as being the reason why FGM is performed. Table 13.1 lists some of the myths that are used to justify FGM.

FGM is often thought to be a Muslim practice and the phrase "sunnah" is sometimes used to describe Type 1 and Type 2 FGM implying a religious obligation. However, no religious texts prescribe the practice (1). Furthermore, FGM has been found amongst Ethiopian Falasha Jews, as well as in many Christian communities in Egypt, Eritrea, Nigeria, and elsewhere, and in other religious groups (2).

Women report that carrying out FGM was required to avoid them being excluded from their community. To perpetuate the practice, village elders would pass down traditional beliefs; for example, claiming that the clitoris will continue growing if it is not cut and that this could render the female daughter infertile or lead to the death of a child during childbirth [7]. There remains much secrecy surrounding the practice and sometimes children are told that they will die if they tell anyone that they have had FGM [7].

13.4   Incidence

A UNICEF report highlighted in 2021 that: -

The practice of FGM has been declining over the last three decades. In the 30 countries with nationally representative prevalence data, around 1 in 3 girls aged 15 to 19 today have undergone the practice versus 1 in 2 in the late-1980s. However, not all countries have made progress and the pace of decline has been uneven. [8]

FGM is becoming less common in some countries where it was historically universal such as Egypt, Eritrea, Sierra Leone and Kenya; however, in other countries such as Somalia, Guinea and Mali, little has changed over the last 30 years [6]. Thankfully, UNICEF reports that *"in most countries in Africa and the Middle East, the majority of girls and women think FGM should end"* [8].

Nevertheless, despite United Nations goals to achieve gender equality empower all women and girls and eradicate FGM by 2030 [3], overall, it is estimated that the prevalence of FGM may rise over the next 15 years as the world population grows [9].

FGM is performed on female babies as well as grown women, but is most common in girls aged 6–15 years. Population Council research carried out from 2015 to 2019 in Somaliland, Kenya, Ethiopia and Senegal found that FGM is being performed on younger girls in less public cere-

Table 13.1 Common myths used to justify FGM

Custom & tradition	Family honour
Religion	Preparation and eligibility for marriage and right to inherit
Cut genitals perceived as 'clean' and 'beautiful'	Enhancing fertility
Virginity & chastity	A sense of belonging to the group or conversely a fear of social exclusion
Increasing sexual pleasure for men	Peer pressure
Social pressure/norms	Preservation of virginity prior to marriage and ensure fidelity after marriage
Clitoris seen as masculine and so removal increases perceived femininity	Rite of passage from childhood to womanhood
Male coercion and control	Reducing female promiscuity

monies; it was also determined that while there may be less Type 3 FGM occurring, (see below) it is increasingly carried out by healthcare professionals [10]. According to the World Health Organization (WHO), this growing medicalisation of FGM is of great universal concern [11].

13.5 Classification of FGM Types

There are four types of FGM classified by the WHO (Table 13.2). In practice, women rarely know what type of FGM they have undergone. A genital examination is always preferable when assessing presenting symptoms using a sensitive, culturally competent, trauma-informed approach. The WHO commissioned visual reference guides [12, 13] are a useful

Table 13.2 WHO classification of FGM types

FGM type	Description
Type 1	Partial or total removal of the clitoral glans and/or prepuce. Sometimes known as clitoridectomy. **Type Ia**: Removal of the clitoral hood or prepuce only. **Type Ib**: Removal of the clitoral glans with the prepuce.
Type 2	Partial or total removal of the clitoral glans and labia minora, with or without excision of the labia majora. Sometimes known as excision. **Type IIa**: Removal of the labia minora only. **Type IIb**: Partial or total removal of the clitoral glans and labia minora. **Type IIc**: Partial or total removal of the clitoral glans, labia minora and labia majora.
Type 3	Narrowing of the vaginal orifice with creation of a covering seal by cutting and appositioning the labia minora and/or the labia majora, with or without excision of the clitoral glans. Sometimes known as infibulation or pharaonic circumcision. **Type IIIa**: Removal and apposition of the labia minora. **Type IIIb**: Removal and apposition of the labia majora.
Type 4	All other harmful procedures to the female genitalia for non-medical purposes, including Gishiri cuts, pricking, piercing, incising, scraping and cauterisation and labial elongation.

Adapted from WHO [1]

resource for healthcare professionals who have not come across FGM before.

13.6 Type 3 FGM

FGM Type 3 is mostly found in the Horn of East Africa and performed on girls between 5 and 10 years old. It is estimated that eight million women worldwide have suffered Type 3 FGM [1]. The practice is usually carried out by traditional circumcisers, however, in urban areas midwives and doctors may be involved. Typically, the child is physically restrained in her own home by senior, female members of the family. Without anaesthesia, the clitoral glans, prepuce and variable amounts of labia majora or minora are removed (usually cut with a non-sterilised razor blade or knife). The raw edges are then sewn across the midline to produce a fibrous barrier of scar tissue, leaving only a small orifice for the passage of urine and menses. Thorns are sometimes used instead of sutures, especially in remote areas. Traditionally, the girls' legs are bound for several days to restrict movement and promote healing [5]. Women have spoken of their circumciser boasting of the introitus size being equivalent to a grain of rice [7] (Fig. 13.1).

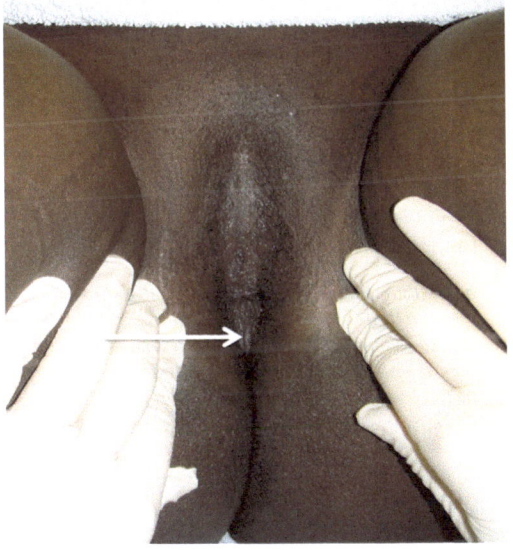

Fig. 13.1 Woman with Type 3 FGM. Arrow points to pinhole size introitus – difficult to visualize

Infections, psychosexual complications, coital problems and apareunia are common, and infertility is an issue if normal penetrative sexual intercourse is not possible (Table 13.2). An intact Type 3 'circumcision' is regarded as a sign of virginity and uncircumcised women may be regarded as unmarriageable. Once married, the FGM will need to be reversed, to permit intercourse. In parts of Somalia, after marriage, it is common for the bridegroom's mother to inspect and confirm "virginity" and arrange for the traditional circumciser to attend on the wedding night and open the scar. In other regions of Somalia, the husband is expected to open the introitus by forceful intercourse; women have reported subsequent years of excruciating pain [5].

When presenting, women with Type 3 may say that they have not experienced any health problems from their FGM, as they have never known anything different. They may believe that difficulty passing urine or painful intercourse is 'normal'. However, patients often describe the urine 'dribbling out slowly', sometimes taking 10–20 minutes to empty the bladder, and 'having to go backwards and forwards to the toilet' to urinate, passing blood clots when menstruating, and needing repeated trips to the general practicioner (GP) for antibiotics to treat genitourinary infections [7].

13.7   FGM Type 4

Gordon described some examples of FGM Type 4 which includes other unclassified mutilations. For example, these injuries have been described as follows:

Scraping and burning the genital area (or) the introduction of corrosive substances into the vagina. Some of these procedures have serious long-term complications. Gynaetresia is recorded in Ibadan, Nigeria, mainly in relation to the use of caustic vaginal pessaries prescribed by tradi-

tional healers. The caustic pessaries are prescribed for the treatment of amenorrhoea, infertility, fibroids and vaginal discharge. They are also used in an attempt to procure abortion. Of the 148 cases documented at University College Hospital, Ibadan, between 1967 and 1996, 106 required extensive vaginoplasty [14]. Gishiri cuts are another potentially dangerous form of FGM Type 4. These are incisions into (usually) the anterior vagina carried out by traditional healers to treat a variety of conditions including obstructed labour, infertility, dyspareunia, amenorrhoea, goitre and backache. In one study from Nigeria, 13% of vesico-vaginal fistulae were caused by Gishiri cuts. [5, 15]

13.8   Classification Challenges

The WHO definitions formerly described partial or total removal of the clitoris with Type 1, 2, and 3 FGM. In 2020 the definitions were updated to align with improved knowledge of clitoral anatomy, highlighting that during FGM the whole clitoris is never removed as the clitoral body and crux remain deep below the level of the skin layer. It is important to sharee with women who have been victimised by this practice that some clitoral tissue always remains intact despite FGM. In fact, sometimes women with Type 3 FGM find that beneath the scar there may be a fully intact clitoral glans.

13.9   Difficulties Associated with Classification of FGM

- Specific forms of FGM vary from one geographical area to another.
- Girls and women rarely know which type they have been subjected to and may not associate their health problems with the practice.
- There may be significant variation in the extent of cutting because of the poor conditions in which FGM is performed. For exam-

ple, the circumciser may use rudimentary instruments and have no medical training.

- Type 4 FGM, which may comprise only a prick or a small scratch, may heal completely leaving no scar or only a small scar; this mutilation may be impossible to detect years later.
- Because a genital examination cannot exclude type 4 FGM/C, a true diagnosis should be based on the woman's history along with genital assessment.
- It is impossible to deduce a timeline for an FGM procedure unless it is visualized within 2–4 weeks of being carried out.

13.10 Differential Diagnosis

- Labial adhesions due to an inflammatory process or lichen sclerosis
- Small irregularities in the skin of the vulva or clitoris due to congenital variation (Table 13.3)

Table 13.3 Summary of short and long term complications of FGM

Short term complications	Long term complications
Severe pain and injury to genitals	Scarring/keloid formation, Epidermoid cysts/abscesses, Neuroma formation, Vesicovaginal fistula formation
Haemorrhage and haemorrhagic shock	Haematocolpos and dysmenorrhoea
Systemic Infection e.g. tetanus, sepsis	Dysuria and recurrent urinary tract infections
Urinary retention	Pelvic inflammatory disease
Trauma to adjacent tissue	Infertility
Transmission of blood borne viruses (Hepatitis B, HIV)	Morbidity during pregnancy and childbirth
Bone fractures secondary physical restraining during the procedure	Psychological and psychosexual problems including post-traumatic stress disorder, dyspareunia, apareunia, decreased satisfaction
Death	Mortality during pregnancy and childbirth

13.11 Clinical Presentation, Management and Complications

The management, clinical presentation and incidence of serious complications varies with the type (extent) of the mutilation. The severity of the mutilation also varies according to the available medical facilities. The European experience for example may differ markedly from the African experience. Within Africa, the results for rural and urban populations may also differ and there may be significant unreported mortality and morbidity [5]. Table 13.4 describes some of the most common consequences of FGM. In the UK women with FGM often present for the first time to a healthcare professional during pregnancy.

Table 13.4 Surgical procedures associated with FGM

Deinfibulation	This involves opening the sealed introitus of a woman who has been infibulated/Type 3. It is carried out to expose the vaginal opening and urinary meatus, to allow sexual intercourse to facilitate childbirth. This may take place either before marriage, pre-conception, during pregnancy, intrapartum, or during caesarean section.
Simple deinfibulation	This version of the procedure as defined above is carried out (often by a Midwife or Nurse) using only local anaesthesia. It can be done on the same day in an outpatient or community setting. There is no attempt to expose the clitoral glans and prepuce.
Complex deinfibulation	Where Type 3 FGM is accompanied by cyst formation, a fused anterior scar, or keloid scar, complex deinfibulation is required. This surgery should be done by a suitably trained doctor and usually involves epidural, spinal or general anaesthesia in theatre as day case surgery. There may be an attempt to expose clitoral tissue [16].
Reinfibulation	This is the re-closing of a woman who has had previous Type 3 FGM. This often is performed after childbirth. This is illegal in many countries of the global North.
Reconstruction Surgery	This involves any procedures attempting to restore original genital appearance. This is available in some countries in Europe, Africa and in parts of USA. It is currently not recommended by Royal College of Obstetricians and Gynaecologists (RCOG) or WHO [3, 4] as there is not enough evidence to recommend it.

13.12 FGM and Psychological Consequences

Women with FGM are at increased risk of developing psychological disorders such as post-traumatic stress disorder (Table 13.4), anxiety, depression and low self-esteem [1]. Psychological trauma may be severe with all FGM Types. Women report problems such as touch and needle phobia, flashbacks, nightmares, distorted body image, and "not feeling whole" [7]. Psychosexual issues include suffering pain during sexual intercourse, lower desire and reduced sexual satisfaction when compared to uncut women [17]. Even women with FGM Type 1 and 2 may suffer long-term psychological and psychosexual complications [5].

13.13 Women with FGM Presenting to a Gynaecological Setting

Clitoral pain, vulvodynia and epidermoid inclusion cysts (requiring excision and draining under general anaesethetic) are common presentations of women with FGM seeking gynaecologic care. Some of the phrases used by women to describe their symptoms upon presentation include: *'severe pain and bleeding during sex'; 'rashes and swelling of genitals'; 'very dry and itchy and burning sensation after intercourse'; 'sore, stuck, itchy labia'; 'can't relax, tense, no lubrication, can't feel anything'; 'unable to have sexual penetration'; 'incontinence.'; 'never experienced pleasure'; 'don't feel whole'* [7]. Treatments such as physiotherapy, hormonal creams, dilators, or nerve blocks may be helpful. However, it is important to screen these women not only for gynaecologic issues, but also for HIV, hepatitis B and C, as the use of non-sterile equipment during the original procedure places women with FGM at higher risk for these infections.

At the Sunflower Clinic, Imperial College Healthcare NHS Trust in London, UK, approximately 100 non-pregnant women with FGM are seen annually. Data from over a decade in the clinic shows the age range of women presenting from 18 years to over 60 years. The main reasons for women attending this specialist service were to access either one or a combination of the following services: (1) deinfibulation (often for women who have recently, or are about to, get married); (2) clinical documentation to confirm FGM in support of an asylum application; (3) complex perineal trauma requiring uro-gynaecology referral; (4) counselling; (5) difficulty in taking cervical smears; and/or (6) diagnosis of FGM type to find out exactly what has been cut [18].

Clinicians should be aware that FGM survivors are predominantly women from Black, Asian and minority ethnic groups. They are more likely to have suffered other intersectional violence (such as forced early marriage, domestic violence, witchcraft/juju, trafficking or enslavement), are often refugees/asylum seekers, have greater health inequalities and are less likely to be offered, or have access to healthcare.

13.14 Deinfibulation

Deinfibulation is sometimes termed a 'reversal' of FGM, however, it does not replace genital tissue or restore genital anatomy and function. The need for deinfibulation can be determined on inspection of the external genitals by an experienced health professional. If the introitus is sufficiently open to permit vaginal examination and if the urethral meatus is visible, then deinfibulation is unlikely to be necessary. Gordon [19] reported from his experiences leading an FGM service that in over 70% of cases, the clitoris was revealed present and undamaged during deinfibulation.

Deinfibulation is recommended, however, if the introitus is not sufficiently open to permit normal urinary and menstrual flow, comfortable vaginal penetrative intercourse, to permit cervical smears, sexual health screens and gynaeco-

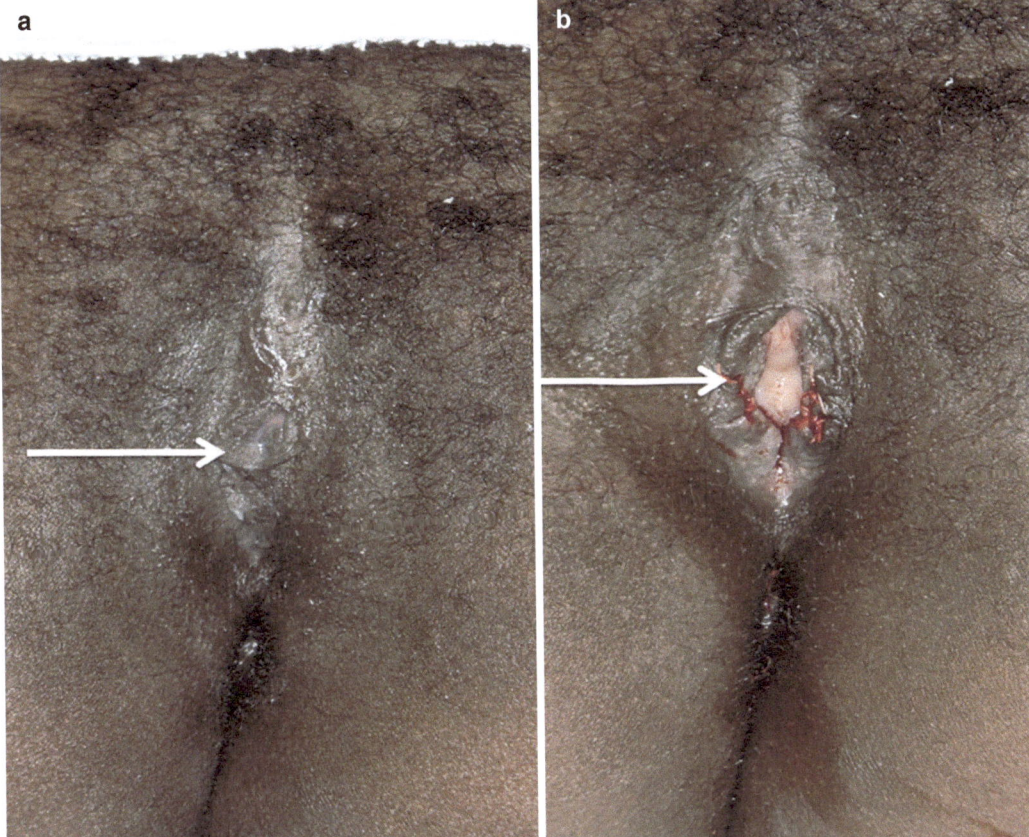

Fig. 13.2 (**a**) Woman with Type 3 FGM. Small central hole visible, for passing urine and menstrual blood, of approximately 0.5 cm diameter. Pre deinfibulation. (**b**) Post deinfibulation. Posterior incision made to open introitus. Clitoral glans and prepuce mostly intact

logical surgery such as surgical management of miscarriage or termination of pregnancy, hysteroscopy or endometrial biopsy [20]. Table 13.4 describes surgical procedures associated with FGM.

As previously explained, extent of mutilation varies considerably. Figure 13.2a and b is an example of Type 3 FGM, where a posterior incision was required to 'open' the introitus. Figure 13.3a and b depict thick, fused scar tissue that remains anterior to the urinary meatus post deinfibulation; no labia minora or majora or clitoral glans and prepuce remain. Figure 13.4a and b depict a buttonhole appearance, where scar dehiscence may have been caused by repeated, attempted penetration or the skin may have been closed with thorns, thus leaving a perforated scar.

Figure 13.5 shows a piece of detritus lodged within the scar.

Deinfibulation can usually be performed under local anaesthetic as a minor procedure in an outpatient setting. Emla cream can be used to numb the scar prior to administering Xylocaine 1% (Lidocaine 1% with adrenaline). Scissors or a blade are used to then incise the scar. Bleeding is usually minimal. Once the urethral meatus has been exposed, the incision may be extended with care into the clitoral region; this would occur if it appears that the remaining anterior scar is still tight and will prevent comfortable sexual intercourse. The raw edges should be closed with fine (3/0–4/0) absorbable sutures using continuous sutures where possible. The edges should not be left unsutured, as there is a tendency for the scar

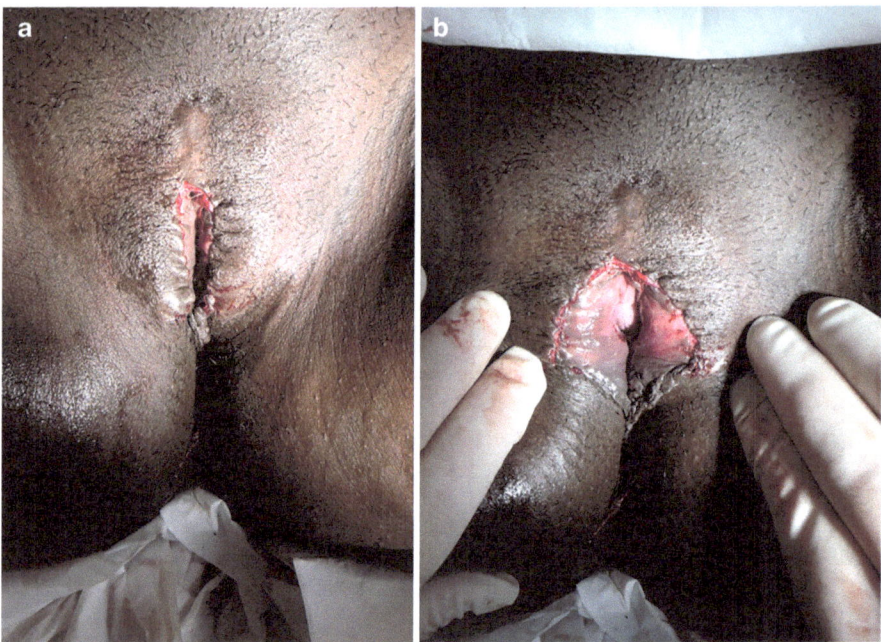

Fig. 13.3 (**a** and **b**) Woman with Type 3 FGM post dein-fibulation procedure. Continuous sutures visible along edges where anterior scar has been incised. Densely fused scar tissue anteriorly (where clitoral glans and prepuce were removed during original FGM procedure). Thus, the introitus could not be "opened" any further. Introitus visu-alized to reveal 2 cm thick incised scar

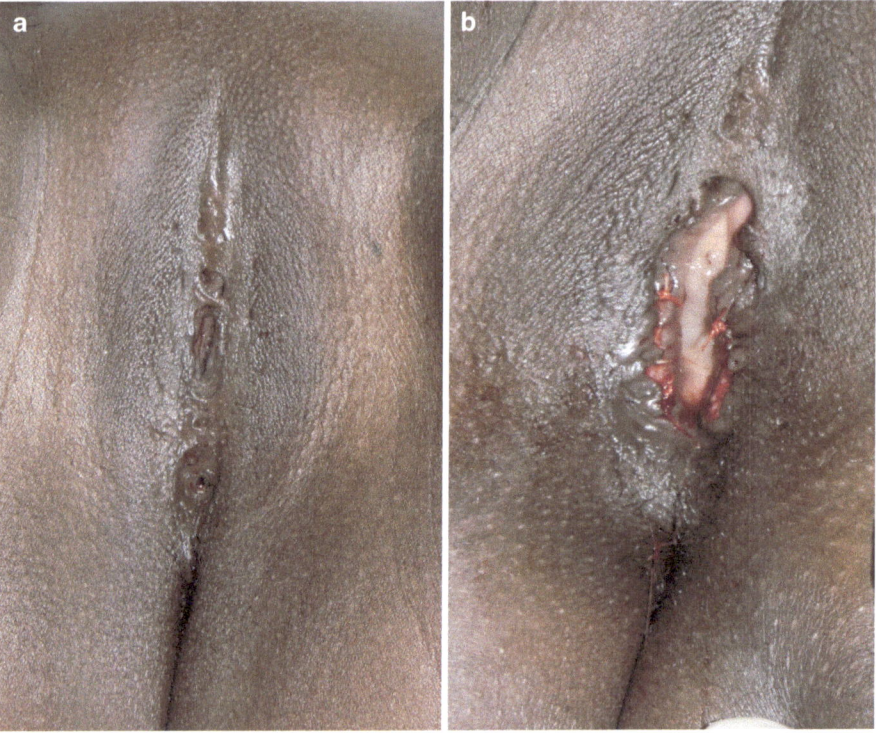

Fig. 13.4 (**a**) Woman with Type 3 FGM 'buttonhole' appearance. This is secondary to possible repeated attempted sexual penetration causing scar dehiscence or secondary to the skin having been closed with thorns, thus leaving a perforated scar. (**b**) Post deinfibulation

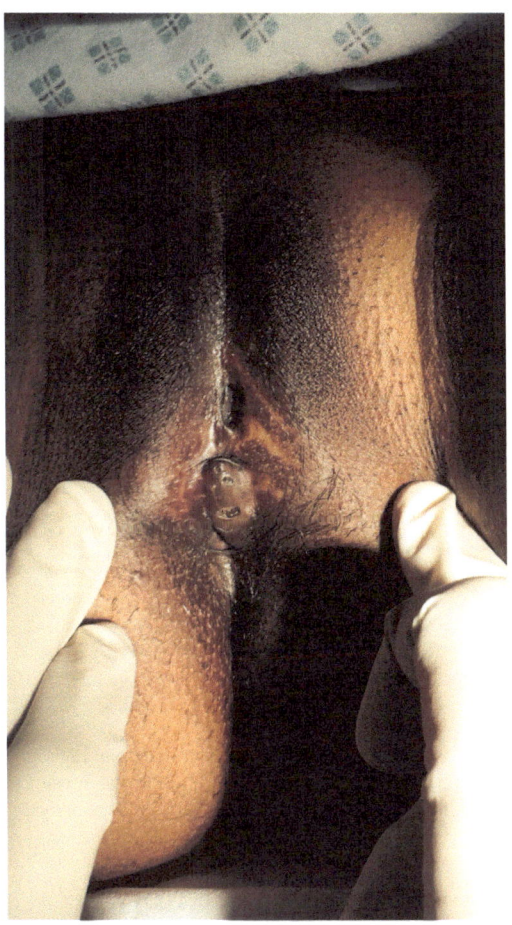

Fig. 13.5 Somali woman presented with Type 3 FGM and piece of detritus lodged within scar, measuring approximately 2 cm × 1 cm. The patient presented with urine dribbling out of several tiny holes, severe dysuria and dysmenorrhea. She was referred for deinfibulation under general anaesthetic

to re-fuse. Postoperative analgesia, such as a long-acting local anaesthetic, is injected under the sutured edges (e.g. bupivacaine 0.5%) or via the use of a voltarol suppository.

Spinal or general anaesthetic should be offered if the FGM presentation is more complex, for example, if the patient is (1) presenting with a para-clitoral cyst (see Fig. 13.6a and b); (2) touch or needle phobic; (3) if there is a risk of the deinfibulation procedure triggering psychological flashbacks or distress; or (4) this is simply the woman's preference. Fig. 13.7a and b depict an Eritrean woman who presented with both inner labia minora and outer labia majora stitched; and Fig. 13.8a–f depicts a Sudanese woman who presented with extensive Type 3 scar with both anterior, central and posterior holes.

It is critical that women be counselled preoperatively about the physical and physiologic changes to expect post deinfibulation. These include change to vulval appearance, urinary flow, the appearance of menstrual flow rather than just blood clots, increased vaginal discharge, and what to expect when having sexual intercourse for the first time.

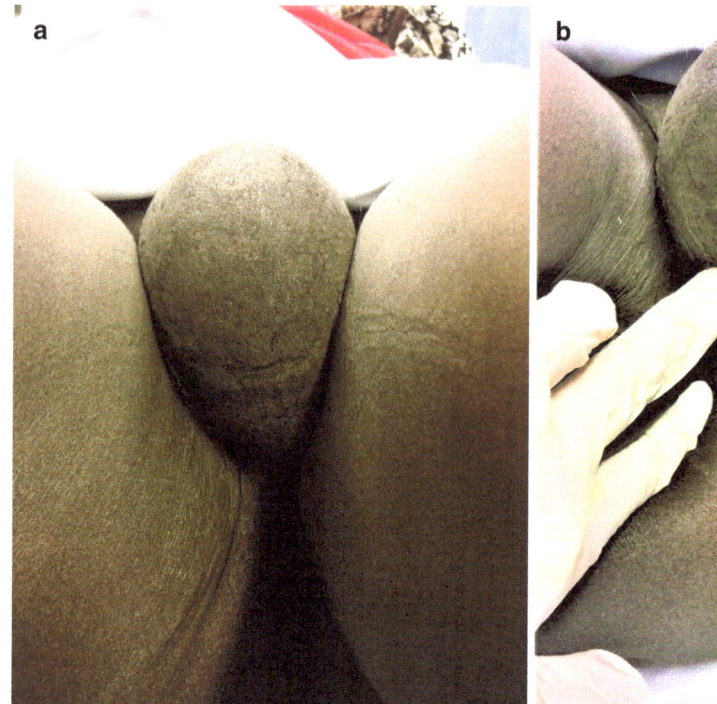
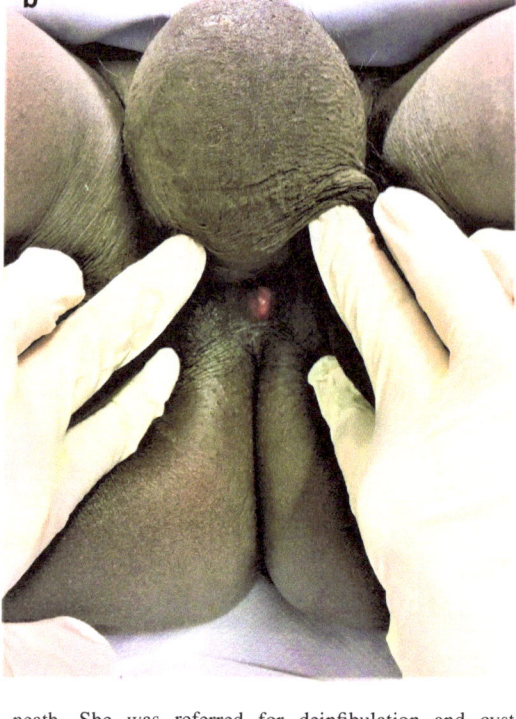

Fig. 13.6 (**a**) Somali woman presented with Type 3 FGM and large epidermoid inclusion cyst approximately 10 cm × 4 cm × 3 cm. Her introitus was almost obscured under-neath. She was referred for deinfibulation and cyst removal under general anaesthetic. (**b**) Introitus appears to be approximately 0.5 cm diameter beneath edge of cyst

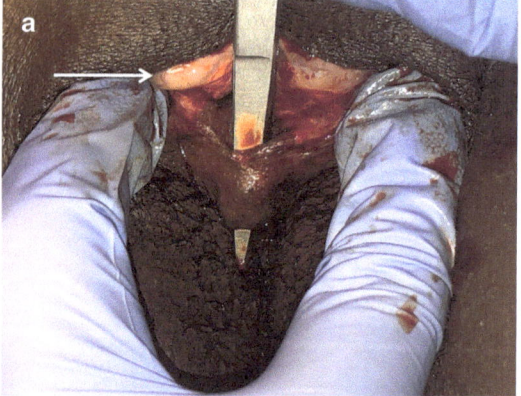
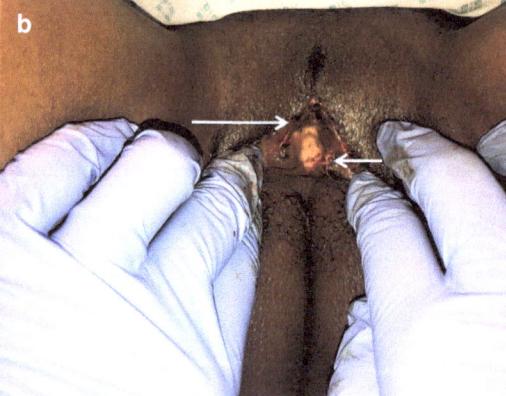

Fig. 13.7 (**a**) Eritrean woman presented with two layers of scar tissue. The arrow shows where labia majora has been incised (during deinfibulation procedure) to reveal another bridge of scar tissue underneath where labia minora edges have also been closed. This required incis-ing to facilitate sexual intercourse, taking cervical smears, passing of menstrual blood and urine. (**b**) The top arrow shows where continuous sutures of vicryl rapide 3/0 were used to oversew the edges of scar tissue from the labia major. The bottom arrow points to the interrupted sutures used to close edges of scar tissue from the labia minora. The introitus was opened to reveal the vaginal opening and urinary meatus

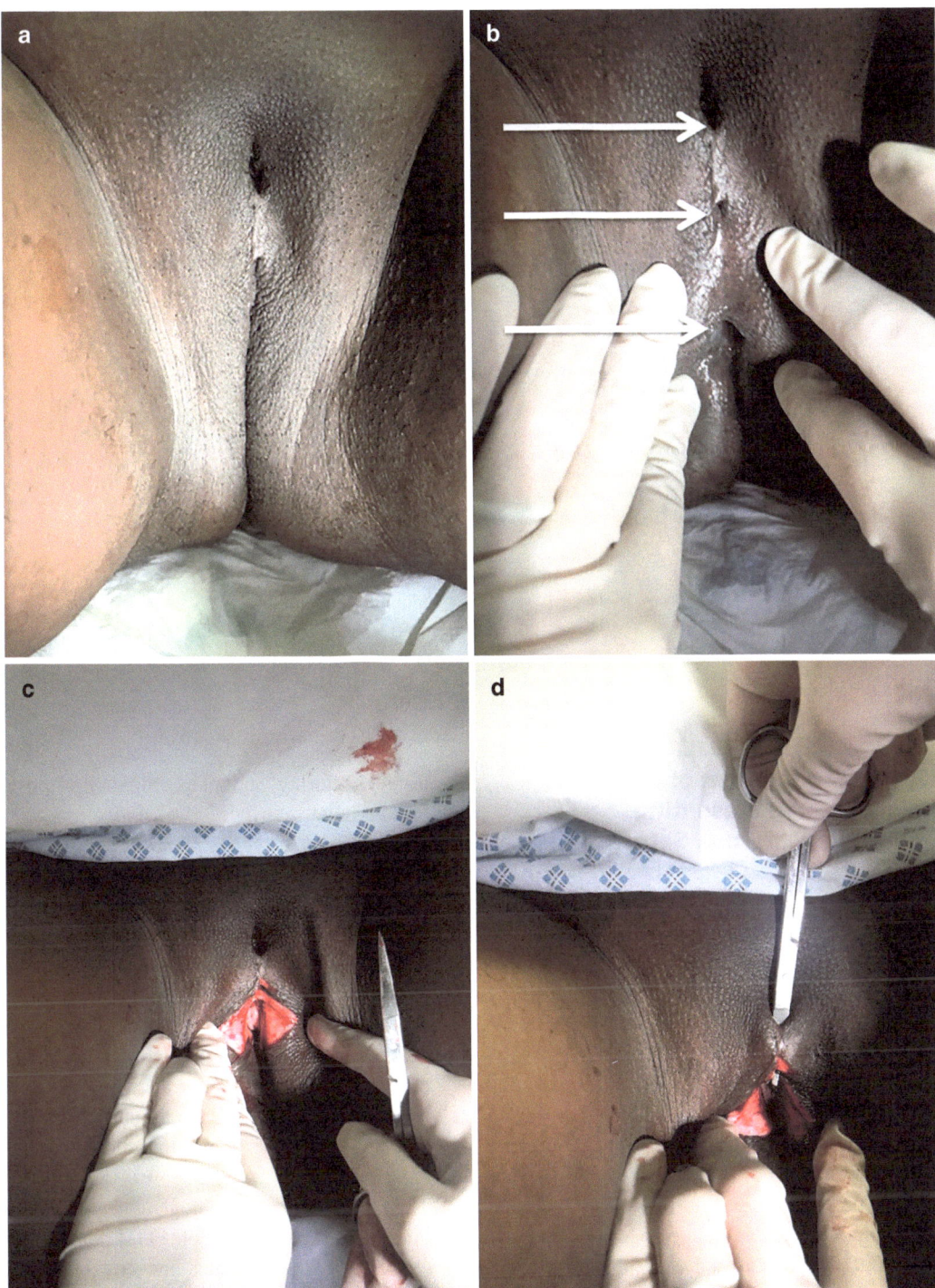

Fig. 13.8 (a) A Sudanese woman presented with Type 3 FGM with extensive scar tissue. (b) The skin was stretched to reveal anterior, central and posterior holes. (c) An incision was made to open scar tissue between the central and posterior holes. (d) The anterior scar was lifted prior to opening. (e) The introitus was opened. The arrow pointing to clitoral glans revealed intact anatomy beneath scar tissue. (f) This is the patient 2 weeks post deinfibulation

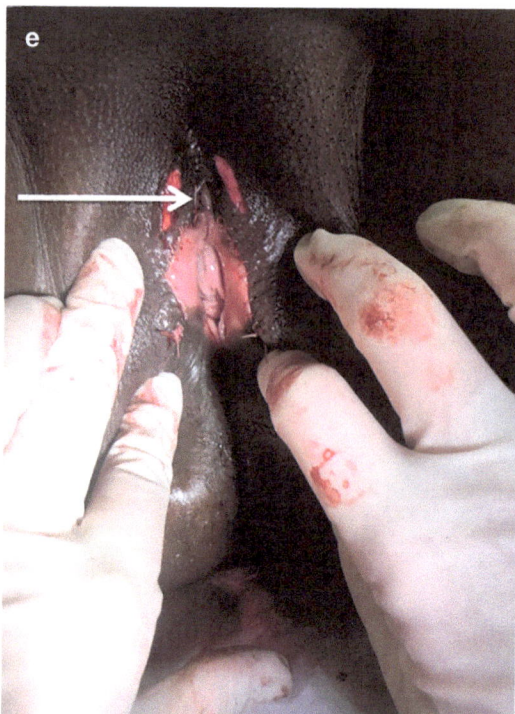 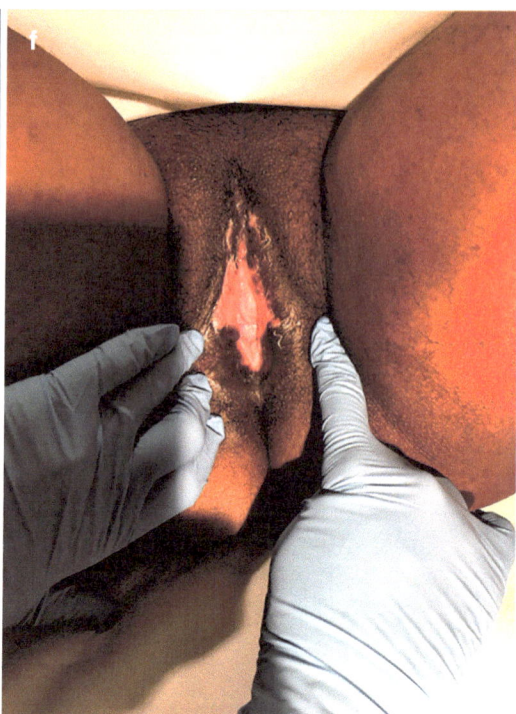

Fig. 13.8 (continued)

13.15 Management of Pregnant Women Presenting in a Maternity Setting

All pregnant women should be asked at their initial visit whether they have been subjected to FGM. As women have often never spoken of their FGM, translation/interpretation support by a female attendant is imperative. Ideally FGM survivors should be referred to an FGM expert (Midwife or Doctor), preferably in a specialist clinic setting where she can also access FGM health advocates, counsellors, and interpreters. Women should be informed that they are at higher risk of postpartum haemorrhage and perineal trauma than women without FGM due to scarring and reduced skin elasticity of the introitus. In addition, women with Type 3 FGM can suffer additional complications during vaginal delivery than women with other FGM Types [21]. Clinicians should be aware that flashbacks may be triggered during vaginal examination or postpartum perineal suturing.

A holistic, best-practice prenatal consultation should include the following:

1. Gentle and sensitive questioning using a trauma-informed culturally competent approach to ascertain whether the woman has had FGM. The terms 'cut' or 'circumcision' are usually understood internationally. The presence of a suitably qualified specialist or community/health advocate who is herself from an FGM practising community is preferable to reassure the woman that she is in a safe environment.

2. The physical and psychological health consequences of each type of FGM should be explained in detail using line drawings. For example, the infographic from Barnardo's National FGM Centre could be used [6].

3. There should be a discussion around the law, explaining that FGM is a human rights

violation and a form of child sexual abuse which removes a woman's right to bodily integrity and sexual pleasure. Barnardo's National FGM Centre world map can be used to explain the prevalence and legal status of FGM in the woman's country of origin [7].

4. A detailed medical history should be taken, documenting any symptoms related to FGM. A genital assessment to diagnose the FGM type should be offered. A mirror can be used if the woman wants to know exactly what has been cut. Questions should include the following:

(a) Who performed the FGM and did they use pain relief?
(b) Were there any complications afterwards?
(c) Has FGM caused you any health problems, such as difficulty passing urine?
(d) Have you ever suffered nightmares or flashbacks?

5. Data should be recorded. In the UK, prevalence data is recorded in accordance with the NHS Digital FGM Enhanced Dataset [8]. These include age at FGM, country where FGM was performed, date of entry to UK (if applicable) and past history of deinfibulation and/or reinfibulation.

6. A safeguarding assessment should be performed. The patient should be asked the following questions:

(a) How old were you when you were cut?
(b) Where was it carried out?
(c) Were other girls cut at the same time, such as siblings or cousins?
(d) Who arranged the cut or circumcision and do you know why?
(e) Does your family still practice FGM?
(f) How does your partner feel about FGM?
(g) Does your partner's family believe in practising FGM?
(h) Do you have female children or younger female siblings who have been had FGM?

13.16 Management of Pregnant Women with Type 3 FGM

Antenatal discussion of the benefits of deinfibulation prior to labour should be undertaken. Patients should be informed that antenatally, they are at higher risk of urinary tract and vaginal infections. Similarly, intrapartum risks are higher and include difficulty in intrapartum monitoring (including application of fetal scalp electrodes and fetal blood sampling), difficulty in catheterisation during labour, increased risk of prolonged labour and higher incidence of stillbirth, neonatal death, wound infection and retention of lochia [11, 20]. The patient and her partner should be counselled about the risks of a precipitate delivery or unattended birth including fetal asphyxia or anoxia, and/or extensive maternal perineal damage including fistulae.

Simple deinfibulation may be performed either antenatally, in the first stage of labour or at the time of delivery under local anaesthetic. It can also be performed perioperatively after caesarean birth. In Africa, women would usually be deinfibulated in the second stage of labour by a traditional birth attendant or a midwife. Deinfibulation is usually recommended in the second trimester, typically at around 20 weeks of gestation [20]. The advantage of antenatal deinfibulation is that an experienced clinician is present, and the area will be well healed before the onset of labour. If vaginal examination, intrapartum procedures and urinary catheterisation are not possible because of the introitus size, then deinfibulation in the first stage of labour is recommended. At delivery the incision should be made with scissors (rather than a scalpel) just before crowning of the fetal head. Lidocaine should be used. Once the procedure has been performed, the need for episiotomy should be assessed. Medio-lateral episiotomy should only be carried out after an anterior incision is made, as it may not be required. Bilateral episiotomy is never indicated in these cases.

It is important for clinicians to know that some women will refuse antenatal deinfibulation, wishing to follow the traditional practice or because they fear pain, while others will be lost to follow-up. Where possible a detailed plan for intrapartum care should be documented and discussed in detail with the woman and her partner.

13.17 Safeguarding and Law

FGM is condemned by several international treaties and conventions, as well as by national legislation in many countries. Article 25 of the Universal Declaration of Human Rights states that "everyone has the right to a standard of living adequate for health and well-being," and this statement has been used to argue that FGM violates the right to health and bodily integrity. With FGM considered as a form of violence against women, the UN Convention on the Elimination of All Forms of Discrimination against Women can be invoked. Similarly, defining it as a form of torture brings it under the rubric of the Convention against Torture and Other Cruel, Inhuman, or Degrading Treatment or Punishment. Moreover, since FGM is regarded as a traditional practice prejudicial to the health of children and is, in most cases, performed on minors, it violates the Convention on the Rights of the Child. [8]

In the UK, most women present with historic cases of FGM. Few have been cut in the UK, and those that were, underwent the mutilation over 15 years ago. In the Sunflower clinic several cases of women that were either born in the UK or who came to the UK when very young but were taken abroad for FGM to be performed have been seen. The UK's "Failure to Protect Clause of the Serious Crime Act 2015" is an attempt to close this loophole by making it a criminal offence if parents fail to prevent their daughters from undergoing FGM by extended family/community members. In 2018, FGM remained legal in the six African countries of Sudan, Somalia, Chad, Mali, Sierra Leone and Liberia. In July 2020, Sudan passed legislation banning the practice across the whole country, however, recent unrest has raised concerns that the law may yet go unenforced.

A report by 28 Too Many in 2021 estimates that more than 600,000 women and girls in Europe have experienced FGM (of which 45% are living in the UK and France) and a further 130,000 are at risk of FGM [22]. However, prevalence data is sparse, particularly in countries of Eastern Europe.

As of 2022, only 25 out of 32 European countries have ratified the Istanbul Convention [9] which states the intention to eliminate violence against women [10]. However, all 32 countries have criminalised FGM either explicitly (through a specific FGM law as in Ireland, Sweden and UK) or implicitly, through national legal frameworks criminalizing FGM as a form of sexual assault [22].

13.18 Safeguarding

Some countries have laws to ensure that relevant professionals and institutions are obliged to report FGM cases. In England and Wales, the Mandatory Reporting duty was introduced in October 2015. Currently, all regulated health and social care professionals and teachers are mandated by law to report 'known' cases of FGM in girls under 18 years of age to the police. 'Known' cases are those where a girl herself discloses that she has undergone FGM or where a professional observes evidence on a girl's genitals that she may have been cut [23].

The Department of Health's FGM risk assessment guidance can be used to inform safeguarding discussions. For example, children who have had FGM may become withdrawn and alteration in micturition habits may be noticed. Children may spend longer amounts of time in the toilet or suddenly become reluctant to join in with physical education. Girls talking of attending a coming-of-age ceremony or special party (usually during school holidays) or being absent from school for prolonged periods may require careful enquiry.

FGM Type 1 or clitoridectomy is sometimes regarded as a less traumatic alternative to other forms of mutilation. Women are reported to sometimes say their FGM was "just a bleed" or "just a little cut". It is important that healthcare professionals are clear that no type of FGM is permissible.

13.19 Conclusion

Female genital mutilation is a danger to women's and girls' health and an abuse of young women and children. Every effort is being made by the WHO, governments and other organisations to eliminate FGM in all its forms, with variable success. The complications are significant, and it is important that health professionals are aware of the best therapeutic options available.

Take Home Messages

- FGM is a form of child sexual abuse and a human rights violation.
- FGM is an illegal form of gender-based violence.
- Women and girls who have suffered FGM should always be treated sensitively using a trauma-informed and culturally safe approach.
- Consultation with a woman who is a victim of FGM is an opportunity to explain the health consequences of FGM and to help prevent the continuation of the practice.
- Globally, at least 200 million women and girls (or 5% of the global female population) are living with the consequences of FGM.
- There are no health benefits of FGM and all women and girls who have experienced FGM are likely to report some health problems related to it, including physical and psychological complications.
- FGM is usually performed by traditional cutters but rates of medicalised cutting are increasing.
- FGM is performed for a range of different reasons including cultural, religious and psychosexual.
- FGM is illegal in at least 59 countries, including the UK

Appendix: MCQ

Mark each item TRUE or FALSE

Questions

1. The WHO definition of Type 3 FGM is:-
   (A) Partial or total removal of the clitoral glans and/or the prepuce, sometimes called clitoridectomy
   (B) Narrowing of the vaginal orifice with creation of a covering seal by cutting and appositioning the labia minora and/ or labia majora, with or without excision of the clitoral glans
   (C) Partial or total removal of the clitoral glans and labia minora, with or without excision of the labia majora, sometimes called excision
   (D) All other harmful procedures to the female genitalia for non-medical purposes, for example: pricking, piercing, incising, scraping and cauterization

2. The number of women and girls worldwide estimated to have been affected by FGM is:-
   (A) 200 million
   (B) 50 million
   (C) 120 million
   (D) 500million
   (E) 10million

3. Pharaonic circumcision is usually associated with: -
   (A) Difficulty passing menstrual blood
   (B) Difficulty passing stools
   (C) Difficulty passing urine
   (D) Difficulty having sexual intercourse
   (E) Difficulty taking a cervical smear

4. What is reinfibulation?
   (A) Opening the sealed introitus of a woman who has been infibulated to expose the vaginal opening and urinary meatus.
   (B) Cyst removal for woman with Type 3 FGM
   (C) Where FGM is performed by a medically trained health professional
   (D) Procedure to narrow the vaginal opening in a woman after she has been deinfibulated
   (E) Surgical procedure where skin is grafted to restore original genital appearance.

5. Which of the following statements is false regarding the long term consequences of FGM?
   (A) Women may suffer touch and needle phobia.
   (B) Women with FGM are more likely to suffer endometriosis

(C) Women with FGM may suffer with nightmares and flashbacks.

(D) Pelvic inflammatory disease and infertility are possible long term complications of FGM.

(E) FGM can cause vaginal/ urinary/reproductive tract infections.

Answers

1. The WHO definition of Type 3 FGM is:-
   (A) FALSE
   (B) TRUE
   (C) FALSE
   (D) FALSE

2. The number of women and girls worldwide estimated to have been affected by FGM is:-
   (A) TRUE
   (B) FALSE
   (C) FALSE
   (D) FALSE
   (E) FALSE

3. Pharaonic circumcision is usually associated with: -
   (A) TRUE
   (B) FALSE
   (C) TRUE
   (D) TRUE
   (E) TRUE

4. What is reinfibulation?
   (A) FALSE
   (B) FALSE
   (C) FALSE
   (D) TRUE
   (E) FALSE

5. Which of the following statements is false regarding the long term consequences of FGM?
   (A) TRUE
   (B) FALSE

(C) TRUE
(D) TRUE
(E) TRUE

References

1. WHO. Female genital mutilation. Key Facts. [Internet]. WHO webpage. 2021 [cited 2020 Feb 24]. p. 1–5. Available from: https://www.who.int/en/news-room/fact-sheets/detail/female-genital-mutilation
2. WHO. Eliminating female genital mutilation: an interagency statement UNAIDS, UNDP, UNECA, UNESCO, UNFPA, UNHCHR, UNHCR, UNICEF, UNIFEM, WHO. 2008. Available from: http://apps.who.int/iris/bitstream/handle/10665/43839/9789241596442_eng.pdf.;jsessionid=996E4B151551E5B1C8D31AFC670234BE?sequence=1
3. United Nations. Transforming our world: the 2030 agenda for sustainable development. 2015. Available from: https://sustainabledevelopment.un.org/content/documents/21252030 Agenda for Sustainable Development web.pdf.
4. Elchalal U, Ben-Ami B, Gillis R, Brzezinski A. Ritualistic female genital mutilation. Obstet Gynecol Surv. 1997;52(10):643–51.
5. Gordon H. Female genital mutilation. In: Perineal and anal sphincter trauma. 2007. p. 80–8.
6. United Nations Children's Fund. Female genital mutilation: a new generation calls for ending an old practice. New York: UNICEF; 2020. https://data.unicef.org/resources/female-genital-mutilation-a-new-generation-calls-for-ending-an-old-practice/.
7. Albert J, Wells M. The acton model: support for women with female genital mutilation. Br J Midwifery. 2020;28(10):697–708. Available from: http://www.magonlinelibrary.com/doi/10.12968/bjom.2020.28.10.697
8. UNICEF. Female genital mutilation [Internet]. 2021. Available from: https://data.unicef.org/topic/child-protection/female-genital-mutilation/
9. UNICEF. Female genital mutilation/cutting: a global concern [Internet]. 2016 [cited 2020 Dec 1]. Available from: https://www.who.int/en/news-room/fact-sheets/detail/female-genital-mutilation
10. Population Council. Evidence to end FGM/C: research to help girls and women thrive [Internet]. 2020. Available from: file:///C:/Users/44773/Documents/research articles/2020RH_FGMC_ReflectionsFiveYears.pdf
11. WHO. Care of women and girls living with female genital mutilation: a clinical handbook. [Internet].

2018. Available from: file:///C:/Users/44773/Downloads/9789241513913-eng.pdf

12. Abdulcadir J, Catania L, Hindin MJ, Say L, Petignat P, Abdulcadir O. Female genital mutilation: a visual reference and learning tool for health care professionals. Obstet Gynecol. 2016;128(5):958–63. Available from: http://www.ncbi.nlm.nih.gov/pubmed/27741194

13. Abdulcadir J, Marras S, Catania L, Abdulcadir O, Petignat P. Defibulation: a visual reference and learning tool. J Sex Med. 2018;15(4):601–11. Available from: https://doi.org/10.1016/j.jsxm.2018.01.010

14. Arowojolu O, Okunlola MA, A. O. A. Three decades of acquired gynaetresia in Ibadan: clinical presentation and management. J Obstet Gynaecol (Lahore). 2001;21(4):375–8. Available from: http://www.tandfonline.com/doi/full/10.1080/01443610120059923

15. Tahzib F. Epidemiological determinants of vesicovaginal fistulas. Br J Obstet Gynaecol. 1983;90(5):387–91.

16. Abdulcadir J, Rodriguez M, Say L. Research gaps in the care of women with female genital mutilation: an analysis. BJOG An Int J Obstet Gynaecol. 2015;122(3):294–303. Available from: http://doi.wiley.com/10.1111/1471-0528.13217

17. Berg RC, Taraldsen S, Said MA, Sørbye IK, Vangen S. Reasons for and experiences with surgical interventions for Female Genital Mutilation/Cutting (FGM/C): a systematic review. J Sex Med. 2017;14(8):977–90.

Available from: https://linkinghub.elsevier.com/retrieve/pii/S1743609517312663

18. Albert J, Evans C, Wells M. Analysis of a specialist service for nonpregnant women with female genital mutilation: 2008–2019. Br J Midwifery. 2023;31(11):610–21.

19. Gordon H, Comerasamy H, Morris NH. Female genital mutilation: experience in a West London clinic. J Obs Gynaecol. 2007;27(4):416–9.

20. RCOG. RCOG Green-top Guideline No. 53 [Internet]. 2015. Available from: https://www.rcog.org.uk/globalassets/documents/guidelines/gtg-53-fgm.pdf

21. Banks E, Meirik O, Farley T, Akande O, Bathija H, Ali M. Female genital mutilation and obstetric outcome: WHO collaborative prospective study in six African countries. Lancet. 2006;367(9525):1835–41. Available from: https://linkinghub.elsevier.com/retrieve/pii/S0140673606688053

22. 28 Too Many. The law and FGM in Europe [Internet]. 2021. Available from: https://www.28toomany.org/static/media/uploads/LawReports/EULaw/the_law_and_fgm_in_europe.pdf

23. Department of Health. Female genital mutilation risk and safeguarding; guidance for professionals. 2016. https://assets.publishing.service.gov.uk/media/5a8041f3ed915d74e622d655/FGM_safeguarding_report_A.pdf.

Anorectal Pathophysiology and Investigations

14

S. Mark Scott

Overview

Test your learning and check your understanding of this book's contents: use the "Springer Nature Flashcards" app to access questions using ▶ https://sn.pub/wqrf89. To use the app, please follow the instructions in Chap. 1.

Learning Points

- Obstetric trauma is a major risk factor for the development of FI. However, in the general population, diarrhoea (loose stools), frequency of defaecation, faecal urgency and evacuatory dysfunction may pose greater risk in some sufferers.
- Faecal continence is dependent upon a morphologically intact gastrointestinal tract and the complex interplay between several physiological systems including: neural (both sensory and motor domains), muscular (smooth and striated), hormonal (endocrine and paracrine) and cognitive.

- The pathophysiology of FI does not only involve damage to the anal sphincters and pelvic floor and their innervation. Multiple other mechanisms are now recognised, including the following: loss of anal 'seal' function, compromised 'barrier' function, rectal 'reservoir' dysfunction, incomplete rectal evacuation, impaired sigmoid 'brake' function and colonic dysmotility.
- In patients with symptoms refractory to conservative management, specialist diagnostic testing is indicated. These include tests of anorectal motor and sensory function, imaging of the anal sphincters and pelvic floor, investigation of evacuatory function, and assessment of gut motility and transit.

14.1 Introduction

Obstetric trauma is recognised as a major risk factor for the development of FI in women [1–3]. However, epidemiological studies have shown that FI is almost as prevalent in men [4, 5]. Further, recent data show a comparable prevalence of FI in nulliparous women [6, 7]. Clearly, therefore, factors other than obstetric-related ones play a vital (and perhaps *more* important) role in some sufferers. Diarrhoea (or loose stools) is the strongest risk factor for FI in the community [8–11]. Other important bowel-related factors are faecal urgency [8] and increased

S. M. Scott (✉)
National Bowel Research Centre and GI Physiology Unit, Blizard Institute, Centre for Neuroscience, Surgery & Trauma, Queen Mary University of London, London, UK
e-mail: m.scott@qmul.ac.uk

frequency of defaecation (>3 bowel movements/day) [8, 9]. Conversely, there is increasing recognition of the frequent coexistence of significant symptoms of chronic constipation and evacuatory dysfunction and FI [8, 11, 12] (>40% of patients at tertiary-care level) [13], with FI proposed to occur as a secondary phenomenon (as is widely acknowledged in paediatric and geriatric practice). Other identified risk factors include increased body mass index, smoking, cholecystectomy and poor general health [10]. Anal intercourse may also be a risk factor [14, 15]. The prevalence of FI is much greater in both quiescent and active ulcerative colitis than in the general background population [16].

Historically, damage to the anal sphincters and their innervation [3] have been seen as the principal pathophysiological mechanisms leading to FI. Although these factors may indeed hold primacy in parous women, a more contemporary understanding of the pathophysiology of FI now recognises a multifactorial process involving several other, often overlapping, 'upstream' mechanisms. The relative importance of each individual factor, or combinations of factors, remains unclear. Nevertheless, given a limited and relatively non-specific symptom repertoire of the gut, reliance on clinical symptoms alone to guide therapy in patients with FI refractory to standard conservative management (lifestyle and medication) is now considered obsolete [17]. Thus, akin to other areas of modern scientific medicine, further specialist diagnostic testing may be used to identify the pathophysiological basis of FI with the aim of guiding therapy. Several complementary investigations now exist to routinely evaluate pelvic floor, colonic and anorectal structure and function.

14.2 Physiology of Defaecation and Continence

Before considering the pathophysiology of FI, a prior understanding of the mechanisms contributing to human defaecation is essential. Defaecation is a fundamental physiological process resulting in the evacuation of faeces and is inextricably linked to bowel continence, which, in turn, is dependent upon the voluntary (and involuntary) control of defaecation. Dysfunction or disruption of one or (usually) more of the multiple factors contributing to the process of defaecation may lead to FI or constipation/evacuation disorders which may themselves coexist [13, 18]. Both defaecation and continence are dependent on a morphologically intact gastrointestinal tract and the coordination and integration of multiple physiological systems including: neural (principally the enteric nervous system, modulated by the peripheral somatic, autonomic and central nervous systems, and involving both sensory and motor domains); muscular (smooth and striated); hormonal (endocrine and paracrine); and cognitive (behavioural and psychosocial) [19, 20].

The various factors required for normal bowel continence are listed in Table 14.1. Bowel continence requires a complex balance between pelvic floor and anal canal 'barrier' function, rectal reservoir and evacuatory function, neurological function, colorectal motility, stool volume and consistency and ultimately conscious control [20]. Simplistically, an appropriate, coordinated interplay between these factors results in anal canal pressure being greater than that in the rectum and allows continence to be maintained [21].

It is important to appreciate that although the lowest sphincter of the gastrointestinal tract is the structure most threatened by obstetric trauma, the ability of an individual to retain rectal contents and only allow their passage when desired, results from a multitude of factors *in addition* to the anal sphincter complex. The idea that involuntary contraction of the internal anal sphincter (IAS) is the primary mechanism of continence and that the external anal sphincter (EAS) supports continence only by voluntary contraction is outdated [22].

Bowel continence, for the majority of our days and nights, is largely controlled by subconscious processes, with a myriad of reflexes occurring at multiple levels; it is only when recruitment reaches a threshold that awareness of lower gut activity reaches consciousness, enabling the owner to make decisions about whether to respond by visiting the toilet, or whether it may be possible to defer defaecation until more socially convenient. Western patterns of living have somewhat interfered with such a balanced process. For example, firstly, our eating habits may not be conducive to

Table 14.1 Factors contributing to the maintenance of continence

Sphincteric components
  Structural
    Internal anal sphincter
    External anal sphincter
    Conjoined longitudinal muscle
    Vascular anal cushions
    Longitudinal anal muscle folds
  Functional
    Anal resting tone
    Anal canal/high-pressure zone length
    Resting anal pressure gradient
    Voluntary anal squeeze pressure
    Anal sensation
    Anal motility
    Recto-anal inhibitory ("sampling") reflex
    Recto-anal contractile reflex
  Neurological
    Pudendal nerve
    Sympathetic (hypogastric) nerves
    Parasympathetic (pelvic) nerves
Supra-sphincteric components
  Structural
    Levator ani
      Puborectalis
      Iliococcygeus
      Pubococcygeus
    Perineal resting position/level of descent
    Rectal
      Capacity
      Curvatures/transverse folds
      Flap valve effect of the anterior wall
    Endopelvic musculofascial support
    Rectosigmoid sphincter
  Functional
    Tonic levator ani contraction
    Anorectal angle
    Rectosigmoid angle
    Postural pelvic floor reflex
    Rectal sensation
    Rectal tone
    Rectal compliance
    Rectosigmoid motility/sigmoid 'brake'
    Anorectal pressure gradient
    Rectosigmoid pressure gradient
    Rectosigmoid high pressure zone
    Stool consistency
    Stool volume
    GI/colonic motility
  Neurological
    Pudendal nerve
    Sympathetic nerves
    Parasympathetic nerves
    Afferent nerves
    Intrinsic (enteric) nerves
Other components
    Normal rectal evacuation
    Psycho-behavioural factors

optimal gut motor activity. Secondly, the perceived necessity of ridding the bowel of its contents (through straining) before important activities such as work (and before defaecation has been triggered from the bowel itself), or repeatedly suppressing the natural desire to defaecate until one's own toilet at home is reached, may, over time, have a detrimental effect upon the efficiency of such a complex process.

14.3 Pathophysiology of Faecal Incontinence

FI occurs when one or more of the mechanisms that maintain continence are disrupted to an extent that other mechanisms are unable to compensate [23]. The principal pathophysiological mechanisms are detailed below and outlined in Fig. 14.1.

14.3.1 Anal Canal: Impaired 'Seal' Function

The thick and highly vascular anal lining has blood vessels grouped in 3 anal 'cushions'. These are superimposed by the vertical mucosal folds of the columns of Morgagni [24, 25] which together interdigitate to provide a hermetic seal to the anal canal. Lesions which mechanically interfere with, or prevent complete closure of the anus may result in FI to liquid stool or a mucus discharge. These include prolapsing haemorrhoids, which may displace the anal cushions and secondary mucosal folds, or following haemorrhoidectomy [26]. Other lesions include anal fissures, cancer or fistulae, as well as congenital malformations of the anus.

14.3.2 Anus and Pelvic Floor: Impaired 'Barrier' Structure/ Function

Structural integrity of the pelvic floor and anal musculature (and their innervation) provides the final 'barrier' function with regard to faecal continence. The levator ani muscle complex comprises the striated coccygeus, pubococcygeus and

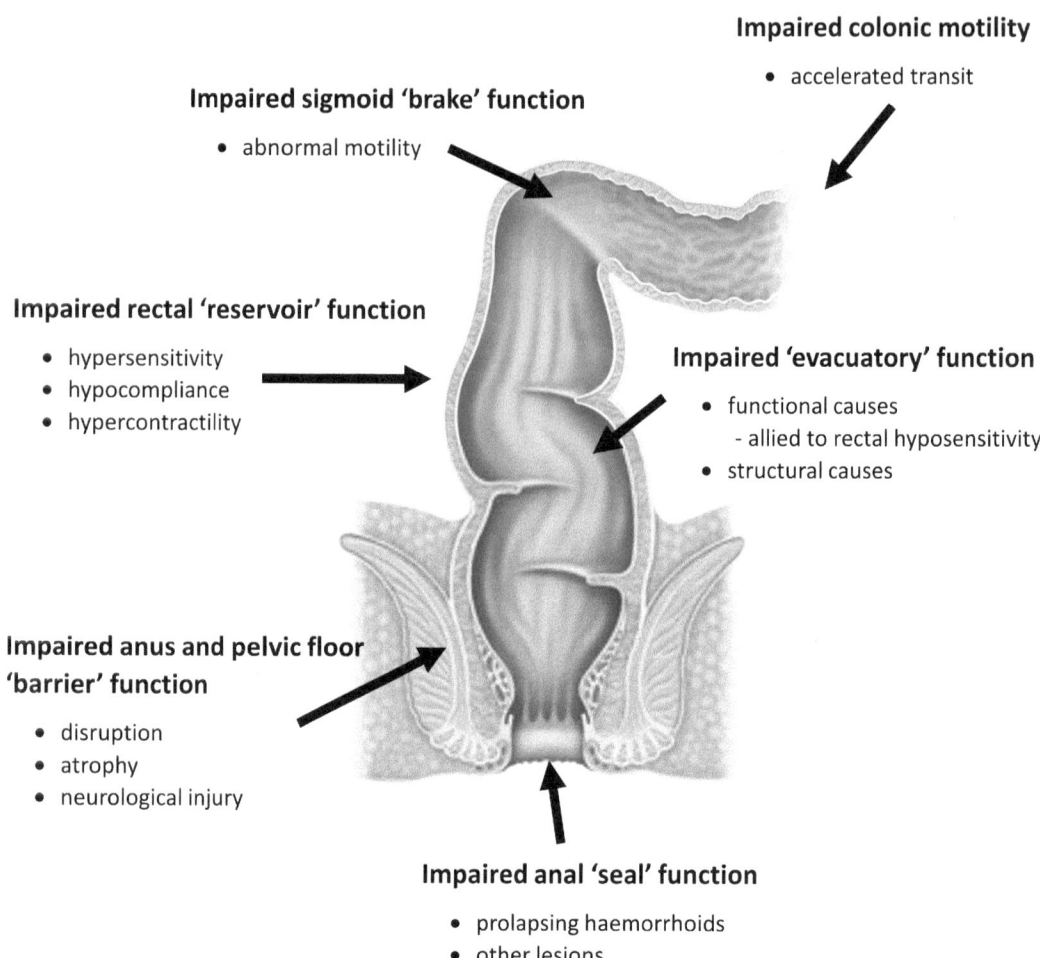

Fig. 14.1 Overlapping pathophysiological mechanisms contributing to faecal incontinence

iliococcygeus muscles, which form the majority of the funnel-shaped pelvic floor through which the pelvic organs pass. These muscles are uniquely maintained in a state of tonic contraction by the autonomic pelvic floor postural reflex [27] to help maintain continence. Muscle activity increases dynamically according to reflex activation of stretch receptors in the pelvic floor muscles themselves, consequent to coughing, laughing, moving etc. [27]. Endopelvic fascia and ligamentous attachments support the pelvic viscera and provide attachments to the pelvic wall as well. The puborectalis muscle (PRM) is best considered the deep part of the EAS, and constitutes the inferior margin of the pelvic hiatus. It forms a U-shaped sling around the anorectal junction with the direction of contraction towards the pubis, creating a 60–105° angulation between the anal canal and rectum at rest. Intra-abdominal pressure is hypothesised to seal the anterior rectal wall as a 'flap valve' over the underlying anal canal [28]. Through voluntary contraction, the anorectal angle becomes more acute, further closing the upper anal canal, vagina and urethra [29]. The pelvic floor muscles receive dual innervation via branches of the pudendal nerve (the perineal nerve and inferior rectal nerve), and directly from sacral nerve roots S3 and S4. The PRM is primarily innervated by pudendal nerve branches, but may also receive direct innervation via the sacral nerves [29, 30].

The anal canal arises at the anorectal junction where the rectum passes through the pelvic hiatus; it is surrounded by the inner, tubular smooth muscle IAS, the outer striated EAS (which extends from the PRM) and the (often overlooked) conjoint longitudinal muscle, which is a continuation of the longitudinal muscle of the rectum and binds and braces the sphincters. The anal canal is tightly closed at rest, with resting tone provided by the anal cushions, IAS and EAS. The major contributor is the IAS [31, 32], which is contemporaneously considered a phasically-active muscle that generates tonic activity [33]. The EAS is predominantly composed of slow-twitch muscle fibres allowing it to maintain a sustained tonic contraction. The EAS is further supported by the action of the transverse perineii and bulbospongiosus musculature, to create a "purse string" closure at the perineal body [34]. Other fast-twitch fibres allow the EAS (and PRM) to contract rapidly with voluntary squeeze to supplement continence control (e.g. when stool enters the upper part of the anal canal) [35], or during rapid changes in intra-abdominal pressure (e.g. on lifting, coughing, sneezing) through a polysynaptic reflex [22, 36].

The IAS is innervated by postganglionic sympathetic nerves, via the hypogastric and inferior mesenteric plexuses, which provide a tonic excitatory discharge [37] and by inhibitory preganglionic parasympathetic nerves travelling with the sacral nerves [26]. Innervation to the IAS is also supplied by nerve fibres coursing in the intersphincteric space; these are derived from the myenteric plexus of the distal rectum [38, 39]. Innervation of the EAS is distinct from that of the levator ani muscles; it receives bilateral innervation via the pudendal nerves [40], and may also receive an additional direct branch from the fourth sacral nerve [41].

The anal canal mucosa contains numerous free and organised nerve endings that convey proprioceptive, mechanoreceptive (tactile and nociceptive) and thermal information via pudendal afferents [42, 43]. Periodic transient reflex relaxations of the IAS enable rectal content to come into contact with these sensory receptors, allowing discrimination between flatus and solid or liquid stool, which is essential to maintaining continence [44]. Such 'sampling' reflexes usually occur secondary to a rectal pressure increase, sometimes concomitant with colonic contractile activity moving stool or gas into the rectum [45].

All structures of the pelvic floor and anal canal are susceptible to damage from obstetric trauma. This damage is caused via neural traction injury, bladder compression, stretching of the vaginal wall, stretching and tearing of the rectovaginal septum and fascia, stretching and avulsion of the levator ani muscles, compression of the pudendal (Alcock's) canal, and ligamentous injury and tearing of the anal sphincter complex.

14.3.2.1 Structural Damage to the Anal Canal and Pelvic Floor

Thirty years ago, the seminal study by Sultan et al. [46] reported a 13% incidence of FI or faecal urgency in 79 primiparous women following vaginal delivery and a 4% incidence of new symptoms among 48 multiparous mothers [46]. Of perhaps greater significance was the incidence of sphincter defects observed at endo-anal ultrasound following childbirth; 35% of primiparous and 4% of multiparous women were noted to have defects resulting from vaginal delivery (with only two women having recognised tears of the anal sphincter at the time of delivery). Not surprisingly, a strong association was demonstrated between presence of a defect and development of symptoms [46]. Subsequent systematic reviews and meta-analyses show that the incidence of ultrasonographic-confirmed sphincter injury in primiparous women is 26–27% [47, 48]. Bayesian calculation has suggested that for a woman presenting with faecal incontinence postpartum, the probability of her having a sphincter defect is ~80% [47].

Obstetric-related disruption of the IAS or EAS may be associated with differing symptom presentation. While IAS disruption is usually allied to passive faecal incontinence, EAS disruption is typically associated with symptoms of urge or stress faecal incontinence [49, 50]. However, this is not an absolute relationship, symptoms of urge and passive leakage very commonly coexist [1], and both sphincters may be affected. Obstetric trauma can also lead to damage or avulsion of the levator ani (including the PRM) [51, 52]. Levator ani failure is recognised as being of aetiological importance in the development of pelvic organ prolapse and FI [53–55].

The impact of obstetric-related injury to the anal sphincters and pelvic floor muscles is explored in much greater detail in Chaps. 2–5, 15, and 16.

14.3.2.2 Compromised Anal Canal and Pelvic Floor Function

Normative manometric reference data show that mean anal squeeze pressures (primarily reflecting EAS and PRM function) are lower in asymptomatic parous women compared to nulliparous women [56]. Large prospective studies of anal sphincter function in women giving birth show that first vaginal delivery, particularly if instrumental, causes a permanent lowering of anal squeeze pressures and also resting tone, irrespective of postpartum continence status or sphincter integrity [57–59].

In women with FI, anal sphincter weakness (as measured by manometry) is the most widely recognized anorectal disturbance. Anal hypocontractility (squeeze pressures *below* the lower limit of normal) is found in the majority (~75%) [60] of sufferers (Fig. 14.2b), principally due to obstetric-related anal sphincter injury [46]. Other causes, which may be additive or contributory, are congenital abnormalities (e.g. imperforate anus, rectal agenesis) [61] and iatrogenic injury, notably after surgery for fistula-in-ano [62]. Anal sphincter function continues to deteriorate with age [63] and with subsequent vaginal deliveries [64–66].

Anal hypotension (resting tone below the lower limit of normal: Fig. 14.2c) is found in ~45% of women [60]. It is principally caused by IAS disruption, typically through obstetric injury [67]. With further regard to vaginal delivery, some suggest that reduced anal tone is confined to those who have had an instrumental delivery [58], or in only those who become incontinent [68]. Other causes of anal hypotension include iatrogenic injury [61, 62], myopathy (e.g. scleroderma), atrophy or degeneration [50] or as a complication of radiotherapy [69]. Altered IAS morphology (such as a thickened and asymmetric muscle ring) [70] and hypotension are also seen in patients with FI due to a high-grade rectal intussusception or rectal prolapse [71, 72].

Weakness of the pelvic floor musculature through obstetric injury (e.g. levator ani avulsion;

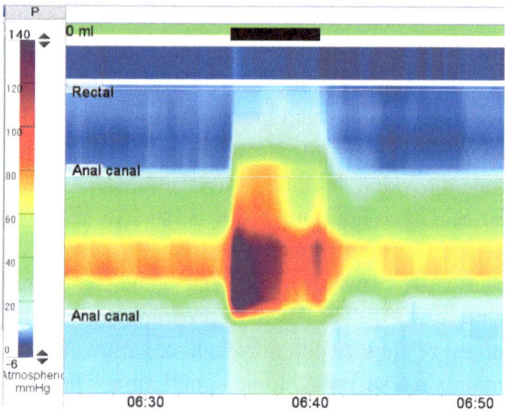
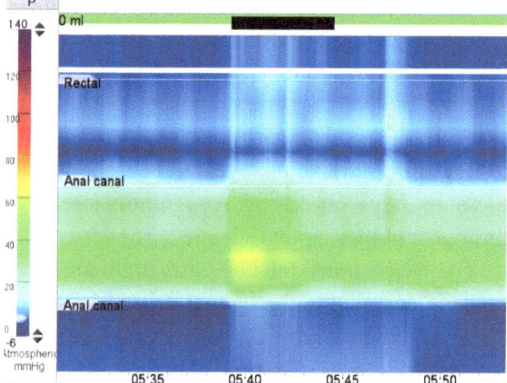
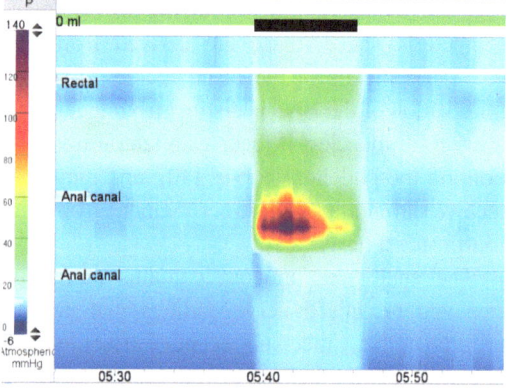

Fig. 14.2 Manometric representation of anal sphincter function. High-resolution anorectal manometry images at rest and during a 5 s squeeze manoeuvre. (**a**) Anal normotension and normal voluntary contractility. (**b**) Anal normotension with profound voluntary anal hypocontractility in a female with FI and a history of obstetric trauma. (**c**) Profound anal hypotension with normal voluntary contractility in a patient with passive FI allied to rectal prolapse—anal tone is almost indistinguishable at rest

enlargement of the levator hiatus) [51, 73] or atrophy, together with laxity of ligamentous attachments [74] as well as rectovaginal septal and endopelvic fascia tears, are other fundamental contributors to loss of barrier function.

It is important to note, however, that patients with very poor sphincter or pelvic floor function may be totally continent, whereas those with normal sphincter function may be incontinent. This again highlights the multifactorial nature of FI.

14.3.2.3 Neurological Injury

Injury to the pudendal or perineal nerves, as evidenced by external anal sphincter and puborectalis denervation [75], with subsequent muscle reinnervation [76], was proposed as the principal cause of FI in the late 1970's. Subsequent studies confirmed that such denervation/reinnervation injury occurred following vaginal delivery [77, 78], and hence the majority of patients with FI were labelled as having 'neurogenic' incontinence [79]. However, although pudendal neuropathy is commonly found in FI [3, 23], with the advent of endoanal ultrasound in the early to mid-1990's, it is now known that *isolated* pudendal neuropathy (unilateral or bilateral) as a cause of FI is rare (~10%) [80].

The dense neural network of the pelvic floor and anal canal is also susceptible to traction injury (such as with obstetric trauma or chronic straining at stool). The pudendal nerve, which contains both motor and sensory fibres, is particularly vulnerable during childbirth [77, 81–83], when descent of the pelvic floor and progression of the foetal head toward the pelvic outlet may stretch the nerve as it emerges from Alcock's canal; there, its course is relatively fixed along the pelvic sidewall.

In most prospective studies, first vaginal delivery appears to be the most injurious to sphincter [64, 84, 85] and neural [64, 82] integrity alike, with damage to the pudendal nerves being cumulative with subsequent deliveries [64, 81, 86, 87]. Caesarean birth, performed as an emergency procedure after the onset of labour (especially during the later stages) does not protect against neural damage [46, 78, 88].

Anal hyposensitivity (a marker of pudendal nerve afferent dysfunction) can manifest as increased sensory thresholds to mucosal electrostimulation [89] and has been reported in patients with FI [90]. Anal hyposensitivity following childbirth has been shown in some studies [91], but not others [58].

More recent studies have demonstrated both afferent and efferent neural *pathway* dysfunction in response to stimulation from multiple sources (end organ, transcranial, trans-sacral, translumbar and anal) [92–95]. Indeed, translumbosacral anorectal magnetic stimulation has revealed significant lumbar and sacral plexus neuropathy in the majority of FI patients [96]. Global pelvic floor weakness, manifest as descending perineum syndrome (>4 cm perineal descent) may also lead to progressive denervation.

14.3.3 Rectum: Impaired 'Reservoir' Function

The rectum commences at the sigmoid mesocolic-mesorectal junction ('sigmoid takeoff'), corresponding to the point of the coalescence of the taenia coli, and extends to the level of the PRM [97]. It consists of an inner, circular, smooth muscle layer surrounded by an outer longitudinal muscle layer. The luminal wall typically forms two or three transverse folds (valves of Houston), which are hypothesized to slow stool, but also to compartmentalise the rectum and assist in separating solid and gaseous content to allow for sensory sampling [98].

The rectum is usually empty [99]. Under normal circumstances, the rectum's capacity and compliance (and hence, its distensibility) are crucial in allowing the rectum to accommodate and store stool (the rectal 'reservoir') during filling without significant increases in intraluminal pressure, until defaecation is socially convenient [100]. However, when distended beyond a critical threshold (believed to be related to perception of rectal sensation), rectal smooth muscle contracts reflexively [101], which may empty the rectum (e.g. by defaecation) unless opposed by strong both involuntary and voluntary contraction of the EAS and PRM. The sense of urgency then wanes, together with relaxation of the rectum to accommodate more stool [102].

Rectal sensory innervation involves visceral afferents of the enteric nervous system which communicate with enteric motor neurons to effect local reflexes, and also with extrinsic sacral afferents via interneurons. The extrinsic spinal sensory fibres follow the path of somatic and efferent autonomic nerves to the spine, with cell bodies in the sacral dorsal root ganglia (S1–S2) [19]. The lower rectum is supplied by visceral afferents as well as sensory somatic nerves arising from the pudendal nerve. Intact rectal sensory function allows for graded perception of filling, leading to the conscious urge to defaecate.

Heightened (hypersensitivity) [103] or blunted (hyposensitivity) [104] rectal sensation can be associated with FI. For example, if rectal reservoir function is impaired, a small volume of stool can generate high intra-rectal pressures which can overwhelm anal resistance and result in FI [23]. Impaired reservoir function (Fig. 14.3) is characterised by decreased rectal size and hypocompliance (i.e. a "stiffer" rectum, e.g. after rectal surgery or with inflammatory disease) [105]. This is often allied to rectal hypersensitivity (and

perhaps rectal hypercontractility) [106, 107], as well as increased faecal urgency and frequency of defaecation [103, 107]. Overall, rectal hypersensitivity is found in a small minority of women with FI (~10%) [60] and may also be associated with the irritable bowel syndrome.

Rectal hyposensitivity is allied to an attenuated 'call to stool' and may be 'primary' (due to direct impairment of afferent pathway function), 'secondary' (due to altered biomechanical properties, e.g. an oversized and hypercompliant, or 'lax' reservoir: Fig. 14.3), or both [108]. Causes of impaired sensation include multiple sclerosis, diabetes mellitus, or spinal cord injury. In patients with FI, elevated rectal sensory thresholds have been shown to be independently associated with incontinence after multivariate analysis [109], where faecal leakage may be secondary to 'overflow' allied to an inappropriate 'compensatory' reflex sphincteric response [110–112].

The pivotal role that the rectum plays in FI should not be understated. The barrier-centric containment model is insufficient to explain FI, including the origin of the symptom of urgency and development of incontinence over the life course. A recent revisionist theory presents reflex control of rectal contractility as central to FI pathogenesis, with the anorectum considered a single functional unit that cooperates with the colon and central nervous system to maintain continence [113].

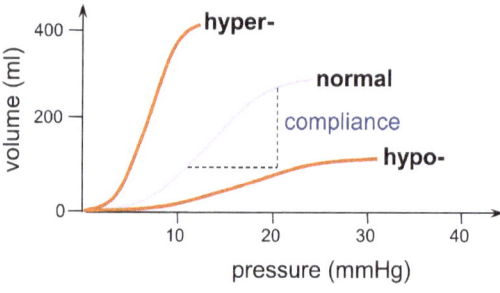

Fig. 14.3 Rectal compliance. During rectal distension, intrarectal volumes and pressures are recorded concomitantly, allowing rectal compliance to be calculated from the derived sigmoid-shaped pressure-volume curve. With a *hypo*compliant ('stiff') rectum, the slope of the pressure-volume curve is reduced (i.e. it is closer to the horizontal position: greater increase in pressure with applied volume); this reflects loss of rectal 'reservoir' function, and is often allied to rectal hypersensitivity and rectal hypercontractility. With a *hyper*compliant ('lax') rectum, the slope of the pressure-volume curve is increased (i.e. displaced towards the vertical position: smaller pressure change with applied volume); this is typically allied to a large capacity, hyposensitive rectum

14.3.4 Impaired Evacuatory Function

Effective rectal evacuation is vital to maintaining continence. Incomplete emptying of stool may predispose to FI (for example as post-defaecation faecal leakage) [104, 114, 115] if other continence mechanisms are compromised. There is a growing body of literature that supports the frequent (up to 69%) coexistence of constipation/evacuatory dysfunction in the general adult population [12, 13, 18, 116–118] which also extends to the obstetric field [119, 120]; this relationship is frequently overlooked by the referring clinician [13]. A unifying concept to explain combined pelvic floor disorders (including evacuatory dysfunction) and FI has long been proposed. This mechanism begins with damage to the pelvic floor and anal sphincter innervation through vaginal birth. The injury is further exacerbated through chronic straining during defaecation which leads to pelvic floor weakness, pelvic organ descent, worsening of evacuatory difficulties, progression of the neurogenic lesion, and ultimately to faecal incontinence [121].

Incomplete evacuation can be due to several mechanisms. For example, it may be due to 'functional' causes (e.g. dyssynergia or ineffective rectal propulsion. Fig. 14.4b), often allied to rectal hyposensitivity [23, 122, 123]. Conversely, it may be due to structural obstructive phenomena such as a rectocoele (Fig. 14.4c), intussusception (Fig. 14.4d) or enterocoele. Acknowledgment of coexisting FI and constipation has major implications regarding management. If FI is indeed secondary to an underlying evacuation disorder, then intervention directed to improving constipation symptoms and efficacy of evacuation should be considered first-line treatments. Several studies have demonstrated significant improvements or resolution of symptoms of FI when causes of evacuatory dysfunction have been addressed (e.g. after surgical repair of rectocoele and/or intussusception [124–126] and following colorectal irrigation [127, 128].

14.3.5 Sigmoid: Impaired 'Brake' Function

The sigmoid colon contributes to continence through specialised motility patterns (predominant cyclic retrograde propulsive activity: Fig. 14.5) which likely act as a 'brake' mechanism to govern passage of stool into the rectum [129]. The presence of a true 'rectosigmoid sphincter' has long been debated [130–132]. Retrograde sigmoid motility (and hence 'brake' function) may be reduced in FI [133, 134].

14.3.6 Colon: Impaired Motility

While obstetric factors are rated most important for the development of FI by healthcare professions (particularly colorectal surgeons) [135], community-based studies have shown diarrhoea and loose stools to be the primary risk factor [8–11]. This is underscored by disordered colonic motility leading to accelerated colonic transit. High-amplitude propulsive contractions (HAPC) of the colon allow for progression of stool into the rectum. However, increased HAPC activity may lead to too-rapid progression of loose stool. This can then overwhelm the reservoir capacity of the rectum and the resistance of the anal and pelvic floor barrier function [136, 137]. This may be compounded by loss of the sigmoid 'brake' [134, 138].

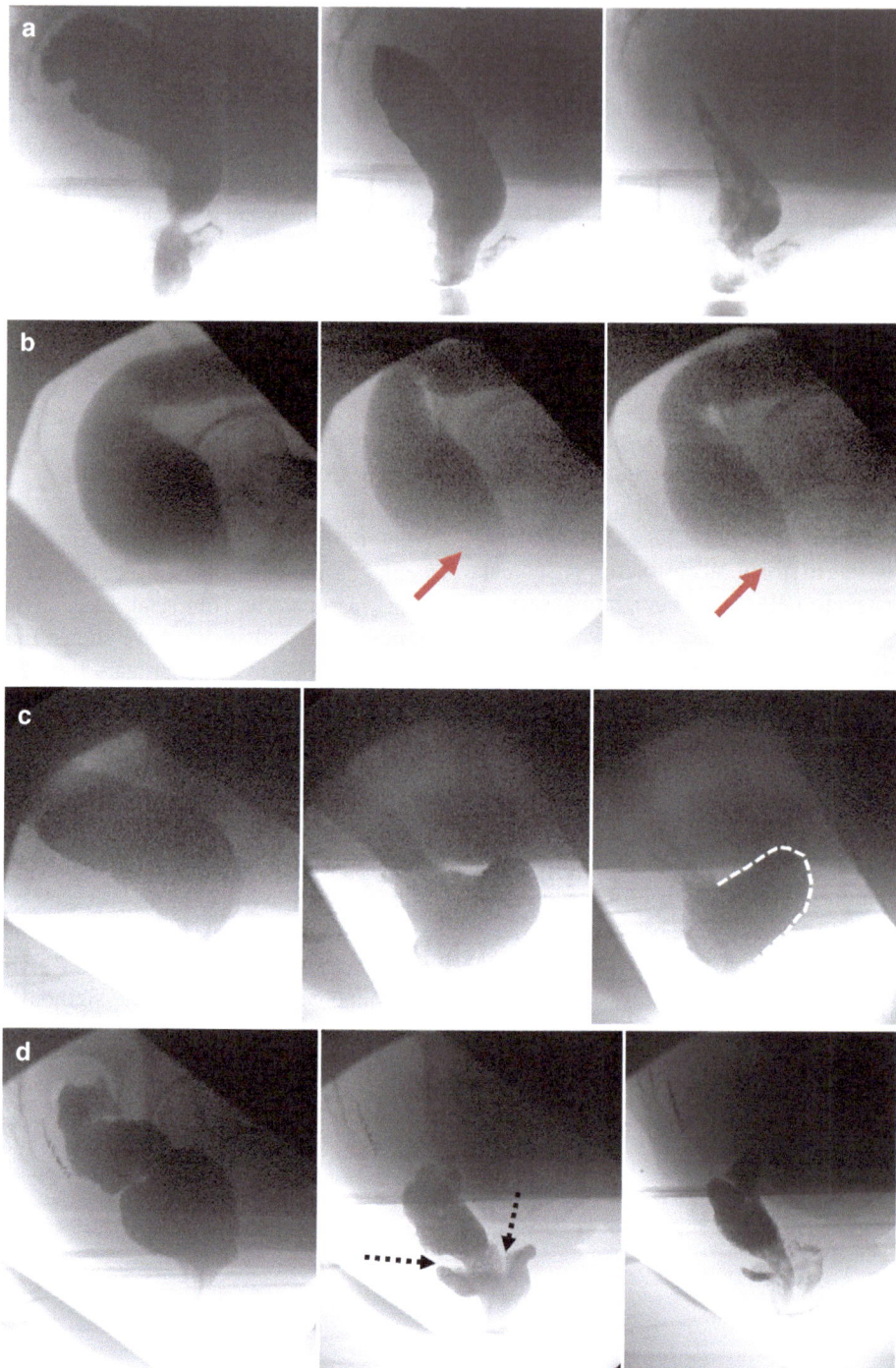

Fig. 14.4 Structural and functional abnormalities impeding defaecation. Each row shows three representative defaecographic images (lateral view) from an individual patient at start, mid and end-evacuation. (**a**) Normal evacuation: there is a good opening of the anorectal angle and the majority of instilled contrast is expelled. (**b**) 'Functional' evacuation disorder: there is no opening of the anorectal angle (a persistent impression of puborectalis is evident, indicated by solid black arrow) and little opening of the anal canal, and only a small percentage of contrast is successfully expelled. (**c**) 'Structural' evacuation disorder due to a large rectocoele in which all residual contrast is retained (delineated by dashed white line). (**d**) 'Structural' evacuation disorder allied to a full-thickness rectal intussusception which originates in the mid rectum (dashed black arrows) and descends to the anal verge at end evacuation

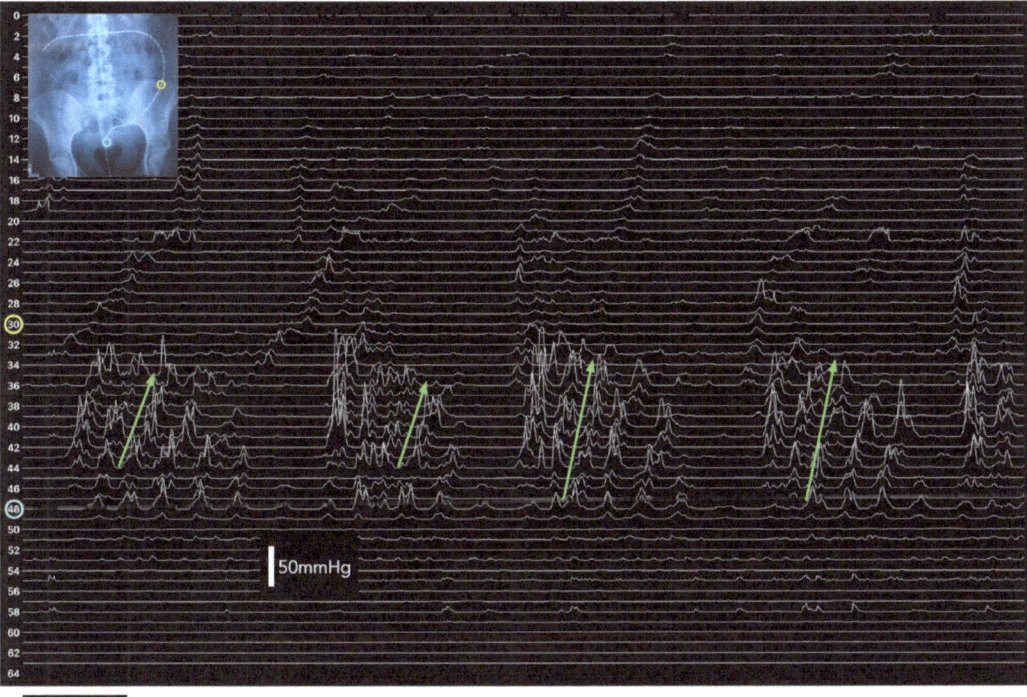

Fig. 14.5 Sigmoid 'brake' function. A 64 channel high-resolution manometry catheter, with 1 cm spacing between sensors, has been introduced into the colon (x-ray, top left inlay). Data over 10 min from a ~17 cm segment of the sigmoid colon (between the two dots) are displayed. Bursts of repetitive contractions, occurring at 2–3 cycles per minute, propagating *away* from the direction of the rectum (i.e. retrograde cyclic motility pattern) can be clearly observed. *Thanks to Professor Phil Dinning, Flinders University, South Australia, for providing the images*

14.4 Investigations

A comprehensive clinical evaluation of patients, with integration of findings from the clinical history, physical examination and other investigations, allows (1) the pathoaetiology of FI to be deduced, (2) co-existing pathology to be excluded, and (3) a decision regarding choice of suitable therapy to be made on an individual basis.

A detailed clinical history should be obtained to assess the following:

1. duration and severity of symptoms, including frequency and nature of FI;
2. likely aetiology and risk factors, with focus on any precipitating events;
3. impact of FI on quality of life (QoL), such as the patient's ability to leave the house and social activities, and also use of pads, plugs and constipating agents;
4. secondary problems and associated pathologies [139–141].

Several validated questionnaires exist that can be incorporated into history taking and may aid assessment of FI severity and impact on QoL, though no system has been universally adopted in clinical practice. However, it is well-accepted that stool form is best assessed through the Bristol stool form scale [142]. A thorough physical examination should then be performed and should include external inspection, digital anorectal examination and basic instrumentation e.g. proctoscopy [139–141].

14.4.1 Diagnostic Testing

Diagnostic testing is indicated in patients with FI in whom conservative measures have failed, concurrent disease has been excluded, and have a significant impact of symptoms on quality of life. The aim of investigation is to explain the cause of symptoms and to establish a diagnosis that can guide rational and effective treatment. Several complementary investigations exist to assess the functional and structural competency of several measureable components of continence and defaecation (Table 14.2), carried out in the context of a *global* pelvic floor evaluation which include the following: (1) anorectal motor and sensory function; (2) anal and pelvic floor morphology/structure; (3) evacuatory function; and (4) colonic motility (transit and contractility) [143].

A comprehensive assessment is recommended, performed in a systematic manner. No single investigation can fully assess either struc-

ture or function. The general rationale for testing is to: (1) confirm the clinical impression and provide the basis for therapy; (2) acquire objective test results, which enable accurate phenotyping of the patient; (3) provide information to the patient. Disease-responsive biomarkers may be provided that can help monitor or explain the outcome of intervention (especially if this is suboptimal) [144].

14.4.1.1 Tests of Anorectal Motor and Sensory Function

Anorectal Manometry
The human finger is a poor pressure measuring device, and digital examination alone is not accurate enough for the diagnostic assessment of anal sphincter function [145]. In addition, it is not possible to assess other important components of the continence mechanism by this method.

Anorectal manometry (ARM) is the best established and the most widely available diag-

Table 14.2 Diagnostic testing for faecal incontinence

Structure/function	Investigation	Relevant possible diagnoses
(A) Baseline recommendations		
Anal sphincter structure	Endo-anal ultrasound	Sphincter disruption/atrophy/degeneration/hypertrophy
Anal sphincter function	High-resolution anorectal manometry	Anal hypotension; anal hypercontractility; abnormal cough-anorectal reflex response
Rectal sensory function	Balloon distension	Rectal hypersensitivity; rectal hyposensitivity
Rectal evacuatory function[a]	Defaecography (X-ray or MRI)	Impaired evacuation; 'functional' evacuation disorder; 'structural' evacuation disorder (e.g. rectocoele; high-grade intussusception)
(B) Specialist investigations		
Anal sphincter structure	Endo-anal/pelvic MRI	Sphincter disruption/atrophy/degeneration/hypertrophy
Pelvic floor structure/function	Transperineal/transvaginal ultrasound	Levator avulsion; pelvic organ prolapse (e.g. rectocoele; intussusception; enterocoele; cystocoele)
Anal sensation	Mucosal electrosensitivity	Anal hyposensitivity
Rectal biomechanical and sensory function	Barostat	Rectal hypocompliance; rectal hypercompliance; rectal hypersensitivity; rectal hyposensitivity; enlarged or reduced rectal capacity
Pelvic floor neurophysiology	EMG; pudendal nerve terminal motor latencies	Anal sphincter defects; anal sphincter/pelvic floor denervation; pudendal neuropathy
Anorectal afferent pathway	Cortical evoked potentials	Afferent pathway dysfunction/abnormal cortical processing
Anorectal efferent pathway	Magnetic stimulation of cortex or lumbar/sacral region	Efferent pathway dysfunction/peripheral neuropathy
Whole-gut transit	Scintigraphy or ingested telemetry capsules	Accelerated regional gut transit
Colonic motility	High-resolution colonic manometry	Increased propulsive contractile activity abnormal sigmoid 'brake'

[a] If symptoms suggest concomitant evacuation disorder

nostic tool in routine clinical practice, providing objective evaluation of various parameters of anorectal function [146].

Manometric equipment consists of four major components: (1) an intraluminal pressure-sensing catheter (either solid-state or water-perfused) to span the anorectum; (2) pressure transducers; (3) a balloon for inflation within the rectum to enable assessment of sensation and recto-anal reflexes; and (4) an amplification, recording, and display system [147].

Over the last decade, there has been a shift towards technology [148] which has the ability to record and display detailed information simultaneously from the whole anal canal and distal rectum [149]. Two technologies exist: (1) 'high-resolution anorectal manometry' (HRAM: Fig. 14.2) records luminal pressures circumferentially from closely-spaced sensors mounted on a flexible catheter, with data presented either topographically in colour plots or as an average circumferential pressure at different longitudinal levels of the anorectum; and (2) 'high-definition anorectal manometry/topography', which records point pressures longitudinally and radially from 256 sensors mounted on a rigid probe, with morphology represented in both two and three-dimensions.

Although lack of standardisation has previously been recognised as the major pitfall of ARM [148], a landmark contemporary consensus guideline document has now been published through the International Anorectal Physiology Working Group (IAPWG) [150]. This provides a framework for the indications, application (through use of a standardised protocol) and clinical interpretation of ARM (via the London classification of anorectal disorders) applicable to equipment produced by any manufacturer.

Employing the IAPWG protocol, a series of pre-defined manoeuvres are performed sequentially during the ARM investigation [146, 150], allowing for the interrogation of a number of functions of the anorectal unit, namely:

1. anal tone at rest (primarily assessing internal anal sphincter function);
2. voluntary anal contraction ['squeeze'], primarily assessing external anal sphincter function;
3. prolonged voluntary anal contraction ['endurance squeeze'], primarily assessing fatigability of the external anal sphincter;
4. recto-anal activity (to coughing), assessing integrity of the reflex pathway (Rasijeff);
5. recto-anal co-ordination during simulated defaecation ('push'), giving consideration to those patients with coexistent constipation/evacuatory dysfunction;
6. rectal sensation (to mechanical distension).

A combination of qualitative and quantitative measurements for describing manoeuvre outcomes are recommended [150]. For quantitative assessment, recorded values need to be referenced to appropriate normative ranges (the endpoint of any useful clinical test). Several large (>100 subjects) normative datasets exist [56, 151].

In patients with FI, the following clinically relevant features can be diagnosed:

1. anal hypotension (low anal resting pressure: Fig. 14.2c), primarily associated with passive FI [60, 107];
2. a short functional anal canal length [152, 153], though the clinical impact of this measure remains unclear
3. anal hypocontractility (impaired ability to voluntarily contract the anal sphincter: Fig. 14.2b) primarily associated with faecal urgency [49, 60].
4. reduced anal squeeze duration, indicating increased fatigability of the external anal sphincter [154, 155]. It should be noted that though attenuated or poorly sustained voluntary anal squeeze pressures imply external anal sphincter weakness, ARM alone cannot differentiate between compromised muscle integrity, impaired innervation, or both (or indeed a poorly compliant patient [156] as a cause of that weakness]
5. altered cough-anorectal reflex response [157], suggestive of subclinical neuropathy or neural damage to the sacral reflex arc.

Anorectal Sensory Testing

Rectal sensory testing is most conveniently and cost-effectively assessed as part of a manometric investigation; the patient is instructed to volunteer a range of sensations to increasing distension of the intra-rectal balloon and can allow diagnosis of:

1. rectal hypersensitivity (reduced thresholds to distension), often allied to impaired rectal reservoir function [106, 107].
2. rectal hyposensitivity (elevated reduced thresholds to distension), commonly associated with impaired evacuation [23, 122, 123].

Nevertheless, evaluation of both rectal sensory *and* motor function (sensory thresholds, compliance, capacity, tone) is best performed with a computerized barostat that enables distension at a specified and precise rate, thereby minimizing observer bias and measurement error [147]. An 'oversized', non-elastic bag is used (which can be regarded as infinitely compliant and whose properties have no influence on internal pressure). However, this test is time-consuming and reserved for highly selected patients in specialised practice.

Anal sensation can be quantified through mucosal electrostimulation via a catheter-mounted bipolar ring electrode inserted into the anal canal. Rectal sensation can also (as an alternative to mechanical distension) be assessed using this method. Anal mucosal sensitivity thresholds elevated beyond the normal range (i.e. anal hyposensitivity) have been reported in patients with FI [89, 90]. However, although such findings have contributed to our understanding of the pathophysiology of FI, assessment of mucosal electrosensitivity is not currently considered routine.

Neurophysiological Tests

It has long been recognised that anal sphincter dysfunction may be related to denervation injury [75], and thus neurophysiological assessment of the pelvic floor is indicated in patients with FI. Diagnostic neurophysiological tests can enable characterisation of nerve, muscle and neuromuscular junction integrity, help localise the nerve injury, and may also provide a measure of severity. The mainstay of investigation in the 1980s and 1990s was electromyography and evaluation of pudendal nerve terminal motor latencies [143, 146, 147].

Electromyography (EMG)

Recording of pelvic floor EMG (from both the EAS and puborectalis) enables: (1) mapping of the EAS to identify sphincter defects; (2) determination of striated muscle function; and (3) assessment of denervation-reinnervation potentials, indicative of neural injury [143]. Studies of EMG activity can be performed using a needle (either a concentric needle, which samples approximately 30 motor units simultaneously, or a single-fibre electrode, which samples only one motor unit at a time), skin, or anal plug electrodes. Disposable needle electrodes are usually favoured, and are inserted transcutaneously with or without topical anaesthesia into the four quadrants of the external anal sphincter and also through the EAS into the deeper puborectalis, by a midline approach between the anus and tip of the coccyx.

Concentric needle electrodes enable measurement of insertional and spontaneous activities, and also motor unit action potential morphology (duration, amplitude, percentage polyphasia) and recruitment during voluntary or reflex (e.g. cough) muscle contraction [158, 159]. With single-fibre electrodes, fibre density can be calculated, which is an index of motor unit grouping, a consequence of denervation and subsequent reinnervation [158].

Despite its recognised utility, the routine use of EMG studies is diminishing in clinical practice, as it has been superseded by endo-anal ultrasonography for the identification of muscle defects. More commonly now, EMG signals derived from an anal plug electrode are used to facilitate biofeedback for pelvic floor retraining.

Pudendal Nerve Terminal Motor Latencies (PNTML)

PNTML is a measurement of the conduction time from stimulation of the pudendal nerve to EAS contraction and hence allows evaluation of neuromuscular integrity. Stimulation of the pudendal nerve generates a compound muscle action potential (CMAP) response of the EAS which can be recorded by surface electrodes [143]. This is achieved using a disposable bipolar electrode (St. Mark's pudendal electrode) consisting of flexible printed circuits and pairs of stimulating and recording electrodes attached to a suitable EMG machine. The electrode is mounted on the index finger of a gloved hand which is then inserted into the anorectum so that the recording electrodes, located at the base of the finger, are sited within the anus at the level of the EAS. The electrodes, located at the tip of the finger, can stimulate the pudendal nerve as it courses around the pelvic brim through palpation of the ischial spines on either side and application of intermittent electrical pulses; to ensure that all motor fibres within the nerve are stimulated, a supramaximal stimulus should be used. A number of CMAP responses should be elicited bilaterally to provide reproducibility of the response. Prolonged latencies are used as a surrogate marker of pudendal motor neuropathy [145] and are commonly found in patients with FI who have suffered obstetric trauma [81, 82]. Nevertheless, given concerns over test validity, assessment of PNTML is now not routinely advocated [3, 160].

Contemporary Neurophysiological Investigation

The integrity of cortico- and spino-anorectal descending (efferent) neuronal pathways governing anorectal function can be assessed by magnetic stimulation of the cortex and lumbosacral regions overlying the nerve plexi, and recording motor evoked potentials from the rectum or EAS [93]. Peripheral neuropathy may be better delineated using this technique than assessment of PNTML alone [93]. However, combining measurement of PTNML and sacral root terminal motor latencies allows study of both the proximal and distal pudendal nerve, thus enabling better localisation of neuropathy [161].

Somatosensory evoked potentials (EP) allow interrogation of the whole afferent pathway and higher centre processing; these are measured by applying a peripheral stimulus and recording evoked potentials from the central nervous system [143]. The transmission and processing of sensory information from the anus and/or rectum to the brain may be assessed using cortical evoked potentials (CEP). These are measurements of the electrical potentials generated by cortical neurons in response to a series of repeated sensory stimuli. Both mechanical [162, 163] and electrical stimulation [94, 162] has been used, with the former being more reliable for recording CEPs [162]. In patients with FI, both rectal [163] and anal EP latencies [94, 163] have been shown to be prolonged, indicating anorectal afferent pathway dysfunction, along with reduced area of cortical activation [94].

Greater detail on pelvic floor and anal sphincter neuropathy after childbirth is given in Chap. 17.

14.4.1.2 Imaging of Anal and Pelvic Floor Structure

Several diagnostic imaging modalities are available to study anorectal and pelvic floor *structure*. However, it must be acknowledged that the incorporation of protocols that detect dynamic changes in structure with time or provocation (e.g. defaecography) means that they are also, *de facto*, tests of function.

Ultrasound

Endo-anal ultrasonography (EAUS) [164] is a simple and well-tolerated technique recognised as the gold-standard imaging modality for the diagnosis and assessment of anal sphincter injury. It has substantially increased our understanding of the pathogenesis of FI. Contemporary scanners primarily utilise a rotating ultrasound crystal to acquire cross-sectional 360° axial images of the tubular anal canal. Modern systems allow continuous capturing of images as the EAUS transducer is withdrawn through the anal canal with *post hoc* multiplanar 3D image reconstruction.

On EAUS scanning, the IAS may be classified as normal or pathological, with the latter defined by: (1) sphincter discontinuity (defect); (2) atrophy or degeneration (diffuse thinning of the sphincter [thickness $\leq$ 1 mm]) [165]; or (3) hypertrophy (as seen with rectal intussusception or prolapse) [70]. The EAS may be characterized as normal or with a sphincter discontinuity (defect) or interruption of its fibrillar echotexture manifest as focal thinning, scarring, or atrophy. All abnormalities may be described in cross-section according to a clock face (e.g. defect between 1 and 3 o'clock), and also in the longitudinal plane. EAS disruption is a characteristic feature of obstetric anal sphincter injury, often associated with anal hypocontractility [146].

A more detailed description of anal sphincter ultrasonographic imaging allied to obstetric trauma is provided in Chap. 15.

More recently, pelvic floor ultrasound (integrating endoanal, transvaginal and transperineal ultrasound) has been used to also assess pelvic organ prolapse (i.e. rectocoele, enterocoele, intussusception, cystocoele, perineal descent) and levator plate integrity [73, 166, 167]. Transperineal ultrasound is performed with the patient placed in the dorsal lithotomy position with the hips flexed using a curved array probe. Assessment is in real time and dynamic but more operator-dependent than the alternative methods of imaging.

Magnetic Resonance Imaging (MRI)

Endoanal or pelvic MRI are alternative imaging modalities available in specialist centres that enable high-resolution imaging, particularly of the EAS. For example, MRI can differentiate between defects, scaring and atrophy, and can also visualise surrounding structures pertinent to pelvic organ prolapse and FI (e.g. pubovisceral avulsion) [107, 168].

14.4.1.3   Tests of Evacuatory Function

As an evacuation disorder and incomplete rectal emptying may predispose to FI [12], assessment of defaecatory function in patients with coexistent symptoms of FI and constipation should be considered [12, 13]. The goal of testing is to diagnose underlying cause(s) of evacuatory dysfunction; this can be broadly categorised as 'functional' (e.g. dyssynergia, poor propulsive force) or 'structural' (e.g. retaining rectocoele, obstructing intussusception, enterocoele etc.) [143]. Several modalities are available and can be grouped as the following:

1. direct tests (balloon expulsion test and defaecography), which employ evacuation of a stool surrogate;
2. indirect tests (manometry and transperineal/pelvic floor ultrasound), which measure variables deemed to be biologically relevant to the process of defaecation. Unfortunately, it is unclear which test can be regarded as the 'gold standard', and agreement between results of testing is poor [169].

Direct Tests

Balloon Expulsion Test

The balloon expulsion test (BET) is a simple, inexpensive, office-based investigation for the diagnosis of impaired evacuation. With the patient lying in the left lateral position, a lubricated, preferably non-latex balloon attached to a plastic catheter is inserted into the rectum and inflated with 50 ml of warm water. The patient is then transferred to a private commode and asked to expel the balloon. Inability to expel the balloon within a given timeframe is indicative of evacuatory dysfunction. However, the method is poorly standardised (cut-offs for "normality" vary greatly from 22 s to 5 min [170–174]), and the BET cannot provide information regarding functional or anatomical phenomena that may impair evacuation [143, 146]. Further, the use of a small balloon is criticised as a poor analogue for stool as it may not generate a normal urge to defaecate [175].

Defaecography

Defaecography provides a real-time anatomical and dynamic study of the act of (simulated) defaecation (Fig. 14.4). It is the only direct test of evacuation which provides detail of structural features (Fig. 14.4c and d) that may impede rectal emptying, and identifies 'functional' obstructive causes (Fig. 14.4b) [176]. It may be performed using fluoroscopy or MRI, with a contrast paste inserted into the rectum to act as a stool surrogate [176].

For fluoroscopic or barium defaecography, the patient is asked to evacuate the contrast paste while seated on a private commode while representative images are acquired. Rectal dimensions, anorectal angles, rectal wall morphological features, perineal descent and evacuatory efficacy (rate, percentage of contrast expelled) can all be measured. Similarly, the ability to co-ordinate the pelvic floor musculature during evacuatory manoeuvres is assessed [176]. Truly pathological obstructive features (e.g. rectocoele >4 cm in size, enterocoele, high-grade intussusception: Fig. 14.4c and d) have now been defined [176, 177]. In comparison with other tests of evacuatory function (as above), defaecography, when performed in the sitting position with a native urge to defaecate, provides better overall evaluation of the defaecatory process and the structure and function of the anorectum [143, 146, 178]. Nevertheless, barium defaecography does not image soft tissues and requires the use of ionising radiation. Further, there is significant variability in measures used for reporting of results which limits transferability of data [176]. Additionally, there is some overlap of findings between symptomatic and control subjects, especially in parous women [177, 179].

MRI defaecography involves semi-filling the rectum with a stool substitute (e.g. ultrasound gel) mixed with contrast agent if necessary. It can be performed either with the patient supine, within a closed-configuration magnet, or upright (sitting) within an open-configuration system. Lack of widespread availability of the latter, however, means that the majority of studies are performed with the patient in a non-physiological supine position; this certainly has limitations. However, MR imaging has advantages over barium defaecography in that it lacks exposure to ionising radiation and provides excellent multiplanar soft tissue resolution of all pelvic floor compartments and supporting structures, enabling assessment of coexisting utero-vaginal prolapse [180].

Various grading systems exist for defining structural abnormalities and pelvic organ descent, both for barium [181–183] and MRI modalities [184, 185]. These may be used as a basis for guiding therapy, particularly with regard to abnormalities deemed amenable to surgical repair. However, anatomical findings such as a small rectocele or minor intussusception are frequently found in healthy control subjects [177, 181] and failure to recognize such normal variants can lead to over diagnosis. Barium defaecography better detects intussusceptions than MR, either using supine [186] or upright imaging [187], and is more sensitive for identifying retentive rectocoeles [188, 189]. Upright MR defaecography is superior to dynamic supine MR imaging in imaging intussusceptions; diagnostic utility is otherwise equivalent [190].

Indirect Tests (Manometry and Transperineal/Pelvic Floor Ultrasound)

Manometry

As part of the IAPWG standardised manometric protocol [150], the ('push') manoeuvre is widely used to assess rectoanal co-ordination through simultaneous measurement of both anal and rectal pressures during simulated defaecation [146]. However, ARM is not, de facto, a test of evacuation. Abnormal patterns of recto-anal co-ordination on ARM (manifest as poor rectal propulsion and/or anal dyssynergia), should be considered in conjunction with an abnormal direct test of evacuation such as BET or defaecography) to diagnose dyssynergic defaecation, as recognised in the London classification [150]. Nevertheless, interpretation can still be very challenging, as there is a wide overlap of findings between symptomatic and control subjects. In particular, blinded diagnostic accuracy studies suggest that the specificity of previously well-accepted manometric patterns of dyssynergia may be as low as 13% [191].

Pelvic Floor Ultrasound

As above, pelvic floor ultrasound can be used to assess pelvic organ prolapse and has been validated in comparison to defaecography [192–194]. Akin to manometry, however, pelvic floor ultrasound as an indirect test of evacuation cannot determine the *functional* consequences of an observed anatomical 'abnormality'. Therefore, its role in the diagnostic algorithm remains, as yet, undefined. Nevertheless, recent studies show pelvic floor ultrasound to be a reliable assessment tool for defaecatory disorders, and it may be as good as barium defaecography for surgical planning [195].

14.4.1.4   Other Tests

Gut transit studies are usually performed in the context of diagnosing *delayed* transit. In routine clinical practice, this is typically done using radio-opaque markers, although in specialist centres, radionuclide scintigraphy is an alternative [143]. Scintigraphy also lends itself to the assessment of suspected *rapid* gut transit, which may contribute to diarrhoea in FI. Although cut-offs do exist for diagnosing accelerated transit based on the progression of the ingested radionuclide marker [196, 197], this test is limited to tertiary-care centres and patient compliance is an issue (geographic and time constraints, need for repeated daily scans [143]). Another option is ingestible telemetric capsule devices which have been shown to accurately diagnose rapid regional gut transit in conditions characterised by diarrhoea [198, 199]. Large normative reference datasets exist [200, 201], though no studies have been performed to date in FI.

14.5   Conclusion

The maintenance of bowel continence is complex and is the result of a balance between pelvic floor and anal canal 'barrier' function, rectal reservoir storage and evacuatory function, neurological function (both motor and sensory domains), colorectal motility, stool volume and consistency, as well as cognitive function. The pathophysiology of faecal incontinence is usually multifactorial. Although anal sphincter dysfunction may hold primacy in women with early-onset FI following obstetric-related injury, the much higher prevalence of female FI in later life reflects the additive effects of other 'upstream' pathophysio-

logical mechanisms, further insults (often surgical) and ageing.

The majority of patients with mild to moderate symptoms of FI will successfully respond to simple medical or conservative management. However, in those patients in whom such measures have failed, rigorous clinical evaluation incorporating a comprehensive assessment of anorectal structure and function is warranted. Several diagnostic tests with proven clinical utility exist; accurate and objective measurements can identify disease phenotypes, allowing definitive diagnoses that can have a direct impact on treatment decisions in clinical practice.

Take Home Messages
- Diarrhoea (loose stools) is the primary risk factor for the development of FI in the general population.
- Coexistent constipation/evacuatory dysfunction may underlie FI in a significant proportion of patients; management may be better directed at improving completeness of evacuation.
- The pathophysiology of FI involves multiple overlapping mechanisms, not only obstetric-related damage to the anal sphincters and their innervation.
- Complementary diagnostic tests are indicated In patients with refractory symptoms of FI to assess anorectal motor and sensory function, anal and pelvic floor structure and rectal evacuation.

Appendix: MCQ

Mark each item TRUE or FALSE

Questions

1. In the general population, what is the principal recognised risk factor for the development of faecal incontinence?
   (A) Obstetric-related injury to anal sphincters and pelvic floor.
   (B) Anoreceptive sex.
   (C) Diarrhoea/loose stools.
   (D) Obesity.
   (E) Low socioeconomic status.

2. Which anatomical element is *not* involved in closure of the anal canal at rest?
   (A) Anal cushions.
   (B) Myogenic internal anal sphincter activity.
   (C) Nerve-induced internal anal sphincter activity.
   (D) Perianal skin.
   (E) Tonic external anal sphincter activity.

3. Which pathophysiological feature do the majority of women with FI, who have a history of obstetric trauma, exhibit?
   (A) Anal hypotension.
   (B) Voluntary anal hypocontractility.
   (C) Rectal hypersensitivity.
   (D) Accelerated colonic transit.
   (E) Disrupted internal anal sphincter.

4. In a patient with refractory symptoms of faecal urgency and post-defaecation faecal leakage, what is the minimum recommended combination of diagnostic tests that should be undertaken (given that resources allow)?
   (A) High-resolution anorectal manometry and endo-anal ultrasound.
   (B) Conventional anorectal manometry, endo-anal ultrasound and transperineal ultrasound.
   (C) High-resolution anorectal manometry, rectal sensory testing and the balloon expulsion test.
   (D) High-resolution anorectal manometry, rectal sensory testing, pelvic floor EMG, pudendal nerve terminal motor latencies, total pelvic floor ultrasound and MRI defaecography.
   (E) High-resolution anorectal manometry, rectal sensory testing, endo anal ultrasound and defaecography

5. In patients with coexistent faecal incontinence and symptoms of difficulty in rectal evacuation, which test can best discriminate between a 'functional' or 'structural' evacuation disorder?
   (A) x-ray defaecography.
   (B) Transvaginal/transperineal ultrasound.

(C) Balloon expulsion test.
(D) High-definition anorectal manometry in a seated position.
(E) Pelvic MRI

Answers

1. In the general population, what is the principal recognised risk factor for the development of faecal incontinence?
   (A) FALSE
   (B) FALSE
   (C) TRUE
   (D) FALSE
   (E) FALSE

2. Which anatomical element is *not* involved in closure of the anal canal at rest?
   (A) FALSE
   (B) FALSE
   (C) FALSE
   (D) TRUE
   (E) FALSE

3. Which pathophysiological feature do the majority of women with FI, who have a history of obstetric trauma, exhibit?
   (A) FALSE
   (B) TRUE
   (C) FALSE
   (D) FALSE
   (E) FALSE

4. In a patient with refractory symptoms of faecal urgency and post-defaecation faecal leakage, what is the minimum recommended combination of diagnostic tests that should be undertaken (given that resources allow)?
   (A) FALSE
   (B) FALSE
   (C) FALSE
   (D) FALSE
   (E) TRUE

5. In patients with coexistent faecal incontinence and symptoms of difficulty in rectal evacuation, which test can best discriminate between

a 'functional' or 'structural' evacuation disorder?

(A) TRUE
(B) FALSE
(C) FALSE
(D) FALSE
(E) FALSE

References

1. Lunniss PJ, Gladman MA, Hetzer FH, Williams NS, Scott SM. Risk factors in acquired faecal incontinence. J R Soc Med. 2004;97:111–6.
2. Cattani L, Neefs L, Verbakel JY, Bosteels J, Deprest J. Obstetric risk factors for anorectal dysfunction after delivery: a systematic review and meta-analysis. Int Urogynecol J. 2021;32:2325–36.
3. Bharucha AE, Knowles CH, Mack I, Malcolm A, Oblizajek N, Rao S, Scott SM, Shin A, Enck P. Faecal incontinence in adults. Nat Rev Dis Primers. 2022;8:53.
4. Ditah I, Devaki P, Luma HN, Ditah C, Njei B, Jaiyeoba C, Salami A, Ditah C, Ewelukwa O, Szarka L. Prevalence, trends, and risk factors for fecal incontinence in United States adults, 2005-2010. Clin Gastroenterol Hepatol. 2014;12:636–43.e1-2.
5. Ng KS, Sivakumaran Y, Nassar N, Gladman MA. Fecal incontinence: community prevalence and associated factors—a systematic review. Dis Colon Rectum. 2015;58:1194–209.
6. Okeahialam NA, Thakar R, Ilczyszyn A, Sultan AH. Anal and urinary incontinence in nulliparous women—prevalence and associated risk factors. Post Reprod Health. 2021;27:89–97.
7. Al-Mukhtar Othman J, Åkervall S, Nilsson IEK, Molin M, Milsom I, Gyhagen M. Fecal incontinence in non-pregnant nulliparous women aged 25 to 64 years-a randomly selected national cohort prevalence study. Am J Obstet Gynecol. 2022;226:706.e1–706.e23.
8. Bharucha AE, Seide BM, Zinsmeister AR, Melton LJ 3rd. Relation of bowel habits to fecal incontinence in women. Am J Gastroenterol. 2008;103:1470–5.
9. Whitehead WE, Borrud L, Goode PS, Meikle S, Mueller ER, Tuteja A, Weidner A, Weinstein M, Ye W, Pelvic Floor Disorders Network. Fecal incontinence in US adults: epidemiology and risk factors. Gastroenterology. 2009;137:512–7.
10. Bharucha AE, Zinsmeister AR, Schleck CD, Melton LJ 3rd. Bowel disturbances are the most important risk factors for late onset fecal incontinence: a population-based case-control study in women. Gastroenterology. 2010;139:1559–66.
11. Menees SB, Almario CV, Spiegel BMR, Chey WD. Prevalence of and factors associated with fecal incontinence: results from a population-based survey. Gastroenterology. 2018;154:1672–81.e3.
12. Scott SM, Simrén M, Farmer AD, Dinning PG, Carrington EV, Benninga MA, Burgell RE, Dimidi E, Fikree A, Ford AC, Fox M, Hoad CL, Knowles CH, Krogh K, Nugent K, Remes-Troche JM, Whelan K, Corsetti M. Chronic constipation in adults: contemporary perspectives and clinical challenges. 1: epidemiology, diagnosis, clinical associations, pathophysiology and investigation. Neurogastroenterol Motil. 2021;33:e14050.
13. Vollebregt PF, Wiklendt L, Dinning PG, Knowles CH, Scott SM. Coexistent faecal incontinence and constipation: a cross-sectional study of 4027 adults undergoing specialist assessment. EClinicalMedicine. 2020;27:100572.
14. Markland AD, Dunivan GC, Vaughan CP, Rogers RG. Anal intercourse and fecal incontinence: evidence from the 2009-2010 National Health and Nutrition Examination Survey. Am J Gastroenterol. 2016;111:269–74.
15. Gana T, Hunt LM. Young women and anal sex. BMJ. 2022;378:o1975.
16. Vasant DH, Nigam GB, Bate S, Hamdy S, Limdi JK. The prevalence and burden of Rome IV faecal incontinence in ulcerative colitis: a cross-sectional study. Aliment Pharmacol Ther. 2023;58:26–34.
17. Camilleri M, Talley NJ. Pathophysiology as a basis for understanding symptom complexes and therapeutic targets. Neurogastroenterol Motil. 2004;16:135–42.
18. Cauley CE, Savitt LR, Weinstein M, Wakamatsu MM, Kunitake H, Ricciardi R, Staller K, Bordeianou L. A quality-of-life comparison of two fecal incontinence phenotypes: isolated fecal incontinence versus concurrent fecal incontinence with constipation. Dis Colon Rectum. 2019;62:63–70.
19. Brookes SJ, Dinning PG, Gladman MA. Neuroanatomy and physiology of colorectal function and defaecation: from basic science to human clinical studies. Neurogastroenterol Motil. 2009;21(Suppl 2):9–19.
20. Heitmann PT, Vollebregt PF, Knowles CH, Lunniss PJ, Dinning PG, Scott SM. Understanding the physiology of human defaecation and disorders of continence and evacuation. Nat Rev Gastroenterol Hepatol. 2021;18:751–69.
21. Rasmussen OO, Sorensen M, Tetzschner T, Christiansen J. Anorectal pressure gradient in patients with anal incontinence. Dis Colon Rectum. 1992;35:8–11.
22. Trzpis M, Sun G, Chen JH, Huizinga JD, Broens P. Novel insights into physiological mechanisms underlying fecal continence. Am J Physiol Gastrointest Liver Physiol. 2023;324(1):G1–9.
23. Rao SS. Pathophysiology of adult fecal incontinence. Gastroenterology. 2004;126(Suppl 1):S14–22.
24. Thomson H. The anal cushions—a fresh concept in diagnosis. Postgrad Med J. 1979;55:403–5.

25. Gibbons CP, Trowbridge EA, Bannister JJ, Read NW. Role of anal cushions in maintaining continence. Lancet. 1986;1:886–8.

26. Rasmussen OØ. Anorectal function. Dis Colon Rectum. 1994;37:386–403.

27. Parks AG, Porter NH, Melzak J. Experimental study of the reflex mechanism controlling the muscle of the pelvic floor. Dis Colon Rectum. 1962;5:407–14.

28. Parks AG. President's Address. Anorectal incontinence. Proc R Soc Med. 1975;68:681–90.

29. Grigorescu BA, Lazarou G, Olson TR, Downie SA, Powers K, Greston WM, Mikhail MS. Innervation of the levator ani muscles: description of the nerve branches to the pubococcygeus, iliococcygeus, and puborectalis muscles. Int Urogynecol J Pelvic Floor Dysfunct. 2008;19:107–16.

30. Raizada V, Mittal RK. Pelvic floor anatomy and applied physiology. Gastroenterol Clin N Am 2008;37:493–509.

31. Frenckner B, Euler CV. Influence of pudendal block on the function of the anal sphincters. Gut. 1975;16:482–9.

32. Lestar B, Penninckx F, Kerremans R. The composition of anal basal pressure. An in vivo and in vitro study in man. Int J Color Dis. 1989;4:118–22.

33. Keef KD, Cobine CA. Control of motility in the internal anal sphincter. J Neurogastroenterol Motil. 2019;25:189–204.

34. Mittal RK, Bhargava V, Sheean G, Ledgerwood M, Sinha S. Purse-string morphology of external anal sphincter revealed by novel imaging techniques. Am J Physiol Gastrointest Liver Physiol. 2014;306:G505–14.

35. Duthie HL, Watts JM. Contribution of the external anal sphincter to the pressure zone in the anal canal. Gut. 1965;6:64–8.

36. Chan CLH, Ponsford S, Swash M. The anal reflex elicited by cough and sniff: validation of a neglected clinical sign. J Neurol Neurosurg Psychiatry. 2004;75:1449–51.

37. Frenckner B, Ihre T. Influence of autonomic nerves on the internal and sphincter in man. Gut. 1976;17:306–12.

38. Hieda K, Cho KH, Arakawa T, Fujimiya M, Murakami G, Matsubara A. Nerves in the intersphincteric space of the human anal canal with special reference to their continuation to the enteric nerve plexus of the rectum. Clin Anat. 2013;26:843–54.

39. Kinugasa Y, Arakawa T, Murakami G, Fujimiya M, Sugihara K. Nerve supply to the internal anal sphincter differs from that to the distal rectum: an immunohistochemical study of cadavers. Int J Color Dis. 2014;29:429–36.

40. Snooks SJ, Swash M. The innervation of the muscles of continence. Ann R Coll Surg Engl. 1986;68:45–9.

41. Gagnard C, Godlewski G, Prat D, Lan O, Cousineau J, Maklouf Y. The nerve branches to the external anal sphincter: the macroscopic supply and microscopic structure. Surg Radiol Anat. 1986;8:115–9.

42. Duthie HL, Gairns FW. Sensory nerve-endings and sensation in the anal region of man. Br J Surg. 1960;47:585–95.

43. Gould RP. Sensory innervation of the anal canal. Nature. 1960;187:337–8.

44. Miller R, Lewis GT, Bartolo DC, Cervero F, Mortensen NJ. Sensory discrimination and dynamic activity in the anorectum: evidence using a new ambulatory technique. Br J Surg. 1988;75:1003–7.

45. Huizinga JD, Liu L, Barbier A, Chen JH. Distal colon motor coordination: the role of the coloanal reflex and the rectoanal inhibitory reflex in sampling, flatulence, and defecation. Front Med (Lausanne). 2021;8:720558.

46. Sultan AH, Kamm MA, Hudson CN, Thomas JM, Bartram CI. Anal-sphincter disruption during vaginal delivery. N Engl J Med. 1993;329:1905–11.

47 Oberwalder M, Dinnewitzer A, Baig MK, Thaler K, Cotman K, Nogueras JJ, Weiss EG, Efron J, Vernava AM 3rd, Wexner SD. The association between late-onset fecal incontinence and obstetric anal sphincter defects. Arch Surg. 2004;139:429–32.

48. Sideris M, McCaughey T, Hanrahan JG, Arroyo-Manzano D, Zamora J, Jha S, Knowles CH, Thakar R, Chaliha C, Thangaratinam S. Risk of obstetric anal sphincter injuries (OASIS) and anal incontinence: a meta-analysis. Eur J Obstet Gynecol Reprod Biol. 2020;252:303–12.

49. Engel AF, Kamm MA, Bartram CI, Nicholls RJ. Relationship of symptoms in faecal incontinence to specific sphincter abnormalities. Int J Color Dis. 1995;10:152–5.

50. Vaizey CJ, Kamm MA, Bartram CI. Primary degeneration of the internal anal sphincter as a cause of passive faecal incontinence. Lancet. 1997;349:612–5.

51. Friedman T, Eslick GD, Dietz HP. Delivery mode and the risk of levator muscle avulsion: a meta-analysis. Int Urogynecol J. 2019;30:901–7.

52. Pipitone F, Miller JM, DeLancey J. Injury-associated levator ani muscle and anal sphincter ooedema following vaginal birth: a secondary analysis of the EMRLD study. BJOG. 2021;128:2046–53.

53. Fernandez-Fraga X, Azpiroz F, Malagelada JR. Significance of pelvic floor muscles in anal incontinence. Gastroenterology. 2002;123:1441–50.

54. Handa VL, Blomquist JL, Roem J, Muñoz A, Dietz HP. Pelvic floor disorders after obstetric avulsion of the levator ani muscle. Female Pelvic Med Reconstr Surg. 2019;25:3–7.

55. Melendez-Munoz J, Subramanian N, Friedman T, Dietz HP. Is levator trauma an independent risk factor for anal incontinence? Color Dis. 2020;22:298–302.

56. Carrington EV, Brokjaer A, Craven H, Zarate N, Horrocks EJ, Palit S, Jackson W, Duthie GS, Knowles CH, Lunniss PJ, Scott SM. Traditional measures of normal anal sphincter function using high-resolution anorectal manometry (HRAM) in 115 healthy volunteers. Neurogastroenterol Motil. 2014;26:625–35.

57. Wynne JM, Myles JL, Jones I, Sapsford R, Young RE, Hattam A, Cantamessa SE. Disturbed anal sphincter function following vaginal delivery. Gut. 1996;39:120–4.

58. Chaliha C, Sultan AH, Bland JM, Monga AK, Stanton SL. Anal function: effect of pregnancy and delivery. Am J Obstet Gynecol. 2001;185:427–32.

59. Yilmaz E, Nas T, Korucuoglu U, Guler I. Manometric evaluation of anal sphincter function after vaginal and cesarean delivery. Int J Gynaecol Obstet. 2008;103:162–5.

60. Rasijeff AM, García-Zermeño K, Di Tanna GL, Remes-Troche JM, Knowles CH, Scott SM. Systematic review and meta-analysis of anal motor and rectal sensory dysfunction in patients undergoing anorectal manometry for symptoms of fecal incontinence. Color Dis. 2022;24:562–76.

61. Athanasakos EP, Ward HC, Williams NS, Scott SM. Importance of extrasphincteric mechanisms in the pathophysiology of faecal incontinence in adults with a history of anorectal anomaly. Br J Surg. 2008;95:1394–400.

62. Scott SM, Lunniss PJ. Risk factors in faecal incontinence. In: Ratto C, Doglietto GB, editors. Fecal incontinence. Diagnosis and treatment. London, UK: Springer-Verlag London Ltd; 2007. p. 43–66.

63. Boyle DJ, Knowles CH, Murphy J, Bhan C, Williams NS, Scott SM, Lunniss PJ. The effects of age and childbirth on anal sphincter function and morphology in 999 symptomatic female patients with colorectal dysfunction. Dis Colon Rectum. 2012;55:286–93.

64. Fynes M, Donnelly V, Behan M, O'Connell PR, O'Herlihy C. Effect of second vaginal delivery on anorectal physiology and faecal continence: a prospective study. Lancet. 1999;354:983–6.

65. Fornell EU, Matthiesen L, Sjodahl R, Berg G. Obstetric anal sphincter injury ten years after: subjective and objective long term effects. BJOG. 2005;112:312–6.

66. Jordan PA, Naidu M, Thakar R, Sultan AH. Effect of subsequent vaginal delivery on bowel symptoms and anorectal function in women who sustained a previous obstetric anal sphincter injury. Int Urogynecol J. 2018;29:1579–88.

67. Zetterstrom J, Mellgren A, Jensen LL, Wong WD, Kim DG, Lowry AC, Madoff RD, Congilosi SM. Effect of delivery on anal sphincter morphology and function. Dis Colon Rectum. 1999;42:1253–60.

68. Damon H, Henry L, Bretones S, Mellier G, Minaire Y, Mion F. Postdelivery anal function in primiparous females: ultrasound and manometric study. Dis Colon Rectum. 2000;43:472–7.

69. Loos M, Quentmeier P, Schuster T, Nitsche U, Gertler R, Keerl A, Kocher T, Friess H, Rosenberg R. Effect of preoperative radio(chemo)therapy on long-term functional outcome in rectal cancer patients: a systematic review and meta-analysis. Ann Surg Oncol. 2013;20:1816–28.

70. Dvorkin LS, Chan CL, Knowles CH, Williams NS, Lunniss PJ, Scott SM. Anal sphincter morphology in patients with full-thickness rectal prolapse. Dis Colon Rectum. 2004;47:198–203.

71. Harmston C, Jones OM, Cunningham C, Lindsey I. The relationship between internal rectal prolapse and internal anal sphincter function. Color Dis. 2011;13:791–5.

72. Tsunoda A, Takahashi T, Kusanagi H. Absence of a rectocele may be correlated with reduced internal anal sphincter function in patients with rectal intussusception and fecal incontinence. Int J Color Dis. 2019;34:1681–7.

73. van Delft K, Sultan AH, Thakar R, Schwertner-Tiepelmann N, Kluivers K. The relationship between postpartum levator ani muscle avulsion and signs and symptoms of pelvic floor dysfunction. BJOG. 2014;121:1164–71.

74. Petros PE, Swash M. The musculoelastic theory of anorectal function and dysfunction. J Pelviperineology. 2008;27:89–93.

75. Parks AG, Swash M, Urich H. Sphincter denervation in anorectal incontinence and rectal prolapse. Gut. 1977;18:656–65.

76. Neill ME, Swash M. Increased motor unit fibre density in the external anal sphincter muscle in ano-rectal incontinence: a single fibre EMG study. J Neurol Neurosurg Psychiatry. 1980;43:343–7.

77. Snooks SJ, Setchell M, Swash M, Henry MM. Injury to innervation of pelvic floor sphincter musculature in childbirth. Lancet. 1984;2:546–50.

78. Allen RE, Hosker GL, Smith AR, Warrell DW. Pelvic floor damage and childbirth: a neurophysiological study. Br J Obstet Gynaecol. 1990;97:770–9.

79. Kiff ES, Swash M. Slowed conduction in the pudendal nerves in idiopathic (neurogenic) faecal incontinence. Br J Surg. 1984;71:614–6.

80. Donnelly V, Fynes M, Campbell D, Johnson H, O'Connell PR, O'Herlihy C. Obstetric events leading to anal sphincter damage. Obstet Gynecol. 1998;92:955–61.

81. Snooks SJ, Swash M, Mathers SE, Henry MM. Effect of vaginal delivery on the pelvic floor: a 5-year follow-up. Br J Surg. 1990;77:1358–60.

82. Sultan AH, Kamm MA, Hudson CN. Pudendal nerve damage during labour: prospective study before and after childbirth. Br J Obstet Gynaecol. 1994;101:22–8.

83. Tetzschner T, Sorensen M, Jønsson L, Lose G, Christiansen J. Delivery and pudendal nerve function. Acta Obstet Gynecol Scand. 1997;76:324–31.

84. Richter HE, Brumfield CG, Cliver SP, Burgio KL, Neely CL, Varner RE. Risk factors associated with anal sphincter tear: a comparison of primiparous patients, vaginal births after cesarean deliveries, and patients with previous vaginal delivery. Am J Obstet Gynecol. 2002;187:1194–8.

85. Christianson LM, Bovbjerg VE, McDavitt EC, Hullfish KL. Risk factors for perineal injury during delivery. Am J Obstet Gynecol. 2003;189:255–60.

86. Rieger N, Wattchow D. The effect of vaginal delivery on anal function. Aust N Z J Surg. 1999;69:172–7.

87. Pollack J, Nordenstam J, Brismar S, Lopez A, Altman D, Zetterstrom J. Anal incontinence after vaginal delivery: a five-year prospective cohort study. Obstet Gynecol. 2004;104:1397–402.

88. Fynes M, Donnelly VS, O'Connell PR, O'Herlihy C. Cesarean delivery and anal sphincter injury. Obstet Gynecol. 1998;92:496–500.

89. Roe AM, Bartolo DC, Mortensen NJ. New method for assessment of anal sensation in various anorectal disorders. Br J Surg. 1986;73:310–2.

90. Vasudevan SP, Scott SM, Gladman MA, Lunniss PJ. Rectal hyposensitivity: evaluation of anal sensation in female patients with refractory constipation with and without faecal incontinence. Neurogastroenterol Motil. 2007;19:660–7.

91. Cornes H, Bartolo DC, Stirrat GM. Changes in anal canal sensation after childbirth. Br J Surg. 1991;78:74–7.

92. Paris G, Chastan N, Gourcerol G, Verin E, Menard JF, Michot F, Weber J, Leroi AM. Evoked pressure curves from the external anal sphincter following transcranial magnetic stimulation in healthy volunteers and patients with faecal incontinence. Color Dis. 2013;15:e732–40.

93. Rao SS, Coss-Adame E, Tantiphlachiva K, Attaluri A, Remes-Troche J. Translumbar and transsacral magnetic neurostimulation for the assessment of neuropathy in fecal incontinence. Dis Colon Rectum. 2014;57:645–52.

94. Mundet L, Cabib C, Ortega O, Rofes L, Tomsen N, Marin S, Chacón C, Clavé P. Defective conduction of anorectal afferents is a very prevalent pathophysiological factor associated to fecal incontinence in women. J Neurogastroenterol Motil. 2019;25:423–35.

95. Xiang X, Patcharatrakul T, Sharma A, Parr R, Hamdy S, Rao SSC. Cortico-anorectal, spino-anorectal, and cortico-spinal nerve conduction and locus of neuronal injury in patients with fecal incontinence. Clin Gastroenterol Hepatol. 2019;17:1130–7.e2.

96. Rao SSC, Yan Y, Xiang X, Sharma A, Ayyala D, Hamdy S. Effects of translumbosacral neuromodulation therapy on gut and brain interactions and anorectal neuropathy in fecal incontinence: a randomized study. Neuromodulation. 2021;24:1269–77.

97. D'Souza N, de Neree Tot Babberich MPM, d'Hoore A, Tiret E, Xynos E, RGH B-T, Nagtegaal ID, Blomqvist L, Holm T, Glimelius B, Lacy A, Cervantes A, Glynne-Jones R, West NP, Perez RO, Quadros C, Lee KY, Madiba TE, Wexner SD, Garcia-Aguilar J, Sahani D, Moran B, Tekkis P, Rutten HJ, Tanis PJ, Wiggers T, Brown G. Definition of the rectum: an International, expert-based Delphi consensus. Ann Surg. 2019;270:955–9.

98. Shafik A, Doss S, Ali YA, Shafik AA. Transverse folds of rectum: anatomic study and clinical implications. Clin Anat. 2001;14:196–203.

99. McNeil NI, Rampton DS. Is the rectum usually empty? A quantitative study in subjects with and without diarrhea. Dis Colon Rectum. 1981;24:596–9.

100. Sagar PM, Pemberton JH. Anorectal and pelvic floor function. Relevance of continence, incontinence, and constipation. Gastroenterol Clin N Am. 1996;25:163–82.

101. Andrews C, Bharucha AE, Seide B, Zinsmeister AR. Rectal sensorimotor dysfunction in women with fecal incontinence. Am J Physiol Gastrointest Liver Physiol. 2007;292:G282–9.

102. Bharucha AE. Fecal incontinence. Gastroenterology. 2003;124:1672–85.

103. Chan CL, Scott SM, Williams NS, Lunniss PJ. Rectal hypersensitivity worsens stool frequency, urgency, and lifestyle in patients with urge fecal incontinence. Dis Colon Rectum. 2005;48:134–40.

104. Gladman MA, Scott SM, Chan CL, Williams NS, Lunniss PJ. Rectal hyposensitivity: prevalence and clinical impact in patients with intractable constipation and fecal incontinence. Dis Colon Rectum. 2003;46:238–46.

105. Rao SS, Read NW, Davison PA, Bannister JJ, Holdsworth CD. Anorectal sensitivity and responses to rectal distention in patients with ulcerative colitis. Gastroenterology. 1987;93:1270–5.

106. Chan CL, Lunniss PJ, Wang D, Williams NS, Scott SM. Rectal sensorimotor dysfunction in patients with urge faecal incontinence: evidence from prolonged manometric studies. Gut. 2005;54:1263–72.

107. Bharucha AE, Fletcher JG, Harper CM, Hough D, Daube JR, Stevens C, Seide B, Riederer SJ, Zinsmeister AR. Relationship between symptoms and disordered continence mechanisms in women with idiopathic faecal incontinence. Gut. 2005;54:546–55.

108. Gladman MA, Aziz Q, Scott SM, Williams NS, Lunniss PJ. Rectal hyposensitivity: pathophysiological mechanisms. Neurogastroenterol Motil. 2009;21:508–16.

109. Nordenstam JF, Altman DH, Mellgren AF, Rothenberger DA, Zetterström JP. Impaired rectal sensation at anal manometry is associated with anal incontinence one year after primary sphincter repair in primiparous women. Dis Colon Rectum. 2010;53:1409–14.

110. Buser WD, Miner PB Jr. Delayed rectal sensation with fecal incontinence. Successful treatment using anorectal manometry Gastroenterology. 1986;91:1186–91.

111. Sun WM, Read NW, Miner PB. Relation between rectal sensation and anal function in normal subjects and patients with faecal incontinence. Gut. 1990;31:1056–61.

112. Lubowski DZ, Nicholls RJ. Faecal incontinence associated with reduced pelvic sensation. Br J Surg. 1988;75:1086–8.

113. Knowles CH, Dinning P, Scott SM, Swash M, de Wachter S. New concepts in the pathophysiology of fecal incontinence. Ann Laparosc Endosc Surg. 2022;7:15.

114. Rex DK, Lappas JC. Combined anorectal manometry and defecography in 50 consecutive adults with fecal incontinence. Dis Colon Rectum. 1992;35:1040–5.

115. Rao SS, Ozturk R, Stessman M. Investigation of the pathophysiology of fecal seepage. Am J Gastroenterol. 2004;99:2204–9.

116. Damon H, Guye O, Seigneurin A, Long F, Sonko A, Faucheron JL, Grandjean JP, Mellier G, Valancogne G, Fayard MO, Henry L, Guyot P, Barth X, Mion F. Prevalence of anal incontinence in adults and impact on quality-of-life. Gastroenterol Clin Biol. 2006;30:37–43.

117. Nurko S, Scott SM. Coexistence of constipation and incontinence in children and adults. Best Pract Res Clin Gastroenterol. 2011;25:29–41.

118. Brochard C, Chambaz M, Ropert A, l'Héritier AM, Wallenhorst T, Bouguen G, Siproudhis L. Quality of life in 1870 patients with constipation and/or fecal incontinence: constipation should not be underestimated. Clin Res Hepatol Gastroenterol. 2019;43:682–7.

119. Shatari T, Hayes J, Pretlove S, Toosz-Hobson P, Radley S, Keighley MR. Importance of evacuatory disturbance in evaluation of faecal incontinence after third degree obstetric tear. Color Dis. 2005;7:18–21.

120. Speksnijder L, Oom DMJ, de Leeuw JW, Steensma AB. Which factors are associated with anal incontinence after obstetric anal sphincter injury? Ultrasound Obstet Gynecol. 2021;58:476–82.

121. Swash M, Snooks SJ, Henry MM. Unifying concept of pelvic floor disorders and incontinence. J R Soc Med. 1985;78:906–11.

122. Gladman MA, Lunniss PJ, Scott SM, Swash M. Rectal hyposensitivity. Am J Gastroenterol. 2006;101:1140–51.

123. Vollebregt PF, Burgell RE, Hooper RL, Knowles CH, Scott SM. Clinical impact of rectal hyposensitivity: a cross-sectional study of 2,876 patients with refractory functional constipation. Am J Gastroenterol. 2021;116:758–68.

124. Slawik S, Soulsby R, Carter H, Payne H, Dixon AR. Laparoscopic ventral rectopexy, posterior colporrhaphy and vaginal sacrocolpopexy for the treatment of recto-genital prolapse and mechanical outlet obstruction. Color Dis. 2008;10:138–43.

125. Sung VW, Rardin CR, Raker CA, LaSala CA, Myers DL. Changes in bowel symptoms 1 year after rectocele repair. Am J Obstet Gynecol. 2012;207:423.e1–5.

126. Formijne Jonkers HA, Poierrié N, Draaisma WA, Broeders IA, Consten EC. Laparoscopic ventral rectopexy for rectal prolapse and symptomatic rectocele: an analysis of 245 consecutive patients. Color Dis. 2013;15:695–9.

127. Koch SM, Melenhorst J, van Gemert WG, Baeten CG. Prospective study of colonic irrigation for the treatment of defaecation disorders. Br J Surg. 2008;95:1273–9.

128. Woodward S. Treating chronic constipation and faecal incontinence using transanal irrigation. Br J Nurs. 2017;26:1220–2.

129. Lin AY, Du P, Dinning PG, Arkwright JW, Kamp JP, Cheng LK, Bissett IP, O'Grady G. High-resolution anatomic correlation of cyclic motor patterns in the human colon: evidence of a rectosigmoid brake. Am J Physiol Gastrointest Liver Physiol. 2017;312:G508–15.

130. Ballantyne GH. Rectosigmoid sphincter of O'Beirne. Dis Colon Rectum. 1986;29:525–31.

131. Wadhwa RP, Mistry FP, Bhatia SJ, Abraham P. Existence of a high pressure zone at the rectosigmoid junction in normal Indian men. Dis Colon Rectum. 1996;39:1122–5.

132. Chen JH, Nirmalathasan S, Pervez M, Milkova N, Huizinga JD. The sphincter of O'Beirne—part 1: study of 18 normal subjects. Dig Dis Sci. 2021;66:3516–28.

133. Patton V, Wiklendt L, Arkwright JW, Lubowski DZ, Dinning PG. The effect of sacral nerve stimulation on distal colonic motility in patients with faecal incontinence. Br J Surg. 2013;100:959–68.

134. Lin AY, Varghese C, Paskaranandavadivel N, Seo S, Du P, Dinning P, Bissett IP, O'Grady G. Faecal incontinence is associated with an impaired rectosigmoid brake and improved by sacral neuromodulation. Color Dis. 2022;24:1556–66.

135. Chaichanavichkij P, Hartmann M, Scott SM, Fenton N, Knowles CH. Evaluating the risk factors for the development of benign disorders of defaecation: a surgical perspective. Tech Coloproctol. 2023;27(10):847–57.

136. Bouchoucha M, Devroede G, Faye A, Arsac M. Importance of colonic transit evaluation in the management of fecal incontinence. Int J Color Dis. 2002;17:412–7.

137. Chey WY, Jin HO, Lee MH, Sun SW, Lee KY. Colonic motility abnormality in patients with irritable bowel syndrome exhibiting abdominal pain and diarrhea. Am J Gastroenterol. 2001;96:1499–506.

138. Wiklendt L, Mohd Rosli R, Kumar R, Paskaranandavadivel N, Bampton PA, Maslen L, Costa M, Brookes SJ, O'Grady G, Dinning PG. Inhibited postprandial retrograde cyclic motor pattern in the distal colon of patients with diarrhea predominant irritable bowel syndrome. Am J Physiol Gastrointest Liver Physiol. 2023;325(1):G62–79.

139. Madoff RD, Parker SC, Varma MG, Lowry AC. Faecal incontinence in adults. Lancet. 2004;364:621–32.

140. Gladman MA, Scott SM, Williams NS. An overview. Assessing the patient with fecal incontinence. In: Zbar AP, Pescatori M, Wexner SD, editors. Complex anorectal disorders—investigation and management. London, UK: Springer-Verlag, London Ltd; 2005. p. 547–94.

141. Paquette IM, Varma MG, Kaiser AM, Steele SR, Rafferty JF. The American Society of Colon and

Rectal Surgeons' Clinical Practice Guideline for the treatment of fecal incontinence. Dis Colon Rectum. 2021;64:995–1002.

142. Heaton KW, Radvan J, Cripps H, Mountford RA, Braddon FE, Hughes AO. Defecation frequency and timing, and stool form in the general population: a prospective study. Gut. 1992;33:818–24.

143. Scott SM, Williams AB. Specialist investigation of anorectal and colonic structure and functions. In: Keighley MR, Williams NS, Knowles CH, editors. Surgery of the anus, rectum and colon. 2nd ed. Boca Raton, FL: CRC Press, Taylor Francis Group; 2018. p. 271–304.

144. Shim LS, Jones M, Prott GM, Morris LI, Kellow JE, Malcolm A. Predictors of outcome of anorectal biofeedback therapy in patients with constipation. Aliment Pharmacol Ther. 2011;33:1245–51.

145. Diamant NE, Kamm MA, Wald A, Whitehead WE. American Gastroenterological Association medical position statement on anorectal testing techniques. Gastroenterology. 1999;116:732–60.

146. Carrington EV, Scott SM, Bharucha A, Mion F, Remes-Troche JM, Malcolm A, Heinrich H, Fox M, Rao SS, International Anorectal Physiology Working Group and the International Working Group for Disorders of Gastrointestinal Motility and Function. Expert consensus document: advances in the evaluation of anorectal function. Nat Rev Gastroenterol Hepatol. 2018;15:309–23.

147. Scott SM, Gladman MA. Manometric, sensorimotor, and neurophysiologic evaluation of anorectal function. Gastroenterol Clin N Am. 2008;37:511–38.

148. Carrington EV, Heinrich H, Knowles CH, Rao SS, Fox M, Scott SM, International Anorectal Physiology Working Party Group (IAPWG). Methods of anorectal manometry vary widely in clinical practice: results from an international survey. Neurogastroenterol Motil. 2017;29:e13016.

149. Dinning PG, Carrington EV, Scott SM. Colonic and anorectal motility testing in the high-resolution era. Curr Opin Gastroenterol. 2016;32:44–8.

150. Carrington EV, Heinrich H, Knowles CH, Fox M, Rao S, Altomare DF, Bharucha AE, Burgell R, Chey WD, Chiarioni G, Dinning P, Emmanuel A, Farouk R, RJF F-B, Jung KW, Lembo A, Malcolm A, Mittal RK, Mion F, Myung SJ, O'Connell PR, Pehl C, Remes-Troche JM, Reveille RM, Vaizey CJ, Vitton V, Whitehead WE, Wong RK, Scott SM, All members of the International Anorectal Physiology Working Group. The international anorectal physiology working group (IAPWG) recommendations: standardized testing protocol and the London classification for disorders of anorectal function. Neurogastroenterol Motil. 2020;32:e13679.

151. Oblizajek NR, Gandhi S, Sharma M, Chakraborty S, Muthyala A, Prichard D, Feuerhak K, Bharucha AE. Anorectal pressures measured with high-resolution manometry in healthy people—normal values and asymptomatic pelvic floor dysfunction. Neurogastroenterol Motil. 2019;31:e13597.

152. Nivatvongs S, Stern HS, Fryd DS. The length of the anal canal. Dis Colon Rectum. 1981;24:600–1.

153. Vollebregt PF, Rasijeff AMP, Pares D, Grossi U, Carrington EV, Knowles CH, Scott SM. Functional anal canal length measurement using high-resolution anorectal manometry to investigate anal sphincter dysfunction in patients with fecal incontinence or constipation. Neurogastroenterol Motil. 2019;31:e13532.

154. Chiarioni G, Scattolini C, Bonfante F, Vantini I. Liquid stool incontinence with severe urgency: anorectal function and effective biofeedback treatment. Gut. 1993;34:1576–80.

155. Cattle KR, Telford K, Kiff ES. Changes in fatigability of the striated anal canal after childbirth. Color Dis. 2010;12:880–4.

156. Azpiroz F, Enck P, Whitehead WE. Anorectal functional testing: review of collective experience. Am J Gastroenterol. 2002;97:232–40.

157. Rasijeff AMP, Garcia-Zermeno K, Carrington EV, Knowles C, Scott SM. Systematic evaluation of cough-anorectal pressure responses in health and in fecal incontinence: a high-resolution anorectal manometry study. Neurogastroenterol Motil. 2021;33:e13999.

158. Swash M. Electromyography in pelvic floor disorders. In: Henry MM, Swash M, editors. Coloproctology and the pelvic floor. 2nd ed. Oxford: Butterworth-Heinemann Ltd; 1992. p. 84–195.

159. Lefaucheur JP. Neurophysiological testing in anorectal disorders. Muscle Nerve. 2006;33:324–33.

160. Hill J, Hosker G, Kiff ES. Pudendal nerve terminal motor latency measurements: what they do and do not tell us. Br J Surg. 2002;89:1268–9.

161. Morren GL, Walter S, Lindehammar H, Hallböök O, Sjödahl R. Evaluation of the sacroanal motor pathway by magnetic and electric stimulation in patients with fecal incontinence. Dis Colon Rectum. 2001;44:167–72.

162. Hobday DI, Hobson A, Furlong PL, Thompson DG, Aziz Q. Comparison of cortical potentials evoked by mechanical and electrical stimulation of the rectum. Neurogastroenterol Motil. 2000;12:547–54.

163. Haas S, Brock C, Krogh K, Gram M, Lundby L, Drewes AM, Laurberg S. Abnormal neuronal response to rectal and anal stimuli in patients with idiopathic fecal incontinence. Neurogastroenterol Motil. 2015;27:954–62.

164. Abdool Z, Sultan AH, Thakar R. Ultrasound imaging of the anal sphincter complex: a review. Br J Radiol. 2012;85:865–75.

165. Albuquerque A, Macedo G. Idiopathic internal anal sphincter degeneration: how common is it? Does size really matter? Color Dis. 2017;19:396–7.

166. Hainsworth AJ, Solanki D, Schizas AM, Williams AB. Total pelvic floor ultrasound for pelvic floor defaecatory dysfunction: a pictorial review. Br J Radiol. 2015;88:20150494.

167. Hainsworth A, Solanki D, Ferrari L, Igbedioh C, Johnston L, Morris SJ, Igualada-Martinez P, Schizas AMP, Williams AB. The association between levator plate integrity and pelvic floor defaecatory dysfunction. Neurourol Urodyn. 2023;42:690–8.

168. Heilbrun ME, Nygaard IE, Lockhart ME, Richter HE, Brown MB, Kenton KS, Rahn DD, Thomas JV, Weidner AC, Nager CW, Delancey JO. Correlation between levator ani muscle injuries on magnetic resonance imaging and fecal incontinence, pelvic organ prolapse, and urinary incontinence in primiparous women. Am J Obstet Gynecol. 2010;202:488.e1–6.

169. Palit S, Thin N, Knowles CH, Lunniss PJ, Bharucha AE, Scott SM. Diagnostic disagreement between tests of evacuatory function: a prospective study of 100 constipated patients. Neurogastroenterol Motil. 2016;28:1589–98.

170. Rao SS, Patel RS. How useful are manometric tests of anorectal function in the management of defecation disorders? Am J Gastroenterol. 1997;92:469–75.

171. Rao SS, Azpiroz F, Diamant N, Enck P, Tougas G, Wald A. Minimum standards of anorectal manometry. Neurogastroenterol Motil. 2002;14:553–9.

172. Chiarioni G, Kim SM, Vantini I, Whitehead WE. Validation of the balloon evacuation test: reproducibility and agreement with findings from anorectal manometry and electromyography. Clin Gastroenterol Hepatol. 2014;12:2049–54.

173. Ratuapli S, Bharucha AE, Harvey D, Zinsmeister AR. Comparison of rectal balloon expulsion test in seated and left lateral positions. Neurogastroenterol Motil. 2013;25:e813–20.

174. Chedid V, Vijayvargiya P, Halawi H, Park SY, Camilleri M. Audit of the diagnosis of rectal evacuation disorders in chronic constipation. Neurogastroenterol Motil. 2019;31:e13510.

175. Minguez M, Herreros B, Sanchiz V, Hernandez V, Almela P, Añon R, Mora F, Benages A. Predictive value of the balloon expulsion test for excluding the diagnosis of pelvic floor dyssynergia in constipation. Gastroenterology. 2004;126:57–62.

176. Grossi U, Di Tanna GL, Heinrich H, Taylor SA, Knowles CH, Scott SM. Systematic review with meta-analysis: defecography should be a first-line diagnostic modality in patients with refractory constipation. Aliment Pharmacol Ther. 2018;48:1186–201.

177. Palit S, Bhan C, Lunniss PJ, Boyle DJ, Gladman MA, Knowles CH, Scott SM. Evacuation proctography: a reappraisal of normal variability. Color Dis. 2014;16:538–46.

178. Bharucha AE. Update of tests of colon and rectal structure and function. J Clin Gastroenterol. 2006;40:96–103.

179. Tirumanisetty P, Prichard D, Fletcher JG, Chakraborty S, Zinsmeister AR, Bharucha AE. Normal values for assessment of anal sphincter morphology, anorectal motion, and pelvic organ prolapse with MRI in healthy women. Neurogastroenterol Motil. 2018;30:e13314.

180. Mortele KJ, Fairhurst J. Dynamic MR defecography of the posterior compartment: indications, techniques and MRI features. Eur J Radiol. 2007;61:462–72.

181. Shorvon PJ, McHugh S, Diamant NE, Somers S, Stevenson GW. Defecography in normal volunteers: results and implications. Gut. 1989;30:1737–49.

182. Collinson R, Cunningham C, D'Costa H, Lindsey I. Rectal intussusception and unexplained faecal incontinence: findings of a proctographic study. Color Dis. 2009;11:77–83.

183. Morandi C, Martellucci J, Talento P, Carriero A. Role of enterocele in the obstructed defecation syndrome (ODS): a new radiological point of view. Color Dis. 2010;12:810–6.

184. Roos JE, Weishaupt D, Wildermuth S, Willmann JK, Marincek B, Hilfiker PR. Experience of 4 years with open MR defecography: pictorial review of anorectal anatomy and disease. Radiographics. 2002;22:817–32.

185. Piloni V, Tosi P, Vernelli M. MR-defecography in obstructed defecation syndrome (ODS): technique, diagnostic criteria and grading. Tech Coloproctol. 2013;17:501–10.

186. Pilkington SA, Nugent KP, Brenner J, Harris S, Clarke A, Lamparelli M, Thomas C, Tarver D. Barium proctography vs magnetic resonance proctography for pelvic floor disorders: a comparative study. Color Dis. 2012;14:1224–30.

187. Dvorkin LS, Hetzer F, Scott SM, Williams NS, Gedroyc W, Lunniss PJ. Open-magnet MR defaecography compared with evacuation proctography in the diagnosis and management of patients with rectal intussusception. Color Dis. 2004;6:45–53.

188. van Iersel JJ, Formijne Jonkers HA, Verheijen PM, Broeders IA, Heggelman BG, Sreetharan V, Fütterer JJ, Somers I, van der Leest M, Consten EC. Comparison of dynamic magnetic resonance defaecography with rectal contrast and conventional defaecography for posterior pelvic floor compartment prolapse. Color Dis. 2017;19:O46–53.

189. Zafar A, Seretis C, Feretis M, Karandikar S, Williams SC, Goldstein M, Chapman M. Comparative study of magnetic resonance defaecography and evacuation proctography in the evaluation of obstructed defaecation. Color Dis. 2017;19:O204–O20.

190. Bertschinger KM, Hetzer FH, Roos JE, Treiber K, Marincek B, Hilfiker PR. Dynamic MR imaging of the pelvic floor performed with patient sitting in an open-magnet unit versus with patient supine in a closed-magnet unit. Radiology. 2002;223:501–8.

191. Grossi U, Carrington EV, Bharucha AE, Horrocks EJ, Scott SM, Knowles CH. Diagnostic accuracy study of anorectal manometry for diagnosis of dyssynergic defecation. Gut. 2016;65:447–55.

192. Steensma AB, Oom DM, Burger CW, Schouten WR. Assessment of posterior compartment pro-

lapse: a comparison of evacuation proctography and 3D transperineal ultrasound. Color Dis. 2010;12: 533–9.

193. Martellucci J, Naldini G. Clinical relevance of transperineal ultrasound compared with evacuation proctography for the evaluation of patients with obstructed defaecation. Color Dis. 2011;13:1167–72.

194. Murad-Regadas SM, dos Santos D, Soares G, Regadas FS, Rodrigues LV, Buchen G, Kenmoti VT, Surima WS, Fernandes GO. A novel three-dimensional dynamic anorectal ultrasonography technique for the assessment of perineal descent, compared with defaecography. Color Dis. 2012;14:740–7.

195. Hainsworth AJ, De Robles MS, Ferrari L, Solanki D, Williams AB, Schizas A. Total pelvic floor ultrasound can reliably predict long-term treatment outcomes for patients with pelvic floor defaecatory dysfunction. Neurourol Urodyn. 2023;42:90–7.

196. Manabe N, Wong BS, Camilleri M, Burton D, McKinzie S, Zinsmeister AR. Lower functional gastrointestinal disorders: evidence of abnormal colonic transit in a 287 patient cohort. Neurogastroenterol Motil. 2010;22:293–e82.

197. Maurer AH. Gastrointestinal motility, part 2: small-bowel and colon transit. J Nucl Med. 2015;56:1395–400.

198. Gregersen T, Haase AM, Schlageter V, Gronbaek H, Krogh K. Regional gastrointestinal transit times in patients with carcinoid diarrhea: assessment with the novel 3D-Transit system. J Neurogastroenterol Motil. 2015;30(21):423–32.

199. Sangnes DA, Dimcevski G, Frey J, Søfteland E. Diabetic diarrhoea: a study on gastrointestinal motility, pH levels and autonomic function. J Intern Med. 2021;290:1206–18.

200. Wang YT, Mohammed SD, Farmer AD, Wang D, Zarate N, Hobson AR, Hellström PM, Semler JR, Kuo B, Rao SS, Hasler WL, Camilleri M, Scott SM. Regional gastrointestinal transit and pH studied in 215 healthy volunteers using the wireless motility capsule: influence of age, gender, study country and testing protocol. Aliment Pharmacol Ther. 2015;42:761–72.

201. Nandhra GK, Mark EB, Di Tanna GL, Haase AM, Poulsen J, Christodoulides S, Kung V, Klinge MW, Knudsen K, Borghammer P, Andersen KO, Fynne L, Sutter N, Schlageter V, Krogh K, Drewes AM, Birch M, Scott SM. Normative values for region-specific colonic and gastrointestinal transit times in 111 healthy volunteers using the 3D-Transit electromagnet tracking system: influence of age, gender, and body mass index. Neurogastroenterol Motil. 2020;32:e13734.

Anal Sphincter Imaging of Obstetric Trauma

15

Giulio A. Santoro, Patrizia Pelizzo, and Abdul H. Sultan

Overview

Test your learning and check your understanding of this book's contents: use the "Springer Nature Flashcards" app to access questions using ▶ https://sn.pub/wqrf89. To use the app, please follow the instructions in Chap. 1.

Learning Objectives

- To understand the normal ultrasonographic anatomy of the anal canal
- To understand endoanal ultrasound assessment of obstetrical anal sphincter injuries
- To understand the evaluation of levator ani damage by endovaginal ultrasound, transperineal ultrasound and magnetic resonance imaging
- To understand the role of imaging in the management of obstetric anal sphincter injuries

G. A. Santoro (✉) · P. Pelizzo
Tertiary Referral Pelvic Floor Center, 2nd Division of General Surgery, ULSS2 Marca Trevigiana, University of Padua, Treviso, Italy
e-mail: patrizia.pelizzo@aopd.veneto.it

A. H. Sultan
Croydon University Hospital, London, UK

15.1 Introduction

The most frequent cause of anal incontinence (AI) is childbirth injury to the anal sphincter muscles. Obstetric anal sphincter injury (OASI) is a term used to include third- and fourth-degree tears that occur during vaginal birth and is described in detail in Chap. 3. The incidence of any degree of anal sphincter defects in primiparous women is reported to be as high as 27–33% [1]. Of all women who delivered vaginally, OASIS were diagnosed on ultrasound in 26% (95%CI, 21–30) [2]. Between 4% and 8.5% of multiparous women have a new sphincter defect after subsequent births. In the last two decades, the mean rate of AI following primary repair of OASIs has fallen from 39% [1] to 18% between 22% and 29% depending on the grade of tear [3].

A careful evaluation of OASIs is fundamental to assess the underlying muscular defects and determine the appropriate treatment. Endoanal ultrasonography (EAUS) is the "gold standard" technique for the assessment of anal sphincter integrity [4]. EAUS can identify sphincter lesions (defects, scarring, thinning, thickening, and atrophy) [4, 5] associated with AI after OASIs. In addition, EAUS can demonstrate undiagnosed sphincter tears (previously referred to as occult tears), which are reported in upwards of 33% of primiparous females after vaginal birth [6]. High-resolution three-dimensional (3D) US with multiplanar reconstruction (MPR) has further improved the accuracy of this modality [4, 5]. On the other hand, obstetric damage of the levator ani (LA) and puborectalis (PR) muscles is best assessed by Magnetic Resonance Imaging (MRI) [7, 8], endovaginal (EVUS) [9, 10] or transperineal (TPUS) [11, 12] ultrasound to identify detachment of the muscle fibres from the pubic rami.

Imaging has a crucial role in the management of OASIs [13]. In a study by Faltin et al., when primary repair was performed after EAUS assessment, it was associated with a reduction in severe AI. However, some injuries identified by ultrasound could not be located clinically [14]. The role of TPUS immediately after OASIS repair has also been explored, but its value was found to be limited [15]. Imaging also has a role in the evaluation of persistent sphincter defects after repair and in the decision of mode of birthing subsequent pregnancies [16] (Level of evidence: 3).

15.2 Three-Dimensional Endoanal Ultrasound (3D EAUS)

EAUS is performed with the patient placed in dorsal lithotomy, prone or, more commonly, the left lateral position by a mechanical rotating 360-degree (9–16 MHz frequencies) transducer (Fig. 15.1). On the screen, the image is oriented with the anterior at 12 o'clock, left lateral at 3 o'clock, posterior at 6 o'clock and right lateral at

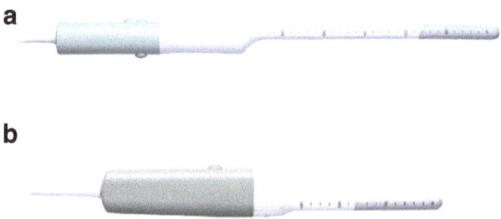

Fig. 15.1 Endocavitary 3D 20R3 (9052) mechanical transducer (**a**) and 3D X14L4 (9038) electronic transducer (**b**) (BK Medical) for endovaginal, endoanal and endorectal imaging with built-in-high resolution 3D

9 o'clock position. Automatic 3D acquisition provides a 3D cube formed by 300 transaxial 2D images over a distance of 60 mm, with a distance of 0.2–0.3 mm between two adjacent slices. Multiplanar reconstruction allows visualisation of the images in the axial, coronal and sagittal planes, as well as any other oblique plane [5]. Newer linear electronic transducers provide high-resolution images and also allow for the evaluation of the elastic properties of the tissues by elastography, based on the strain ratio calculation [13] (Fig. 15.1).

The optimal cut-off number of slices on tomographic ultrasound imaging for the EAS and IAS allows for standardization of a significant defect. Significant OASIs have been defined as visible defects of at least 30° in at least 4/6 slices using tomographic ultrasound imaging (TUI) with TPUS [17, 18]. TPUS without TUI has proven to be effective as well [18]. OASIs have been graded as 3a tear if the EAS was abnormal in <4/6 slices, 3b tear if it was abnormal in ≥4/6 slices and 3c/4 tear if both the EAS and the IAS were abnormal in ≥4/6 slices (Fig. 15.2).

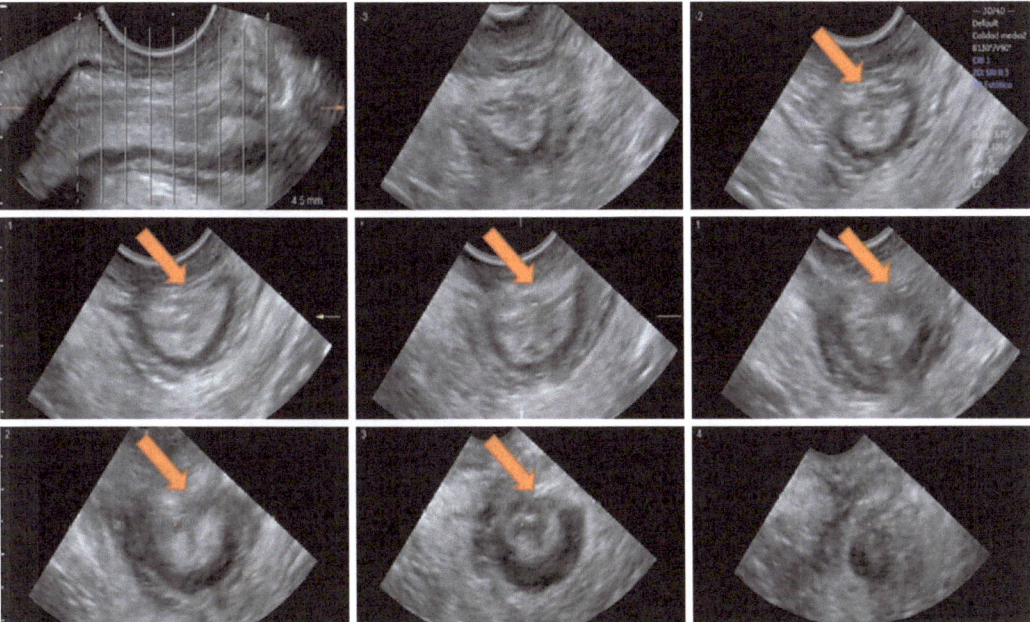

Fig. 15.2 OASIs have been defined as visible defects of at least 30° in at least 4/6 slices using tomographic ultrasound imaging

15.3   Normal Ultrasound Anatomy

The anal canal is 2–4 cm in length. In the upper third of the anal canal, EAUS visualises the PR muscle as a U-shaped hyperechoic structure. This muscle is part of the levator ani complex and it is contiguous with the EAS posteriorly. The submucosa layer is adjacent to the probe. The IAS appears as a dark, hypoechoic ring. Between the IAS and EAS there is a hyperechoic layer, that represents the conjoint longitudinal muscle (LM), in continuity with the longitudinal fibres of muscularis propria of the rectal wall. The LM extends through the anal canal within the intersphinteric space and traverses the subcutaneous EAS. The EAS is visualized as a mixed echogenic ring, larger but less distinct than the IAS [5]. In the lower third of the anal canal, the IAS is anatomically absent and therefore only the subcutaneous part of the EAS is visualised (Fig. 15.3). In the axial plane, normal measurements of IAS range from 1.5 to 4 mm in thickness and those of the EAS range from 7.7 to 8.6 mm [19]. On the coronal plane, the anterior length of EAS is on average 15.8 mm (range 14.9–22 mm) in women [14, 19] (Fig. 15.4).

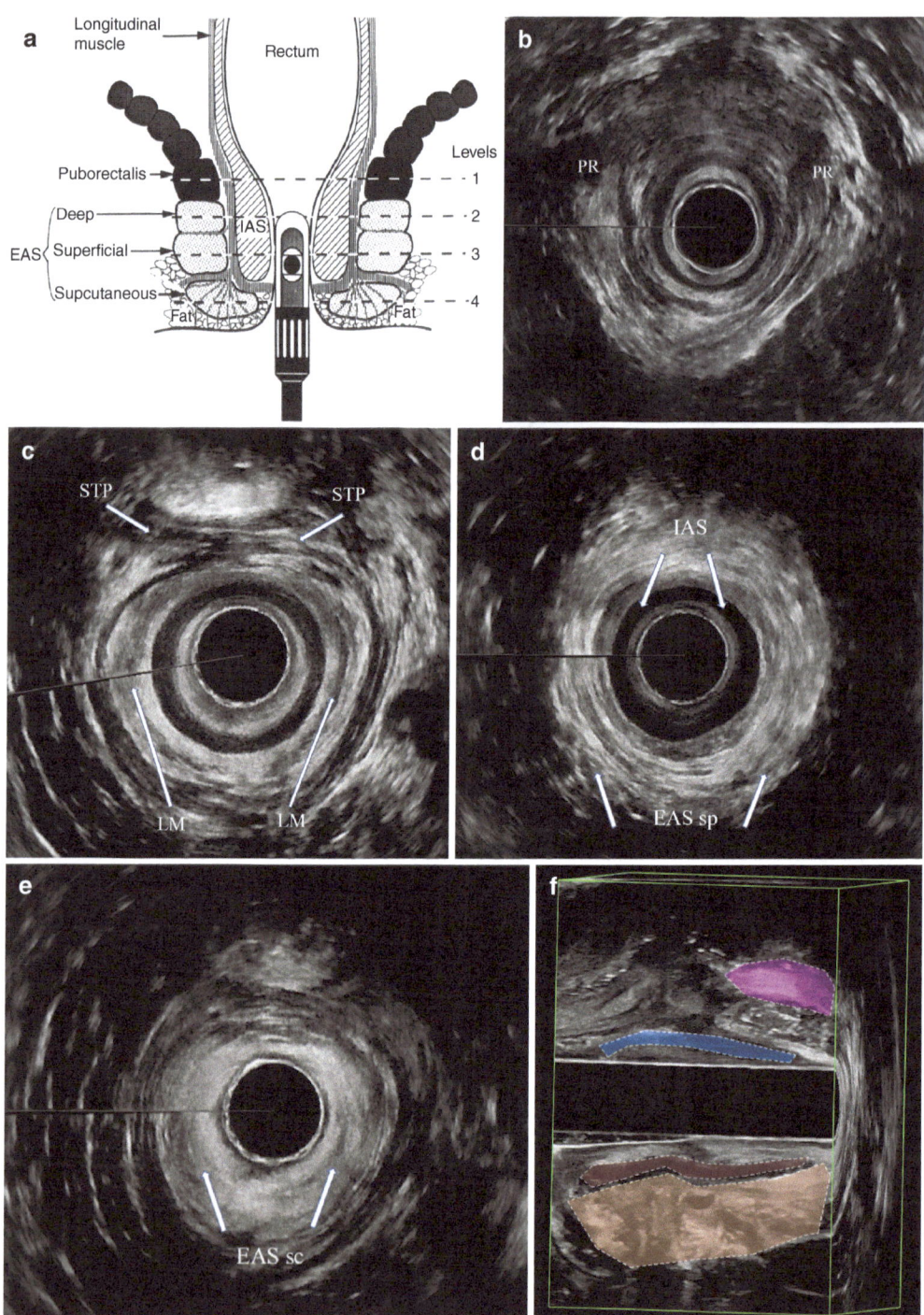

Fig. 15.3 (a) Schematic representation of the anorectum demonstrating levels of imaging (EAS: external anal sphincter; IAS: internal anal sphincter). Endoanal ultrasound with linear electronic probe (type 9038, BK Medical); (b) Upper level with the puborectalis muscle (PR); (c) Middle level with the deep external anal sphincter, the superficial transverse perineii muscle (STP) and the longitudinal muscle (LM); (d) Middle level with the internal anal sphincter (IAS) and the superficial external anal sphincter (EASsp); (e) Lower level with the subcutaneous external anal sphincter (EASsc); (f) Longitudinal reconstruction of the anal canal in female: the external anal sphincter is shorter anteriorly (violet) than the posteriorly (beige). The internal anal sphincter has a similar length anteriorly (blue) and posteriorly (brown)

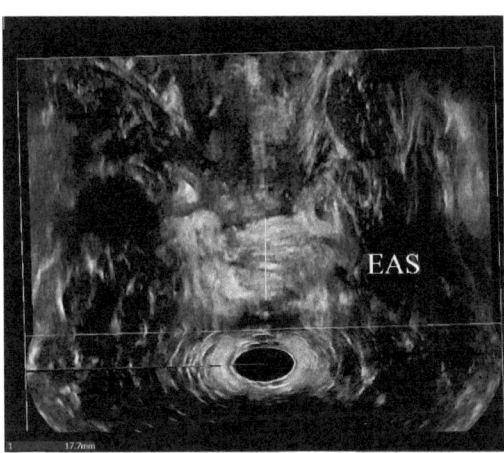

Fig. 15.4 Three-dimensional endoanal ultrasound with linear electronic probe (type 9038, BK Medical). Normal anterior thickness (17.7 mm) of the external anal sphincter (EAS) measured in the coronal plane

15.4 Endoanal Ultrasound in OASIs

15.4.1 Evaluation of OASIS

The ultrasonographic classification of OASI adopts the clinical classification by Sultan et al. described in detail in Chap. 3 [1]. Following OASI, the haematoma is initially replaced by granulation tissue and later by avascular collagenous scar tissue. This tissue appears on EAUS as homogeneous and of low reflectivity and crosses normal tissue planes. It is important to differentiate the natural gap of the EAS in the upper third of the anal canal (hypoechoic area with smooth, regular edges) and a sphincter rupture (mixed echogenicity area due to scarring, with irregular edges and loss of symmetry) [5] (Fig. 15.5). Visible alterations of the anal sphincters after vaginal birth include also thinning of the anterior part of the EAS with thickening of the LM [20]. Williams et al. reported a shortening of the anterior length of the EAS from 21.7 to 20.5 mm and a greater angle, from 10° to 13.8° in the axial plane of the anal canal [21]. Tears of the puboanalis muscle appear as loss of symmetry within the EAS in the upper third of the anal canal, associated with low and inhomogeneous reflectivity

and a failure of confluence of fibres into the midline. Isolated tears of the transverse perineii are often difficult to demonstrate because these muscles cannot be easily distinguished from the EAS [22].

15.4.2 Missed Tears

Missed tears (previously believed to be occult injuries) are OASIs that had been undiagnosed at childbirth. Endosonography is useful to detect these missed tears [23] which are found in up to 33% of primiparous [1, 6]. 71.5% of patients with missed anal sphincter injury demonstrated at least moderate AI in the early postpartum phase [24] (Level of evidence: 1b). All missed tears that involved the EAS only, were graded 3a or 3b [25]. Currently, there is no recommendation about screening women after vaginal birth for undiagnosed sphincter defects. There are no cost-benefit studies of EAUS in this setting, neither data on whether asymptomatic patients could benefit from imaging [9].

Missed OASIs had worse functional outcomes than primary repair immediately following childbirth [20, 26]. In a matched retrospective cohort study [20], comparing missed to recognized and repaired OASIs, the consequences of undiagnosed tears were higher anal and urinary incontinence symptoms. All missed OASIs had a shorter perineal body and larger sphincter defect on EAUS (Level of evidence 1b). Roper et al. recently reported that OASIs that are under-classified at childbirth are likely to be inadequately repaired, resulting in a persistent anal sphincter defect [23].

15.4.3 Evaluation After OASI

After repair of OASI, EAUS has a role in the evaluation of residual injury or recurrent OASIs [27]. There are a few systematic reviews or randomised controlled trials to define the best method of follow-up after OASIs. Roper et al. reviewed 13 national guidelines and reported a need for an agreed international guideline [28].

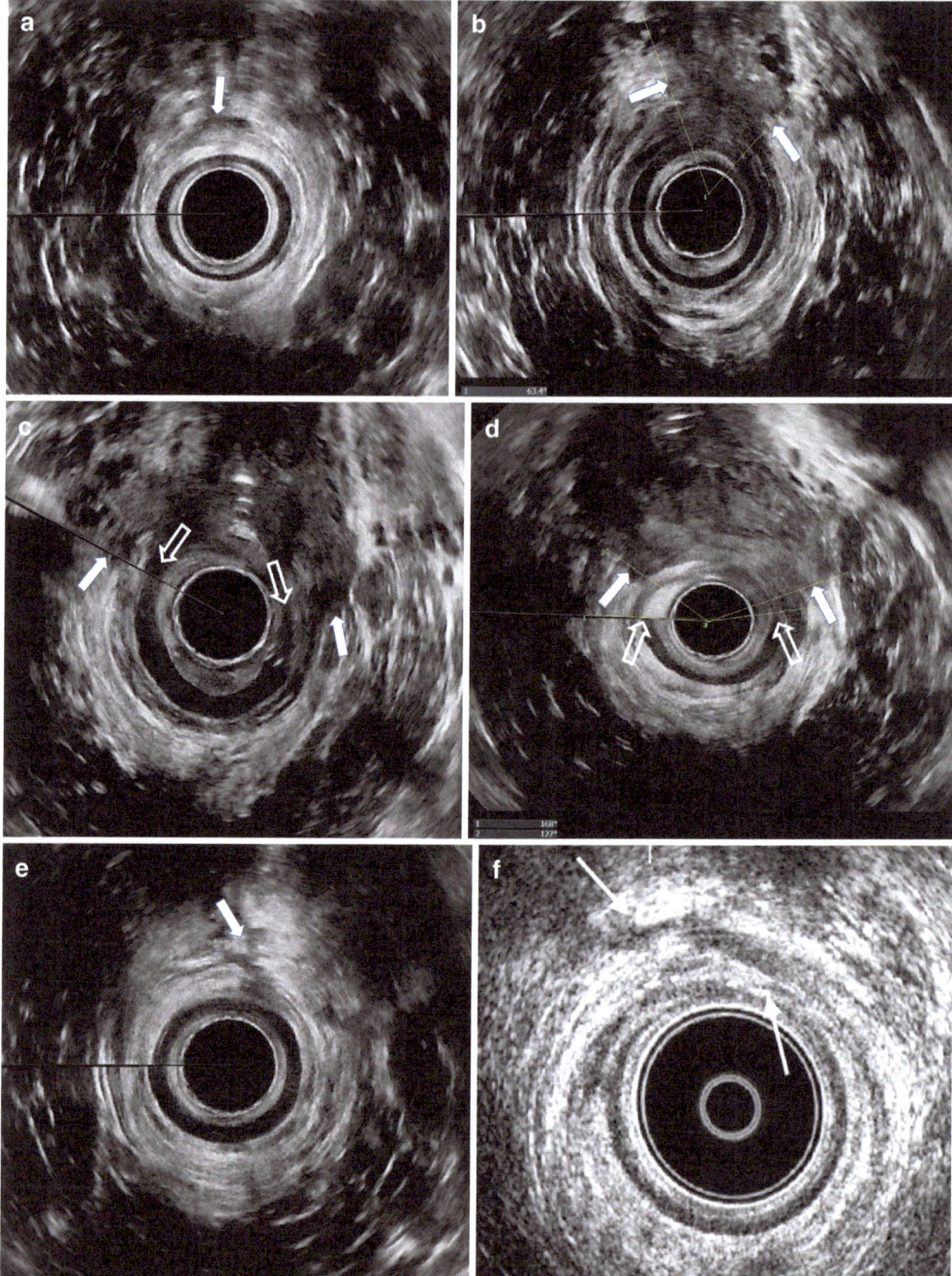

Fig. 15.5 Obstetrical anal sphincter injuries (OASIs) detected by endoanal ultrasound with linear electronic probe (type 9038, BK Medical)

(**a**) A repaired grade 3a tear. Note EAS partial thickness residual scarring at the 12 o'clock position (arrow).

(**b**) An inadequately repaired grade 3b tear with a persistent full thickness EAS defect between 11 and 1 o'clock (63.4°) (arrows).

(**c**) An inadequately repaired grade 3c tear. There is a large defect of the EAS between 10 o'clock and 3 o'clock

(128°) (filled arrows) and a defect of the IAS between 11 and 2 o'clock (96°) (empty arrows). Note the retraction effect of the residual IAS between 2 and 11 o'clock.

(**d**) A poorly repaired fourth degree tear with a EAS defect between 10 and 3 o'clock (122°) (filled arrows) and an IAS defect between 9 and 3 o'clock (168°) (empty arrows).

(**e**) Normal scar tissue (arrow) after end-to-end repair of OASI 3b at 2 month follow-up.

(**f**) Normal overlapping repair (arrows) of OASI 3b at 2 months follow-up.

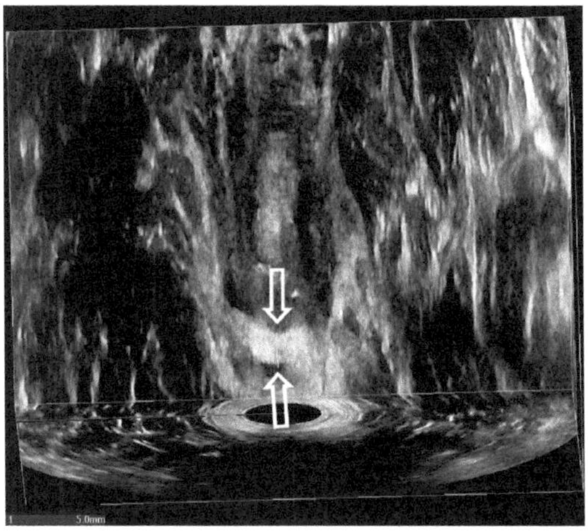

Fig. 15.6 Three-dimensional endoanal ultrasound with linear electronic probe (type 9038, BK Medical). Shorter anterior EAS length in the coronal plane of 5 mm (arrows)

Sideris et al. in a meta-analysis on 16,110 women from 103 studies found a strong association between ultrasound diagnosed OASIS and AI (RR 3.74, 2.17–6.45, $I^2 = 98\%$) (Level of evidence: 1a) [2]. Other studies have shown a high frequency of endosonographic sphincter defects after primary repairs in 54–93% of women [29, 30]. These data emphasize the importance of complete OASIs repair. The role of ultrasound imaging of the anal sphincter immediately after repair has its limitations and therefore focused training of obstetricians is of paramount importance [15]. However, if a woman is experiencing AI at follow-up after repair, referral for EAUS should be considered.

In IUGA/ICS 2017 joint report on female anorectal dysfunction terminology, EAUS, TPUS and EVUS were recommended as imaging modalities for pelvic investigation [25].

It is well-known that persistent ultrasound-detected defects in the anal sphincter muscles after OASIs are associated with AI [20]. Therefore, reconstruction of the entire length of the EAS is crucial. Anal incontinence after primary repair of OASIs is directly related to the relative length of the reconstructed EAS (Fig. 15.6) as well as to the extent of the ultrasonographic defects demonstrated by 3D-EAUS [31] (Fig. 15.5). In a prospective study that assessed long term function and morphology of

the anal sphincters and the pelvic floor after primary repair of OASIs, women who experienced deterioration of continence over time had a significantly shorter anterior EAS at 3D-EAUS. EAS length also correlated with increased severity of AI [32].

15.4.4 Management of Subsequent Pregnancy

This is described in detail in Chap. 5. Endoanal ultrasound performed 2 months postpartum has revealed that up to 33% of primiparous women and 44% of multiparous women have evidence of sphincter disruption [6]. Risk factors for both overt and missed sphincter injuries include forceps-assisted vaginal births, a prolonged second stage of labour, larger birth weight, midline episiotomy, and occipito-posterior presentation [1].

Subsequent vaginal birth is associated with increased risk of sustaining a further OASI. Whilst caesarean section is protective against new sphincter defects, there is also a risk of associated morbidity. The decision on the mode of childbirth after OASIs is multifactorial and should be based on symptoms, anal manometry and EAUS; this helps in preserving anal sphincter function and avoiding unnecessary caesarean sections [16, 31]. In a descriptive study of women who had OASIs from 2006 to 2013, vaginal birth was recommended to asymptomatic women with normal investigations (EAUS and anal manometry); caesarean section was recommended for women with AI, anal sphincter defects of more than 30° or low resting or incremental anal pressures. Caesarean section was done in 22 women and 28 women had vaginal births. Worsening of incontinence symptoms and reduction in anal pressures were not observed in the planned vaginal birth or elective caesarean birth groups. There were no new sphincter defects or recurrent OASIs in any of the women in the study group [33]. In a prospective study by Jordan et al. [16], pregnant women who had sustained previous OASIs were assessed both in the antenatal and postnatal period. Mode of childbirth was either vaginal or elective caesarean section. Vaginal birth was recommended if symptoms were minor (flatus incontinence or occasional passive soiling) or the woman was asymptomatic, and the EAS scar extended for less than 1 h on the clock face (30° angle) and the squeeze incremental pressure was >20 mmHg. Caesarean section was recommended for all others. No significant worsening of anorectal symptoms was observed following subsequent delivery in the vaginal birth group (99 women). In the EPIC multicenter randomized controlled trial [34], women with asymptomatic OASIs diagnosed by EAUS were randomised to a planned caesarean birth or a vaginal birth. At 6 months after the second birth, there were no significant differences in anal and urinary continence or in sexual functions between the two groups. These results thus do not support recommending caesarean birth for this indication (Level of evidence: 1b). However, there were concerns raised regarding the methodology and definitions of a sphincter defect in this study [35].

15.4.5 Selection of Patient for Rehabilitation

Ultrasound assessment can also be useful in the selection of patients who might benefit from rehabilitation. Pelvic floor physical therapy is likely less effective in patients with sphincter lesion, as there is a linear relationship between post-rehabilitative scores of AI severity and extent of sphincter defects [36]. According to the protocol proposed by Sultan et al. [25], pelvic floor exercises or biofeedback should be recommended in symptomatic females with a history of OASIs and a normal anorectal manometry and EAUS. They can also be recommended as conservative management in symptomatic women with a defect >1 h at EAUS and an incremental of maximal squeeze pressure <20 mmHg in females who desire further pregnancies. If family is complete, the best treatment in these cases remain a secondary sphincter repair.

Currently, there is no evidence to support the use of real time elastography in the diagnostic workup of AI. There was no correlation in elastogram colour distributions of the IAS and EAS with major clinical and functional parameters [37].

15.5 Transperineal Ultrasonography (TPUS) and Introital Ultrasonography (IUS)

Transperineal US has been evaluated as an alternative imaging modality of sphincter integrity in patients with AI [22, 38] (Level of Evidence: 3). Advantages of this approach include the availability of transducers, absence of anal canal distortion, better patient acceptability, and the possibility for functional studies [39]. 2D-TPUS is performed with conventional convex transducers (with frequencies between 3 and 6 MHz and field of view at least 70°), applied in a trans-labial fashion or on the perineum between the mons pubis and the anal margin [39] (Fig. 15.7). It can also be performed with the end-fire transducer positioned at the vaginal introitus (introital US) [40] (Fig. 15.8).

2D ultrasound provides an overall assessment of the pelvic organs in the midsagittal plane (bladder, urethra, vaginal walls, anal canal and rectum) between the posterior surface of the sym-

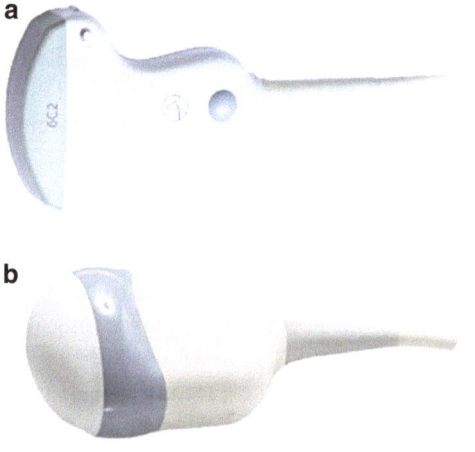

Fig. 15.7 (**a**) 6C2 (9040) curved array transducer (BK Medical) and GE RAB 4–8-D 3D/4D convex transducer (GE Medical) (**b**) for transperineal ultrasound

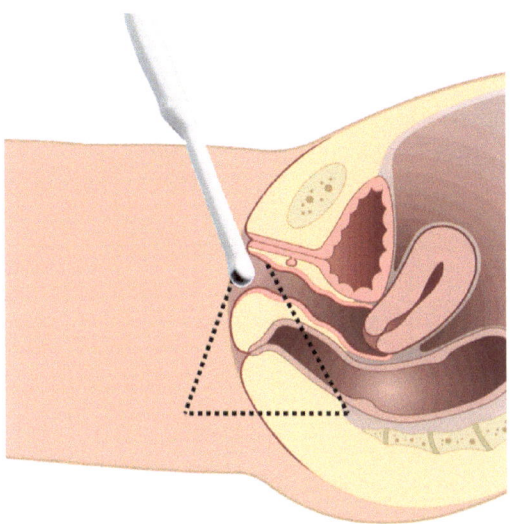

Fig. 15.8 Schematic representation of introital ultrasound with an endfire transducer (E13C2 BK Medical)

physis pubis (SP) and the posterior part of the LA. In the transverse plane, the IAS and EAS may also be visualised and OASIs detected (Fig. 15.9). Imaging is usually performed at rest, on maximal Valsalva maneuver, and on pelvic floor maximal contraction (dynamic assessment). 3D/4D TPUS is performed with a volumetric probe (Fig. 15.7).

The most important clinical application of 3D-TPUS is the assessment of LA injuries [41]. The disconnection of the muscle from its insertion on the inferior pubic ramus and the pelvic sidewall, a consequence of overstretching during the second stage of labour, is defined as LA avulsion [7, 8] (Fig. 15.10). In a study on 215 women

who sustained OASIs, TPUS-based grading of OASIs showed 70% of agreement with the Sultan clinical classification [40].

There are only a few studies that compared TPUS to EAUS [42, 43]. Taithongchai et al. compared 3-D IUS, TPUS and EAUS imaging in 250 women with OASIs: IUS and TPUS were not suitable for the identification of sphincter defects but they were associated with less discomfort; EAUS was the most accurate diagnostic imaging modality for diagnosis of obstetric tears with the greatest sensitivity and specificity [44]. Although the sensitivity for the detection of sphincter defects is only 50% for TPUS, this tool can be used in combination with EAUS, to provide additional information on pelvic floor muscles and the levator hiatus (LH) damage. It is well documented that during childbirth, the LH is distended massively [11] and the PR muscle, can be permanently damaged, either due to irreversible overdistension or muscle disconnection (avulsion) from its insertion on the pubis bone [41, 45]. Both forms of trauma seem to be risk factors for pelvic organ prolapse (POP) and recurrence after reconstructive surgery [12, 46].

Like EAUS, TPUS may be used as screening modality for the detection of clinically undiagnosed anal sphincter injuries after vaginal birth. In a prospective, randomised controlled trial, the missed tear rate increased from 3.5% (clinically detected) to 11.5% with TPUS using an end-fire probe [24]. However, there are no guidelines that recommend the screening of OASIs in clinical practice.

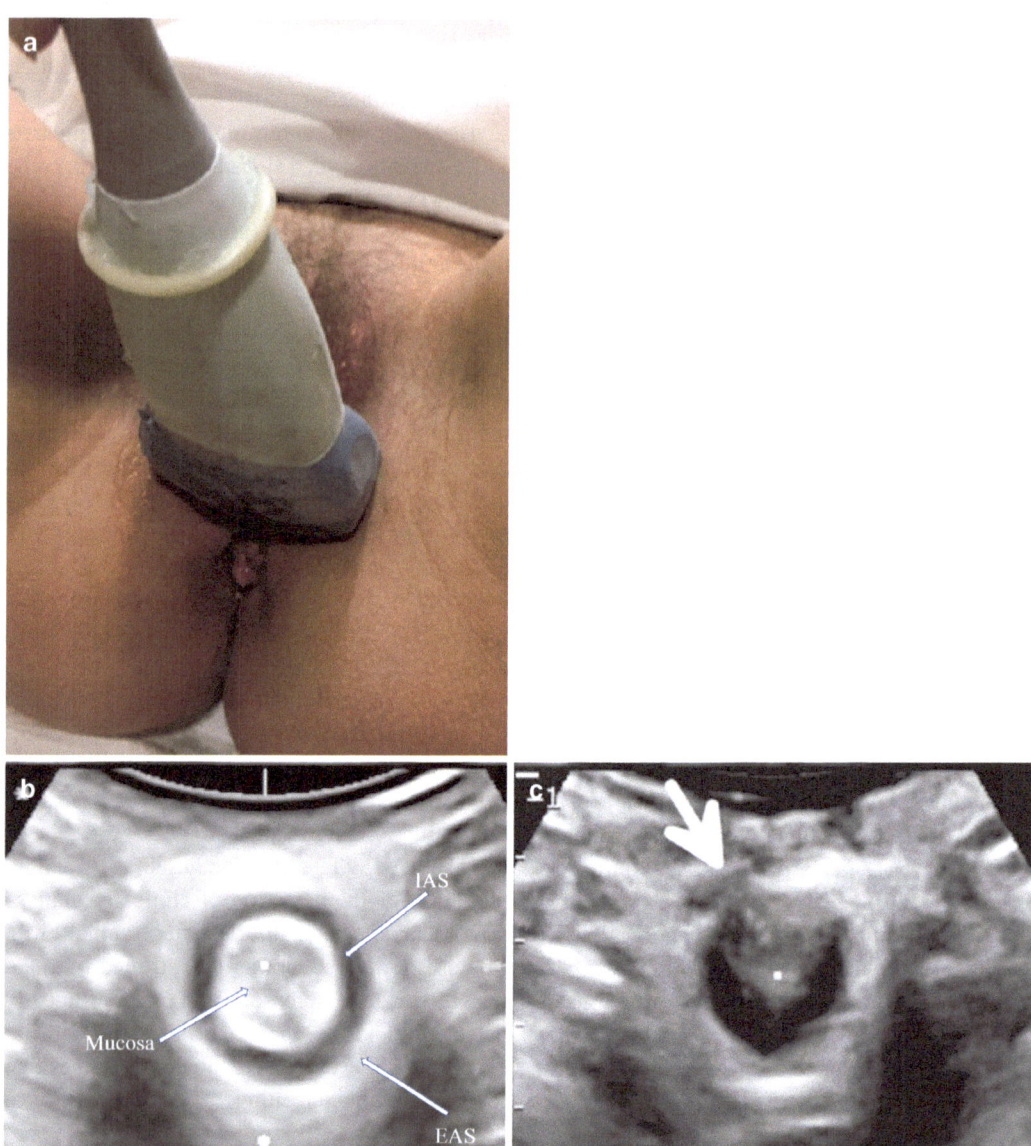

Fig. 15.9 (a) Transperineal ultrasound with transverse position of the convex transducer (BK Medical); (b) Normal anatomy at the middle level of the anal canal with the mucosa, the internal anal sphincter (IAS) and the external anal sphincter (EAS); (c) OASI grade 3c (arrow indicating the lesion)

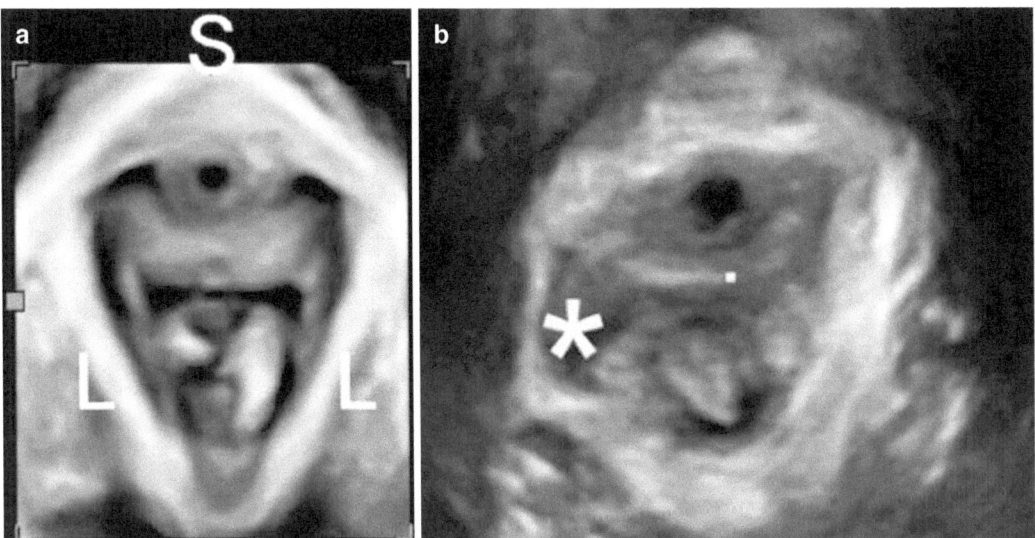

Fig. 15.10 Three-dimensional transperineal ultrasound with volumetric probe (type RAB 4–8, GE Medical). (**a**) Normal attachment of the levator ani (L) at the symphysis pubis (S); (**b**) Avulsion of the LA on the right side (*)

15.6 Endovaginal Ultrasonography (EVUS)

3D-EVUS is performed with the same transducers used for 3D-EAUS and represents an alternative modality for the evaluation of the anal sphincters [47] (Fig. 15.1). Sultan et al. described that the IAS was significantly thicker measured by EVUS and attributed this to possible stretching and thinning of the muscle by the endoanal probe [47] (Level of evidence: 2). Overall, there was an agreement between the two approaches in the evaluation of OASIs [48]. EVUS enables visualization of the anal sphincters and the LA and measurements of the LH dimensions (Fig. 15.11).

The sensitivity of EVUS for the detection of sphincter defects is 44%. In a prospective, observational study, defects of the LA muscle were identified by 3D-EVUS in 27% of women with AI after vaginal birth. Severity of incontinence was related to the extent of damage of the LA and to the enlargement of the LH [9]. These findings were not confirmed in a retrospective study where worsening of LA deficiency among patients with major AI, did not reach statistical significance [49]. 2D-TPUS and 3D-EVUS are not accurate modalities for the assessment of anal sphincters after repair of OASIS. 3D-TPUS shows good agreement with the gold standard 3D-EAUS and a high sensitivity in detecting residual defects [48]. EAUS has the strongest association with AI after OASIs compared to IUS or TPUS [44, 49].

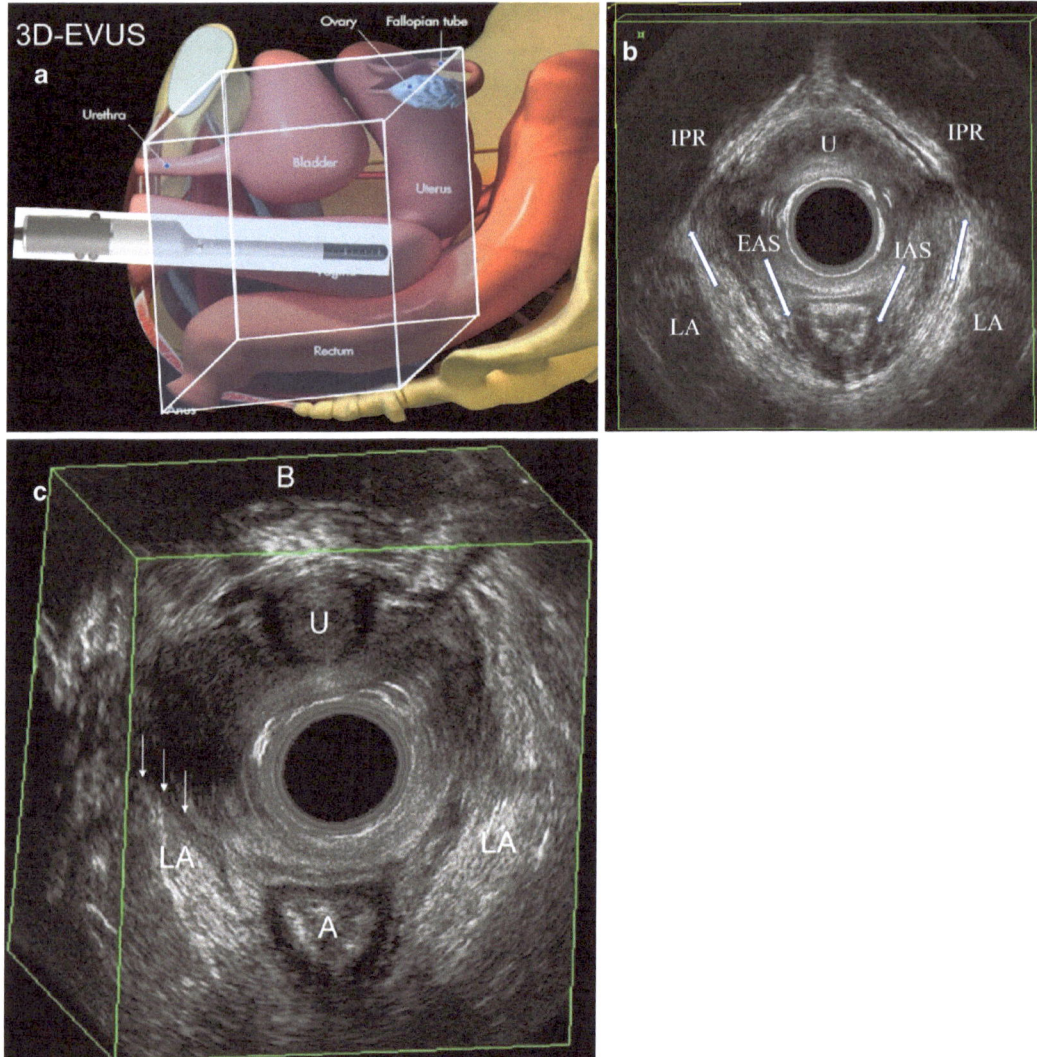

Fig. 15.11 (**a**) Schematic representation of three-dimensional endovaginal ultrasound (type 9052, BK Medical). (**b**) Normal ultrasonographic anatomy of the pelvic floor in a nulliparous female; (**c**) Avulsion of the LA on the right side (arrows) (A anal canal, B bladder, EAS external anal sphincter; IAS internal anal sphincter, IPR inferior pubic rami, LA levator ani, U urethra)

15.7   Magnetic Resonance Imaging

MRI provides detailed information of the anal sphincters and pelvic floor anatomy [25]. MRI can be performed with endoluminal (endoanal or endovaginal) coils or surface phased-array coils placed external to the patient (Fig. 15.11). The spatial resolution of MRI, however, is lesser than EAUS and therefore, accuracy for detecting OASIs is reported to be slightly below that of EAUS [50, 51]. The role of MRI for the assessment of AI is limited in clinical practice and it remains a second line investigation after EAUS for the evaluation of anal sphincter integrity [52, 53]. MRI is superior to EAUS for quantifying anal sphincter and pelvic floor muscles and delineating the presence of atrophy [54, 55] (Fig. 15.12). The association between a poor visualisation of EAS and a thinning of IAS is

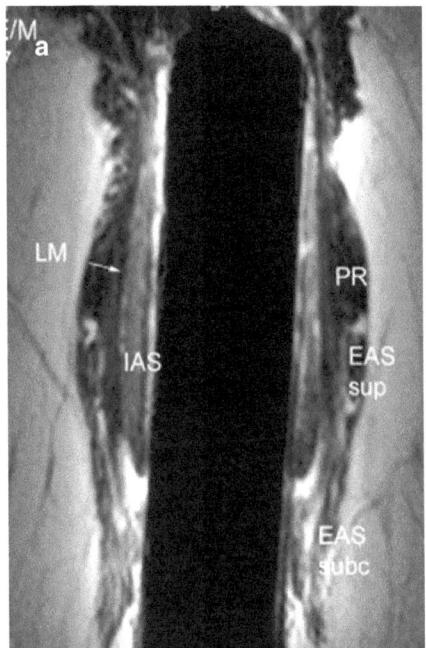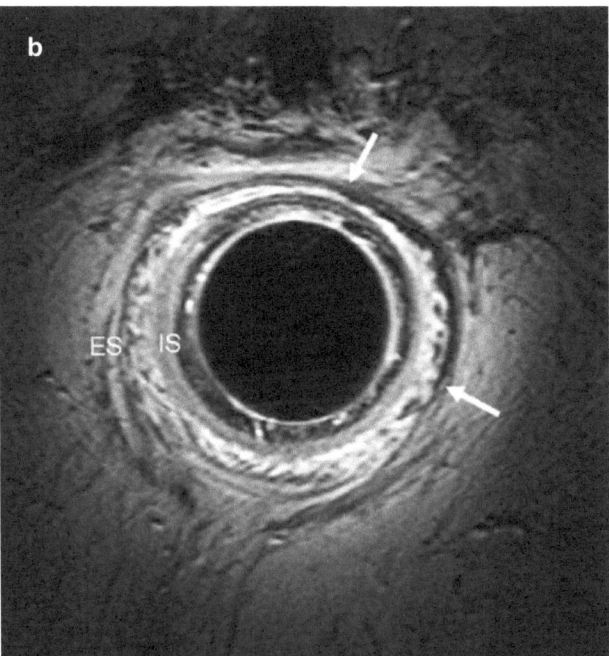

Fig. 15.12 MRI with endoanal coil. (**a**) Coronal section in a normal female showing the internal sphincter (IAS) to be of moderate signal, and the striated muscle of the puborectalis (PR) and external sphincter (EAS) to be of low signal (LM: longitudinal muscle). The deep part of the EAS is fused with the PR, but the superficial (sup) and subcutaneous parts (subc) are clearly separate. (**b**) Axial section T2-weighted turbo spin-echo in a female patient with anal incontinence due to severe atrophy of the external sphincter (ES) at 12 and at 3 o'clock position (arrows). There is also atrophy of the internal sphincter (IS) the thickness of the IAS and EAS are not clear. What are the arrows showing? (indication of atrophy, see the legend now)

suggestive of atrophy (positive predictive value 74%) [56]. MRI is also more useful in detecting LA muscle avulsions, which could be associated with AI after vaginal birth [57].

15.8 Conclusions

3D EAUS remains the most accurate diagnostic imaging modality for the diagnosis and classification of OASIs. 3D TPUS, 3D EVUS and MRI are used to demonstrate LA avulsion and LH enlargement after childbirth. MRI is superior to EAUS for assessing EAS atrophy which may correlate with symptoms of AI and predicts poorer outcome after anal sphincteroplasty.

Take Home Messages
- 3D EAUS is the gold standard investigation to evaluate OASIs

- 3D EAUS may be used to detect missed tears at birth or recurrent OASIs after repair
- 3D EAUS may guide mode of birth in subsequent pregnancy after OASIs and select patient for rehabilitation
- EVUS and TPUS provide additional information on trauma to the LA muscle
- MRI remains second line for the evaluation of OASIs

Appendix: MCQ

Questions

1. Which description is the normal ultrasonographic configuration of the anal canal?
   (A) PR muscle has a U-shaped hyperechoic structure; IAS appears as a dark, hypoechoic ring; the conjoint longitudi-

nal muscle is a hyperechoic layer; EAS is visualized as a mixed echogenic ring
- (B) PR muscle as a U-shaped hypoechoic structure; IAS appears as a dark, hypoechoic ring; the conjoint longitudinal tendon is a hyperechoic layer; EAS is visualized as a mixed echogenic ring
- (C) PR muscle as a U-shaped hyperechoic structure; IAS appears as a sharp, hyperechoic ring; the conjoint longitudinal muscle is a hypoechoic layer; EAS is visualized as a mixed echogenic ring
- (D) PR muscle as a U-shaped hyperechoic structure; IAS appears as a dark, hypoechoic ring; the conjoint longitudinal muscle is a hypoechoic layer; EAS is visualized as a dark, hypoechoic ring

2. Which of the following is correct regarding the clinical relevance of EAUS in the evaluation of OASIS?
- (A) Ultrasonographic residual defects after repair of OASIS are not related to anal incontinence
- (B) EAUS has a limited role in planning the mode of delivery after a previous OASIS
- (C) EAUS and manometry have a relevant role in planning the mode of delivery after a previous OASIS
- (D) EAUS is not able to identify anal sphincter lesions clinically undiagnosed at the delivery

3. Which is the most important clinical application of 3D-TPUS?
- (A) The assessment of perineal body damage
- (B) The assessment of transverse perineii muscle damage
- (C) The assessment of rectovaginal fascia damage
- (D) The assessment of levator ani damage

Answers

1. Which description is the normal ultrasonographic configuration of the anal canal?

- (A) TRUE
- (B) FALSE
- (C) FALSE
- (D) FALSE

2. Which of the following is correct regarding the clinical relevance of EAUS in the evaluation of OASIS?
- (A) FALSE
- (B) FALSE
- (C) TRUE
- (D) FALSE

3. Which is the most important clinical application of 3D-TPUS?
- (A) FALSE
- (B) FALSE
- (C) FALSE
- (D) TRUE

References

1. Sultan AH, Thakar R. Third and fourth degree tears. In: Sultan AH, Thakar R, Fenner D, editors. Perineal and anal sphincter trauma. London: Springer; 2007. p. 33–51.
2. Sideris M, McCaughey T, Hanrahan JG, Arroyo-Manzano D, Zamora J, Jha S, et al. Risk of obstetric anal sphincter injuries (OASIS) and anal incontinence: a meta-analysis. Eur J Obstet Gynecol Reprod Biol. 2020;252:303–12.
3. Haylen BT, de Ridder D, Freeman RM, Swift SE, Berghmans B, Lee J, et al. An International Urogynecological Association (IUGA)/International Continence Society (ICS) joint report on the terminology for female pelvic floor dysfunction. Int Urogynecol J. 2010;21:5–26.
4. Santoro GA, Fortling B. New technical developments in endoanal and endorectal ultrasonography. In: Santoro GA, Di Falco G, editors. Benign anorectal diseases. Milano: Springer Milan; 2006. p. 13–26.
5. Santoro GA, Fortling B. The advantages of volume rendering in three-dimensional endosonography of the anorectum. Dis Colon Rectum. 2007;50:359–68.
6. Sultan AH, Kamm MA, Hudson CN, Thomas JM, Bartram CI. Anal-sphincter disruption during vaginal delivery. N Engl J Med. 1993;329:1905–11.
7. DeLancey JOL, Kearney R, Chou Q, Speights S, Binno S. The appearance of levator ani muscle abnormalities in magnetic resonance images after vaginal delivery. Obstet Gynecol. 2003;101:46–53.

8. Lien KC, Mooney B, DeLancey JOL, Ashton-Miller JA. Levator ani muscle stretch induced by simulated vaginal birth. Obstet Gynecol. 2004;103:31–40.
9. Murad-Regadas SM, Fernandes GO da S, Regadas FSP, Rodrigues LV, Pereira J de JR, Dealcanfreitas ID, et al. Assessment of pubovisceral muscle defects and levator hiatal dimensions in women with faecal incontinence after vaginal delivery: is there a correlation with severity of symptoms? Colorectal Dis. 2014;16:1010–8.
10. Rostaminia G, White D, Hegde A, Quiroz LH, Davila GW, Shobeiri SA. Levator ani deficiency and pelvic organ prolapse severity. Obstet Gynecol. 2013;121:1017–24.
11. Svabík K, Shek KL, Dietz HP. How much does the levator hiatus have to stretch during childbirth? BJOG. 2009;116:1657–62.
12. Vergeldt TFM, Notten KJB, Weemhoff M, van Kuijk SMJ, Mulder FEM, Beets-Tan RG, et al. Levator hiatal area as a risk factor for cystocele recurrence after surgery: a prospective study. BJOG. 2015;122:1130–7.
13. Walsh KA, Grivell RM. Use of endoanal ultrasound for reducing the risk of complications related to anal sphincter injury after vaginal birth. Cochrane Database Syst Rev. 2015;2015:CD010826.
14. Faltin DL, Boulvain M, Irion O, Bretones S, Stan C, Weil A. Diagnosis of anal sphincter tears by postpartum endosonography to predict fecal incontinence. Obstet Gynecol. 2000;95:643–7.
15. Wong KW, Thakar R, Andrews V, Sultan AH. Is there a role for transperineal ultrasound imaging of the anal sphincter immediately after primary repair of third degree tears? Eur J Obstet Gynecol Reprod Biol. 2022;271:260–4.
16. Jordan PA, Naidu M, Thakar R, Sultan AH. Effect of subsequent vaginal delivery on bowel symptoms and anorectal function in women who sustained a previous obstetric anal sphincter injury. Int Urogynecol J. 2018;29:1579–88.
17. Stuart A, Ignell C, Örnö AK. Comparison of transperineal and endoanal ultrasound in detecting residual obstetric anal sphincter injury. Acta Obstet Gynecol Scand. 2019;98:1624–31.
18. Martínez Franco E, López Negre JL, Parés D, Ros Cerro C, Amat Tardiu L, Cuadras D, et al. Anatomic and functional evaluation of the levator ani muscle after an obstetric anal sphincter injury. Arch Gynecol Obstet. 2019;299:1001–6.
19. Norderval S, Pedersen TK, Collinson RJ. Anal sphincter length as determined by 3-dimensional endoanal ultrasound and anal manometry. J Ultrasound Med. 2021;40:331–9.
20. Taithongchai A, Veiga SI, Sultan AH, Thakar R. The consequences of undiagnosed obstetric anal sphincter injuries (OASIS) following vaginal delivery. Int Urogynecol J. 2020;31:635–41.
21. Williams A, Bartram C, Halligan S, Marshall MM, Spencer J, Nicholls R, et al. Alteration of anal sphincter morphology following vaginal delivery revealed by multiplanar anal endosonography. BJOG. 2002;109:942–6.
22. Santoro GA, Wieczorek AP, Dietz HP, Mellgren A, Sultan AH, Shobeiri SA, et al. State of the art: an integrated approach to pelvic floor ultrasonography. Ultrasound Obstet Gynecol. 2011;37:381–96.
23. Roper JC, Thakar R, Sultan AH. Under-classified obstetric anal sphincter injuries. Int Urogynecol J. 2022;33:1473–9.
24. Ozyurt S, Aksoy H, Gedikbasi A, Yildirim G, Aksoy U, Acmaz G, et al. Screening occult anal sphincter injuries in primigravid women after vaginal delivery with transperineal use of vaginal probe: a prospective, randomized controlled trial. Arch Gynecol Obstet. 2015;292:853–9.
25. Sultan AH, Monga A, Lee J, Emmanuel A, Norton C, Santoro G, et al. An International Urogynecological Association (IUGA)/International Continence Society (ICS) joint report on the terminology for female anorectal dysfunction. Int Urogynecol J. 2017;28:5–31.
26. Ramage L, Yen C, Qiu S, Simillis C, Kontovounisios C, Tan E, et al. Does a missed obstetric anal sphincter injury at time of delivery affect short-term functional outcome? Ann R Coll Surg Engl. 2018;100:26–32.
27. Fitzpatrick M, Cassidy M, Barassaud ML, Hehir MP, Hanly AM, O'Connell PR, et al. Does anal sphincter injury preclude subsequent vaginal delivery? Eur J Obstet Gynecol Reprod Biol. 2016;198:30–4.
28. Roper JC, Amber N, Wan OYK, Sultan AH, Thakar R. Review of available national guidelines for obstetric anal sphincter injury. Int Urogynecol J. 2020;31:2247–59.
29. Reid AJ, Beggs AD, Sultan AH, Roos AM, Thakar R. Outcome of repair of obstetric anal sphincter injuries after three years. Int J Gynaecol Obstet. 2014;127:47–50.
30. Oude Lohuis EJ, Everhardt E. Outcome of obstetric anal sphincter injuries in terms of persisting endoanal ultrasonographic defects and defecatory symptoms. Int J Gynaecol Obstet. 2014;126:70–3.
31. Norderval S, Røssaak K, Markskog A, Vonen B. Incontinence after primary repair of obstetric anal sphincter tears is related to relative length of reconstructed external sphincter: a case-control study. Ultrasound Obstet Gynecol. 2012;40:207–14.
32. Soerensen MM, Pedersen BG, Santoro GA, Buntzen S, Bek K, Laurberg S. Long-term function and morphology of the anal sphincters and the pelvic floor after primary repair of obstetric anal sphincter injury. Color Dis. 2014;16:O347–55.
33. Karmarkar R, Bhide A, Digesu A, Khullar V, Fernando R. Mode of delivery after obstetric anal sphincter injury. Eur J Obstet Gynecol Reprod Biol. 2015;194:7–10.
34. Abramowitz L, Mandelbrot L, Bourgeois Moine A, Tohic AL, Carne Carnavalet C, Poujade O, et al. Caesarean section in the second delivery to prevent anal incontinence after asymptomatic obstetric anal sphincter injury: the EPIC multicentre randomised trial. BJOG. 2021;128:685–93.

35. Okeahialam NA, Wong KW, Roper J, Thakar R, Sultan AH. Re: cesarean section in the second delivery to prevent anal incontinence after asymptomatic obstetrical anal sphincter injury: the EPIC multicentre randomised trial. BJOG. 2021;128:770–1.

36. Pucciani F, Raggioli M, Gattai R. Rehabilitation of fecal incontinence: what is the influence of anal sphincter lesions? Tech Coloproctol. 2012;17:299–306.

37. Allgayer H, Ignee A, Zipse S, Crispin A, Dietrich CF. Endorectal ultrasound and real-time elastography in patients with fecal incontinence following anorectal surgery: a prospective comparison evaluating short- and long-term outcomes in irradiated and non-irradiated patients. Z Gastroenterol. 2012;50:1281–6.

38. Meriwether KV, Hall RJ, Leeman LM, Migliaccio L, Qualls C, Rogers RG. The relationship of 3-D translabial ultrasound anal sphincter complex measurements to postpartum anal and fecal incontinence. Int Urogynecol J. 2015;26:1191–9.

39. Dietz HP. Ultrasound imaging of the pelvic floor. Part II: three-dimensional or volume imaging. Ultrasound Obstet Gynecol. 2004;23:615–25.

40. Cattani L, Van Schoubroeck D, Housmans S, Callewaert G, Werbrouck E, Verbakel JY, et al. Exoanal imaging of the anal sphincter: a comparison between introital and transperineal image acquisition. Int Urogynecol J. 2020;31:1107–13.

41. Dietz HP, Lanzarone V. Levator trauma after vaginal delivery. Obstet Gynecol. 2005;106:707–12.

42. Oom DMJ, West RL, Schouten WR, Steensma AB. Detection of anal sphincter defects in female patients with fecal incontinence: a comparison of 3-dimensional transperineal ultrasound and 2-dimensional endoanal ultrasound. Dis Colon Rectum. 2012;55:646–52.

43. Meriwether KV, Hall RJ, Leeman LM, Migliaccio L, Qualls C, Rogers RG. Anal sphincter complex: 2D and 3D endoanal and translabial ultrasound measurement variation in normal postpartum measurements. Int Urogynecol J. 2015;26:511–7.

44. Taithongchai A, van Gruting IMA, Volløyhaug I, Arendsen LP, Sultan AH, Thakar R. Comparing the diagnostic accuracy of 3 ultrasound modalities for diagnosing obstetric anal sphincter injuries. Am J Obstet Gynecol. 2019;221:134.e1–9.

45. Shek KL, Dietz HP. Intrapartum risk factors for levator trauma. BJOG. 2010;117:1485–92.

46. Dietz HP, Chantarasorn V, Shek KL. Levator avulsion is a risk factor for cystocele recurrence. Ultrasound Obstet Gynecol. 2010;36:76–80.

47. Sultan AH, Loder PB, Bartram CI, Kamm MA, Hudson CN. Vaginal endosonography. New approach to image the undisturbed anal sphincter. Dis Colon Rectum. 1994;37:1296–9.

48. Ros C, Martínez-Franco E, Wozniak MM, Cassado J, Santoro GA, Elías N, et al. Postpartum two- and three-dimensional ultrasound evaluation of anal sphincter complex in women with obstetric anal sphincter injury. Ultrasound Obstet Gynecol. 2017;49:508–14.

49. Volløyhaug I, Taithongchai A, Van Gruting I, Sultan A, Thakar R. Levator ani muscle morphology and function in women with obstetric anal sphincter injury. Ultrasound Obstet Gynecol. 2019;53:410–6.

50. Fletcher JG, Busse RF, Riederer SJ, Hough D, Gluecker T, Harper CM, et al. Magnetic resonance imaging of anatomic and dynamic defects of the pelvic floor in defecatory disorders. Am J Gastroenterol. 2003;98:399–411.

51. Beets-Tan RG, Morren GL, Beets GL, Kessels AG, el Naggar K, Lemaire E, et al. Measurement of anal sphincter muscles: endoanal US, endoanal MR imaging, or phased-array MR imaging? A study with healthy volunteers. Radiology. 2001;220:81–9.

52. Morren GL, Beets-Tan RG, van Engelshoven JM. Anatomy of the anal canal and perianal structures as defined by phased-array magnetic resonance imaging. Br J Surg. 2001;88:1506–12.

53. Rao SSC, Tetangco EP. Anorectal disorders: an update. J Clin Gastroenterol. 2020;54:606–13.

54. West RL, Dwarkasing S, Briel JW, Hansen BE, Hussain SM, Schouten WR, et al. Can three-dimensional endoanal ultrasonography detect external anal sphincter atrophy? A comparison with endoanal magnetic resonance imaging. Int J Colorectal Dis. 2005;20:328–33.

55. Williams AB, Bartram CI, Modhwadia D, Nicholls T, Halligan S, Kamm MA, et al. Endocoil magnetic resonance imaging quantification of external anal sphincter atrophy. Br J Surg. 2001;88:853–9.

56. Cazemier M, Terra MP, Stoker J, de Lange-de Klerk ESM, Boeckxstaens GEE, Mulder CJJ, et al. Atrophy and defects detection of the external anal sphincter: comparison between three-dimensional anal endosonography and endoanal magnetic resonance imaging. Dis Colon Rectum. 2006;49:20–7.

57. Lammers K, Fütterer JJ, Inthout J, Prokop M, Vierhout ME, Kluivers KB. Correlating signs and symptoms with pubovisceral muscle avulsions on magnetic resonance imaging. Am J Obstet Gynecol. 2013;208(148):e1–7.

Obstetric Pelvic Floor Trauma

16

Ingrid Volløyhaug

Overview

Test your learning and check your understanding of this book's contents: use the "Springer Nature Flashcards" app to access questions using ▶ https://sn.pub/wqrf89. To use the app, please follow the instructions in Chap. 1.

Learning Objectives

- To be able to define levator trauma and describe its prevalence
- To be able to diagnose levator trauma on ultrasound and MRI
- To describe risk factors for and prevention of levator trauma
- To describe the consequences of levator trauma
- To be able to describe the definition, prevalence and consequences of connective tissue and nerve injury

I. Volløyhaug (✉)
Clinic of Obstetrics and Gynecology, St. Olav's Hospital, Trondheim University Hospital, Trondheim, Norway

Department of Clinical and Molecular medicine, Norwegian University of Science and Technology, Trondheim, Norway
e-mail: ingrid.volloyhaug@ntnu.no

16.1 Introduction

Clinical diagnosis of levator injury after birth was first described in 1942 by the American obstetrician Gainey [1]. He used palpation to diagnose detachment of the levator ani muscle and the urethra. For many years, pelvic floor trauma involving the levator ani muscle, connective tissue, and nerves was not given much interest, possibly because it is usually occult or hidden under intact vaginal mucosa and difficult to diagnose at the time of birth.

In the early 2000s, DeLancey and coworkers demonstrated how levator trauma could be diagnosed with magnetic resonance imaging (MRI) [2, 3], and Dietz et al. introduced 3D/4D transperineal ultrasonographical diagnosis of levator avulsion [4, 5]. Subsequently, we have gained more knowledge about risk factors for obstetric pelvic floor trauma and its consequences. Women delivered by cesarean birth have virtually no injuries, whereas forceps birth is associated with a higher risk of injury than spontaneous vaginal and vacuum assisted birth [6].

Levator injuries result in larger opening (or hiatus) of the pelvic floor and weaker muscles, thereby contributing to pelvic organ descent over time [7]. Some women develop pelvic floor disorders soon after childbirth [8–11], but there is usually a delay of many years between the injury and the desire for prolapse-correcting reconstructive surgery [12].

16.2 Functional Anatomy of the Pelvic Floor

The levator ani muscles provide contractile tone at rest and can be activated to contract further. Together with the connective tissue fascia and ligaments, they provide support for the female pelvic organs [13]. The muscles are innervated by S2-S4 nerve roots via the pudendal nerve and direct branches from the motor roots [14].

The *levator hiatus* is the opening in the muscles for the passage of the urethra, vagina and rectum [15]. The puborectalis muscle constitutes the inner margin of the opening, attaching to the pubic bone at both sides and surrounding the urethra, vagina and rectum. Computer models have shown that the medial aspect of the levator muscle undergoes the largest stretch during vaginal birth and is at the greatest risk for injury [16, 17]. Connective tissue and nerves are also stretched and prone to injury at birth. Obstetric pelvic floor trauma can result in a larger levator hiatus and less support to the pelvic organs [7].

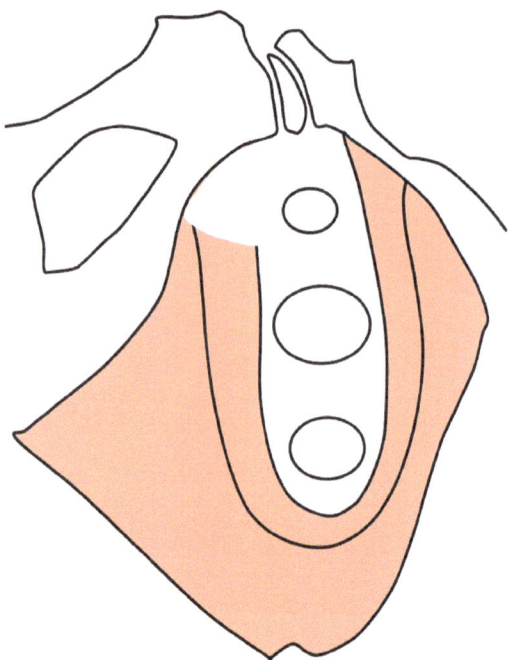

Fig. 16.1 Levator avulsion (macrotrauma). The puborectalis muscle is detached from its insertion at the symphysis pubis

16.3 Definition and Prevalence of Obstetric Pelvic Floor Trauma

Levator avulsion (macrotrauma) is defined as an injury to the inferomedial aspects of the pubovisceral/puborectalis muscle of the levator ani muscle complex. The muscle fibers are detached from their insertion on the arcus tendineus fasciae pelvis at the symphysis, see Fig. 16.1 [3, 18]. The injury can be unilateral or bilateral. By definition, an injury must have a certain extension to be significant or complete (>5 mm on ultrasound), whereas smaller injuries are considered incomplete and not clinically relevant [19]. (See also Ultrasound diagnosis).

Levator microtrauma occur when the muscle is over-stretched and does not recover to pre-birth size (see Fig. 16.2). The pathophysiology of irreversible overdistension is not fully understood. It may be due to physical alterations in the muscle itself or to changes in the neuromuscular pathways [20].

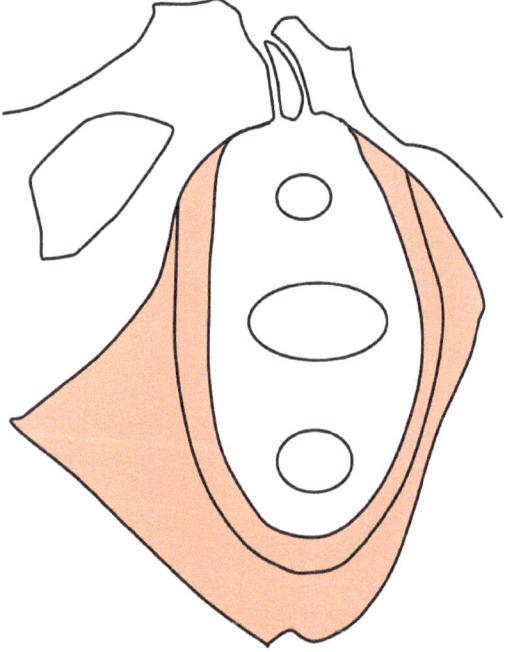

Fig. 16.2 Levator microtrauma. The muscle is over stretched and does not recover to pre-delivery size after delivery

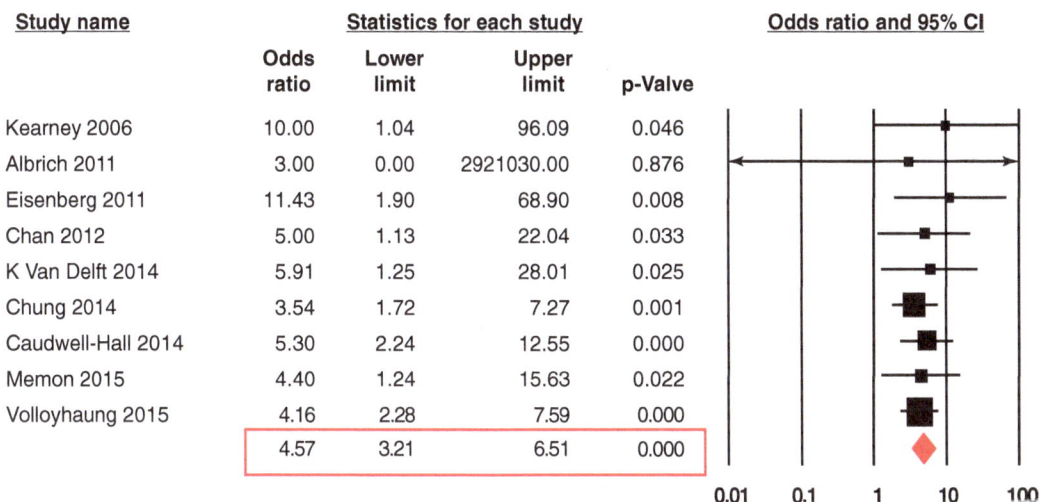

Study name	Statistics for each study				Odds ratio and 95% CI
	Odds ratio	Lower limit	Upper limit	p-Valve	
Kearney 2006	10.00	1.04	96.09	0.046	
Albrich 2011	3.00	0.00	2921030.00	0.876	
Eisenberg 2011	11.43	1.90	68.90	0.008	
Chan 2012	5.00	1.13	22.04	0.033	
K Van Delft 2014	5.91	1.25	28.01	0.025	
Chung 2014	3.54	1.72	7.27	0.001	
Caudwell-Hall 2014	5.30	2.24	12.55	0.000	
Memon 2015	4.40	1.24	15.63	0.022	
Volloyhaung 2015	4.16	2.28	7.59	0.000	
	4.57	3.21	6.51	0.000	

Fig. 16.3 Forest plot from a meta-analysis of the association between mode of delivery and levator avulsion showing an overall odds ratio of 4.57 for levator avulsion when comparing forceps to vacuum-assisted vaginal birth. (With permission after Friedman et al.)

Macrotrauma and microtrauma can both result in a larger levator hiatus and weaker muscles at contraction [21]. Some women have both types of trauma [22].

The prevalence of *levator avulsion* varies after different modes of birth. Levator injury generally does not occur after cesarean birth, even when performed in the second stage of birth [23]. The prevalence varies between 6–20% after spontaneous vaginal birth [24, 25], 9–41% after vacuum birth [24, 26] and 35–89% after forceps birth [23, 24, 26]. A meta-analysis showed that forceps birth is associated with seven-fold increased risk of levator avulsion compared to spontaneous, and a four-to five-fold increased risk compared to vacuum assisted birth (Fig. 16.3). Vacuum carries a similar risk as spontaneous vaginal birth [6].

Depending on the criteria applied, approximately 15–30% of women have *microtrauma* or levator overdistension after vaginal birth [26]. It is therefore not surprising that levator hiatal areas are larger after forceps than after spontaneous and vacuum assisted births [23].

16.3.1 Connective Tissue Injury

Connective tissue injury has been less studied, probably because this is more difficult to visualize with ultrasound and MRI. Various terms are often used to define the same structure, and the same term is used for more than one structure. This is not helpful in understanding such injuries [27].

The *rectovaginal "fascia"* is the tissue that lies between the vagina and the rectum. It is denser closer to the perineal body and thinner in the upper part of the vagina. This "fascia" can be torn during birth, and it is important to identify and repair such defects, as they can manifest as a posterior wall prolapse later in life. This tissue can be recognized as a thin whitish structure under the injured vaginal mucosa and over the rectum (Fig. 16.4) [28].

The *pubocervical fascia* lies along the anterior vaginal wall and is attached laterally to the arcus tendinous fascia pelvis. Since the anterior vaginal wall is usually intact, injuries to this fascia have not been described in relation to birth. Studies indicate that there are indirect signs of connective tissue trauma, such as "tenting" of the vaginal

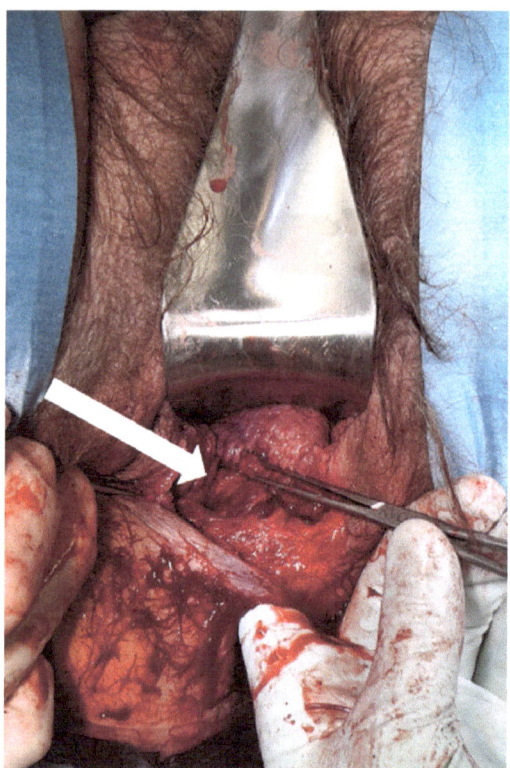

Fig. 16.4 Rectovaginal "fascia" (white arrow) exposed in a vaginal tear at delivery

fornices seen on examination several weeks to months after birth [29].

It is likely that occult connective tissue trauma occurs during birth, but the prevalence is unknown. Pelvic floor connective tissue resilience decreases after vaginal birth [30]. When the pelvic floor muscles are also weakened, decreases in connective tissue resilience around menopause further contribute to development of pelvic organ prolapse.

16.3.2 Nerve Injury

The muscles of the pelvic floor are innervated by the S2-S4 nerve roots via the pudendal nerve and direct branches from the motor roots [14]. Labor and vaginal birth cause partial denervation of the pelvic floor in 80% of primiparous women [20]. The degree of denervation is usually slight, and electromyography (EMG) evidence of reinnervation is common [20]. Abnormally prolonged ter-

minal motor latencies of the pudendal nerve recover to the normal range within 6 months after birth in most women [31]. Usually, pudendal nerve injury causes little or no clinical symptoms, because of reinnervation and subsequent muscle hypertrophy. In some women, however, the denervation is more severe and associated with urinary and fecal incontinence soon after birth. Unfortunately, in a small proportion of women nerve damage is permanent. Denervation may progress with future births and aging and may cause pelvic floor symptoms in later life [32].

Multiparity, forceps birth, increased duration of second stage of labor, obstetric anal sphincter trauma and high birth weight are important factors leading to pudendal nerve injury [33].

16.4 Diagnosis of Levator Trauma

16.4.1 Diagnosis at Birth

Diagnosis of levator avulsion in the birth room is usually impossible. Avulsion is commonly occult, covered by intact vaginal mucosa, and it is difficult to assess even if exposed by vaginal tears [34]. An observant birth attendant may identify such injuries, because levator avulsion can sometimes be evident when the tissues are exposed in deep vaginal tears, typically when fatty tissue is visible under a tear in the posterolateral vaginal wall [35] (Fig. 16.5). However, most injuries are diagnosed later, when women seek help for pelvic floor disorders. Unfortunately, birth attendants are almost never aware of the consequences of such injuries.

Perineal and vaginal tears are clinical markers for occult levator ani trauma [34]. Women with perineal tears have upwards of a three to eight times increased risk of levator trauma; this is something of which the birth attendant should be aware.

On physical exam upon inspection, women with a unilateral levator avulsion often show asymmetry in the axis between the vagina and anus, because the anus is pulled toward the side of the healthy muscle (Fig. 16.6). This will not be evident, however, if there is a bilateral avulsion. Also, measuring the genital hiatus (Gh) and peri-

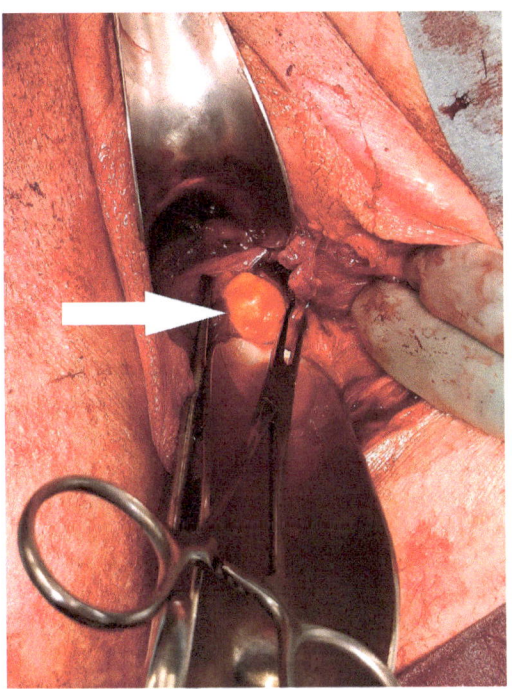

Fig. 16.5 Fatty tissue (white arrow) exposed in a deep vaginal tear implies high suspicion of levator avulsion

neal body (Pb) at Valsalva as defined by the pelvic organ prolapse quantification (POP-Q) system [36], can help identify women with levator avulsion [37]. The measurement of Gh+Pb >8.5 cm at Valsalva has sensitivity and specificity of 70% to diagnose women with avulsion (Fig. 16.7).

Palpation can be used to detect levator trauma by inserting two fingers into the vagina and palpating the lateral vaginal wall at rest and during pelvic floor muscle contraction. If there is a significant muscle injury, there will be no muscle covering the bone, and therefore not possible to feel any contraction at this point. Learning how to palpate and diagnose avulsions might be easier when performing pelvic floor ultrasound to confirm the diagnosis. Even after substantial training, detection of major levator trauma by palpation is less reliable than identification by ultrasound [38].

Muscle contraction can be assessed by palpation or devices inserted into the vagina to measure vaginal pressure (perineometry) or muscle

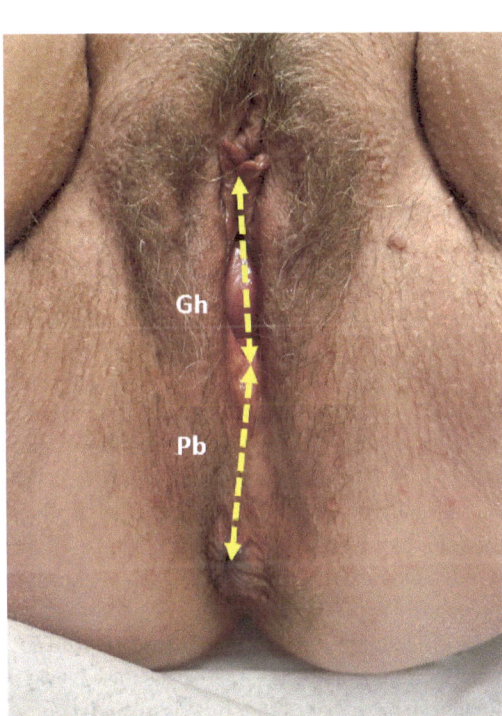

Fig. 16.6 Perineal asymmetry in woman with left levator avulsion. The anus is pulled to the side of the healthy muscle, creating an angle between the genital hiatus (Gh) and the perineal body (Pb)

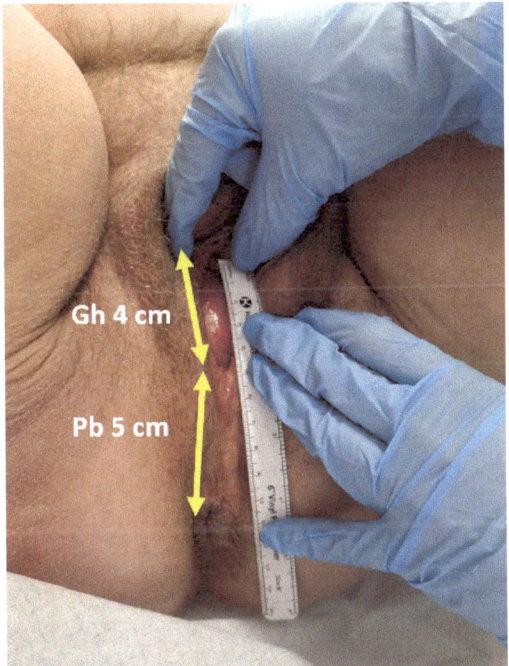

Fig. 16.7 The measurement of genital hiatus (Gh) + perineal body (Pb) >8.5 cm at Valsalva indicates high risk of levator avulsion (sensitivity and specificity 70%). This woman has a Gh+Pb of 11 cm indicating high risk of levator trauma

activity (EMG) [39–41]. Weaker pelvic floor muscle contraction is associated with muscle injury, but some women with intact muscles are not able to contract correctly, and women with injuries often maintain some ability to contract [42, 43]. Palpation of the presence or absence of the muscle bulk at its insertion point or imaging is therefore necessary to confirm the diagnosis.

16.4.2 Ultrasound Diagnosis

Transperineal (translabial) ultrasound via application of a 3D abdominal probe is usually used to diagnose pelvic floor muscle trauma. It is also possible to use a vaginal probe for introital [44] or endovaginal imaging [45]. Diagnosis of levator avulsion on 2D ultrasound has also been described [46]. For *transperineal ultrasound,* we use a 3D curved array abdominal probe covered with gel and an examination glove placed on the woman's introitus and perineum (Fig. 16.8). By convention, the bowel and urinary bladder should

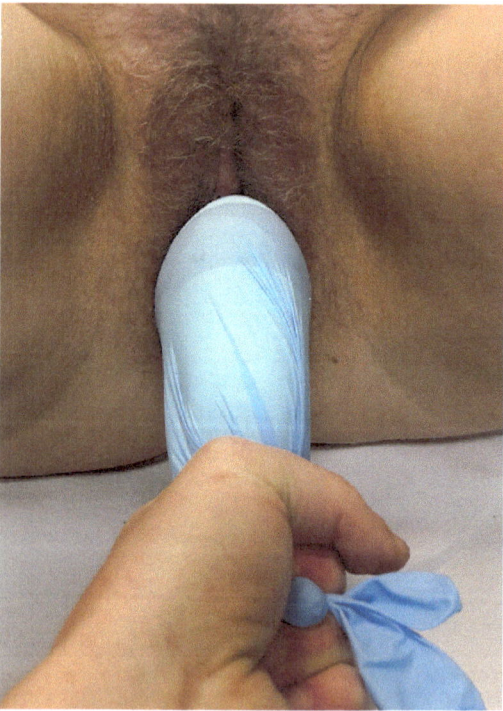

Fig. 16.8 Transperineal ultrasound. The 3D abdominal probe is covered with gel and a glove and is placed in the sagittal plane on the woman's introitus and perineum

be emptied before imaging, and the woman is placed in the dorsal lithotomy position. The standardized criteria for diagnosis of muscle injury apply to 3D/4D imaging and require post processing of the ultrasound volumes either directly on the ultrasound machine (Fig. 16.9) or on a computer using specific programs provided by the manufacturers, such as GE 4D View® (Fig. 16.10).

Levator avulsion (macrotrauma) is diagnosed at pelvic floor muscle contraction or at rest if a woman is unable to contract. We use *tomographic ultrasound imaging* (TUI) and evaluate the insertion of the muscle at the pubic bone at the plane of minimal levator hiatal dimensions and the planes 2.5–5.0 mm cranial to this. *The plane of minimal hiatal dimensions* is the oblique axial plane where we find the shortest distance between the symphysis pubis and the anterior margin of the puborectalis muscle, as this curves behind the rectum (Figs. 16.9 and 16.10). Abnormal muscle insertion in all three central slices is defined as a complete avulsion, which can be uni- or bilateral [19] (Fig. 16.11). Abnormal muscle insertion in one or two planes is regarded as incomplete and is not strongly associated with symptoms or anatomical prolapse. Measurement of the *levator-urethral gap* can be used when there is doubt about avulsion diagnosis. A distance >25 mm between the center of the urethra and the levator insertion on the symphysis is strongly associated with levator avulsion [47] (Fig. 16.11). The optimal cut-off probably varies between different populations [48].

Microtrauma causing abnormal distensibility or *ballooning* of the levator hiatus is diagnosed at Valsalva maneuver. The woman performs a moderately forceful exhalation against a closed airway with simultaneous relaxation of the pelvic floor, for minimum 6 seconds [49]. Hiatal areas are measured in the *rendered image* of 1–2 cm thickness at the plane of minimal hiatal dimensions, as the levator hiatus is slightly curved (Fig. 16.10) [50]. Microtrauma is defined as >20% increased levator hiatal area on Valsalva after birth [26], and requires examination of women before and after birth. Another definition of overdistension requires examination at only one time point, using established cut-offs for hiatal ballooning at Valsalva:

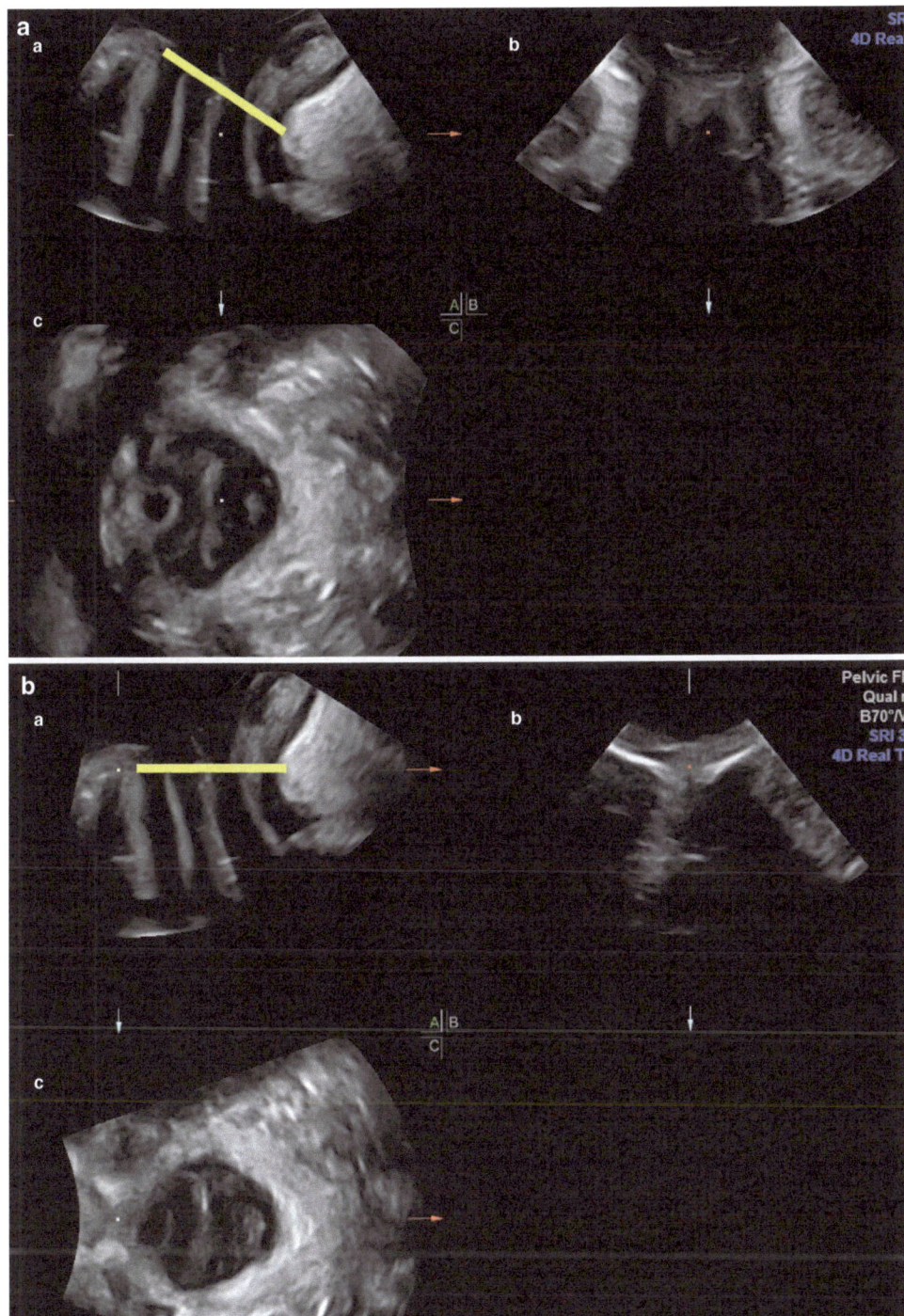

Fig. 16.9 Intact levator. Starting with "sectional planes", the plane of minimal hiatal dimensions (yellow line) is identified in image A (**a**), and rotated to the horizontal plane (**b**). Then, image C is rotated 90° and "tomographic ultrasound imaging" is chosen (**c**). The distance between the slices is adjusted to 2.5 mm. This image shows an intact levator in the three central planes (yellow box): the plane of minimal hiatal dimensions and the planes 2.5–5.0 mm cranial to this. The symphysis pubis is open-closing-closed in the three central planes

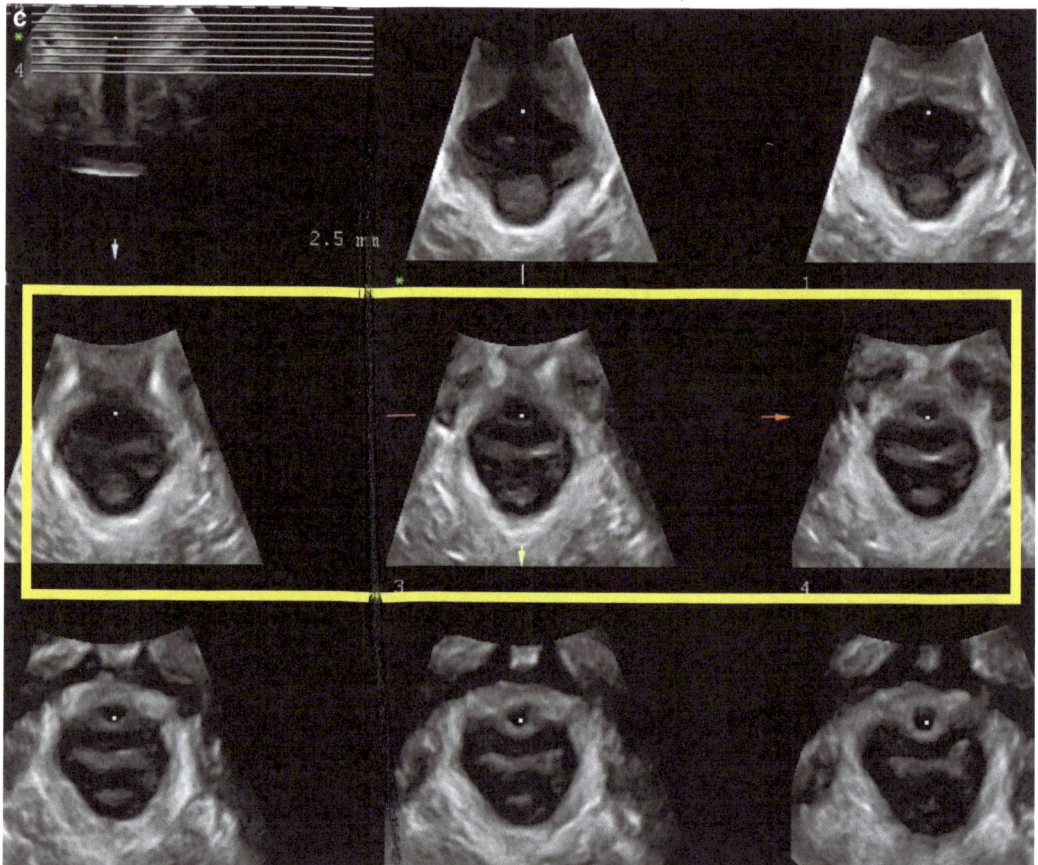

Fig. 16.9 (continued)

25–29.9 cm² is considered 'mild', 30–34.9 cm² is 'moderate', 35–39.9 cm² is 'marked' and ≥40 cm² is 'severe' ballooning or overdistension [51]. These cut-offs are commonly used but have not been validated in different populations. Figure 16.12 demonstrates the difference in levator hiatal areas at Valsalva in a woman with intact levator, one with unilateral avulsion, and one with severe ballooning.

Connective tissue injury is difficult to diagnose with ultrasound [52]. Imaging can indirectly indicate such injuries, e.g. diagnosis of posterior prolapse (rectocele) implies a weakening or defect of the rectovaginal fascia [53]. Vaginal birth is also associated with loss of "tenting" of the vaginal fornices and with impaired anterior vaginal wall support, independent of levator injury [29]. This indicates detachment of the pubocervical fascia from its lateral attachment at the arcus tendineous fascia pelvis.

16.4.3 Magnetic Resonance Imaging Diagnosis

Magnetic resonance imaging (MRI) can be used to diagnose pelvic floor trauma, but due to higher costs and limited availability, MRI is used more often in research than in clinical practice. On MRI, levator ani muscle abnormalities are found after vaginal birth, and the images are analyzed in the axial plane at the level of the mid urethra [3, 54]. The left and right muscles are scored separately, and the total score is the sum of the two sides, categorized as: 0 = normal or no defect, 1–3 = minor defect and 4–6 = major defect, Fig. 16.13. A woman with unilateral score of 3 is considered to have a unilateral minor defect. Hiatal areas can be measured in the angled axial plane to determine the shortest distance between the posterior margin of the symphysis pubis and the anterior margin of the puborectal muscle (plane of minimal hiatal dimensions), then measuring the hiatal area [55].

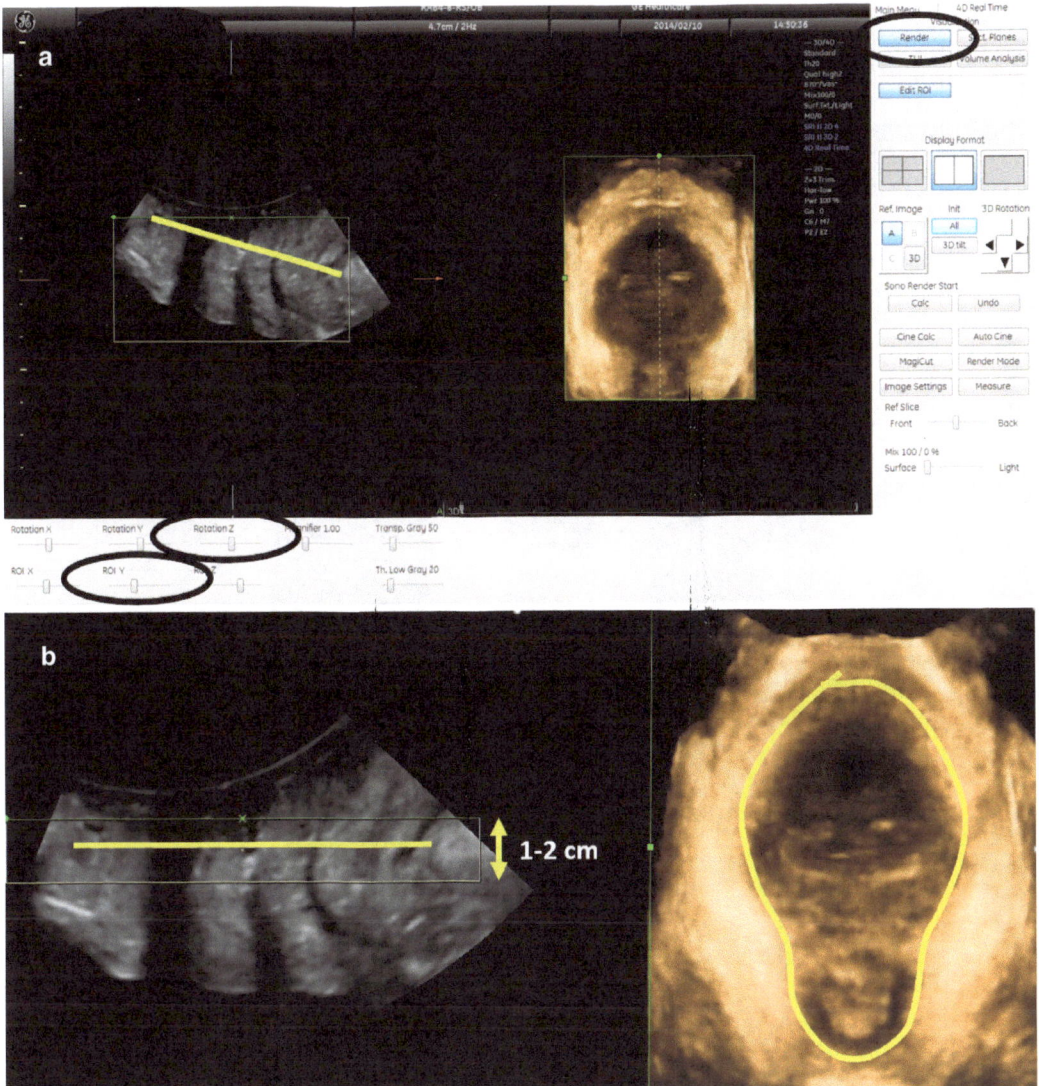

Fig. 16.10 Measurement of levator hiatal area in 4D View®. Starting with "rendered imaging", the plane of minimal hiatal dimensions (yellow line) is identified in image **a**, and rotated to the horizontal plane (**b**). The region of interest (ROI) (box covering the plane of minimal hiatal dimensions) is adjusted to 1–2 cm thickness. The hiatal area is measured in the rendered image

The criteria used for levator avulsion and measurements of hiatal areas on ultrasound and MRI vary slightly. Levator avulsion can be diagnosed reliably by both tomographic ultrasound imaging and MRI [56]. Applying the same diagnostic criteria to ultrasound and MRI showed very good agreement between the two classification systems in diagnosing levator defects [57]. On the other hand, levator hiatal biometry measurements are significantly larger on MRI when compared with ultrasound [55]. The agreement between transperineal ultrasound and MRI for measurement of the levator hiatus at rest is only moderate, most likely because we use a 3D rendered ultrasound image of 1–2 cm thickness to measure the area; on MRI the area is measured in one plane [55]. Ultrasound and MRI measurements can therefore not be used interchangeably in the clinic or in research [55, 58].

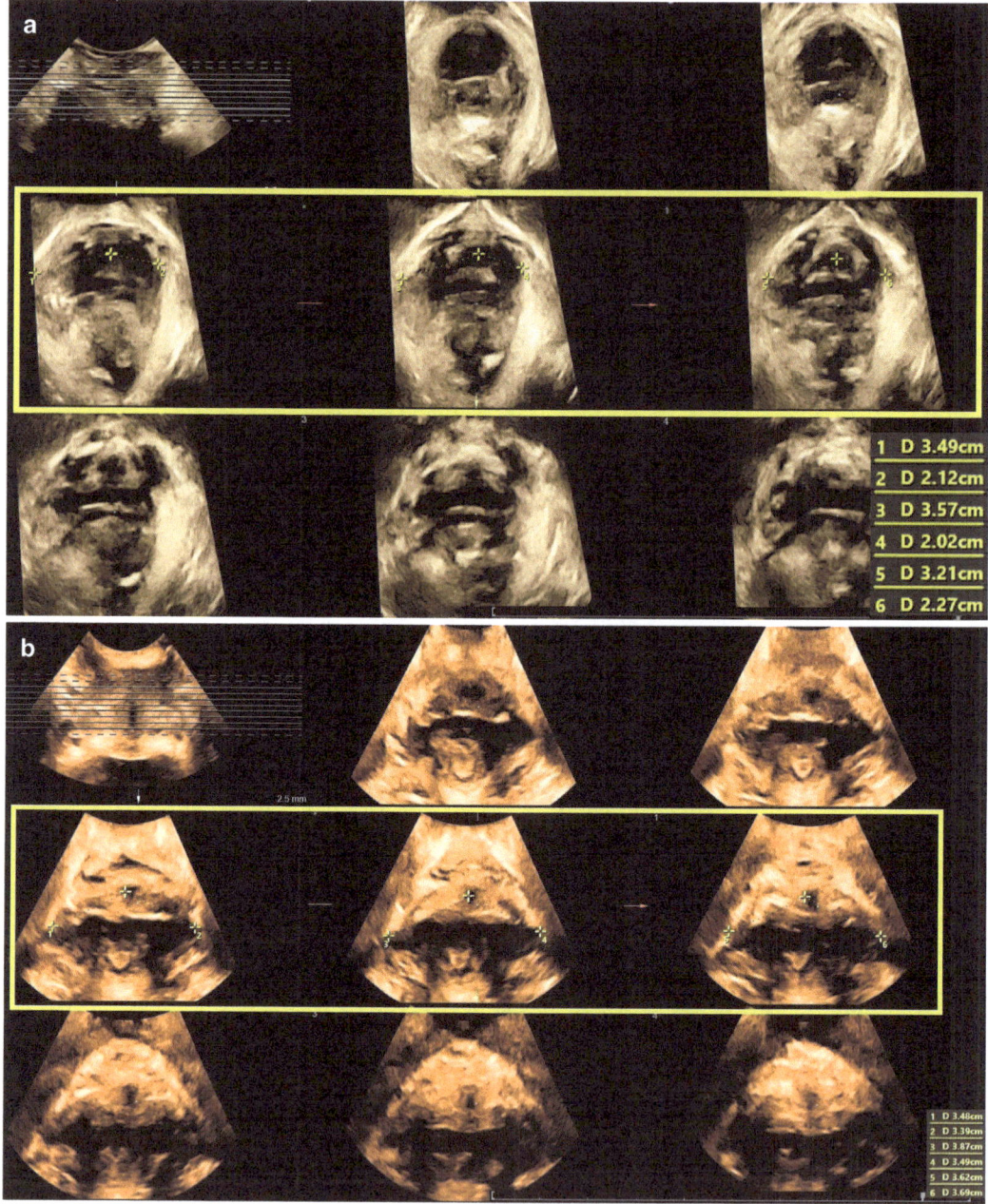

Fig. 16.11 (a) Unilateral levator avulsion. The levator-urethral gap is measured in all three central slices (yellow box) and is >25 mm on the right side, confirming a right-sided avulsion. (b) Bilateral levator avulsion. There is no visible attachment to the pubic bone in the three central slices (yellow box), and the levator urethral gap is >25 mm on both sides

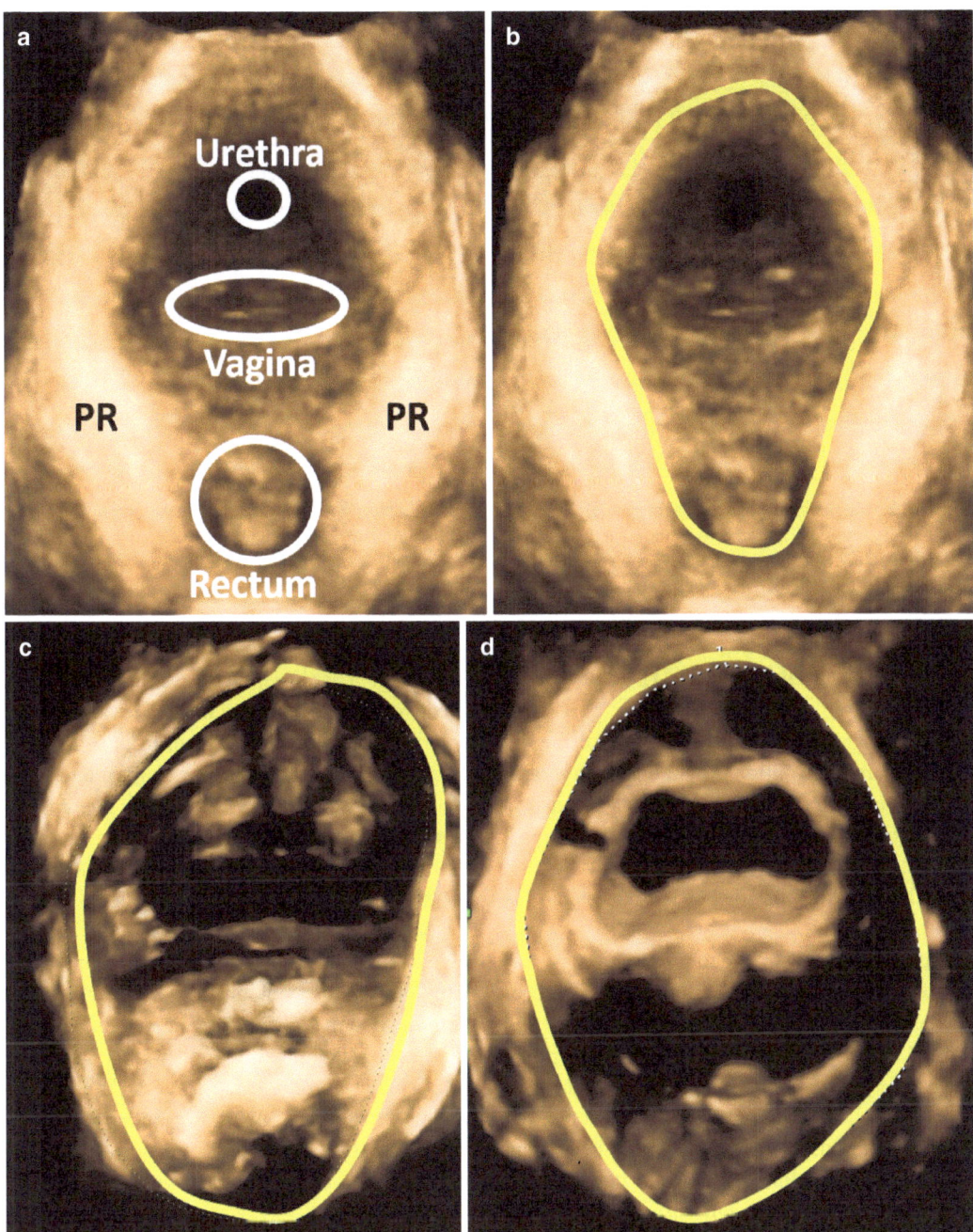

Fig. 16.12 (a) Rendered image showing the puborectalis (PR) muscle surrounding the urethra, vagina and rectum. Hiatal area at Valsalva measured in the rendered image in woman with (b) intact levator (20 cm²), (c) unilateral avulsion (41 cm²) and (d) microtrauma (45 cm²)

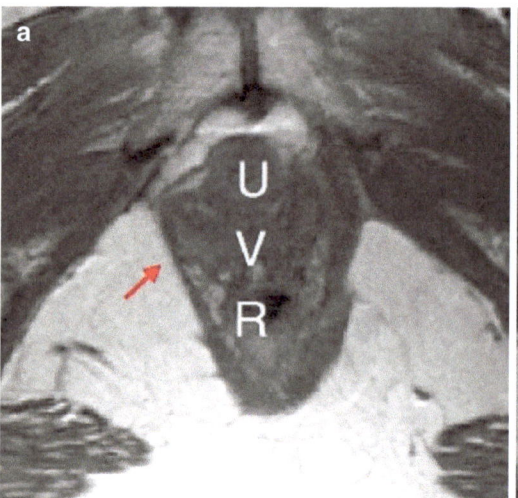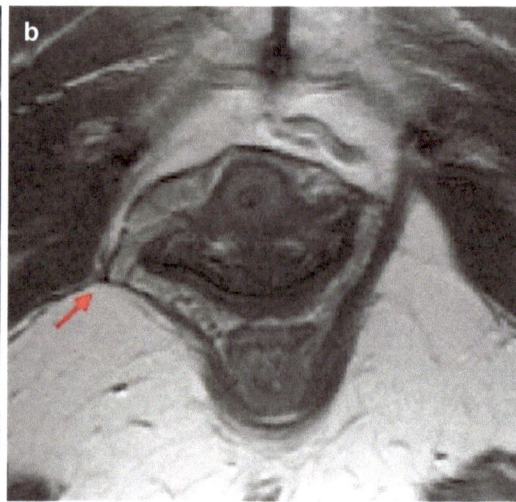

Fig. 16.13 Magnetic resonance imaging of defects in the puborectalis muscle. The red arrows indicate the location of the muscle defect. (**a**) Unilateral levator defect (**b**) Unilateral levator defect and architectural distortion.

(From Larson KA et al 2012: "Measurement of the 3D geometry of the fascial arches in women with a unilateral levator defect and architectural distortion", with permission from Springer Nature)

16.5   Repair of Levator Trauma

Levator repair at birth has not been described in the literature as an option. Re-suturing the levator immediately after birth has been described in a case report, but this was not successful [35]. Since levator trauma usually is occult at the time of birth, access to the muscle is not feasible for repair.

Attempt has been made to *repair levator avulsion* at the time of prolapse surgery. A polypropylene mesh was attached to the muscle and sutured to the medial surface of the inferior pubic ramus [59]. While the surgical procedure was apparently successful, a substantial portion of the cohort experienced recurrent prolapse or pain [59]. The same group of researchers have applied a polypropylene puborectalis sling to *reduce the hiatal area* in women with severe hiatal ballooning at the time of prolapse surgery [60]. The hiatal area was reduced by 30% on average, but 66% of the women had prolapse recurrence within 2 years. A case report found that ultrasound guided surgical repair of bilateral levator avulsions was successful [61], but long-term results are not reported. As such, these surgical techniques remain unproven, and the results are not promising. Therefore, we have no established effective surgical procedure to repair levator avulsions or correct levator overdistension.

Despite the inability to surgically repair levator trauma, studies from different populations have found that the levator muscle can recover after pregnancy and birth, and most of the recovery probably occurs during the first 6 months postpartum [10, 62, 63]. Partial avulsion can recover over time, but this is less common for complete levator avulsion [63]. Healing of *complete levator avulsion* was observed in 13–30% of women reexamined 3–4 years after birth [10, 64]. *Levator hiatal areas* restitute during the first months after birth, but do not decrease to pre-birth level [62]. Some women also have persistently increased hiatal areas when reexamined after 4 years [64].

16.6   Consequences of Levator Trauma

Levator avulsion and microtrauma are independent risk factors for the development of pelvic organ prolapse [65]. The role of avulsion in the pathogenesis of prolapse is not fully explained by its effect on levator hiatal areas. Women with levator avulsions have weaker pelvic floor muscle contraction, and this can be an important mediator in the development of prolapse as well [43]. Levator avulsion implies not only muscular trauma, but is also marker for possible damage to structures difficult to assess clinically or by imaging, such as connective tissue, all of which play an important role in pelvic organ support [65].

A systematic review found that levator avulsion is strongly associated with both symptomatic and anatomical prolapse [66]. A meta-analysis of nine studies confirmed that women with levator avulsions had double the risk of symptomatic prolapse, and prolapse at clinical examination increased almost four times [66]. Severe levator hiatal ballooning with an area >40 cm^2 increased the risk of anatomical prolapse seven-fold and symptomatic prolapse more than three fold [67].

Interestingly, levator trauma is more strongly associated with prolapse in the anterior and middle compartments, resulting in anterior prolapse (cystocele) and apical descent of the uterus, than it is with prolapse in the posterior compartment [65, 67].

Levator avulsion and microtrauma are also associated with reduced contractile function of the muscles [21]. This has been demonstrated in several studies that used different tools to assess contraction, such as palpation, perineometry and ultrasound [43, 68]. Although women with levator injuries have significantly lower muscle strength and endurance than women without such defects, most women with levator injuries are able to contract to some degree. This indicates a potential capacity by non-injured muscle fibres to compensate for loss in muscle strength [69].

From a sexual dysfunction standpoint, women with levator avulsion have lower scores for desire, lubrication, orgasm and satisfaction than women without avulsion when assessed with the Female Sexual Function Index [70] 6 months after birth [71]. During the first months after birth, women with levator trauma are more likely to have a sensation of vaginal laxity [8, 9]. However, hiatal dimensions seem not to be related to sexual dysfunction within the first year after birth [72]. Intestingly, later in life, a larger hiatal area on Valsalva is associated with vaginal laxity and

sexual dysfunction [73, 74]. Reduced pelvic floor muscle strength could be a link between levator trauma and sexual dysfunction [75]. However, a general lack of long-term studies regarding levator trauma and sexual function exists.

In looking at urinary incontinence, a meta-analysis including data from seven studies found no association between levator avulsion and stress urinary incontinence [76]. Only one included study at 3–5 years after birth found that women with levator avulsion reported stress incontinence symptoms more often than those without avulsion; not surprisingly, they had higher symptom scores as well [10].

There are also controversies regarding levator trauma and anal incontinence. Some studies have found that levator avulsion is associated with higher prevalence of fecal incontinence [77–79], but other studies have not confirmed this [80]. Thus, it seems that the effect of levator trauma on urinary and colorectal anal distress is of unclear clinical importance.

Several studies have shown that obstetric anal sphincter injuries are associated with a three to eight times increased risk of levator injuries [34, 81–83], and approximately 30–40% of women with anal sphincter trauma also have a significant levator injury [68, 82]. The high prevalence of anal incontinence in women with combined injuries seems to be caused by the anal sphincter injury, with no additional effect of levator injury on incontinence symptoms few months after delivery [68]. However, more long-term follow-up studies are needed to investigate if levator injury adds to the effect of anal sphincter injuries later in life.

16.7 Conservative Treatment of Women with Levator Trauma

16.7.1 Pelvic Floor Muscle Exercise

While levator ani muscle trauma is associated with weaker pelvic floor muscle contraction, most women with levator avulsion do retain the ability to contract [43, 69]. There is a need for studies to determine if pelvic floor muscle exercise in women with levator trauma can delay or prevent the occurrence of symptomatic pelvic floor disorders. Overall, pelvic floor muscle exercise is effective in the prevention and treatment of stress urinary incontinence and symptoms of mild prolapse [84, 85]. Therefore, pelvic floor muscle exercise should be recommended to women with muscle trauma, understanding that women with injuries will likely benefit less than women without injuries.

16.7.2 Vaginal Pessary Treatment of Pelvic Organ Prolapse

Unfortunately, levator avulsion and microtrauma are associated with failed vaginal pessary treatment for pelvic organ prolapse. Women with levator avulsion are two to three times more likely to expel a pessary, and women with large hiatal areas are two times more likely to have unsuccessful pessary fitting than those with intact pelvic floor muscles [86], thus limiting this as a treatment option for POP in these women.

16.8 Surgical Treatment of Women with Levator Trauma and Prolapse

Women with levator trauma undergoing surgery for pelvic organ prolapse tend to be younger and have lower BMIs compared to women without avulsion [87]. Similalry, women with larger hiatal areas are also younger at surgery [88]. In one study, the time span between first birth and surgery was 8 years shorter for women with levator avulsion (30 vs. 38 years).

Unfortunately, outcomes of surgery are often less optimal in women with levator avulsions. For example, recurrent anatomical prolapse occurred almost three times more often in women with levator avulsion in a meta-analysis including ten studies [89]. A more recent meta-analysis could not confirm levator avulsion as a risk factor for objective prolapse recurrence, except for native tissue repair in the anterior wall [90]. Also, women with a combined anal sphincter and leva-

tor injury are reported to improve less after prolapse surgery and have higher symptom scores related to prolapse, urinary and colorectal-anal distress when assessed 6 months postoperatively [91]. Given these findings, surgical procedure of choice may differ in women with levator trauma. For example, in this population, vaginal mesh surgery was associated with four times reduction in anatomical and symptomatic recurrence of prolapse [92]. While the use of vaginal mesh has been abandoned in most countries, laparoscopic sacrocolpopexy and -uteropexy should be considered in women with avulsions, as prolapse recurrence is similar in women with and without levator trauma for these mesh-augmented repairs [93].

16.9 Prevention of Levator Trauma

It is well-known that risk reduction is essential in the prevention of trauma. A prenatal prediction model of the risk of sustaining pelvic floor muscle trauma during birth would be of great clinical value. Maternal age, advanced maternal age at first birth, BMI, high estimated birth weight, bladder neck descent and family history of cesarean birth are all *antenatal predictors for levator trauma* [23, 94, 95].

In the delivery suite, *forceps birth* is the strongest modifiable obstetric risk factor for levator ani muscle trauma. Forceps carry a seven times higher risk for levator avulsion than spontaneous vaginal birth and a four to five times higher risk of avulsion than vacuum assisted birth (Fig. 16.3) [6]. In fact, vacuum-assistance carries the same risk for levator trauma as spontaenous vaginal birth. In most obstetric situations it is possible to use vacuum interchangeably with forceps, and vacuum should be preferred in order to minimize the risk of levator trauma and pelvic floor disorders later in life. *Episiotomy* is not a risk factor for levator avulsion, and it seems more likely that it has a slightly protective effect [68, 96]. A mediolateral episiotomy only involves the perineal muscles and not the anal sphincters or levator ani muscle. As episiotomy is known to increase the risk of anal sphincter injury, however, judicious use is recommended [97]. Labour dystocia and long duration of second stage of birth are also associated with levator injury [83].

Antenatally, there have been suggestions of various pelvic floor trainers. For example, a vaginal device used to increase elasticity of pelvic floor muscle prior to birth has been tested in a randomized controlled trial [98]. Women in the intervention group were instructed to use the device from 37 weeks of gestation onward, for two daily 20-min sessions. A balloon was inserted two-thirds into the vagina and inflated until causing a stretching sensation. At the end of each session, the inflated balloon was expelled by the woman, simulating birth of the fetal head. There was no difference in levator avulsion or microtrauma between the two groups, indicating that antenatal use of childbirth training devices is unlikely to be clinically beneficial in the prevention of levator injury and perineal trauma [98]. Similarly, while antenatal pelvic floor muscle exercise may be effective at shortening the second stage of labour and reducing severe perineal trauma, little is known about the effect on prevention of pelvic floor muscle trauma [99].

16.10 Management of Subsequent Pregnancy and Birth

It is well-known that a woman's first vaginal birth carries the greatest risk for levator injury. Prospective studies have shown that a second vaginal birth can result in deterioration of a partial levator avulsion, but new avulsions usually do not occur [10, 64, 100]. Moreover, a second pregnancy and birth do not have the same effect on bladder support or levator ani muscle function [100]. Other studies have compared the prevalence of levator avulsion and the size of levator hiatal areas between primiparous and multiparous women. No significant difference in prevalence of levator avulsion or size of hiatal areas was found between primipara and multipara [101, 102]. Levator injury is therefore not an indication for cesarean at subsequent deliveries.

16.11 Conclusions

Obstetric levator ani muscle injury is usually occult at the time of birth, and it is impossible to repair. Levator injury diagnosed with ultrasound or MRI later in life is strongly associated with pelvic organ prolapse, failure of vaginal pessary treatment, need for reconstructive pelvic surgery at a younger age and recurrence of prolapse after surgery. Therefore caution should be taken to prevent such injuries. Forceps assisted birth is the strongest modifiable obstetric risk factor for levator injury, and vacuum should be preferred when possible.

Take Home Messages
- Obstetric levator ani muscle injury and trauma to connective tissue and nerves are risk factors for pelvic floor dysfunction later in life.
- Levator injury is usually occult at the time of birth.
- Levator injury can be visualized with 3D/4D transperineal ultrasound and MRI after birth and is categorized as levator avulsion (macrotrauma) and microtrauma.
- Levator injury is strongly associated with pelvic organ prolapse, failure of vaginal pessary treatment, need for reconstructive pelvic surgery at a younger age and recurrence of prolapse after surgery.
- Levator injury cannot be repaired, and therefore injury prevention is critical
- Forceps delivery is the strongest modifiable obstetric risk factor for levator injury. Vacuum carries the same risk as spontaneous vaginal birth and should be preferred. Episiotomy seems to be protective, however, should be used judiciously.
- An injured muscle still retains its ability to contract, and pelvic floor muscle exercise may protect against pelvic floor disorders in women with levator injuries.
- Levator injury is not an indication for cesarean birth at subsequent deliveries.

Appendix: MCQ

Mark each item TRUE or FALSE

Questions

1. Levator ani muscle avulsion is a strong risk factor for which of the following?
   (A) Stress urinary incontinence
   (B) Fecal urgency
   (C) Anterior compartment prolapse
   (D) Posterior compartment prolapse
   (E) Urge urinary incontinence

2. Minimal criteria for diagnosis of clinically significant levator ani muscle avulsion on tomographic ultrasound include which of the following?
   (A) Unilateral Abnormal muscle insertion in all three central slices
   (B) Bilateral Abnormal muscle insertion in all three central slices
   (C) Unilateral Abnormal muscle insertion in at least one of three central slices
   (D) Bilateral Abnormal muscle insertion in at least one of three central slices

3. The most important risk factor for levator ani muscle trauma is
   (A) Mediolateral episiotomy
   (B) Forceps delivery
   (C) Vacuum delivery
   (D) High BMI
   (E) High maternal age

4. Obstetric nerve injury is usually associated with
   (A) Urinary incontinence
   (B) Pelvic organ prolapse
   (C) Persistent vulvodynia
   (D) Sexual dysfunction
   (E) Little or no clinical symptoms

5. Pelvic floor disorders caused by pelvic floor muscle trauma can be prevented by
   (A) Surgically repair of the levator muscle immediately after childbirth
   (B) Pelvic floor muscle exercise
   (C) Surgical repair of the levator muscle after menopause

   (D) Treatment with vaginal pessary until 6 months after childbirth
   (E) Cesarean section at subsequent childbirths

6. Typical signs of connective tissue injury are
   (A) "Tenting" of the vaginal fornices
   (B) Increased retrovesical angle on ultrasound
   (C) Weakened pelvic floor muscle contraction
   (D) Inability to relax the pelvic floor muscles
   (E) Expulsion of vaginal pessary

Answers

1. Levator ani muscle avulsion is a strong risk factor for which of the following?
   (A) FALSE
   (B) FALSE
   (C) TRUE
   (D) FALSE
   (E) FALSE

2. Minimal criteria for diagnosis of clinically significant levator ani muscle avulsion on tomographic ultrasound include which of the following?
   (A) TRUE
   (B) FALSE
   (C) FALSE
   (D) FALSE

3. The most important risk factor for levator ani muscle trauma is
   (A) FALSE
   (B) TRUE
   (C) FALSE
   (D) FALSE
   (E) FALSE

4. Obstetric nerve injury is usually associated with
   (A) FALSE
   (B) FALSE
   (C) FALSE
   (D) FALSE
   (E) TRUE

5. Pelvic floor disorders caused by pelvic floor muscle trauma can be prevented by
   (A) FALSE
   (B) TRUE
   (C) FALSE
   (D) FALSE
   (E) FALSE

6. Typical signs of connective tissue injury are
   (A) TRUE
   (B) FALSE
   (C) FALSE
   (D) FALSE
   (E) FALSE

References

1. Gainey HL. Postpartum observation of pelvic tissue damage: further studies. Am J Obstet Gynecol. 1955;70(4):800–7. https://doi.org/10.1016/s0002-9378(16)37836-x.
2. Tunn R, DeLancey JO, Howard D, Thorp JM, Ashton-Miller JA, Quint LE. MR imaging of levator ani muscle recovery following vaginal delivery. Int Urogynecol J Pelvic Floor Dysfunct. 1999;10(5):300–7. https://doi.org/10.1007/s001929970006.
3. DeLancey JO, Kearney R, Chou Q, Speights S, Binno S. The appearance of levator ani muscle abnormalities in magnetic resonance images after vaginal delivery. Obstet Gynecol. 2003;101(1):46–53. https://doi.org/10.1016/s0029-7844(02)02465-1.
4. Dietz HP. Ultrasound imaging of the pelvic floor. Part II: three-dimensional or volume imaging. Ultrasound Obstet Gynecol. 2004;23(6):615–25. https://doi.org/10.1002/uog.1072.
5. Dietz HP, Shek C, Clarke B. Biometry of the pubovisceral muscle and levator hiatus by three-dimensional pelvic floor ultrasound. Ultrasound Obstet Gynecol. 2005;25(6):580–5. https://doi.org/10.1002/uog.1899.
6. Friedman T, Eslick GD, Dietz HP. Delivery mode and the risk of levator muscle avulsion: a meta-analysis. Int Urogynecol J. 2019;30(6):901–7. https://doi.org/10.1007/s00192-018-3827-8.
7. Siahkal SF, Iravani M, Mohaghegh Z, Sharifipour F, Zahedian M, Nasab MB. Investigating the association of the dimensions of genital hiatus and levator hiatus with pelvic organ prolapse: a systematic review. Int Urogynecol J. 2021;32(8):2095–109. https://doi.org/10.1007/s00192-020-04639-0.
8. Thibault-Gagnon S, Yusuf S, Langer S, Wong V, Shek KL, Martin A, et al. Do women notice the impact of childbirth-related levator trauma on pelvic floor and sexual function? Results of an observational ultrasound study. Int Urogynecol J. 2014;25(10):1389–98. https://doi.org/10.1007/s00192-014-2331-z.
9. van Delft K, Sultan AH, Thakar R, Schwertner-Tiepelmann N, Kluivers K. The relationship between postpartum levator ani muscle avulsion and signs and symptoms of pelvic floor dysfunction. BJOG. 2014;121(9):1164–71; discussion 72. https://doi.org/10.1111/1471-0528.12666.
10. Chan SSC, Cheung RYK, Lee LL, Choy RKW, Chung TKH. Longitudinal follow-up of levator ani muscle avulsion: does a second delivery affect it? Ultrasound Obstet Gynecol. 2017;50(1):110–5. https://doi.org/10.1002/uog.16009.
11. Chan SS, Cheung RY, Yiu KW, Lee LL, Chung TK. Effect of levator ani muscle injury on primiparous women during the first year after childbirth. Int Urogynecol J. 2014;25(10):1381–8. https://doi.org/10.1007/s00192-014-2340-y.
12. Thomas V, Shek KL, Guzmán Rojas R, Dietz HP. Temporal latency between pelvic floor trauma and presentation for prolapse surgery: a retrospective observational study. Int Urogynecol J. 2015;26(8):1185–9. https://doi.org/10.1007/s00192-015-2677-x.
13. Klutke CG, Siegel CL. Functional female pelvic anatomy. Urol Clin North Am. 1995;22(3):487–98.
14. Percy JP, Neill ME, Swash M, Parks AG. Electrophysiological study of motor nerve supply of pelvic floor. Lancet. 1981;1(8210):16–7. https://doi.org/10.1016/s0140-6736(81)90117-3.
15. Herschorn S. Female pelvic floor anatomy: the pelvic floor, supporting structures, and pelvic organs. Rev Urol. 2004;6(Suppl 5(Suppl 5)):S2–s10.
16. Lien KC, Mooney B, DeLancey JO, Ashton-Miller JA. Levator ani muscle stretch induced by simulated vaginal birth. Obstet Gynecol. 2004;103(1):31–40. https://doi.org/10.1097/01.Aog.0000109207.22354.65.
17. Sindhwani N, Bamberg C, Famaey N, Callewaert G, Dudenhausen JW, Teichgräber U, et al. In vivo evidence of significant levator ani muscle stretch on MR images of a live childbirth. Am J Obstet Gynecol. 2017;217(2):194.e1–8. https://doi.org/10.1016/j.ajog.2017.04.014.
18. Dietz HP, Lanzarone V. Levator trauma after vaginal delivery. Obstet Gynecol. 2005;106(4):707–12. https://doi.org/10.1097/01.aog.0000178779.62181.01.
19. Dietz HP, Bernardo MJ, Kirby A, Shek KL. Minimal criteria for the diagnosis of avulsion of the puborectalis muscle by tomographic ultrasound. Int Urogynecol J. 2011;22(6):699–704. https://doi.org/10.1007/s00192-010-1329-4.
20. Allen RE, Hosker GL, Smith AR, Warrell DW. Pelvic floor damage and childbirth: a neurophysiological study. Br J Obstet Gynaecol. 1990;97(9):770–9. https://doi.org/10.1111/j.1471-0528.1990.tb02570.x.
21. Guzmán Rojas R, Wong V, Shek KL, Dietz HP. Impact of levator trauma on pelvic floor muscle function. Int Urogynecol J. 2014;25(3):375–80. https://doi.org/10.1007/s00192-013-2226-4.

22. Shek KL, Dietz HP. The effect of childbirth on hiatal dimensions. Obstet Gynecol. 2009;113(6):1272–8. https://doi.org/10.1097/AOG.0b013e3181a5ef23.

23. Volløyhaug I, Mørkved S, Salvesen Ø, Salvesen K. Forceps delivery is associated with increased risk of pelvic organ prolapse and muscle trauma: a cross-sectional study 16–24 years after first delivery. Ultrasound Obstet Gynecol. 2015;46(4):487–95. https://doi.org/10.1002/uog.14891.

24. Eisenberg V, Brecher S, Kalter A, Achiron R, Schiff E, Alklay M. The birthmark of instrumental deliveries. Ultrasound Obstet Gynecol. 2011;38(Suppl 1):153–4.

25. Kearney R, Fitzpatrick M, Brennan S, Behan M, Miller J, Keane D, et al. Levator ani injury in primiparous women with forceps delivery for fetal distress, forceps for second stage arrest, and spontaneous delivery. Int J Gynaecol Obstet. 2010;111(1):19–22. https://doi.org/10.1016/j.ijgo.2010.05.019.

26. Shek KL, Dietz HP. Intrapartum risk factors for levator trauma. BJOG. 2010;117(12):1485–92. https://doi.org/10.1111/j.1471-0528.2010.02704.x.

27. Roch M, Gaudreault N, Cyr MP, Venne G, Bureau NJ, Morin M. The female pelvic floor fascia anatomy: a systematic search and review. Life (Basel). 2021;11(9) https://doi.org/10.3390/life11090900.

28. Zone G. Second-degree perineal tear incl. the rectovaginal fascia_. https://my.gynzone.com/courses/64-diagnostics/chapters/258-second-degree-perineal-tear/watch/908-second-degree-perineal-tear-incl-the-rectovaginal-fascia. (2020). Accessed 28 Jan 2022.

29. Cassadó-Garriga J, Wong V, Shek K, Dietz HP. Can we identify changes in fascial paravaginal supports after childbirth? Aust N Z J Obstet Gynaecol. 2015;55(1):70–5. https://doi.org/10.1111/ajo.12261.

30. Reay Jones NH, Healy JC, King LJ, Saini S, Shousha S, Allen-Mersh TG. Pelvic connective tissue resilience decreases with vaginal delivery, menopause and uterine prolapse. Br J Surg. 2003;90(4):466–72. https://doi.org/10.1002/bjs.4065.

31. Sultan AH, Kamm MA, Hudson CN. Pudendal nerve damage during labour: prospective study before and after childbirth. Br J Obstet Gynaecol. 1994;101(1):22–8. https://doi.org/10.1111/j.1471-0528.1994.tb13005.x.

32. Van Geelen H, Ostergard D, Sand P. A review of the impact of pregnancy and childbirth on pelvic floor function as assessed by objective measurement techniques. Int Urogynecol J. 2018;29(3):327–38. https://doi.org/10.1007/s00192-017-3540-z.

33. Snooks SJ, Swash M, Henry MM, Setchell M. Risk factors in childbirth causing damage to the pelvic floor innervation. Int J Color Dis. 1986;1(1):20–4. https://doi.org/10.1007/bf01648831.

34. Shek KL, Green K, Hall J, Guzman-Rojas R, Dietz HP. Perineal and vaginal tears are clinical markers for occult levator ani trauma: a retrospective observational study. Ultrasound Obstet Gynecol.

2016;47(2):224–7. https://doi.org/10.1002/uog.14856.

35. Dietz HP, Gillespie AV, Phadke P. Avulsion of the pubovisceral muscle associated with large vaginal tear after normal vaginal delivery at term. Aust N Z J Obstet Gynaecol. 2007;47(4):341–4. https://doi.org/10.1111/j.1479-828X.2007.00748.x.

36. Bump RC, Mattiasson A, Bo K, Brubaker LP, DeLancey JO, Klarskov P, et al. The standardization of terminology of female pelvic organ prolapse and pelvic floor dysfunction. Am J Obstet Gynecol. 1996;175(1):10–7.

37. Volloyhaug I, Wong V, Shek KL, Dietz HP. Does levator avulsion cause distension of the genital hiatus and perineal body? Int Urogynecol J. 2013;24(7):1161–5. https://doi.org/10.1007/s00192-012-1993-7.

38. Dietz HP, Shek C. Validity and reproducibility of the digital detection of levator trauma. Int Urogynecol J Pelvic Floor Dysfunct. 2008;19(8):1097–101. https://doi.org/10.1007/s00192-008-0575-1.

39. Laycock J. Clinical evaluation of the pelvic floor. In: Pelvic floor re-education, principles and practice. London: Springer; 1994. p. 42–28.

40. Bø K, Kvarstein B, Hagen RR, Larsen S. Pelvic floor muscle exercise for the treatment of female stress urinary incontinence: II. Validity of vaginal pressure measurements of pelvic floor muscle strength and the necessity of supplementary methods for control of correct contraction. Neurourol Urodyn. 1990;9:479–87.

41. Siroky MB. Electromyography of the perineal floor. Urol Clin North Am. 1996;23(2):299–307.

42. Dietz HP, Shek C. Levator avulsion and grading of pelvic floor muscle strength. Int Urogynecol J Pelvic Floor Dysfunct. 2008;19(5):633–6. https://doi.org/10.1007/s00192-007-0491-9.

43. Nyhus M, Salvesen K, Volløyhaug I. Association between pelvic floor muscle trauma and contraction in parous women from a general population. Ultrasound Obstet Gynecol. 2019;53(2):262–8. https://doi.org/10.1002/uog.19195.

44. Cassadó Garriga J, Pessarrodona Isern A, Espuña Pons M, Durán Retamal M, Felgueroso Fabregas A, Rodriguez-Carballeira M. Tridimensional sonographic anatomical changes on pelvic floor muscle according to the type of delivery. Int Urogynecol J. 2011;22(8):1011–8. https://doi.org/10.1007/s00192-011-1413-4.

45. van Delft K, Shobeiri SA, Thakar R, Schwertner-Tiepelmann N, Sultan AH. Intra- and interobserver reliability of levator ani muscle biometry and avulsion using three-dimensional endovaginal ultrasonography. Ultrasound Obstet Gynecol. 2014;43(2):202–9. https://doi.org/10.1002/uog.13193.

46. Dietz HP, Shek KL. Levator defects can be detected by 2D translabial ultrasound. Int Urogynecol J Pelvic Floor Dysfunct. 2009;20(7):807–11. https://doi.org/10.1007/s00192-009-0839-4.

47. Dietz HP, Abbu A, Shek KL. The levator-urethra gap measurement: a more objective means of determining levator avulsion? Ultrasound Obstet Gynecol. 2008;32(7):941–5. https://doi.org/10.1002/uog.6268.

48. Greenbaum H, Klein L, Alcalay M, Kassif E, Weisz B, Eisenberg VH. The optimal cutoff value for levator-urethra gap measurements using tomographic ultrasound imaging in avulsion diagnosis is population specific. Neurourol Urodyn. 2020;39(5):1401–9. https://doi.org/10.1002/nau.24353.

49. Orejuela FJ, Shek KL, Dietz HP. The time factor in the assessment of prolapse and levator ballooning. Int Urogynecol J. 2012;23(2):175–8. https://doi.org/10.1007/s00192-011-1533-x.

50. Dietz HP, Wong V, Shek KL. A simplified method for determining hiatal biometry. Aust N Z J Obstet Gynaecol. 2011;51(6):540–3. https://doi.org/10.1111/j.1479-828X.2011.01352.x.

51. Dietz HP, Shek C, De Leon J, Steensma AB. Ballooning of the levator hiatus. Ultrasound Obstet Gynecol. 2008;31(6):676–80. https://doi.org/10.1002/uog.5355.

52. Dietz HP. Can the rectovaginal septum be visualized by transvaginal three-dimensional ultrasound? Ultrasound Obstet Gynecol. 2011;37(3):348–52. https://doi.org/10.1002/uog.8896.

53. Dietz HP, Beer-Gabel M. Ultrasound in the investigation of posterior compartment vaginal prolapse and obstructed defecation. Ultrasound Obstet Gynecol. 2012;40(1):14–27. https://doi.org/10.1002/uog.10131.

54. DeLancey JO, Morgan DM, Fenner DE, Kearney R, Guire K, Miller JM, et al. Comparison of levator ani muscle defects and function in women with and without pelvic organ prolapse. Obstet Gynecol. 2007;109(2 Pt 1):295–302. https://doi.org/10.1097/01.AOG.0000250901.57095.ba.

55. Vergeldt TF, Notten KJ, Stoker J, Fütterer JJ, Beets-Tan RG, Vliegen RF, et al. Comparison of translabial three-dimensional ultrasound with magnetic resonance imaging for measurement of levator hiatal biometry at rest. Ultrasound Obstet Gynecol. 2016;47(5):636–41. https://doi.org/10.1002/uog.14949.

56. Zhuang RR, Song YF, Chen ZQ, Ma M, Huang HJ, Chen JH, et al. Levator avulsion using a tomographic ultrasound and magnetic resonance-based model. Am J Obstet Gynecol. 2011;205(3):232.e1–8. https://doi.org/10.1016/j.ajog.2011.03.052.

57. Vergeldt TF, Weemhoff M, Notten KJ, Kessels AG, Kluivers KB. Comparison of two scoring systems for diagnosing levator ani muscle damage. Int Urogynecol J. 2013;24(9):1501–6. https://doi.org/10.1007/s00192-013-2052-8.

58. Nardos R, Thurmond A, Holland A, Gregory WT. Pelvic floor levator hiatus measurements: MRI versus ultrasound. Female Pelvic Med Reconstr Surg. 2014;20(4):216–21. https://doi.org/10.1097/spv.0000000000000079.

59. Dietz HP, Shek KL, Daly O, Korda A. Can levator avulsion be repaired surgically? A prospective surgical pilot study. Int Urogynecol J. 2013;24(6):1011–5. https://doi.org/10.1007/s00192-012-1984-8.

60. Wong V, Shek KL, Korda A, Benness C, Pardey J, Dietz HP. A pilot study on surgical reduction of the levator hiatus-the puborectalis sling. Int Urogynecol J. 2019;30(12):2127–33. https://doi.org/10.1007/s00192-019-04062-0.

61. Rostaminia G, Shobeiri SA, Quiroz LH. Surgical repair of bilateral levator ani muscles with ultrasound guidance. Int Urogynecol J. 2013;24(7):1237–9. https://doi.org/10.1007/s00192-012-1912-y.

62. Stær-Jensen J, Siafarikas F, Hilde G, Benth J, Bø K, Engh ME. Postpartum recovery of levator hiatus and bladder neck mobility in relation to pregnancy. Obstet Gynecol. 2015;125(3):531–9. https://doi.org/10.1097/aog.0000000000000645.

63. van Delft KW, Thakar R, Sultan AH, IntHout J, Kluivers KB. The natural history of levator avulsion one year following childbirth: a prospective study. BJOG. 2015;122(9):1266–73. https://doi.org/10.1111/1471-0528.13223.

64. van Gruting IMA, van Delft KWM, Sultan AH, Thakar R. Natural history of levator ani muscle avulsion 4 years following childbirth. Ultrasound Obstet Gynecol. 2021;58(2):309–17. https://doi.org/10.1002/uog.23120.

65. Dietz HP, Franco AV, Shek KL, Kirby A. Avulsion injury and levator hiatal ballooning: two independent risk factors for prolapse? An observational study. Acta Obstet Gynecol Scand. 2012;91(2):211–4. https://doi.org/10.1111/j.1600-0412.2011.01315.x.

66. Cattani L, Decoene J, Page AS, Weeg N, Deprest J, Dietz HP. Pregnancy, labour and delivery as risk factors for pelvic organ prolapse: a systematic review. Int Urogynecol J. 2021;32(7):1623–31. https://doi.org/10.1007/s00192-021-04724-y.

67. Volløyhaug I, Mørkved S, Salvesen K. Association between pelvic floor muscle trauma and pelvic organ prolapse 20 years after delivery. Int Urogynecol J. 2016;27(1):39–45. https://doi.org/10.1007/s00192-015-2784-8.

68. Volløyhaug I, Taithongchai A, Van Gruting I, Sultan A, Thakar R. Levator ani muscle morphology and function in women with obstetric anal sphincter injury. Ultrasound Obstet Gynecol. 2019;53(3):410–6. https://doi.org/10.1002/uog.20115.

69. Hilde G, Staer-Jensen J, Siafarikas F, Gjestland K, Ellström Engh M, Bø K. How well can pelvic floor muscles with major defects contract? A cross-sectional comparative study 6 weeks after delivery using transperineal 3D/4D ultrasound and manometer. BJOG. 2013;120(11):1423–9. https://doi.org/10.1111/1471-0528.12321.

70. Rosen R, Brown C, Heiman J, Leiblum S, Meston C, Shabsigh R, et al. The Female Sexual Function Index (FSFI): a multidimensional self-report instrument for the assessment of female sexual function.

J Sex Marital Ther. 2000;26(2):191–208. https://doi.org/10.1080/009262300278597.

71. García-Mejido JA, Idoia-Valero I, Aguilar-Gálvez IM, Borrero González C, Fernández-Palacín A, Sainz JA. Association between sexual dysfunction and avulsion of the levator ani muscle after instrumental vaginal delivery. Acta Obstet Gynecol Scand. 2020;99(9):1246–52. https://doi.org/10.1111/aogs.13852.

72. Roos AM, Speksnijder L, Steensma AB. Postpartum sexual function; the importance of the levator ani muscle. Int Urogynecol J. 2020;31(11):2261–7. https://doi.org/10.1007/s00192-020-04250-3.

73. Aydin S, Bakar RZ, Arioğlu Aydin Ç, Ateş S. Correlation between transperineal 3-dimensional ultrasound measurements of levator hiatus and female sexual function. Female Pelvic Med Reconstr Surg. 2017;23(6):433–7. https://doi.org/10.1097/spv.0000000000000407.

74. Manzini C, Friedman T, Turel F, Dietz HP. Vaginal laxity: which measure of levator ani distensibility is most predictive? Ultrasound Obstet Gynecol. 2020;55(5):683–7. https://doi.org/10.1002/uog.21873.

75. Omodei MS, Marques Gomes Delmanto LR, Carvalho-Pessoa E, Schmitt EB, Nahas GP, Petri Nahas EA. Association between pelvic floor muscle strength and sexual function in postmenopausal women. J Sex Med. 2019;16(12):1938–46. https://doi.org/10.1016/j.jsxm.2019.09.014.

76. Smeets CFA, Vergeldt TFM, Notten KJB, Martens FMJ, van Kuijk SMJ. Association between levator ani avulsion and urinary incontinence in women: a systematic review and meta-analysis. Int J Gynaecol Obstet. 2021;153(1):25–32. https://doi.org/10.1002/ijgo.13496.

77. Heilbrun ME, Nygaard IE, Lockhart ME, Richter HE, Brown MB, Kenton KS, et al. Correlation between levator ani muscle injuries on magnetic resonance imaging and fecal incontinence, pelvic organ prolapse, and urinary incontinence in primiparous women. Am J Obstet Gynecol. 2010;202(5):488.e1–6. https://doi.org/10.1016/j.ajog.2010.01.002.

78. Lewicky-Gaupp C, Brincat C, Yousuf A, Patel DA, Delancey JO, Fenner DE. Fecal incontinence in older women: are levator ani defects a factor? Am J Obstet Gynecol. 2010;202(5):491.e1–6. https://doi.org/10.1016/j.ajog.2010.01.020.

79. Melendez-Munoz J, Subramanian N, Friedman T, Dietz HP. Is levator trauma an independent risk factor for anal incontinence? Colorectal Dis. 2020;22(3):298–302. https://doi.org/10.1111/codi.14864.

80. Mathew S, Guzmán Rojas RA, Salvesen KA, Volløyhaug I. Levator ani muscle injury and risk for urinary and fecal incontinence in parous women from a normal population, a cross-sectional study. Neurourol Urodyn. 2019;38(8):2296–302. https://doi.org/10.1002/nau.24138.

81. Kearney R, Miller JM, Ashton-Miller JA, DeLancey JO. Obstetric factors associated with levator ani muscle injury after vaginal birth. Obstet Gynecol. 2006;107(1):144–9. https://doi.org/10.1097/01.AOG.0000194063.63206.1c.

82. Valsky DV, Cohen SM, Lipschuetz M, Hochner-Celnikier D, Daum H, Yagel I, et al. Third- or fourth-degree intrapartum anal sphincter tears are associated with levator ani avulsion in primiparas. J Ultrasound Med. 2016;35(4):709–15. https://doi.org/10.7863/ultra.15.04032.

83. van Delft K, Thakar R, Sultan AH, Schwertner-Tiepelmann N, Kluivers K. Levator ani muscle avulsion during childbirth: a risk prediction model. BJOG. 2014;121(9):1155–63; discussion 63. https://doi.org/10.1111/1471-0528.12676.

84. Braekken IH, Majida M, Engh ME, Bø K. Can pelvic floor muscle training reverse pelvic organ prolapse and reduce prolapse symptoms? An assessor-blinded, randomized, controlled trial. Am J Obstet Gynecol. 2010;203(2):170.e1–7. https://doi.org/10.1016/j.ajog.2010.02.037.

85. Johannessen HH, Frøshaug BE, Lysåker PJG, Salvesen K, Lukasse M, Mørkved S, et al. Regular antenatal exercise including pelvic floor muscle training reduces urinary incontinence 3 months postpartum-follow up of a randomized controlled trial. Acta Obstet Gynecol Scand. 2021;100(2):294–301. https://doi.org/10.1111/aogs.14010.

86. Manzini C, Morsinkhof LM, van der Vaart CH, Withagen MIJ, Grob ATM. Parameters associated with unsuccessful pessary fitting for pelvic organ prolapse up to three months follow-up: a systematic review and meta-analysis. Int Urogynecol J. 2022. https://doi.org/10.1007/s00192-021-05015-2.

87. Oversand SH, Staff AC, Sandvik L, Volløyhaug I, Svenningsen R. Levator ani defects and the severity of symptoms in women with anterior compartment pelvic organ prolapse. Int Urogynecol J. 2018;29(1):63–9. https://doi.org/10.1007/s00192-017-3390-8.

88. Nyhus N. NTNU Open: Pelvic floor muscle contraction and anatomy in women with pelvic organ prolapse, incontinence and in pregnancy, NTNU Norwegian University of Science and Technology. 2020.

89. Friedman T, Eslick GD, Dietz HP. Risk factors for prolapse recurrence: systematic review and meta-analysis. Int Urogynecol J. 2018;29(1):13–21. https://doi.org/10.1007/s00192-017-3475-4.

90. Yeung E, Malacova E, Maher C. Is levator ani avulsion a risk factor for prolapse recurrence? A systematic review and meta-analysis. Int Urogynecol J. 2022;33(7):1813–26. https://doi.org/10.1007/s00192-022-05217-2.

91. Volløyhaug I NM, Mathew S. Can ultrasound be used to predict symptoms of pelvic floor disorders after prolapse surgery? IUGA. Virtual 2021.

92. Wong NKL, Cheung RYK, Lee LL, Wan OYK, Choy KW, Chan SSC. Women with advanced pelvic organ prolapse and levator ani muscle avulsion would significantly benefit from mesh repair sur-

gery. Ultrasound Obstet Gynecol. 2021;57(4):631–8. https://doi.org/10.1002/uog.23109.

93. Santis-Moya F, Pineda R, Miranda V. Preoperative ultrasound findings as risk factors of recurrence of pelvic organ prolapse after laparoscopic sacrocolpopexy. Int Urogynecol J. 2021;32(4):955–60. https://doi.org/10.1007/s00192-020-04503-1.

94. Caudwell-Hall J, Kamisan Atan I, Brown C, Guzman Rojas R, Langer S, Shek KL, et al. Can pelvic floor trauma be predicted antenatally? Acta Obstet Gynecol Scand. 2018;97(6):751–7. https://doi.org/10.1111/aogs.13315.

95. Rahmanou P, Caudwell-Hall J, Kamisan Atan I, Dietz HP. The association between maternal age at first delivery and risk of obstetric trauma. Am J Obstet Gynecol. 2016;215(4):451.e1–7. https://doi.org/10.1016/j.ajog.2016.04.032.

96. Cassadó J, Pessarrodona A, Rodriguez-Carballeira M, Hinojosa L, Manrique G, Márquez A, et al. Does episiotomy protect against injury of the levator ani muscle in normal vaginal delivery? Neurourol Urodyn. 2014;33(8):1212–6. https://doi.org/10.1002/nau.22488.

97. Jiang H, Qian X, Carroli G, Garner P. Selective versus routine use of episiotomy for vaginal birth.

Cochrane Database Syst Rev. 2017;2(2):Cd000081. https://doi.org/10.1002/14651858.CD000081.pub3.

98. Kamisan Atan I, Shek KL, Langer S, Guzman Rojas R, Caudwell-Hall J, Daly JO, et al. Does the Epi-No(®) birth trainer prevent vaginal birth-related pelvic floor trauma? A multicentre prospective randomised controlled trial. BJOG. 2016;123(6):995–1003. https://doi.org/10.1111/1471-0528.13924.

99. Sobhgol SS, Smith CA, Dahlen HG. The effect of antenatal pelvic floor muscle exercises on labour and birth outcomes: a systematic review and meta-analysis. Int Urogynecol J. 2020;31(11):2189–203. https://doi.org/10.1007/s00192-020-04298-1.

100. Horak TA, Guzman-Rojas RA, Shek KL, Dietz HP. Pelvic floor trauma: does the second baby matter? Ultrasound Obstet Gynecol. 2014;44(1):90–4. https://doi.org/10.1002/uog.13252.

101. Kamisan Atan I, Lin S, Dietz HP, Herbison P, Wilson PD. It is the first birth that does the damage: a cross-sectional study 20 years after delivery. Int Urogynecol J. 2018;29(11):1637–43. https://doi.org/10.1007/s00192-018-3616-4.

102. Volløyhaug I GRR, Mørkved S, Salvesen K Å. Pelvic floor muscle trauma – does vaginal parity matter? ICS. Florence 2017.

Pelvic Floor and Sphincter Neuropathy After Childbirth

17

Conor P. O'Brien

Overview
Test your learning and check your understanding of this book's contents: use the "Springer Nature Flashcards" app to access questions using ▶ https://sn.pub/wqrf89. To use the app, please follow the instructions in Chap. 1.

Learning Points

- Pelvic floor and sphincter neuropathy is a common and often overlooked pathology. This chapter outlines the neuroanatomy of the pelvic floor, evaluates injury patterns with clinical scenarios, describes historical evaluations of the neuromuscular structures in the pelvic floor, and presents the current state of the art techniques for the evaluation of pelvic floor neuropathy.
- Electrodiagnostic (EDX) evaluation of the neuromuscular structure and function of the pelvic floor using verified neurophysiological methods and protocols is an essential element in diagnosing neuropathy and in directing treatment options in women with pudendal and pelvic floor neuropathy.

C. P. O'Brien (✉)
Neurophysiology and Electrodiagnostic Medicine,
National Maternity Hospital, Dublin, Ireland
e-mail: conor.obrien@nmh.ie

17.1 Introduction

Pelvic floor and anal sphincter neuropathy after childbirth is a commonly encountered clinical entity. Neuropathy is intimately related to pelvic floor disorders such as pelvic organ prolapse, anal and urinary incontinence, sexual dysfunction and pelvic pain. A neuropathy may originate in the central or peripheral nervous system, the autonomic and somatic nervous system (through the lumbo-sacral plexus and pudendal nerve, respectively), and can cause a neurological disturbance in the pelvis. Pelvic floor neuroanatomy is complex, and assessment of pelvic neurology is an evolving science with much progress achieved since initial reports of over 40 years ago.

Pelvic floor and anal sphincter neuropathy after childbirth is now more commonly recognised. This, in part, is due to the increased awareness of the condition and its pathophysiology, and a greater understanding the clinical consequences of the neuropathy. Similarly, there have been improvements in the technology of electrodiagnostic medicine (EDX) and neurophysiology to assess for peripheral nerve disease, which has enhanced the ability to diagnose pelvic neuropathies.

A variety of focal and polyneuropathies have been described in pregnancy. These include compression, traction and traumatic neuropathies. Nerves of the lumbo-sacral plexus are usually those being affected.

© The Author(s), under exclusive license to Springer Nature Switzerland AG 2024
A. H. Sultan et al. (eds.), *Pelvic Floor, Perineal, and Anal Sphincter Trauma During Childbirth*,
https://doi.org/10.1007/978-3-031-43095-4_17

Pudendal neuropathy is the most common pelvic neuropathy associated with pregnancy and childbirth. The pudendal nerve can be compromised in up to 1/3 of all pregnancies, with a 1/3 of this group developing clinical symptoms. Other less commonly encountered pregnancy-related neuropathies emanate from the lumbosacral plexus and include injuries to the femoral nerve, the lateral femoral cutaneous nerve, the genitofemoral nerve, and the sciatic nerve. The lumbo-sacral nerve roots can also be affected.

Pudendal neuropathy is associated with a number of clinical presentations: faecal incontinence and bowel dysfunction, urinary incontinence and lower urinary tract dysfunction, sexual dysfunction and pelvic pain. In some individuals, their clinical presentation is a combination of all four entities, namely bowel, bladder and sexual dysfunction and chronic pelvic pain. In other individuals, there are focal clinical entities. Pain, faecal soiling, and urinary incontinence are a cause of great physical and psychological upset that often lead to social isolation in many sufferers [1]. Due to the nature of the complaints associated with pudendal neuropathy, many patients do not volunteer specific information regarding their symptoms. In one epidemiological study, only a 1/3 of people with faecal incontinence had ever discussed the problem with a doctor, due to embarrassment and fear of stigma [2].

This chapter will outline the neuroanatomy of the pelvic floor, evaluate injury patterns with clinical scenarios, describe historical evaluations of the neuromuscular structures in the pelvic floor, and present the current state of the art techniques for the evaluation of pelvic floor and anal sphincter neuropathy.

17.2 Pelvic Floor Neuroanatomy

The anatomy of the pelvic floor has been outlined in Chap. 1. The specifics of the neuroanatomy are important in understanding the aetiology, types of pathology, and diagnosis in cases of neuropathy. The pudendal nerve warrants special knowledge.

17.2.1 Pudendal Nerve

The pudendal nerve is both a motor and sensory nerve. It originates from Onuf's nucleus, a small group of motor neurons located in the ventral horns of the sacral spinal cord. The motor neurons of Onuf's nucleus innervate striated voluntary muscles and are histologically and biochemically similar to other somatic spinal motor neurons; but, unlike other spinal motor neurons, they also show unique autonomic-like features and receive a strong "peptidergic" innervation, where small peptide molecules are used as their neurotransmitter. The nature and function of Onuf's nucleus is not fully understood. It is spared in cases of Anterior Horn cell disease, but is affected in Shy Drager Syndrome and in Parkinson's Disease where incontinence is a clinical feature.

The pudendal nerve is formed by the S2, S3 & S4 nerve roots (Fig. 17.1). The nerve follows a path into the pelvis via the greater sciatic foramen and courses in the posterior hollow of the pelvis, inferior to the piriformis muscle until it exits the pelvis. It travels under the sacrospinous ligament and enters the lesser sciatic foramen, where it travels to the gluteal muscles and medial ischial tuberosity. It then exits the lesser sciatic foramen, where it travels through Alcock's canal to the perineum. It terminates with three branches (Fig. 17.2):

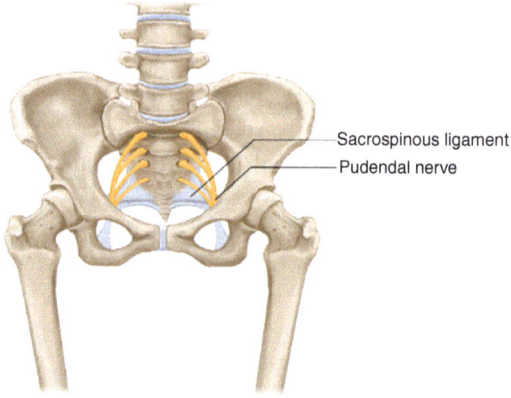

Sacrospinous ligament
Pudendal nerve

Fig. 17.1 Pudendal nerve originating from S2, S3 and S4 nerve root

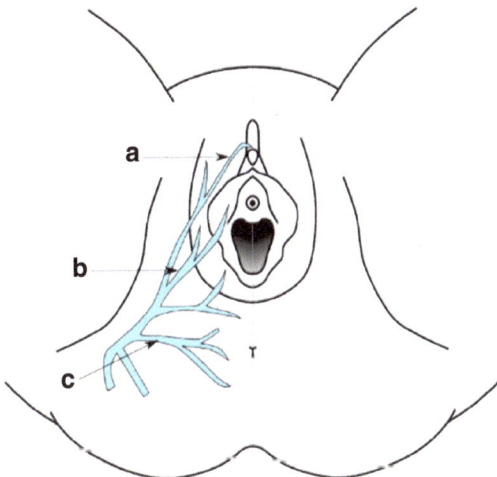

Fig. 17.2 Three Branches of the Pudendal Nerve (a) Clitoral, (b) Perineal (c) Rectal

1. The inferior rectal nerve, which supplies the external anal sphincter
2. The perineal nerve, which supplies the urethral sphincter
3. The dorsal nerve of the penis or clitoris

As a motor and sensory nerve, the pudendal nerve controls critical human functions, such as voluntary control of the external anal sphincter (EAS) and urinary sphincter (US). The nerve also controls pelvic floor muscle activation and the somatic sensation of the clitoris. The pudendal nerve and nerve roots (S2, S3 and S4) contribute the majority of the afferent innervation of the pelvic floor. Afferent sensory mapping has shown that the S2 nerve root contributes 60% of the afferent sensory fibres in comparison to S3, which contributes 35% [3]. The EAS muscle fibres are composed predominantly of small type I fibres, as is the case with most tonically active muscles [4]. The levator muscles, on the other hand, are not innervated by the pudendal nerve, but rather by innervation that originates from the sacral nerve roots directly (S2, S3, S4 and S5) and predominantly S4 [5, 6].

The pudendal nerve supplies cutaneous innervation to a large portion of the pelvic floor (see Fig. 17.6). The dorsal nerve of the clitoris (penis) also supplies afferent fibres that innervate the penile skin, clitoris in females, and also the glans

penis. These afferents propagate sensory signals to the central nervous system that are critical to achieving an erection and sexual function.

17.3 Incidence of Pudendal Neuropathy

Pudendal neuralgia is frequently observed in clinical practice. Its incidence is considered by most clinicians to be higher than reported. The condition often goes unrecognized. Pelvic neuropathy has become of increasing interest to clinicians, as the evidence of the importance of neuromuscular function in maintenance of pelvic floor function and continence accumulates [7]. The pudendal nerve can be compromised in up to a 1/3 of all pregnancies [8, 9].

The true incidence of pudendal neuralgia in the general population is unknown [2, 7]. Spinosa et al. documented the incidence of pudendal neuralgia at 1% in the general population, affecting women more than men; however, it is found in both genders and also occurs in children due to congenital anomalies in the nerve pathway [10].

Women are more commonly affected by this condition, with a female: male ratio of 6:4. An incidence of 4% has been reported in patients undergoing consultations for pain control [11]. Many clinicians who routinely treat pudendal neuralgia believe the actual incidence rates are significantly higher than stated in the existing literature [7, 10, 12].

The significant variability in the reporting of this condition is due to a low index of suspicion by many clinicians and the non-uniformity of diagnosing the condition. Some authors rely on history, others on examination, and even others on different forms and types of neurological assessment, including EDX and histological studies.

In 1977 [13], it was reported that 60% of women with anal incontinence chronicled a difficult childbirth, which prompted the hypothesis that childbirth was a major factor in initiating sphincter denervation. The pudendal nerve was shown to be compromised in 32% of all vaginal deliveries in 1984 [14]. The same year, Kiff and Swash identified the association between pelvic floor nerve injury and faecal incontinence [15]. Two years later, Snook analysed the risk factors in childbirth that caused damage to the pelvic floor neural innervation [8]. EDX single fibre EMG studies and histological studies confirmed evidence of a neuropathy affecting the urethral sphincter [16]. In 1989, further EDX studies were published, confirming the hypothesis of neuropathy. 97% of the women with conduction time delay in the pudendal nerve terminal distal latency were reported to have urinary stress incontinence, thus establishing the first link between pudendal nerve injury and pelvic floor disorders [17].

A 1995 paper [18] identified a 31.4% incidence of pudendal nerve damage in a group of patients with evacuator disorders; this was done with needle EMG using a bi-polar concentric electrode and Pudendal Nerve Terminal Distal Latency (PNTDL) assessment. Of these, 23.8% reported constipation and 37.2% reported faecal incontinence. In 2003, an incidence of 20% of vaginal births having faecal incontinence symptoms requiring medical intervention at 6 weeks was reported, with 80% of these resolving physiologically; the remainder continued to have symptoms [9].

Recognition of pudendal neuropathy has evolved over the past 40 years and has mirrored the advances and improvements in EDX medicine. The variation in reporting of the condition over the past 40 years reflects development of practice in this filed of medicine.

Many authors rely on the Nantes Criteria, which is based on history and nerve block assessment alone with no reference to EDX testing.

In the past, investigators have relied on PNTDL testing. As a single EDX test, it has class 3 evidence (**4E**) in cases of sacral plexopathy and is of less value in cases of pudendal neuropathy. This is so, because while amplitude changes are of assistance, distal latency testing only assess the most distal end of the nerve and fails to evaluate the full length of the nerve. Hence, is now not recommended as a standard test to evaluate pudendal neuropathy. PNTDL testing has been superseded by sacral reflex testing, which evaluates the full length of the nerve.

17.4   Risk Factors

The most common cause of pudendal neuropathy is childbirth and pregnancy, affecting up to 1/3 of new mothers. It is reported in cases of both vaginal and caesarean births [19]. Pregnancy itself can be a risk factor as well. However, pudendal neuropathy is also associated with other specific circumstances. For example, pelvic reconstructive surgery (sacrospinous ligament fixation and mesh procedures) is linked with neuropathy. Similarly, neuropathy with hysterectomy, anterior colporrhaphy and mid-urethral slings is also reported [20]. It is postulated that this may be due to bleeding or vascular congestion in the pudendal neurovascular bundle after these surgeries, resulting in nerve compression.

Interestingly, female athletes are more prone to pudendal neuropathy and frequently report faecal and urinary symptoms. The prevalence of urinary incontinence observed in elite female athletes has been reported to be upwards of 33% [21] and varies according to the sport practised [21, 22] and participation in general pelvic floor exercise programs [22]. Trampolining and high impact activities having the highest incidence of sports-related pudendal neuropathy in both parous and nulliparous women [21–25].

Bicycle riding has been commonly reported as a cause of pudendal neuropathy as well. Compression of the pudendal nerve with this activity was first described in 1987 when it was called Cyclist Syndrome [26]. The neuropathy resulted from mechanical compression of the nerve [26, 27] caused by the cyclist supporting his or her bodyweight on a narrow bicycle seat, thus resulting in transient ischaemic compression of the pudendal nerve between the rigid bicycle seat and the pelvic bones. Wider bike seats decrease pressure on this vulnerable area (Fig. 17.3). Other reported causes of pudendal neuropathy include pelvic trauma, prolonged sitting, constipation and anal intercourse. Medical conditions associated with pudendal-related symptoms include multiple sclerosis, multi sys-

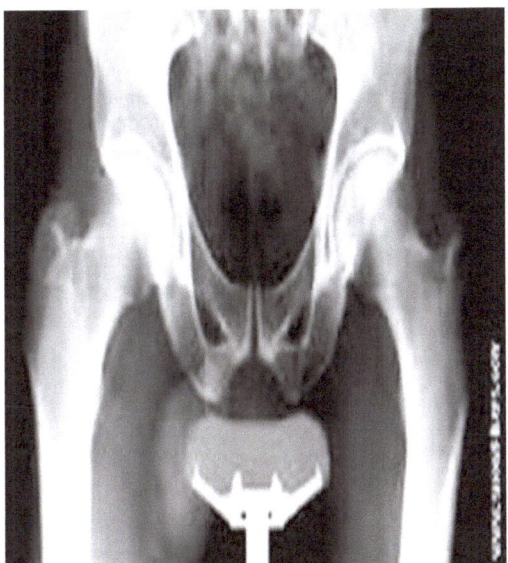

Fig. 17.3 The structure of the new bicycle seats places the supporting struts under pudendal nerve at the level of the ischium, resulting in compression of the nerve between the bony pelvis and the rigid bicycle seat metal struts

tem atrophy, spondylolisthesis and lumbar-sacral spine disease [3, 28].

17.4.1 Childbirth Related Pudendal Neuropathy

Female gender, increasing age, and multiparity are associated with changes in pudendal nerve function [29–31]. Forceps delivery, prolonged second stage of labour, third degree perineal tears and high birth weight are all factors that can lead to an increased incidence of pudendal neuropathy. Age itself is an independent risk factor, as women who deliver by caesarean section are not immune to age-related deterioration of anal sphincter function. Diabetics also appears to have a greater incidence of pregnancy-related pudendal neuropathy [32].

Pre-existing neurological disease of the central or peripheral nervous system increases the likelihood of a pregnancy related pudendal neuropathy [28, 33]. Intra-partum management and

use of epidural pain relief and delayed versus active pushing all also affect pudendal nerve function [34, 35].

17.5 Mechanism of Pudendal Nerve Injury

Injury to the pudendal nerve is classified as a peripheral nerve injury. There are three basic types of peripheral nerve injuries (PNI) commonly seen in clinical practice, resulting in neuronal dysfunction:

1. Stretch related: traction force
2. Lacerations: direct trauma or iatrogenic injury
3. Compressions: compression or entrapment by anatomical structures

There are two commonly used classification for PNI; the Seddon classification and the Sunderland classification. Seddon classified nerve injuries into three major groups: (1) neurapraxia, (2) axonotmesis, and (3) neurotmesis. Sunderland expanded upon Seddon's classification and described five degrees of peripheral nerve injury as described in Fig. 17.4.

The pudendal nerve can be compromised at a number of sites along its full length (Table 17.1).

The pudendal nerve can be injured in a variety of ways (see Table 17.2). The pudendal nerve is subjected to traction forces when straining at stool due to constipation. This can result in perineal decent which can exceed 3 cm. This also can occur with constipation where stretch ranges from 1 to 4 cm [36].

A similar situation occurs and during pregnancy and delivery. In normal subjects, the perineum descends less than 1.5 cm. Stretching of the pudendal nerve by 12% of its length or more than 2 cm can cause injury. Hence excessive perineal descent will compromise the nerve by traction forces.

Studies have shown that excessive straining due to constipation or during the second stage of

Seddon	Sunderland	Injury	Spontaneous recovery	Nerve conduction study	Electromyography
Neurapraxia	Grade I	Focal segmental demyelination	Yes	Partial/complete conduction block proximally Preserved conduction block distally even after 2 weeks	Normal morphology and poor MUAP recruitment
Axonotmesis	Grade II	Damaged axon with intact endoneurium	Yes, slower than neurapraxia	Partial/complete conduction block proximally Preserved conduction block distally until Wallerian degeneration sets in	Abnormal activity
Axonotmesis	Grade III	Damaged axon and endoneurium with intact perineurium	Not very likely, surgical intervention may be needed		
Axonotmesis	Grade IV	Damaged axon, endoneurium, and perineurium with intact epineurium	Highly unlikely, surgical intervention is necessary		
Neurotmesis	Grade V	Complete nerve transection (disruption of myelin sheath, axon, endoneurium, perineurium and epineurium)	No, surgical intervention is necessary	Complete conduction block proximally and distally	Abnormal activity

Fig. 17.4 Classification of peripheral nerve injury (PNI)

Table 17.1 Anatomic Sites for compromise along the pudendal nerve resulting in neuropathy

Nerve root	Spine disease	Degenerative disc
Sacral plexus	Traction injury	Road traffic accident
Piriformis & Coccygeus muscles	Local trauma	Sports related injury
Greater sciatic foramen	Local trauma	Pelvic fractures
Ischial spine	Pressure neuropathy	Sitting/cycling
Alcock's fascia	Traction due to pelvic floor motion	2nd stage of labour/straining Pelvic surgery
Perineum	Local trauma	Sexual intercourse Cycling
External genitalia and rectum	Local trauma/iatrogenic	Haemorrhoidectomy Sexual intercourse Cycling

labour are associated with stretching of up to 20% of the nerve beyond its relatively stable fixed position in Alcock's Canal. These stretch neuropathies are associated with both faecal and urinary incontinence [8, 10, 15].

Table 17.2 Causes of pudendal neuropathy

Local Trauma
    Bike riding
    Herpes simplex infection
    Endometriosis
    Mesh
    Chemoradiation for rectal cancer
    Spinal canal stenosis
Traction injury
    Chronic constipation
    Perineal decent
Iatrogenic
    Pudendal nerve blocks
    Pelvic surgery
    Haemorrhoid surgery
    Sacrospinous ligament fixation
    Spinal surgery

17.6 Other Nerve Injuries in Pregnancy

Any form of polyneuropathy can occur during pregnancy, with compression neuropathies being relatively common. Some of these can result from excessive weight gain, fluid retention and unsuspected trauma. In the upper limb, for example, the median nerve, ulnar nerve and brachial plexus are the most common sites for entrapment neuropathies.

Injury to the nerves of the lumbosacral plexus focally or in combination can result in symptoms of pain, sensory alteration and motor dysfunction. The plexus is a network of nerves formed by the ventral rami of the lumbar and sacral spinal cord; the peripheral nerve emanates from the plexus (Fig. 17.5). They can be injured by direct compression by the foetus, stretch injuries and rarely from forceps application during delivery.

Affected nerves in these injuries can include the (1) femoral, (2) lateral femoral cutaneous, (3) obturator, (4) sciatic, (5) ilio-inguinal, (6) iliohypogastric and (7) genitofemoral (Fig. 17.6). These injuries usually occur due to compression. Lumbosacral neuropathies with focal nerve involvement or selected nerves from the plexus can occur [32]. Each nerve can result in pelvic floor symptoms and can be diagnosed by EDX evaluation.

(1) **Femoral neuropathy:** This can occur due to local trauma or haematoma, which results in nerve compression at the level of the inguinal ligament. A prolonged dorsal lithotomy position, which may be associated with protracted labour, can result in compression of the nerve at this location. Clinically, the patient will present with weakness in her quadriceps muscle function and sensory alteration in the saphenous nerve distribution. A femoral neuropathy can occur in combination with injuries to other elements of the lumbosacral plexus, such as the pudendal nerve. EDX studies will confirm the diagnosis with abnormality in both distal latency and amplitude of response in the femoral motor conduction study. Needle EMG will show evidence of denervation in the vastus medialis, vastus lateralis and rectus femoris muscles [37].

(2) **Lateral femoral cutaneous (LFC) neuropathy of the thigh:** LFC neuropathy (Meralgia paraesthetica) presents with numbness and sensory alteration of the anterolateral thigh. It is reported in association with pregnancy and in overweight patients of both genders. Clinical evaluation reveals numbness and hypersensitivity in the lateral aspect of the thigh and the skin, which is often sensitive to touch. It is caused by kinking of the lateral femoral cutaneous nerve at the lateral pelvis by local compression of an enlarged abdomen.

(3) **Obturator nerve injury:** An obturator nerve injury presents with sensory alteration over the proximal medial aspect of the thigh in association with weakness in thigh adduction. This nerve is injured with compression by the fetal head at the level of the psoas muscle or as it travels through the obturator foramen before supplying the adductor muscles of the hip. Injury to this nerve is a rare occurrence during childbirth.

(4) **Sciatic Neuropathy:** This can occur in cases of prolonged birth. In previous decades, the nerve could be injured by misplaced pain-relieving injections in the gluteal area. Symptoms usually follow a radicular pattern [38].

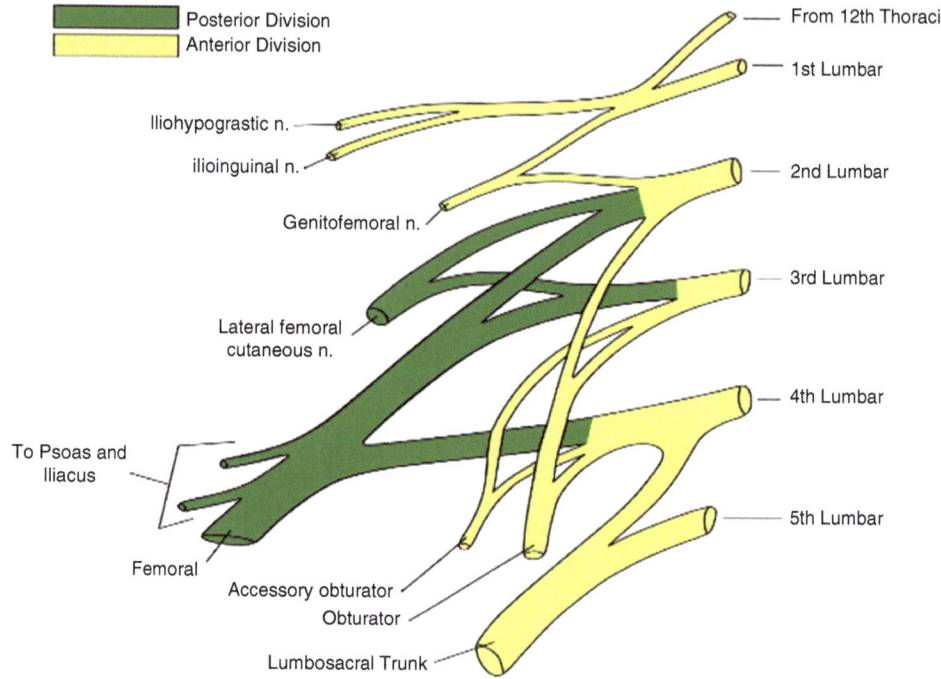

Fig. 17.5 The lumbo-sacral plexus

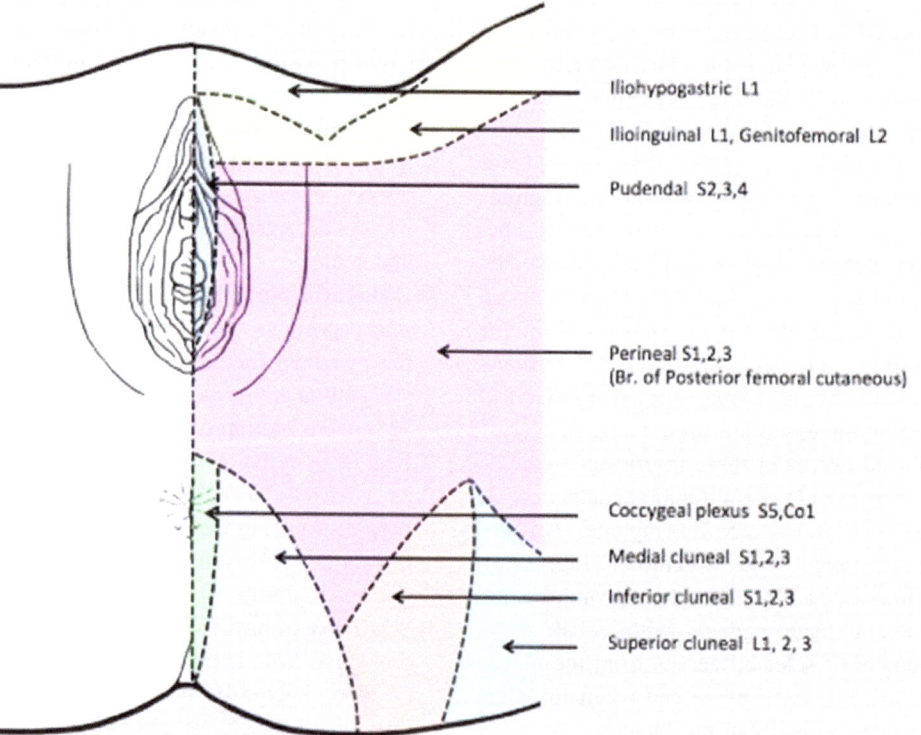

Fig. 17.6 Cutaneous innervation of the pelvic floor

(5) Ilio-inguinal, (6) Ilio-hypogastric and (7) Genitofemoral neuropathy usually result in pelvic pain or sensory alteration. There is a significant overlap in the dermatomal distribution of these nerves and symptoms are usually generalised and non specific.

17.6.1 Levator Ani Syndrome

Levator Ani Syndrome is caused by spasm of part or all of the levator ani muscle complex consisting of the puborectalis, pubococcygeus, and iliococcygeus (see Fig. 1.2). These muscles are composed predominantly of striated muscle, with some smooth muscle elements. The condition presents with a dull ache in the rectum and occasional burning. The pain is often worsened when the stool presses against the muscle while being expelled. The condition is associated with chronic constipation and vaginal delivery. The Levator Ani receives neurological supply directly from the S3 and S4 nerve roots (not from the pudendal nerve), Diagnosis is confirmed by needle EMG to the elements of the Levator Ani. Treatment can involve nerve root

blocking injections or Botulinum Toxin injection directly into the spasmodic element of the muscle complex [39].

17.7 Clinical Presentation of Pudendal Neuropathy

Injury at any site along the course of this motor and sensory nerve can result in some or all of the four cardinal symptoms (Fig. 17.7) of a pudendal neuropathy: bowel incontinence, bladder incontinence, dyspareunia or pain, as described below:

- Faecal incontinence, often described as faecal soiling, which can occur post defecation or after exercise and can be associated with urinary hesitancy
- Stress and/or urge urinary incontinence
- Sexual dysfunction, including persistent arousal, dyspareunia, vulvodynia [40]
- Anal sphincter dysfunction presenting as difficult or painful defecation or tenesmus
- Saddle area dysfunction presenting as pain and/or numbness in the distribution of the

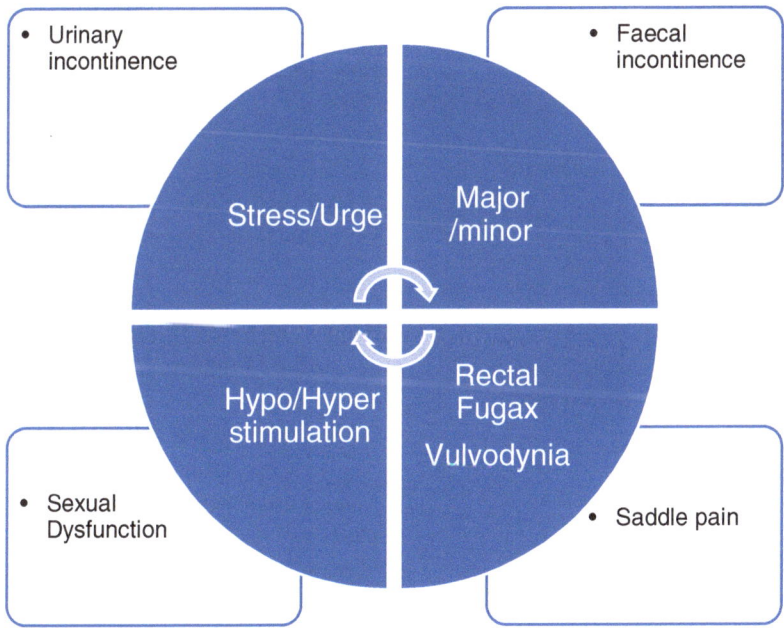

Fig. 17.7 Pudendal Nerve Syndrome, clinical presentation

pudendal nerve that includes genitalia, rectum, and terminal urinary tract
- Foreign body sensation in the anus, rectum, urethra, or vagina

In the female population, there are three patterns of neuropathy that are commonly observed [33]:

1. Acute presentation after childbirth, or in the following 6 month period
2. Progressive presentation (2-to-3-year period post-delivery), which this is thought to be due to evolving sphincter muscle atrophy and
3. Significantly delayed presentation many years after the birth of a last child, likely due to progressive sphincter atrophy and magnified by common age-related sarcopenia and a post menopause reduction in hormones. This third scenario often presents with a sudden onset of faecal and urinary incontinence.

There are frequently non-specific symptoms reported in cases of pudendal neuropathy (Table 17.5) with pain and discomfort in a generalised area. This is a function of the significant over-lap of cutaneous sensory supply to the perineum (Table 17.3).

Table 17.3 Common symptoms of pudendal nerve syndrome

Neuropathic pain in the territory of some or all of the pudendal nerve
Pain aggravated by sitting
Relieved by standing
Worsens during the day
Absent when recumbent
Absent sitting on a toilet seat
No objective sensory impairment {Sacral Roots}
Foreign Body sensation in rectum or vagina
"Sympathalgia"
Constipation
Painful bowel movement
Urinary frequency and urgency
Faecal and Flatus incontinence
Dyspareunia
Painful orgasm

17.8 Historical Evaluation of Pelvic Floor Neuropathy

Evaluation of pelvic floor and anal sphincter neuropathy after childbirth initially commenced in the 1970s and 1980s. Distal latency testing and histochemistry evaluations were deployed in clinical and research practice. Pudendal Nerve Distal latency (PNDL) became popular as a means of assessing the condition, as did needle electromyelography (EMG). Needles have evolved over the past two decades from monopolar electrodes (that required a surface reference electrode) to the currently used concentric electrodes; these yield much better electrical recordings and are easier to manoeuvre. Single fibre EMG has also been utilised. This assessment was helpful in evaluating fibre density of the sphincter, but required sophisticated computer processing and experienced clinicians. Somatosensory testing and central brain stimulation were also employed with varying success. The recurring issue with EDX was the reproducibility of the tests in a clinical setting. These concerns, however, have been overcome by the newer peripheral nerve assessment techniques in modern EMG systems.

Currently, the approach to assessing a case of pudendal neuropathy is to perform a quantitative EMG of the right and left EAS muscle and a clitoro-anal sacral reflex (CAR) for sensory threshold and distal latency. These tests will identify the presence of a neuropathy and give information as to the nature of the pathology: demyelinating or axonal.

17.9 Non -EDX Diagnosis of Pudendal Neuropathy

17.9.1 Nantes Criteria

Many authorities recommend the diagnosis of pudendal neuropathy based on the utilization of Nantes Criteria, in conjunction with clinical history and physical findings. The Nantes Criteria

Table 17.4 Nantes criteria

Pain in the anatomical territory of the pudendal nerve
Pain is worsened by sitting
The patient is not woken at night by the pain.
No objective sensory loss on clinical examination.
Positive anaesthetic pudendal nerve block

originated from the thought that EDX was not specific or sensitive enough for this condition [41–43], with some suggesting that PNMTL and EMG to the EAS and bulbocavernosus was of limited value.

Of note, paravaginal nerve blocking injections have also been used in the past to diagnose the condition, however this is an invasive diagnostic procedure.

The Nantes Criteria [41] is shown (Table 17.4).

This criteria is very helpful in screening patients as part of a surgical work up for with pudendal neuropathy from a "pudendal nerve compression". It is based on a 2008 group of experienced physicians' consensus who treat pudendal neuralgia. Patients meeting all the required criteria have fared better from decompression surgery than patients who only partly meet them [41]. Pudendal neuropathy pudendal neuropathy is a continuum of symptoms with a variety of causes. Merely relying on the Nantes Criteria may preclude symptomatic patients with neuropraxic type pathology (who don't fulfill the Nantes criteria) from receiving modern medical treatment for this disabling condition.

17.10 Under-Utilisation of EDX Medicine in Cases of Pelvic Floor and Sphincter Neuropathy

EDX technologies are under-utilised in many cases of pelvic floor disease due to the following:

1. Lack of knowledge of available EDX evaluations and their clinical relevancy
2. Lack of expertise in this branch of EDX and neurophysiology

Individuals suffering from pelvic floor dysfunction and pain may be referred by their primary care doctor to a variety of specialities (Gynaecology, Urology, Colorectal Surgery, Neurology, Pain and Physiotherapy, Urogynecology). Unfortunately, there has been little collective cross specialty engagement. The International Continence Society and other similar groups have encouraged transdisciplinary collaboration, but more needs to be done to standardise assessment protocols. Many referring physicians are also unaware of the state of the art of EDX medicine; many assume that pudendal motor terminal latency assessments are the current gold standard for assessment of suspected cases. However, this test (performed using the St Mark's electrode method) has been shown to have high intra- and inter-observer variability and only assesses the distal end of the nerve; hence, as noted above, it is inconsistent in its accuracy. But, this is not the case for the currently used battery of EDX tests.

Unfortunately, many institutions lack expertise in pelvic floor EDX medicine. Relatively few centres have trained EDX physicians with the relevant knowledge and access to the commonly performed EDX tests. It is recommended that only trained neurophysiologists should perform these investigations [44].

17.11 Normal Physiology or Pathology

Following childbirth, the pelvic floor neural and muscular structures undergo natural adaptation, which results in physiological changes. In the case of sphincter EMG, the Motor Unit Action Potential (MUAP) parameters change. There are variations in the size of the motor potentials (amplitudes), the length of the potentials (duration), as well as the number of turns and phases of the potentials. When the phases of the MUAP increase above 4, the potential is referred to as "polyphasic." Polyphasic MUAPs are associated with reinnervation of a peripheral nerve injury and also correlate with age and parity. Hence, normal parameters will vary with age and parity. The challenge of pelvic floor neurophysiologic assessment is to establish where the physiologic condition ends and pathologic condition begins [45, 46].

17.12 Modern EDX Evaluation of Pudendal Neuropathy After Childbirth

There are a variety of EDX tests available to assess the integrity and function of the pudendal nerve and its neural pathway (Table 17.5). EDX test sensitivity and specificity will depend on variables such as test reproducibility, normal values and diagnostic criteria. Various academic groups and the World Health Organization guidelines dictate that neurophysiologic assessment of the pelvic floor should include needle EMG of the EAS muscle as well the CAR sacral reflex. This reflex should also measure sensory thresholds or "first sensory response", [3, 29, 44–48].

These studies in Table 17.5 permit the assessment of the full length of the pudendal nerve and its terminal branches. The tests are relatively painless and can be completed in 20 minutes if performed by an experienced clinician. EMG changes take approximately 3 weeks to mature and therefore a neuropathy may be detected within 3 weeks of injury. Using this protocol, the nerve injury may be classified in severity and the degree of progression or recovery of the neuropathy; the presence of resulting muscle atrophy can also be detected.

EDX assists in confirming the presence of a lower motor neuron injury to the pelvic floor. It localises the pathology to a specific peripheral nerve, plexus or nerve root. It also informs the clinician as to the extent and degree of the pathology, the duration, activity and prognosis of the pathophysiological process [46, 48–53]. Early detection of a pudendal nerve injury will ensure appropriate action takes place before muscle atrophy becomes critical. This is of particular important in the treatment of faecal incontinence, where the degree of sphincter atrophy and function can be a deciding factor in treatment selection. Early treatment improves outcomes [53].

There are a variety of EDX test to evaluate the integrity of the pudendal nerve from the pelvic floor to the brain. The combination of concentric needle EMG and CAR sacral reflex have the greatest sensitivity and specificity when used in combination and are the EDX tests of choice in cases of suspected pudendal neuropathy.

Table 17.5 Potential EDX test to evaluate potential pudendal neuropathy

Test	Electrode/Stimulus	Anatomical Pathway	Usage
Concentric needle EMG	Concentric needle	Sacral motor neurones	Clinical screening
CAR Clitoral anal sacral reflex	Concentric needle	Pudendal nerve as afferent and efferent in sacral reflex arc	Clinical screening
PNTDL Pudendal terminal distal latency	St Marks electrode	Distal pudendal nerve	Clinical screening
Surface EMG	Surface electrode	Sacral motor neurones	Kinesiology
pSEP Pudendal somatosensory evoked potential	Surface electrode pelvic stimulation with scalp recording	Somatic afferent pathway from pudendal nerve to the parietal cortex	Research
Trans magnetic stimulation MEP	Transcranial magnetic stimulation	Motor efferents to the pelvic floor	Research
pSSR Perineal sympathetic skin response	Surface electrode	T10-L2 thoracolumbar region of the spinal cord	Research
QST Quantitative sensory testing	Surface electrode, thermal diode and calibrated vibration meter	Small fibre testing of pain temperature and vibration	Small fibre assessment

17.13 Kinesiological EMG of Sphincter Muscles

EMG also allows assessment of the muscle function and recruitment patterns. This method of assessing power output and recruitment pattern is helpful in guiding neuromuscular rehabilitation and is used in other fields of medicine. Observing muscle function and its response to rehabilitation programs can be of great assistance to guide appropriate progression of a neuromuscular rehabilitation program. Kinesiology EMG suggests that faecal continence seems to be maintained at a muscle recruitment pattern of 55% or greater. Functions below this are associated with frank incontinence.

Needle EMG examination also allows this important kinesiological measurement to be made of the sphincter muscles. This is essential if deciding on surgical intervention, as a denervated muscle or atrophic muscle will not recover in the same way as a muscle with normal neurological function. Greater degrees of muscle atrophy identified on EMG and changes in muscle fibre densities are considered to be red flags and associated with poor surgical out-come.

17.14 EDX Test Protocols and Methods for Pudendal Nerve Assessment

17.14.1 Needle EMG of EAS

Needle EMG is performed by inserting a needle electrode into the muscle. Concentric needle electrode are usually employed. These have a recoding component and a reference component. In the past, monopolar electrodes were employed. These required an external reference electrode. The needle electrode picks up bioelectric signal from the muscle which is transferred to an ossciloscope having first been process by amplifiers and an electrical filtering system to create a digital sign and sound wave, which can be read by the EDX physician (see Fig. 17.8).

These waves give an accurate insight to the status of the muscle at rest, or one in a constant firing pattern (such as a sphincter muscle). Care must be taken to establish prior insult to the EAS such as haemorrhoid surgery or surgical repairs which may result in an abnormal signal.

The test is performed with the patient lying in the Sim's position or in a birthing chair. These positions lessen the effect of gravity on the pelvic muscle and improve the quality of the EMG tracing. The concentric electrode is inserted into the rugae of the EAS at the 3-o clock and 9 o clock positions (see Fig. 17.9). The muscle is interrogated with the needle in three directions.

In general, the needle electrode interrogates the muscle in at rest (or dormant, in the case of the sphincter muscles); in cases of denervation there is an increase in spontaneous activity in the muscle with unique potential. These are called positive sharp waves and fibrillation potentials. They are caused by acetylcholine hypersensitivity and are indicative of a neuropathy and a denervated muscle.

The muscle is also interrogated by activation of a voluntary contraction. This produces the MUAPs whose parameters can be observe and quantified. Normal morphological EMG data for sphincter muscles are available (Fig. 17.10) which are utilized to identify pathology. The MUAP parameters or morphology change when the nerve supplying the muscle is damaged result in "pathognomonic" changes in the EMG signal, thus allow the underlying pathophysiology to be determined by the EDX physician. Different patterns exist for individual pathologies. Computer software packages can analyse the MUAP parameters automatically. The multi MUP analysis computer packages, which assist in analysing data obtained from the EMG recording, is the most commonly used in clinical practice [54, 55].

The EMG MUAPs signal can be further analysed and quantified (QEMG). This maximises the data obtained from the EMG signal. The signal is analysed by computer-assisted algorithms. Specific features of the MUAP are analysed such as amplitude, area, phases, turns, duration and

Fig. 17.8 Concentric
and Monopolar needle
electrode recoding from
a skeletal muscle

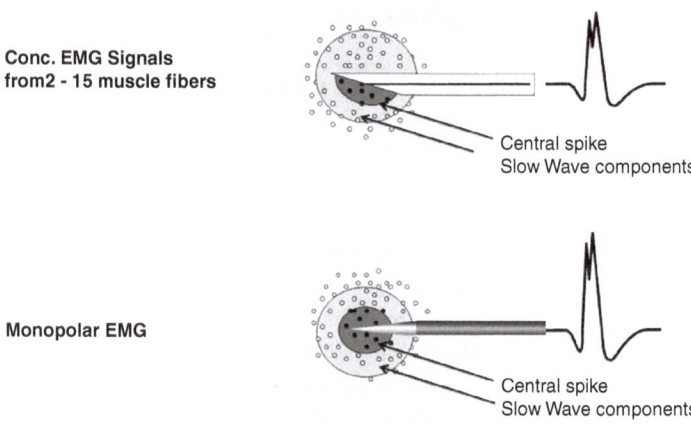

**Conc. EMG Signals
from2 - 15 muscle fibers**

Central spike
Slow Wave components

Monopolar EMG

Central spike
Slow Wave components

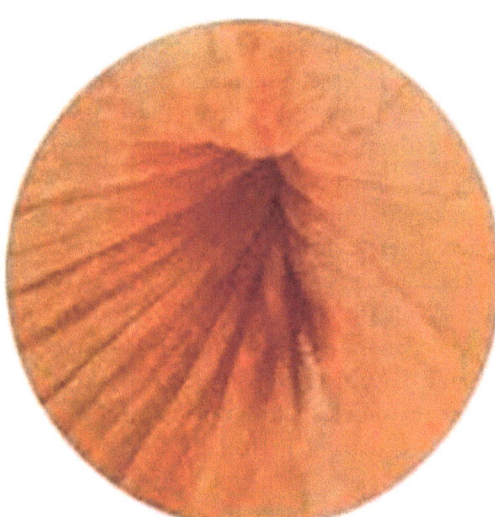

Fig. 17.9 Rugae of External Anal Sphincter

wave form stability (see Fig.17.10). QEMG
assists the EDX examiner in delineating the
extent of the nerve injury and the subsequent pattern of improvement or decline in the sphincter
muscle function (Fig. 17.11).

The EDX physician must be aware of the specific morphology of sphincter MUAPS; they are
of low amplitude ranging from 60 to 600 uV and
of short duration ranging from 3 to 7 ms [3, 50].
Specific values are available for each sphincter
(see Figs. 17.10 and 17.12). The clinician also
has to take into account the constant firing of the
sphincter muscles.

Fig. 17.10 Normal
morphology of external
anal sphincter MUAP of
male or nulliparous
females, showing the
parameters that can be
analysed by EMG
software

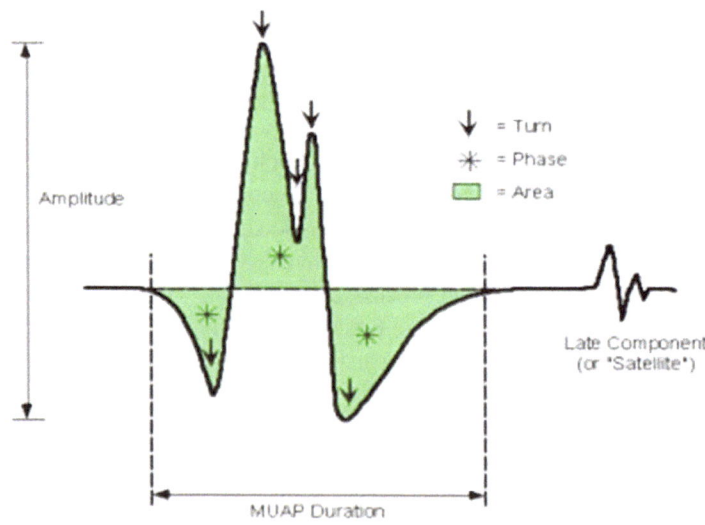

Amplitude

↓ = Turn
✳ = Phase
▢ = Area

Late Component
(or "Satellite")

MUAP Duration

Fig. 17.11 Clitoral Anal (CAR) and Bulbocavernosus (BCR) Sacral Reflexes

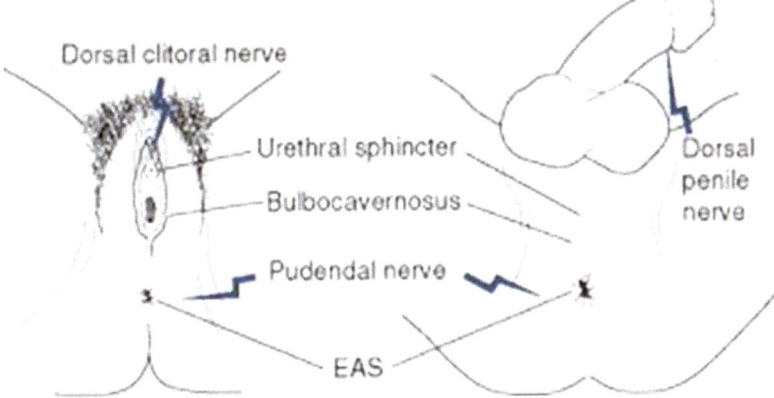

Fig. 17.12 Normal Values for CAR sensory threshold and distal latencies

CAR	Normal Value	Cut off
Sensory Threshold	4.1 +/- 1.6 m A	5.9 m A
Distal Latency	38 +/- 8.8 m s	49 m s

17.15 The Clitoral Anal Reflex (CAR)

Nerve conduction studies (NCS) are performed as part of the EDX work up in all neuromuscular diseases. Standard NCS assess the larger, heavily myelinated nerve fibres of sensory, motor and mixed nerves. This is performed by applying an electrical depolarising stimulus to the nerve and recording the response.

In nerves that are well insulated and difficult to assess (such as the pudendal nerve), indirect tests such as sacral reflexes are used to asses function through sensory thresholds and conduction velocities. The clitoral-anal reflex (CAR) is the sacral reflex most commonly used for pudendal nerve testing and has both afferent and efferent arms. Recording of the CAR is made via electrodes placed in or on the external anal sphincter muscles. Both sides of the sphincter record the muscle reflex. The right and left para clitoral areas are stimulated in sequences which results in an "anal wink". This produces the recordable muscle contraction. Localised slowing of the reflex elicits afferent and efferent pathology, as well as side-to-side differences. Abnormality of the reflex can help recognise sensory and motor pathology and is also useful in identifying the age and severity of a lesion.

In clinical practice, the needle EMG and CAR recording are performed in sequence. A significant amount of data and information is obtained. The needle EMG is performed on the sphincters with a concentric needle electrode. These electrodes are left in situ and the CAR is then performed. The test usually takes less than 20 minutes and the data obtained can be analysed at a later stage.

17.15.1 Other EDX Tests for Pelvic Floor Neuropathies

Following the initial standard tests of EAS EMG and CAR, further investigations may be considered if clinically indicated. These include needle EMG examination of the urethral sphincter muscle, as it is also innervated by the pudendal nerve. The levator ani complex is innervated directly by the S2,S3,S4 and S5 nerve roots and the lower limb and paraspinal muscles may be screened if a plexopathy or radiculopathy is suspected. The urethral-anal sacral reflex (UAR) assess the perineal branch of the pudendal nerve that supplies the urethra and is not routinely performed. But, a UAR sacral reflex can be performed if the CAR is equivocal (see Fig. 17.13 below).

Needle EMG	Recording site	Nerve root	Peripheral nerve
Needle EMG	EAS	S234	Pudendal
CAR	EAS	S234	Pudendal
Needle EMG	Levator Ani	S2345	Nerve root
Needle EMG	Urethra	S234	Pudendal
UAR	Urethra	S234	Pudendal
Needle EMG	Lower limbs and paraspinal muscles	L4, L5, S1	Nerve root
Needle EMG	Quadriceps muscles	L4	Femoral
Femoral MS	Vastus Medialis	L4	Femoral
Needle EMG	Adductor muscles	L4 and L5	Obturator
Needle EMG	Semimembranosus, Tibialis Anterior and Gastrocnemius muscles	L5 and S1	Sciatic
LFCS	Lateral thigh	L2 and L4	Lateral Femoral Cutaneous Nerve

Fig. 17.13 Electrodiagnostic assessment of a potential pelvic floor neuropathy. The first two tests are routinely performed. The other tests are only performed if no specific abnormality is found in the pudendal nerve function

The EMG signal can also be assessed for the kinesiological function of muscle such as the power output and fatiguability of the muscle. This element of EDX can employ both surface and needle EMG data. These kinesiological assessments is often by the sports medicine and rehabilitation medicine practitioners. Knowledge of the physiological power pattern and output of a sphincter can be of clinical importance when following up patients after rehabilitation programs, as it allows quantifying of muscle function, strength and fatiguability.

17.16 The Diagnostic Accuracy and Interpretation of the EDX Tests

The utility of pelvic floor neurophysiological testing is widely recognised and supported by academic evidence [49–57]. Electrodiagnostic tests represent a valid method for studying the functional integrity of neural pathways, localizing the pathological process, and identifying mechanism and severity of injury.

The EDX test showing the highest level of evidence are employed in specific protocols for assessing specific pathologies. Concentric needle EMG of the sphincter muscles and the CAR sacral reflex are the established and recommended tests for pudendal neuropathies, being both sensitive and specific [46, 48].

Other tests not currently supported by high-level evidence should be used in the research setting [44, 54] or as additional tests when assessing possible cases of pudendal neuropathy.

EMG and nerve conduction studies have a high specificity and sensitivity for assessing peripheral nerve disease. Pelvic floor quantitative EMG has sensitivity ranges from 21–70% specificity 74–99%, positive predictive values from 58–99% and negative predictive values from 47–99%; these percentages are dependent on the normative chosen and the number of MUAP parameters chosen to evaluate [58]. The sensitivity of quantitative EMG is significantly increased to 94–96% when the EMG examination is combined with the sacral reflexes [59].

EDX testing however is operator dependent, and the skill and experience level of the electrodiagnostic physician is a critical element to accuracy of the test and its interpretation [44]. Hence, it is also recommended that the EDX tests should be performed by trained neurophysiologists, with experience in pelvic floor evaluation. There is a paucity of trained physicians in pelvic floor EDX medicine and a resulting gap in utilisation of these EDX tests due to the lack of this resource.

Clinician awareness and comprehension of the output of EDX testing if the pelvic floor is also a concern. Some authors have suggested that the EDX examination does not impact clinical outcomes. It is well established that early diagnosis and intervention with any peripheral nerve lesion will prevent muscle atrophy and an acceleration of symptoms. This is probably a function of misapprehension that pudendal neuropathy is a simple trapped nerve at the level of Alcock's fascia. The nerve can be compromised anywhere along is length from Onuf's nuclei to its terminal branches. The EDX examination accesses the full length of this neural structure.

The perceived invasive nature of needle EMG has also restricted some clinicians from EMG examination of the sphincters. Newer concentric needle electrode have reduced much of the discomfort associated with the examination of sphincter muscles.

While surface EMG does not give a full picture of neuromuscular pathology, it has been shown to be useful in diagnosing the neuropathy in cases of faecal incontinence [60, 61], and is also of assistance in assessing the kinesiological function of muscle during rehabilitation.

Needle EMG is still the most powerful tool in diagnosing a neuropathy, providing the clinician information about the severity, duration and prognosis of a pudendal nerve lesion [62]. Sacral reflex such as the clinically used clitoral anal reflex (CAR) also inform the clinician as to the integrity of the nerve. This is a critical piece of information if neuromodulation is a therapeutic option.

Needle EMG can be used in combination with ultrasound and manometry for assessment of cases of pelvic floor disease. Transrectal ultrasound (TRUS) is highly accurate in detection of abnormalities in anal sphincter morphology. Certain TRUS patterns suggest a pudendal neuropathy. Similarly, anal manometry can also show patterns suggestive of a pudendal neuropathy. These findings can be confirmed by EDX testing [63].

17.17 Clinical Utility of EDX Assessment of Pelvic Floor and Sphincter Neuropathy Associated with Childbirth

Pelvic floor neuropathy following childbirth can significantly affect a new mother or older mother who develops symptoms over time. Many women suffer in silence and few discuss the matter with friends, family or their medical providers until symptoms have become unbearable. The condition is a cause of great social isolation secondary to fears of bowel or bladder incontinence. Similarly, sexual activity may be affected due to a lack of the previously normal sensation or a fear of incontinence. The finding of a pelvic floor neuropathy often allows for a great sense of relief when the diagnosis is made; patients are further comforted by the knowledge that many other suffer from a similar problem. In this way, EDX tests can be an opportunity to shine a light on what has been a dark area for many patients.

In general, it is recommend that evaluation of obstetric anal sphincter injuries should include endoanal ultrasound, manometry and pelvic floor EDX; these three elements in concert interrogate the anatomy, physiology and function of the pelvic floor.

Post-partum morbidity is a function of early identification of injury and disease and subsequent timely treatment. Failure of detection of a pudendal neuropathy may result in long term pudendal neuropathy and continence issues [64]. As with all neuropathies, the distal muscle will become atrophied and lose motor function, which is critical in the case of the sphincter muscles supplied by the pudendal nerve. Once a nerve injury has been diagnosed by the EDX assessment, the clinician can offer many treatment options. These include:

1. Targeted rehabilitation of the atrophic muscles
2. Neuromodulation either directly to the sacral plexus, or remotely using the tibial nerve [65]

3. Oral medications for pain relief, reduction in inflammation, augmentation of neuromuscular function and improvement in the blood supply to the injured structures. Phosphodiesterase type 5 (PDE5) inhibitors increase blood supply to pelvic structures and have been shown anecdotally to reduce pain scores [66]
4. Nerve blocking injections for pain relief
5. Growth hormone, gene therapy and stem cell therapy for the atrophic muscles [67].

While most experts generally recommend physical therapy, there is a lack of adequately performed studies to validate its efficacy definitively [68–70].

If the nerve injury can be established at an early-stage, anti-atrophic measures can be taken. It is now recognised that maintaining sensory supply to a denervated structure will prevent the onset of muscle wasting by a phenomenon known as "sensory babysitting", as sensory afferent reinnervation is a fundamental component of recovery after a peripheral nerve injury [71, 72]. If a pudendal nerve injury is suspected, early intervention with local sensory physiotherapy may prevent or reduce sphincter atrophy.

EDX can also give useful information prior to surgical repair. In the case of the obstetric anal sphincter injuries, the degree of denervation and the level of muscle function persisting is often a consideration when deciding on sphincteroplasty. Similarly, the motor function of the urethral sphincter is also a consideration when selecting the type of urinary incontinence surgery, as many require a functioning urethral sphincter.

17.18 Emerging Technologies for Pelvic Floor Neuromuscular Medicine

Automated sphincter QEMG assessment is now available in most EMG systems. This facilitates the identification and quantification of the morphology of MUAPs (Fig. 17.14) The software which analyses the MUAPs are based on a different computer derived algorithm. Cloud computing exists to assist in the diagnosis of other neurological pathologies and therefore, creating analytic software for sphincter physiology is a logical next step, incorporating normative data for different population and levels of parity. The Multi-MUP analysis technique is the fastest and easiest method to use and is employed by most EDX laboratories.

17.18.1 Intra-partum Pudendal Nerve Monitoring

The pudendal nerve an be injured during childbirth as noted above. If clinicians, midwives and obstetricians become aware that the nerve is being compressed during the first, second or third stage of labour, then it may be possible to alter the mother's position, therefore altering the direct effects on the nerve.

A study was undertaken [73] in an effort to establish if the status of the pudendal nerve could be monitored during parturition. Clitoral-anal reflex (CAR) recordings were performed in early cervical dilatation and late cervical dilatation. Of the eight women studied, there was indication that the intrapartum assessment of the pudendal nerve through this sacral reflex was, in fact, possible. Advancing labour had a significant effect on both latency and sensory thresholds, with a demonstrable physiological return to pre-labour levels soon after delivery. It was considered that failure of this post-natal normalisation might be useful as an early indicator of pudendal neuropathy and the subsequent development of faecal incontinence.

Needle EMG evaluation of pudendal nerve function has been proposed in the clinical setting of a delivery suite. However, there has a great degree of reticence among nursing mothers, midwives and ethics committees, reasonably, due to the potential hazards of a needle electrode in this setting. These concerns have been overcome to some degree by the use of surface electrodes and wireless recording of sphincter muscle activity. In this way, the EAS can be monitored non-invasively with the signal being transmitted to a remote oscilloscope for review and recording

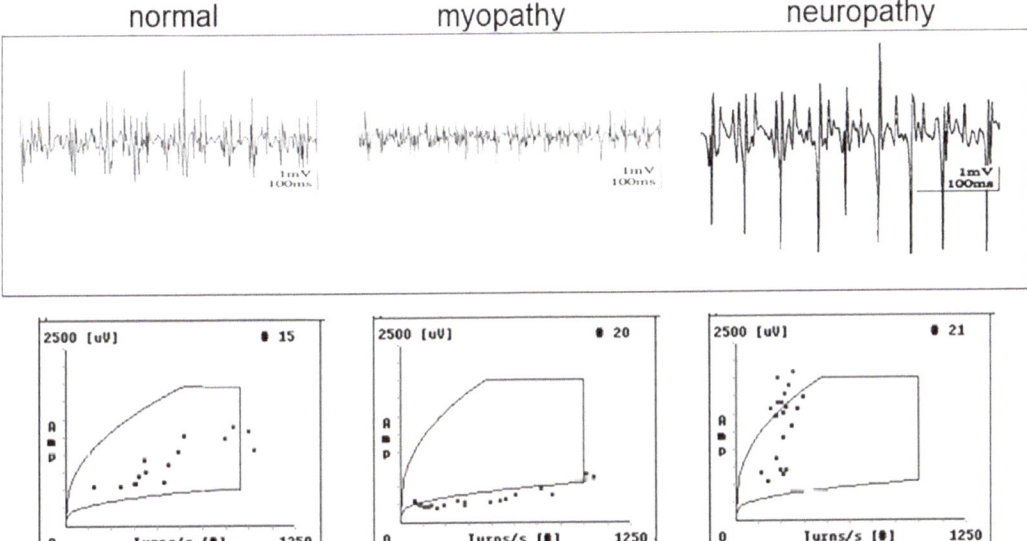

Fig. 17.14 The elements of the Motor Unit Action Potential harvested from the needle EMG recording can be quantified automatically by new EMG software. The data can be collated into "clouds" of normal and abnormal readings based on these elements. In this image, the amplitude of the MUAP is plotted against the number of turns in the MUAP. Normal and pathological recordings have different and specific cloud profiles facilitating diagnosis

[74]. Two studies were conducted at the National Maternity Hospital in Dublin to establish the feasibility of intrapartum monitoring of the pudendal nerve [54, 55]. The studies confirmed that it is possible to (1) record signals from the EAS of mothers in the puerperium, (2) harvest this usable signal, and (3) analyse in real-time the signal for alterations in morphology, thus enabling identification of potential injury to the pudendal nerve. This has borne out in other clinical settings, such as in cases of back surgery and particularly paediatric spina bifida correction surgery. Further study and research are warranted to establish workable protocols ın the electrically hostile environment of a delivery suite.

New non-surgical treatment for pudendal neuropathy have proven to be successful in alleviating symptoms. These include neuropathic pain-relieving medication, prolotherapy such as nerve blocking injections, and stem cell therapy through Platelet Rich Plasma injection (PRP). Botulinum toxin injections as well as the advancing field of neuromodulation have been applied to this setting. In 2021, further advances have been made in this evolving field where the pudendal nerve can be selectively and wireless stimulated to reduce symptoms of pudendal neuropathy [75]. Despite the evolution of knowledge and investigative methodology, pudendal neuropathy is mostly underdiagnosed and causes significant impairment in quality of life [76]. With the availability of new treatments, accurate neuromuscular information is essential. Therefore, pelvic Floor EDX knowledge should be dissipated to referring doctors and be included in their continuing medical education programs. This should also form part of all Neurophysiology and Urogynaecology training programs.

17.19 Conclusion

EDX medicine adds significantly to the diagnosis and treatment of pelvic floor and sphincter neuropathy that occurs in childbirth. Advances in protocols of testing and technology have assisted in accurately diagnosing the neuromuscular elements where are the cause and effect of this common problem. Doctors tasked with treating pelvic floor disease should be conversant with the available EDX tests and the clinical implications and output of their findings.

Take Home Messages

Pelvic floor neuropathies and in particular pudendal neuropathies, are a common but often over looked cause of pelvic dysfunction. Injury to the pudendal nerve can result in a combination of clinical presentations, which have significant physical and psychological consequences. The clinician should have a high index of suspicion for a neuropathic cause when assessing a patient with pelvic floor symptoms. The utility of modern pelvic floor electrodiagnostic testing is widely recognised and supported by academic evidence. These tests represent a valid method for studying the functional integrity of neural pathways. Localizing the pathological process and identifying mechanism and severity. Identification of a neuropathy will assist the clinician in planning treatment. Early recognition and intervention will ameliorate muscle atrophy and progression of symptoms.

Appendix: MCQ

Questions

1. Which of the following is true concerning the anatomy of the pudendal nerve?
   (A) The pudendal nerve has a single S1 nerve root origin
   (B) The pudendal nerve travels through the greater and lesser sciatic foramena
   (C) Alcock's (Pudendal) canal runs the full length of the nerve
   (D) The pudendal nerve has three terminal branches
   (E) The pudendal nerve originates from Onuf's nucleus, which is located in the ventral horns of the sacral spinal cord

2. Which of the following is true concerning the function of the pudendal nerve?
   (A) The pudendal nerve supplies sensation to the buttocks

   (B) The Pudendal nerve supplies the internal anal sphincter
   (C) The pudendal nerve is a pure sensory nerve
   (D) The pudendal nerve supplies sensation to the clitoris
   (E) The pudendal nerve supplies the urethral meatus

3. The clinical presentation of pudendal neuropathy includes which the following?
   (A) Pain on sitting
   (B) Pain that is relieved by sitting on a toilet seat
   (C) Dyspareunia is rare
   (D) Rarely, stymphathalgia of the vagina
   (E) An elevated Wexner score

4. Regarding the assessment of pudendal neuropathy?
   (A) MRI scanning of the pelvic floor is the test of choice in suspected cases of pudendal neuropathy
   (B) Needle EMG is the most accurate diagnostic tool in assessing the severity of pudendal neuropathy
   (C) Cases of Pudendal neuropathy will usually shows conduction slowing through Alcock's canal
   (D) Sphincter Needle EMG can grade the severity of the neuropathy
   (E) Sphincter Needle EMG can be used as a kinesiological tool

5. Regarding the pudendal nerve in clinical practice:
   (A) The Pudendal nerve is spared in cases of Anterior Horn cell disease
   (B) Pudendal Neuropathy commonly occurs in cyclists
   (C) The Pudendal neuropathy is rare in cases of caesarean section
   (D) The pudendal nerve is compromised in cases of Spinal Canal Stenosis
   (E) Trampolining and high impact activities have the highest incidence of neuropathy

Answers

1. Which of the following is true concerning the anatomy of the pudendal nerve?
   - (A) FALSE
   - (B) TRUE
   - (C) FALSE
   - (D) TRUE
   - (E) TRUE

2. Which of the following is true concerning the function of the pudendal nerve?
   - (A) FALSE
   - (B) FALSE
   - (C) FALSE
   - (D) TRUE
   - (E) TRUE

3. The clinical presentation of pudendal neuropathy includes the following?
   - (A) TRUE
   - (B) TRUE
   - (C) FALSE
   - (D) FALSE
   - (E) TRUE

4. Regarding the assessment of pudendal neuropathy?
   - (A) FALSE
   - (B) TRUE
   - (C) FALSE
   - (D) TRUE
   - (E) TRUE

5. Regarding the pudendal nerve in clinical practice:
   - (A) TRUE
   - (B) TRUE
   - (C) TRUE
   - (D) TRUE
   - (E) TRUE.

References

1. Mc CE. Faecal incontinence. Social and economic factors. In: Benson JT, editor. Female pelvic floor disorders. Norton Medical Books; 1992. ISBN 0-393-71013-0.
2. Johanson JF, Lafferty J. Epidemiology of faecal incontinence: the silent affliction. Am J Gastroenterol. 1996;91:33–6.
3. Benson JT. In: Thomas Benson J, editor. Neurophysiology and neuroanatomy in female pelvic floor disorders. Norton Medical Books; 1992. ISBN 0-393-71013-0.
4. Schroder HD, Reske-Nielsen E. Fibre types in the striated urethral and anal sphincters. Acta Neuropathol (Berl). 1983;60:278–82.
5. Barber M, Bremer RE, Thor KB, Dolber PC, et al. Innervation of the female levator ani muscles. Am J Obstet Gynecol. 2002;187(1):64–71.
6. Weidner AC, Saunders DB, Sanjeev D. Quantitative electromyographic analysis of levator ani and external anal sphincter muscles in nulliparous women. Am J Obstet Gynecol. 2000;183:1249–56.
7. Hibner M, Desai N, Robertson LJ, Nour M. Pudendal neuralgia. J Minim Invasive Gynecol. 2010;17(2):148–53. [PubMed].
8. Snook SJ, Henry SM, Setchell MM. Risk factors in childbirth causing damage to the pelvic floor innervation. J Int Colo Rec Dis. 1986;1:20–4.
9. Fitzpatrick M, O'Brien C, O'Connell PR, Herlihy C. Patterns of abnormal pudendal nerve function that are associated with post-partum faecal incontinence. Am J Obst Gynaecol. 2003;189(3):730–5.
10. Spinosa JP, de Bisschop E, Laurençon J, Kuhn G, Dubuisson JB, Riederer BM. Sacral staged reflexes to localize the pudendal compression: an anatomical validation of the concept. Rev Med Suisse. 2006;2(84):2416–8, 2420–1. [PubMed].
11. Guo KK, Wang L, Liu F, Niu JJ, Wang C, You SH, Feng ZG, Lu GJ. Sacral nerve stimulation in patients with refractory pudendal neuralgia. Pain Physician. 2022;25(4):E619–27. [PubMed].
12. Ismael SS, Amarenco B, Bayle B, et al. Postpartum lumbosacral plexopathy limited to autonomic and perineal manifestations, clinical and electrophysiological study of 19 patients. Neuro Neurosurg Psychiatry. 2000;68(60):771–3.
13. Parks AG, Swash M, Urich H. Sphincter denervation in anorectal incontinence and rectal prolapse. Gut. 1977;18:656–65.
14. Snook SH, Swash M. Abnormalities of the innervation of the urethral striated sphincter muscular in incontinence. Br J Urol. 1984;56:401–4051994.
15. Kiff ES, Swash M. Slowed conduction in the pudendal nerves in idiopathic (neurogenic) faecal incontinence. Br J Surg. 1984;71:614–6.
16. Gilphin SA, Gosling JA, Smith ARB, Warrell DW. The patogenises of genitourinary prolapse and

stress incontuinence. A histological and histochemistry study. Br J Obstet Gynaecol. 1989;96:15–23.

17. ARB S, Hosker GL, Warrell DW. The role of pudendal nerve damage in the aetiology of genuine stress incontinence in women. Br J Obstet Gynaecol. 1989;96:29–32.

18. Vaccaro CA, Cheong DMO, Wexner SD, Nogueras JJ, et al. Pudendal neuropathies and evacuatory disorders. DIS Colon Rectum. 1995;32(2)

19. Ramphul M, Corry E, Rowan A, Mahony R, Fitzpatrick M, O'Brien C, McAuliffe F. Pudendal neuropathy after caesarean section in the second stage of labour. AJOG. 2017;216(1):S259–S26.

20. Corona R, De Cicco C, Schonman R, Verguts J, et al. Tension free vaginal tapes and pelvic nerve neuropathy. J Minim Invasive Gynaecol. 2008;15(3):262–6 and Hibner Castellanos et al. 2011.

21. Rodríguez-López ES, Calvo-Moreno SO, García AB, et al. Prevalence of urinary incontinence among elite athletes of both sexes. J Sci Med Sport. 24:338.

22. Goldstick O, Constantini N. Urinary incontinence in physically active women and female athletes. BJSM. 2014;48(4):296–8.

23. Morkeved S, Bo K. Effects of pelvic floor muscle training during pregnancy and after child birth on prevention and treatment of urinary incontinence. BSSM. 2014;48(4):299–310.

24. Almousa S, Van Loon AB. The prevalence of urinary incontinence in nulliparous female sports women: a systematic review. J Sports Sci. 2019;37(14):1663–772.

25. Casey EK. Pelvic floor muscle function and urinary incontinence in the female athlete. The physician and sports medicine. 2017.

26. Leibovitch I, Mor Y. The vicious cycling: bicycling related urogenital disorders. Eur Urol. 2005;47(3):277–86; discussion 86–7.

27. Ramsden CE, McDaniel MC, Harmon RL, Renney KM, Faure A. Pudendal nerve entrapment as source of intractable perineal pain. Am J Phys Med Rehabil. 2003;82(6):479–84.

28. Levesque A, Bautrant E, Quistrebert V, Valancogne G, Riant T, Beer Gabel M, Leroi AM, Jottard K, Bruyninx L, Amarenco G, Quintas L, Picard P, Vancaillie T, Leveque C, Mohy F, Rioult B, Ploteau S, Labat JJ, Guinet-Lacoste A, Quinio B, Cosson M, Haddad R, Deffieux X, Perrouin-Verbe MA, Garreau C, Robert R. Recommendations on the management of pudendal nerve entrapment syndrome: a formalised expert consensus. Eur J Pain. 2022;26(1):7–17. [PubMed].

29. Olsen AL, Ross M, Stansfield RB, Kreiter C. Pelvic floor nerve conduction studies: establishing clinically relevant normative data. Am J Obset Gynecol. 2003;189:1114–9.

30. Eogan M, O'Brien C, Behan M, O'Connell PR, O'Herlihy C. Faecal continence and pudendal nerve function in older women – does vaginal delivery or age have the greatest impact? Joint ICS/IUGA meeting. Paris. 2004.

31. O'Leary BD, Kelly L, O'Brien C, Fitzpatrick M. Pudendal neuropathy associated with postpartum faecal incontinence. Podium presentation at the European Urogynaecological Association virtual annual meeting 2020. Dublin.

32. Mahony R, O'Brien C, O'Connell PR, O'Herlihy C. Evidence of ante partum pudendal neuropathy and the effect of vaginal delivery in pregnant insulin dependent diabetic women. Am J Obstet Gynecol. 2002;S150:331.

33. Fitzpatrick M, O'Brien C, O'Connell PR, O'Herlihy C. Patterns of abnormal pudendal nerve conduction associated with postpartum faecal incontinence. Am J Obstet Gynecol. 2003;189(3):730–5.

34. Snooks J, Swash M, Henry MM. A randomised clinical trial comparing the effects of delayed versus Abnormalities in central and peripheral nerve conduction in patients with anorectal incontinence. J R Soc Med. 1985;78(4):294–300.

35. Fitzpatrick M, Harkin R, McQuillan K, O'Brien C, O'Connell PR, O'Herlihy C. Effect of delayed versus immediate pushing with epidural analgesia on mode of delivery and faecal continence. BJOG. 2002;109(12):1359–65.

36. Feldman M. Sleisenger and Fordtrans gastroenterology and liver disease. 10th ed. ISBN 1455746924 ExpertConsult.com

37. Pierce C, O'Brien C, Herlihy C. Post partum Femoral Neuropathy following spontaneous vaginal delivery. J Obstet Gynaecol. 2010;30(2):203–4.

38. Staal A. Entrapment neuropathies. In: Vink PJ, Bruyn GW, editors. Handbook of clinical neurology. Amsterdam North Holland Publishing Company; 1970. p. 285–325.

39. O'Brien C, Fitzpatrick M, Herlihy C. Levator Ani syndrome. 23rd November 2012, British Society of Clinical Neurophysiology. Joint British & Italian Peripheral Nerve Society Meeting. Queen Square London.

40. Waldinger MD, Venema PL, van Gils AP, Schweitzer DH. New insights into restless genital syndrome: static mechanical hyperesthesia and neuropathy of the nervus dorsalis clitoridis. J Sex Med. 2009;6(10):2778–87.

41. Labatt JJ, Riant T, Roberts R, Amarenco G, Lefaucheur JP, Rigaud J. Diagnostic criteria for pudendal neuralgia by pudendal nerve entrapment (Nantes criteria). Neurourol Urodyn. 2008;27(4):306–10.

42. Paniker J N Manji H. Neuromuscular disorders in pelvic organ dysfunction in neurological disease. 18:278–292. Fowler CJ, Pnicker JN, Emmanuel A, editors. Cambridge Press. ISBN 987-0-52119831-8. 2010.

43. Labatt JJ, Roberts R, Bensignor M, Buzelin JM. Neiuralgia of the pudendal nerve. Anatamo-clinical considerations and therapeutic approach. JUrol (Paris). 1990;96(5):239–44.

44. Bianchi F, Squintani GM, Psio N. Neurophysiology of the pelvic floor in clinical practice: a systematic literature review. Funct Neurol. 2017;32(4):173–93.

45. O'Brien C, Fitzpatrick M. Managing perineal trauma after childbirth. BMJ. 2014;349:6829.

46. O'Brien C, O'Connell PR, Herlihy C. Pudendal neuropathy is best determined by full neurophysiological assessment. AJOG. 2004;191(5):1836.

47. Executive Summary: The International Consultation on Incontinence 2008 – Committee on: "Dynamic Testing"; for urinary or fecal incontinence. Part 3: Anorectal physiology studies, Rosier PF, Hosker GL, Szabó L, Capewell A, Gajewski JB, Sand PK. International Consultation on Incontinence 2008 Committee on Dynamic Testing. Neurourol Urodyn. 2010;29(1):153–8.

48. Podnar S, Vodusek DB. Protocol for clinical neurophysiologic examination of the pelvic floor. Neurourol Urodyn. 2001;20(6):669–82. [PubMed] [Google Scholar].

49. Amarenco G. Electrophysiological of pudendal neuropathy following traction. 1097–4598 line ed. 1097–4598. Muscle Nerve. 2001;24(1):116–9.

50. Benson JT. Pelvic floor neurophysiology workshop. AANEM 1998. Rochester MH 55902..

51. Roberts MM. Neurophysiology in neurology. Muscle Nerve. 2008;38:815–36.

52. Neurophysiology. In: Brams PA, Cardozo L, Khouri S, Wein A, editors. Incontinence: 2nd international consultation on incontinence. World Health Organization; 2002.

53. Irving RK. Faecal incontinence is not irreversible. Br J Med. 1986;292:1618.

54. Podnar S, Vodusek DB. Standardisation of sphincter electromyography, utility of motor unit potential parameters. Muscle Nerve. 2001;24:946–51.

55. Podnar S, Mrkaic M. Predictive power of motorunit potentials parameters in anal sphincter electromyography. Muscle Nerve. 2002;26:389–94.

56. Olsen AL, Rao SS. Clinical neurophysiology and electrodiagnostic testing of the pelvic floor. Gastroenterol Clin N Am. 2001;30(1):33–54. v–vi. [PubMed] [Google Scholar].

57. Dillingham T, Chen S, Andary M, Buschbacher R, Del Toro D, Smith B, Zimmermann K, So Y. Establishing high-quality reference values for nerve conduction studies: a report from the normative data task force of The American Association of Neuromuscular & Electrodiagnostic Medicine Aanem Technology Review, Muscle Nerve. 2016.

58. Podnar S. Predictive values of the anal sphincter electromyography. Neurourol Urodyn. 2009;28(8):1034–5. [PubMed] [Google Scholar].

59. Podnar S. Sphincter electromyography and the penilocavernosus reflex: are both necessary? Neurourol Urodyn. 2008;27(8):813–8. [PubMed] [Google Scholar]

60. Enck P, Hinninghofen H, Merletti R, Azpiroz F. The external anal sphincter and the role of surface electromyography. Neurogastroenterol Motil. 2005;17(Suppl 1):60–7. https://doi.org/10.1111/j.1365-2982.2005.00660.x.PMID. 15836456 Review.

61. Nowakowski M, Tomaszewski KA, Machura Ł, Trybek P, Herman RM. Sensitivity and specificity of multichannel surface electromyography in diagnosing fecal incontinence. Folia Med Cracov. 2017;57(1):29–38.

62. Kraft GH. An approach to electrodiagnostic medicine: The power of needle. In: Electromyography new developments in electrodiagnostic medicine, physical medicine and rehabilitation clinics of North America. WB Saunders and Co; 1994. p. 495–508.

63. Tjandra JJ, Milsom JW, Schroeder T, Fazio VW. Endoluminal ultrasound is preferable to electromyography in mapping anal sphincter defects. Dis Colon Rectum. 1993;36:689–92.

64. Eogan M, O'Brien C, Behan M, O'Connell PR, O'Herlihy C. Long-term effects of childbirth on fecal continence and pudendal nerve function. Am J Obstet Gynecol. 2004;189(6):S72.

65. Peters KM, Carrico DJ, MacDiarmid SA, Wooldridge LS, Khan AU, McCoy CE, Franco N, Bennett JB. Sustained therapeutic effects of percutaneous tibial nerve stimulation: 24-month results of the STEP study. Neurourol Urodyn. 2013;32:24–9.

66. Pineault K, et al. Phosphodiesterase type 5 inhibitor therapy provides sustained relief of symptoms among patients with chronic pelvic pain syndrome. Transl Androl Urol. 2020;9:391–7.

67. Kerns JM, Shott S, Brubaker L, Sakamoto K, Benson JT, Fleischer AE, Coleman ME. Effects of IGF-I gene therapy on the injured rat pudendal nerve. Int Urogynecol J Pelvic Floor Dysfunct. 2003;14(1):2–7.

68. Berghmans B. Physiotherapy for pelvic pain and female sexual dysfunction: an untapped resource. Int Urogynecol J. 2018;29(5):631–8. [PMC free article] [PubMed].

69. Fuentes-Márquez C, P, Cabrera-Martos I, Valenza MC. Physiotherapy interventions for patients with chronic pelvic pain: a systematic review of the literature. Physiother Theory Pract. 2019;35(12):1131–8. [PubMed].

70. FitzGerald MP, Anderson RU, Potts J, Payne CK, Peters KM, Clemens JQ, Kotarinos R, Fraser L, Cosby A, Fortman C, Neville C, Badillo S, Odabachian L, Sanfield A, O'Dougherty B, Halle-Podell R, Cen L, Chuai S, Landis JR, Mickelberg K, Barrell T, Kusek JW, Nyberg LM. Urological pelvic pain collaborative research network Randomized multicenter feasibility trial of myofascial physical therapy for the treatment of urological chronic pelvic pain syndromes. J Urol. 2009;182(2):570–80. [PMC free article] [PubMed].

71. Kazusko A, et al. Sensory neurotization of muscle, past, present and future considerations. J Plast Surg Hand Surg. 2019;53:31–6.

72. Nighiem BT, et al. Sensory protection to enhance functional recovery following proximal nerve injury, current trends. Plast Aesthet Res. 2015;2:202–7.

73. Eogan M, O'Brien C, Daly L, Byrne P, O'Connell PR, O'Herlihy C. Monitoring pudendal nerve conduction

during labour and early puerperium. Am J Obstet Gynaecol. 2005;193:S41.

74. O'Leary BD, O'Brien C, Brennan DJ, Keane DP. Feasibility and patient acceptability of non-invasive intrapartum pudendal nerve monitoring. Post and presentation at the European Urogynaecological Association virtual annual meeting 2020 Dublin.

75. Roberts LH, Vollstedt A, Volin J McCartney T, Peters KM. Initial experiences using a novel nerve stimulator for the management of pudendal neuropathy. Neurol Urodyn. 2021

76. Kaur J, Sing P. Pudendal nerve entrapment syndrome. StarPeals Publishing; 2020.

Physical Therapy After OASIs

18

Hege Hoelmo Johannessen and Siv Mørkved

Overview

Test your learning and check your understanding of this book's contents: use the "Springer Nature Flashcards" app to access questions using ▶ https://sn.pub/wqrf89. To use the app, please follow the instructions in Chap. 1.

Learning Points

- Obstetric anal sphincter injury (OASI) increases the risk of anal incontinence (AI)
- AI involves a complex interplay of muscular function, stool consistency and bowel function thus, a combination of modalities such as PFMT, laxatives and bulking agents may be required

H. H. Johannessen (✉)
Department of Health, Welfare and Organisation, Oestfold University College, Fredrikstad, Norway

Department of Physical Medicine and Rehabilitation, Oestfold Hospital Trust, Sarpsborg, Norway
e-mail: hege.h.johannessen@hiof.no

S. Mørkved
Department of Public Health and Nursing, Norwegian University of Science and Technology, Trondheim, Norway

Central Norway Health Authority, Stjoerdal, Norway
e-mail: siv.morkved@ntnu.no

- Studies focusing on principles of stregth training in postpartum women that have with AI as the main outcome, do, in fact, report reduced AI symptoms

18.1 Introduction

Anal incontinence (AI) involves involuntary loss of gas, and solid or liquid stool, whereas faecal incontinence (FI) involves loss of stool only [1, 2]. The mechanism of maintaining anal continence is a complex interaction between motor and sensory pathways of spinal reflexes, rectal compliance and stool consistency, as well as adequate pelvic floor muscle function [3]. Obstetric anal sphincter injury (OASI) is one of the main risk factors for short- and long-term postpartum pelvic floor disorders (PFDs) such as anal (AI) and urinary incontinence (UI). [4–7] PFDs, and AI in particular, may have a severe impact on quality of life (QoL) and are associated with sexual dysfunction. [8–10] Women with more than one PFD symptom tend to report more severe symptoms, larger reductions in physical activity, and poorer psychosocial well-being and QoL compared to those reporting only one symptom [11, 12]. Health professionals tend to perceive regular loss of solid stool as more severe than occasional loss, [13] however, studies show that patients report experiencing involuntary loss of gas alone to be more embarrassing than loss of stool alone [8, 14]. Furthermore, patients with PFDs following OASI may experience co-existing soiling, constipation and problems with bowel evacuation, resulting in a more complicated presentation, and further impairment of QoL [15]. Thus, these patients may require a combination of treatment modalities in order to achieve symptom relief [16, 17].

18.1.1 Physical Therapy After OASIS

The association between OASIS and postpartum AI is well documented, and optimal postpartum care should include a comprehensive postpartum consultation within the first 6–12 weeks after delivery evaluating mental health, emotional well-being and PFDs [18]. Several national guidelines recommend that women experiencing symptoms of PFDs are referred to women's health physical therapists and PFMT [1, 19]. However, few studies to date have explored the effect of physical therapy and PFMT after OASIS. Recent systematic reviews suggest that targeted interventions including PFMT may be effective among women who have sustained an OASIS or experience postpartum PFDs [20, 21].

18.1.1.1 The Repair Phase: Early Recovery within 3 Weeks Postpartum

Management of the Acute Muscular Injury
With acute muscular and soft tissue injuries in sports, physical therapy is based on well-studied sports science and the physiological principles of soft tissue inflammation and healing [22]. An injury to the pelvic floor muscles (PFM) and the anal sphincter complex may be considered an acute obstetric event affecting the soft tissues in the pelvic floor equivalent to a sports-related muscular injury. Thus, management may follow the same principles.

After primary suturing of the OASI, the *early repair phase* starts within 24 hours, during which soft tissue regenerates, scar tissue is formed with new myofibrils as well as approximation of the ruptured myofibrils through macrophagic phago-

cytosis of the necrotic tissue. Forty-eight hours after injury, the regeneration of myofibrils is dominated by proliferation and differentiation of satellite cells. During the first 3 weeks postpartum, there is simultaneous revascularisation and connective scar tissue formation between the torn myofibrils. From 10 to 12 days after delivery, the newly formed scar tissue is stronger than the adjacent muscular fibres. Beyond 10–12 days a re-rupture of the healing fibres during situations involving excess stretching of the pelvic floor such as deep squatting or bending over forwards to pick up the infant from the floor with knees straight, is more likely to affect the adjacent muscular fibres than the newly formed scar tissue [23].

During the early postpartum and repair phase period, the main aim of physical therapy is to reduce pain, optimize soft tissue healing, facilitate scar tissue formation, prevent excessive strain, re-rupture and further soft tissue injury. In sports science, early management has traditionally been based on applying the principles of RICE; Rest, Ice, Compression and Elevation. However, recent studies propose that the immediate care of an acute muscular injury follow the principles of (1) PEACE; Protect, Elevate, Avoid anti-inflammatory drugs, Compression and Education, followed after a few days with (2) LOVE; Load, Optimism, Vascularisation, and Exercise [22].

Protection encompasses restriction of movement, elevation and de-loading of the injured tissues to minimise bleeding. The level of protection and rest needed in both the acute and subacute phase should be guided by pain [22]. Women who have sustained an OASI are advised to rest regularly in supported horizontal or side-lying positions during the early postpartum period to reduce gravitational stress on the structures of the pelvic floor and perineum (Fig. 18.1a, b) [23]. Complete protection, **elevation** or **compression** of the PFM and soft tissues would be neither possible, nor functionally feasible, as all activities of daily living affect these structures [23]. Despite the recent findings that cold therapy may offer some pain relief in the early postpartum period, [24] standard care should not

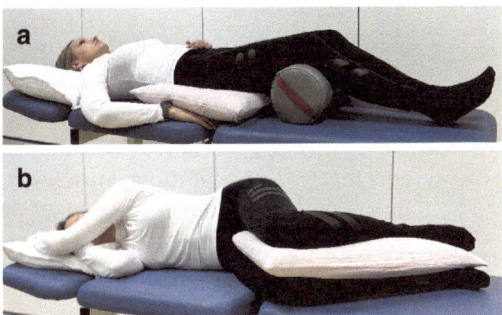

Fig. 18.1 (**a**) Supported supine resting position. (**b**) Supported side-lying position for resting and breastfeeding

include use of cryotherapy due to the potentially harmful effects on the acute and subacute inflammation processes, resulting in subsequent delays of soft tissue repair [22]. However, a systematic review found that women receiving NSAID rectal suppositories experienced less perineal pain and required less additional analgesia up to 48 hours after delivery. Even though the long-term effect on pain relief and use of additional analgesia is unclear, avoiding anti-inflammatory pain relief is not recommended in the early repair phase after OASI [25].

After OASI, an active, pain-guided approach may benefit recovery [22]. Thus, early **education** and promotion of voluntary activation and gentle, pain free, contractions of the PFM (gentle tightening of the pelvic floor muscles followed by complete relaxation) in a comfortable supine or side-lying position [26–28] and relaxation may have a positive impact on the revascularisation process and optimize orientation of the healing muscle fibres [23, 29]. Educating women on the realistic time-frame of recovery may result in better long-term outcomes and reduce unnecessary treatment [22]. Minimizing the strain on the perineum during defaecation may protect the healing perineum and pelvic floor from impaction and re-rupture due to postpartum constipation. Manipulation of stool consistency in the early postpartum period is therefore recommended [1, 30]. A previous study found no effect on pain with first bowel movement and increased risk of AI during the first 10 days after delivery when combining lax-

atives and bulking agents. Thus, laxatives alone can be recommended during the early postpartum period [31].

Physical Therapy and Pelvic Floor Muscle training in the Acute Phase

The effect of early structured postpartum PFMT for PFDs, and AI in particular, is understudied. In general, the published studies are low quality and underpowered to assess the effect of PFMT on postpartum PFDs or AI symptoms [20]. In the retrospective study by Mathé and co-workers [32], physical therapy including PFMT was initiated within the first month of sustaining an OASI. PFMT was continued for 6–8 weeks and AI and UI symptoms were reduced [32]. In the study by Sleep and Grant [33], all participating women received standard postpartum instructions on PFMT for home use prior to discharge. Women in the intervention group received additional home visits within 4 weeks after delivery by a community midwife reinforcing PFMT advise. No assessment of active pelvic floor muscle contractions were conducted, and there were no differences found in UI or AI prevalence between groups 2 months after delivery [33]. In yet another study, women sustaining an OASI were randomized to two daily sessions of PFMT with and without intra-anal biofeedback as instructed prior to discharge home from hospital. No further instructions or follow-up during the 3-month intervention period were included. The main outcome measure was impact of AI on QoL. However, no participating women reported AI symptoms at baseline. No differences in PFM strength, impact on quality of life or AI symptoms were found between groups at follow-up. Seven of the 30 PFMT and biofeedback group women reported not adhering to the biofeedback protocol due to lack of time. In addition, continent women were less willing to perform PFMT with biofeedback [34]. The relevance of assessing the impact of postpartum AI on health-related quality of life among women who report little or no symptoms of AI is questionable. Furthermore, the timing of initiating an invasive intervention using intra-anal biofeedback immediately after primary repair of an OASI may be less than optimal.

Patient Leaflet with Recommendations for women within 3 weeks postpartum

- Manage pain and de-load the injured tissues with regular resting periods in supported horizontal supine and side-lying positions when possible and when breastfeeding [22, 23, 28]
- Avoid straining during defaecation [1, 30]
- Ensure adequate fluid intake particularly if breastfeeding [35, 36]
- Manipulate stool consistency using laxatives [31]

Education

- Review of pelvic floor anatomy and function, and how a pain-guided active approach may benefit recovery [21]

With adequate pain relief, or when pain free

- Re-inforcement of how to perform correct, voluntary activation and gentle contractions of the pelvic floor muscles and ensure adequate relaxation between contractions
  How to do gentle and correct, voluntary contractions of the pelvic floor muscles
  - In a comfortable supine or side-lying position imagine that you are trying to stop passing urine or wind, and **gently** draw or tighten your pelvic floor muscles upwards and inwards. As your muscles contract, you may feel a lifting up and tightening of the muscles. Try to breathe normally, or breathe out through your mouth as you contract. It is normal that the lower part of your tummy may tighten slightly while your pelvic floor muscles contract, but keep your

legs and buttocks relaxed throughout the contraction. After holding the contraction for a few seconds, relax and let go of the contraction and feel your pelvic floor muscles return to the starting position. Repeat 1–5 times or "little and often" during the first days and weeks after delivery [26–28].
  - Pelvic floor muscle contractions should not increase pain during or after contractions
- Some women find it difficult to reconnect with their pelvic floor muscles during the first days and weeks after delivery. If you experience these problems, wait a day or two and try again. If you are not able to voluntarily contract your muscles within 4–6 weeks after delivery you should contact a health care professional [26–28].

18.1.1.2 The Subacute Postpartum Recovery Phase: 3–12 Weeks Postpartum

Management of the Subacute Muscular Injury

Current recommendations suggest that subacute management of soft tissue injuries follow the principles of LOVE; Love, Optimism, Vascularisation, and Exercise, and encompassing the resumption of normal activities as soon as pain allows. Active, pain-free movement enhances muscle regeneration, soft tissue repair, and rebuilds pelvic floor muscle tolerance for mechanical stress through increased vascularisation and blood flow. Painful activities should be avoided, and pain should be used as a guide for optimal loading of the healing tissues in the subacute recovery phase. Patients with optimistic expectations of recovery have better outcomes and prognoses, and known barriers to recovery (such as fear and depression) may result in poorer outcomes [37]. Thus, encouraging physical activity and PFMT as the woman is able is recommended during the subacute phase of recovery. If the woman is able to perform a correct voluntary PFM contraction, the principles of strength training may be applied. The recommendations are to perform three sets of 8–12 repetitions of gentle to submaximal contractions at least 3 days per week [38, 39]. Moreover, applying a holistic approach, rather than just focusing on the injured pelvic floor, may result in more favourable long-term outcomes [22].

Physical Therapy and Pelvic Floor Muscle Training in the Subacute Phase

Despite the recommendations that women should be referred for physical therapy following OASIS, the evidence of what physical therapy should entail is conflicting. The effect of PFMT on postpartum UI is well documented [40]. Several studies documenting this effect have used strength training principles or "resistance training", which is a type of physical exercise recommended to improve a wide range of health-related parameters including neuromuscular fitness, cognitive abilities, insulin sensitivity, bone density, and cardiovascular wellness [41]. Practicing pre-contraction of the PFM (known as "the knack") in situations expected to result in loss of urine, has been shown to reduce the amount of urinary leakage among non-pregnant and pregnant women [42].

Two studies exploring the effect of PFMT in the subacute phase among women following OASIS at delivery have been published. Oakley et al. [44], randomized postpartum women to receiving standard postpartum care between 2 and 4 weeks postpartum (control group), or four individual PFMT sessions reinforced by biofeedback therapy and written information on physical activity, diet and perineal hygiene between 6 and 12 weeks postpartum, (intervention group). The primary outcome was health-related QoL as measured by the Fecal Incontinence Quality of Life Scale (FIQoL) [43].

There were no significant differences between groups in AI symptoms or impact on QoL at 12 weeks postpartum. However, both groups reported improved physical activity, sexual function, and reductions in urinary symptoms [44]. The study was not powered to detect between-group differences in AI symptoms, and adherence to PFMT was not reported. Only two of fifty women reported AI or soiling at baseline, and thus the relevance of assessing impact on health-related QoL using the disease specific FIQL scale is questionable. On the contrary, in the study by von Bargen and co-workers [45] primiparous women sustaining an OASI were randomized 2 weeks after delivery to either standard care (control group) or 12 weekly sessions of standardized physical therapy including PFMT between 2 and 12 weeks postpartum, (intervention group). There was a statistically significant and clinically relevant reduction in PFD symptoms and bother in the intervention group at 12 weeks postpartum, compared to no change in the standard care group. A recent meta-analysis concluded that PFMT may be more beneficial in treating AI among women with OASIS compared to watchful waiting, though the long-term effects are uncertain [21].

Few studies have explored how to prevent postpartum constipation, however, high-fibre diets and adequate fluid intake in the postpartum period is usually recommended [36]. No studies have explored how to treat postpartum constipation [35]. However, studies have looked at improvement in AI symptoms with medications. For example, in a Swedish study of women comparing PFMT and biofeedback with medical treatments such as loperamide or bulking agents, the combination of PFMT and medical treatment was shown to be more effective in relieving AI symptoms than either treatment alone. Among the included women, 80% had defects of the anal sphincter muscles on endoanal ultrasound, and symptom improvement was associated with optimisation of stool consistency, rectal sensory thresholds and reduced urgency [17].

Patient Leaflet Recommendations for women 3–12 weeks postpartum

- Manage pain and reduce oedema of the injured area using pain-free gentle to submaximal aerobic contractions of the pelvic floor muscles with adequate relaxation between contractions [22]
- Avoid straining the pelvic floor during defaecation [1]
- Ensure adequate fluid intake particularly if breastfeeding [35, 36]
- Manipulate stool consistency using a high fibre diet, laxatives or bulking agents if experiencing bowel evacuation problems [17, 31, 35]

Education

- Review pelvic floor anatomy and function and how a pain-guided active approach may benefit recovery [22]
- Re-inforce how to perform correct, gentle to submaximal contractions of the pelvic floor muscles when pain-free [46]
- Initiate a daily PFMT programme of 3 × 8-12 contractions as able [26–28, 47]
- Use "the Knack" prior to activities such as sneezing, coughing and lifting [42]

18.1.1.3 Late Postpartum Recovery: 3–12 Months Postpartum

Late Management of a Muscular Injury 3–12 Months Postpartum

The principles of LOVE are still applicable in the late and long-term management of soft tissue injuries. Therapeutic use of exercise and progressive increases in mechanical loading may stimulate soft tissue repair and remodelling. In soft tissues, the cellular process of mechanotransduction involves converting a physiological mechanical stimulus into a biochemical response. In absence of injury, normal musculoskeletal structures are maintained by way of mechanotransduction through (1) mechanocoupling, where tensile or shearing forces elicit deformation of a soft tis-

sue cell which is transformed into chemical signals within and among cells, (2) intercellular communication, where a single-cell stimulus spreads to neighbouring or distant cells not experiencing the mechanical stimulus, and (3) the on-going physiological process of effector cell response, promoting tissue repair and remodelling. The process of mechanotransduction is best known in bone tissue, where absence of load results in loss of bone density as seen in osteoporosis. Loads above the tissue thresholds increase protein synthesis and regeneration of bone tissue in areas exposed to the increased load. The load-induced signalling process in muscular tissue is not fully understood, though there is strong evidence that overloading muscular tissue using the principles of resistance training result in muscular hypertrophy and mechanotransduction with more rapid and complete regeneration of the muscle fibres [37, 38]. The same principles hold true with pelvic floor muscle injury. When able to perform correct voluntary PFM contractions, it is recommended that three sets of 8–12 submaximal PFM contractions are performed at least 3 days per week [38]. Moreover, when able to perform the recommended PFMT, adding short, intensive contractions at the end of sustained contractions in at least one of the three sets, is advised. In a functional perspective, a gradual progression in starting positions during PFM training, from lying to sitting, standing, walking, jogging or jumping may be of benefit in daily activities.

Physical Therapy and Pelvic Floor Muscle Training in the Late Postpartum Phase

Only one study of women following OASIS examines AI in the late postpartum period as the primary outcome measure; four studies reported on AI as secondary outcome. At 3 months postpartum, Mahony and co-workers [48] randomized women to (1) weekly physical therapy-led PMFT and (2) biofeedback with or without additional electrical stimulation. After the 12-week intervention period, 85% of the participants reported reduced AI symptoms, and 26% were asymptomatic. Anal pressures during voluntary PFM contractions increased in both groups, and health-related QoL scores improved, with coping behaviour showing significant correlation to improvements in incontinence scores [48].

In their recent study, Sigurdadottir and co-workers [49] explored the effect of individual PFMT and gradual progression as instructed by a women's health physical therapist compared to a control group receiving no active follow up [49]. All participants reported UI at baseline 6–10 weeks postpartum. One in seven women reported co-existing AI and bowel-related bother. After the 12-week intervention, there was a significant reduction in UI prevalence and improvements in PFM strength and endurance in the PFMT group. No differences in AI or bowel-related bother were found at the 6 or 12-month follow-up. Long-term adherence to the PFMT protocol was poor, however, the difference in muscle strength and endurance was maintained at 12 months [49]. The study was powered on improvements in UI symptoms, and thus, the reported lack of effect on AI symptoms and bowel-related bother must be interpreted with caution. These results may indicate that symptomatic women with weak, but active PFM may improve PFM strength and endurance through structured PFMT [49]. However, it may be that women with PFDs and AI related to abnormal rectal compliance, stool consistency and spinal reflexes may need additional interventions in combination with PFMT in order to reduce their postpartum symptoms and bother [17].

In 2001, Meyer and co-workers randomized 107 women between 9 and 11 weeks postpartum to either (1) a control group receiving no active follow up or (2) 12 sessions of PFMT augmented by both biofeedback and electrical stimulation during a 6-week intervention period. One in three women reported UI during pregnancy, and there was a significant reduction in UI symptoms in the intervention group at 10 months postpartum. No participants reported AI during pregnancy, only five participants reported AI after delivery and after the intervention period [50].

In 1998, Wilson and Herbison randomized women experiencing UI at 3 months postpartum to either (1) a control group receiving standard care, or one of three intervention groups including either (2) daily PFMT (80–100 contractions at home), (3) PFMT and additional cone weight training (15 minutes twice daily) or (4) cone weight training alone. Drop out during the intervention period was high (85/230) [51]. At 1 year postpartum, there was a significant reduction in UI symptoms in all intervention groups; there were no differences in AI symptoms between control and intervention groups [51]. At 2–4 years postpartum, differences in UI symptoms were no longer significant, and only 8% in total reported regular PFMT [52, 53].

The same extensive PFMT protocol was applied in the study by Glazener and co-workers in 2001 [54]. Women reporting UI symptoms 3 months postpartum received either (1) standard care (control group) or (2) four home visits by a nurse clinician during the first year postpartum including reinforced education on pelvic floor anatomy and function, instructions on PFM contractions, bladder training, and a daily PFMT programme as described by Wilson and Herbison [51] (intervention group). The intervention included no assessment of PFM function or progression of PFMT. Nearly 80% of the intervention group had performed some PFMT, compared to just under half of standard care group women at 12 months; fewer women experienced AI in the intervention group at 12 months. The long-term follow up at 6, and 12 years postpartum show a general increase in prevalence of UI and AI in both groups. Interestingly, 40% of women who experienced UI and co-existing AI on inclusion reported symptoms persisting at the 12-year follow up. Long-term adherence to PFMT was poor and daily PFMT was reported by less than one in ten women at 12 years [10, 52]. Resolved UI was one of the main reasons for non-adherence to the PFMT protocol [54].

In 2020, Bergman and co-workers compared the effect of PFMT to perineorrhapy and distal posterior colporrhaphy among women with PFDs and poorly healed second-degree perineal tears at 6 months postpartum. Surgery was effective and superior to PFMT in relieving PFDs, however, the authors suggest that women with inadequate repairs of the pelvic floor muscles may be unable to perform correct PFMT, limiting the potential effect of PFMT in this population [55].

Patient Leaflet of Recommendations for Women 3–12 Months Postpartum

- Avoid straining the pelvic floor during defaecation [1]
- Manipulate stool consistency using loperamide or bulking agents if experiencing bowel evacuation problems [17]

Education

- Review how to perform correct submaximal contractions of the pelvic floor muscles
- Perform 3 × 8–12 contractions daily, progression as able [26–28, 47]
- Progress with exercises by increasing holding time, adding quick contractions, changing starting positions from lying, sitting, standing, walking to jogging and jumping [26–28, 38]
- Use the "The Knack" prior to activities such as sneezing, coughing and lifting [42]

18.1.1.4 Long-Term Postpartum Recovery– Beyond 12 Months after Delivery

Long-Term Management of a Muscular Injury – From 12 Months Postpartum

Application of the principles of LOVE and resistance training is advised also in the long-term management following OASIS.

Long-Term Postpartum Period – From 12 Months Postpartum

Two studies exploring the effect of PFMT in the late postpartum period have been published. One study included women reporting AI symptoms between 3 and 48 months after sustaining an OASI at delivery, [56] and another included symptomatic postpartum women with and without recognized OASI 12–18 months after delivery [57]. In 1999, Fynes et al. compared the effect of 12-weeks of either (1) vaginal biofeedback or (2) intra-anal biofeedback augmented with electrical stimulation. All women reported AI symptoms following OASI at baseline, and results that show that incontinence scores were reduced in both intervention groups. In the group combining PFMT, intra-anal biofeedback and electrical stimulation more women were asymptomatic after the 12-week intervention, and significant changes in pressures during active contraction and rest were seen in this group only. Not surprisingly, women with large persistent defects in the external anal sphincter had worse improvement rates compared to women with smaller or no persistent defects [56]. These results are similar to those in the study by Johannessen et al. [57] who found that women with higher anal defect scores at baseline reported more severe AI symptoms and had poorer outcomes following PFMT. The intervention consisted of a 6-month individualized PFMT programme with electrical stimulation as needed compared to a control group receiving no active intervention. Reductions in AI symptoms favoured the intervention group, and improvements were associated with performing PFMT regularly [57]. Recommendations for women beyond 12 months postpartum mirror the recommendations at 3–12 months.

Patient Leaflet of Recommendations to women beyond 12 months postpartum

- Avoid straining the pelvic floor during defaecation [1]
- Manipulate stool consistency using medical treatment such as loperamide or bulking agents if experiencing bowel evacuation problems [17]

Education

- Review how to perform correct submaximal contractions of the pelvic floor muscles
- Perform 3 × 8–12 contractions daily, progression as able [26–28, 47]
- Progress with exercises by increasing holding time, adding quick contractions, changing starting positions from lying, sitting, standing, walking to jogging and jumping [38]
- Use the "The Knack" prior to activities such as sneezing, coughing and lifting [42]

The Long-Term Effect of PFMT and Barriers to Physical Therapy

There is limited evidence of the long-term effect of PFMT beyond 12 months of follow up. This may be related to the changes in a women's life from first pregnancy to menopause and beyond. Furthermore, maintenance of strength in any muscle is not achieved unless the muscle is trained regularly over time [38]; thus expecting long-term effects without ensuring adequate adherence to a PFMT protocol is unrealistic [53], as adherence to PFMT over time has proved to be challenging. Similarly, long-term study effects are diluted when women in the control groups start performing PFMT after the intervention period. It has been suggested that if PFMT is to be effective long-term, behavioural as well as physical changes following optimal PFMT are required in order to improve adherence beyond the intervention period [53, 58]. Studies show that most pregnant women are interested in receiving advice on PFMT and are aware of the benefits of PFMT in reducing incontinence symptoms. Factors reported to influence women's willingness to participate in preventative PMFT during pregnancy include symptom severity, travel distance, day/evening hours and good general health. Not surprisingly, acceptance of cost related to PFMT is lower among women who are hesitant or not interested in PFMT during pregnancy when compared to women who are willing to participate in PFMT [59, 60]. Unfortunately, after birth, studies indicate that new mothers may be less attentive to the embarrassment and bother experienced with PFDs than if symptoms persist beyond the early postpartum period. With return to work and resumption of a more regular social life, PFD symptoms may be less tolerated and more likely to impair quality of life, [48] however, it may take years for women to seek medical advice. In a recent review, Salmon and co-workes [61] argue that the recommended implementation of adequate pre- and postpartum follow up, including research on effective management of PFDs, needs to be the responsibility of policymakers at societal level, rather than the individual responsibility of health care providers or the women experiencing PFDs during pregnancy or after delivery [61].

18.2 Conclusions

Though somewhat limited, studies including women with OASI that are powered to detect changes in AI show that PFMT may be effective in treating postpartum AI. The recommendations are such that physical therapy protocols follow the principles of PEACE and LOVE during the acute, subacute and late postpartum periods, in order to optimise tissue repair. Furthermore, PFMT has been found to be more effective among women who are able to actively contract their PFM, and when the principles of strength training are adhered to over a sufficient duration of time (minimum 8–12 weeks). Women with large, persistent defects of the anal sphincter muscles seem to have poorer outcomes with PFMT alone. This may also be applicable to women with large second-degree perineal tears, and potentially among women with occult OASI. In addition, some women experience a combination of different PFDs and symptoms such as constipation and bowel evacuation problems with or without perineal pain. Thus, it is suggested that combining PFMT with medical treatment such as laxatives, loperamide or bulking agents may be superior to PFMT alone. This may possibly be explained by the complex aetiology of AI in general, indicating that optimal physical therapy is based on the individual woman's symptoms, obstetric history and other medical complaints.

Take-Home Message
- Women with OASI should start pelvic floor muscle training as able after delivery, and be referred to physical therapy where available [26–28].
- Physical therapy protocols should follow the principles of PEACE and LOVE during the acute, subacute and late postpartum recovery in order to optimise tissue repair.
- Pelvic floor muscle training should follow the principles of strength training to in order to reduce symptoms of anal incontinence.

Appendix: MCQ

Mark each item TRUE or FALSE

Questions

1. In order to optimise tissue repair, what is the current acronym that physical therapy protocols should follow in the acute, subacute and late postpartum recovery after OASI?
   - (A) RICE; Rest, Ice, Compression, Elevation
   - (B) PRICE; Protection, Rest, Ice, Compression, Elevation
   - (C) POLICE; Protection, Optimal Loading, Ice, Compression, Elevation
   - (D) PEaCE & LOVE; Protection, Elevation, (avoid anti-inflammatory drugs), Compression, Education & Load, Optimism, Vascularisation, Exercise

2. In the acute phase, 0–3 weeks following OASI, how should physical therapists advise women on pain management?
   - (A) Encourage use of NSAID rectal suppositories, regular resting periods in comfortable and supported horizontal or side-lying positions, instruct gentle and pain-free activation of the pelvic floor muscles and ensure adequate relaxation between contractions
   - (B) Encourage women to take brisk walks in fresh air and heavy lifting
   - (C) Encourage 3 × 10 maximal pelvic floor contractions daily
   - (D) Educate women on the benefits of endurance training

3. Few studies have explored the effect of physical therapy and pelvic floor muscle training after OASI, however, recent systematic reviews suggest which of the following:
   - (A) Symptoms of pelvic floor disorders will get better as women grow older, apply watchful waiting
   - (B) All women are at risk of postpartum pelvic floor disorders and should be referred for weekly physical therapy the first year after delivery

   - (C) Targeted intervention including pelvic floor muscle training may be effective among women who have sustained an OASI or experience postpartum pelvic floor disorders
   - (D) Encouragement of low-fibre diets, fluid restriction and monthly pelvic floor muscle training

4. In the subacute postpartum recovery phase 3–12 weeks postpartum, what are the appropriate recommendations for physical therapists to give (select all that apply)?
   - (A) Encourage the patient to do correct, gentle to submaximal contractions of the pelvic floor muscles when pain-free
   - (B) Initiate a daily PFMT programme of 3 × 10 contractions as able
   - (C) Apply watchful waiting
   - (D) Avoid physical activity in general

5. In the late postpartum recovery phase 3–12 months postpartum, what are the appropriate recommendations for physical therapists to give (select all that apply)?
   - (A) Avoid all activities that increase the intra-abdominal pressure
   - (B) nitiate a daily pelvic floor muscle training programme of 3 × 10 contractions
   - (C) Progress pelvic floor muscle training by increasing the holding time, adding quick contractions, and or change starting positions
   - (D) Use the "Knack" prior to activities such as sneezing, coughing and lifting

Answers

1. In order to optimise tissue repair, what is the current acronym that physical therapy protocols should follow in the acute, subacute and late postpartum recovery after OASI?
   - (A) FALSE
   - (B) FALSE
   - (C) FALSE
   - (D) TRUE

2. In the acute phase, 0–3 weeks following OASI, how should physical therapists advise women on pain management?
   (A) TRUE
   (B) FALSE
   (C) FALSE
   (D) FALSE

3. Few studies have explored the effect of physical therapy and pelvic floor muscle training after OASI, however, recent systematic reviews suggest which of the following:
   (A) FALSE
   (B) FALSE
   (C) TRUE
   (D) FALSE

4. In the subacute postpartum recovery phase 3–12 weeks postpartum, what are the appropriate recommendations for physical therapists to give (select all that apply)?
   (A) TRUE
   (B) TRUE
   (C) FALSE
   (D) FALSE

5. In the late postpartum recovery phase 3–12 months postpartum, what are the appropriate recommendations for physical therapists to give (select all that apply)?
   (A) FALSE
   (B) TRUE
   (C) TRUE
   (D) TRUE

References

1. Roper JC, Amber N, Wan OYK, Sultan AH, Thakar R. Review of available national guidelines for obstetric anal sphincter injury. Int Urogynecol J. 2020;31(11):2247–59.
2. Haylen BT, de Ridder D, Freeman RM, Swift SE, Berghmans B, Lee J, et al. An international Urogynecological association (IUGA)/international continence society (ICS) joint report on the terminology for female pelvic floor dysfunction. Int Urogynecol J. 2010;21(1):5–26.
3. Sultan AH, Monga A, Lee J, Emmanuel A, Norton C, Santoro G, et al. An international Urogynecological association (IUGA)/international continence society (ICS) joint report on the terminology for female anorectal dysfunction. Int Urogynecol J. 2017;28(1):5–31.
4. Wan OYK, Taithongchai A, Veiga SI, Sultan AH, Thakar R. A one-stop perineal clinic: our eleven-year experience. Int Urogynecol J. 2020;31(11):2317–26.
5. Johannessen HH, Mørkved S, Stordahl A, Wibe A, Falk RS. Evolution and risk factors of anal incontinence during the first 6 years after first delivery: a prospective cohort study. BJOG. 2020;127(12):1499–506.
6. Jangö H, Langhoff-Roos J, Rosthøj S, Sakse A. Mode of delivery after obstetric anal sphincter injury and the risk of long-term anal incontinence. Am J Obstet Gynecol. 2016;214(6):733.e1–e13.
7. Evans E, Falivene C, Briffa K, Thompson J, Henry A. What is the total impact of an obstetric anal sphincter injury? An Australian retrospective study. Int Urogynecol J. 2020;31(3):557–66.
8. Johannessen HH, Mørkved S, Stordahl A, Sandvik L, Wibe A. Anal incontinence and quality of life in late pregnancy: a cross-sectional study. BJOG. 2014;121(8):978–87.
9. Dean N, Wilson D, Herbison P, Glazener C, Aung T, Macarthur C. Sexual function, delivery mode history, pelvic floor muscle exercises and incontinence: a cross-sectional study six years post-partum. Aust N Z J Obstet Gynaecol. 2008;48(3):302–11.
10. MacArthur C, Wilson D, Herbison P, Lancashire RJ, Hagen S, Toozs-Hobson P, et al. Faecal incontinence persisting after childbirth: a 12 year longitudinal study. BJOG. 2013;120(2):169–79.
11. Espuña-Pons M, Solans-Domènech M, Sánchez E. Double incontinence in a cohort of nulliparous pregnant women. Neurourol Urodyn. 2012;31(8):1236–41.
12. Fialkow MF, Melville JL, Lentz GM, Miller EA, Miller J, Fenner DE. The functional and psychosocial impact of fecal incontinence on women with urinary incontinence. Am J Obstet Gynecol. 2003;189(1):127–9.
13. Rockwood TH, Church JM, Fleshman JW, Kane RL, Mavrantonis C, Thorson AG, et al. Patient and surgeon ranking of the severity of symptoms associated with fecal incontinence: the fecal incontinence severity index. Dis Colon Rectum. 1999;42(12):1525–32.
14. Meyer I, Tang Y, Szychowski JM, Richter HE. The differential impact of Flatal incontinence in women with anal versus fecal incontinence. Female Pelvic Med Reconstr Surg. 2015;21(6):339–42.
15. Keighley MR, Perston Y, Bradshaw E, Hayes J, Keighley DM, Webb S. The social, psychological, emotional morbidity and adjustment techniques for women with anal incontinence following obstetric anal sphincter injury: use of a word picture to identify a hidden syndrome. BMC Pregnancy Childbirth. 2016;16(1):275.

16. ACOG. ACOG Practice Bulletin No. 210 summary: fecal incontinence. Obstet Gynecol. 2019;133(4):837–9.
17. Sjödahl J, Walter SA, Johansson E, Ingemansson A, Ryn AK, Hallböök O. Combination therapy with biofeedback, loperamide, and stool-bulking agents is effective for the treatment of fecal incontinence in women – a randomized controlled trial. Scand J Gastroenterol. 2015;50(8):965–74.
18. McKinney J, Keyser L, Clinton S, Pagliano C. ACOG Committee Opinion No. 736: Optimizing Postpartum Care. Obstet Gynecol. 2018;132(3):784–5.
19. ACOG. ACOG Practice Bulletin No. 198: prevention and Management of Obstetric Lacerations at vaginal delivery. Obstet Gynecol. 2018;132(3):e87–e102.
20. Arkel E, Torell K, Rydhög S, Rikner Å, Neymark Bachmeier H, Gutke A, et al. Effects of physiotherapy treatment for patients with obstetric anal sphincter rupture: a systematic review. Eur J Phys. 2017;19(2):90–6.
21. Wu YM, McInnes N, Leong Y. Pelvic floor muscle training versus watchful waiting and pelvic floor disorders in postpartum women: a systematic review and meta-analysis. Female Pelvic Med Reconstr Surg. 2018;24(2):142–9.
22. Dubois B, Esculier J-F. Soft-tissue injuries simply need PEACE and LOVE. Br J Sports Med. 2020;54(2):72.
23. Tan J-L, Ruane T, Sherburn M. The role of physiotherapy after obstetric anal sphincter injury: an overview of current clinical practice. Aust N Z Continence J. 2013;19(1):6–11.
24. East CE, Dorward EDF, Whale RE, Liu J. Local cooling for relieving pain from perineal trauma sustained during childbirth. Cochrane Database Syst Rev. 2020;(10)
25. Hedayati H, Parsons J, Crowther CA. Rectal analgesia for pain from perineal trauma following childbirth. Cochrane Database Syst Rev. 2003;(3)
26. POGP; Pelvic OaGP, UK. Fit for the Future. – essential advice and exercises following childbirth 2020 [Available from: https://thepogp.co.uk/_userfiles/pages/files/resources/211721pogpfffuture_signed_off.pdf.
27. POGP; Pelvic OaGP, UK. The Pelvic Floor Muscles – a Guide for Women 2020 [Available from: https://thepogp.co.uk/_userfiles/pages/files/resources/20818_pogp_pelvicfloor_for_women_signed_off_1.pdf.
28. Partnership HL. Your Body's Journey during pregnancy and after birth 2022 [Available from: https://myhealth.london.nhs.uk/maternity/pelvic-health-wellbeing.
29. Hendy AM, Spittle M, Kidgell DJ. Cross education and immobilisation: mechanisms and implications for injury rehabilitation. J Sci Med Sport. 2012;15(2):94–101.
30. Mahony R, Behan M, O'Herlihy C, O'Connell PR. Randomized, clinical trial of bowel confinement vs. laxative use after primary repair of a third-degree obstetric anal sphincter tear. Dis Colon Rectum. 2004;47(1):12–7.
31. Eogan M, Daly L, Behan M, O'Connell PR, O'Herlihy C. Randomised clinical trial of a laxative alone versus a laxative and a bulking agent after primary repair of obstetric anal sphincter injury. BJOG. 2007;114(6):736–40.
32. Mathé M, Valancogne G, Atallah A, Sciard C, Doret M, Gaucherand P, et al. Early pelvic floor muscle training after obstetrical anal sphincter injuries for the reduction of anal incontinence. Eur J Obstet Gynecol Reprod Biol. 2016;199:201–6.
33. Sleep J, Grant A. Pelvic floor exercises in postnatal care. Midwifery. 1987;3(4):158–64.
34. Peirce C, Murphy C, Fitzpatrick M, Cassidy M, Daly L, O'Connell PR, et al. Randomised controlled trial comparing early home biofeedback physiotherapy with pelvic floor exercises for the treatment of third-degree tears (EBAPT trial). BJOG. 2013;120(10):1240–7; discussion 6.
35. Turawa EB, Musekiwa A, Rohwer AC. Interventions for treating postpartum constipation. Cochrane Database Syst Rev. 2014;(9)
36. Turawa EB, Musekiwa A, Rohwer AC. Interventions for preventing postpartum constipation. Cochrane Database Syst Rev. 2020;(8)
37. Khan KM, Scott A. Mechanotherapy: how physical therapists' prescription of exercise promotes tissue repair. Br J Sports Med. 2009;43(4):247.
38. ACSM. American College of Sports Medicine position stand. Progression models in resistance training for healthy adults. Med Sci Sports Exerc. 2009;41(3):687–708.
39. Garber CE, Blissmer B, Deschenes MR, Franklin BA, Lamonte MJ, Lee IM, et al. American College of Sports Medicine position stand. Quantity and quality of exercise for developing and maintaining cardiorespiratory, musculoskeletal, and neuromotor fitness in apparently healthy adults: guidance for prescribing exercise. Med Sci Sports Exerc. 2011;43(7):1334–59.
40. Woodley SJ, Lawrenson P, Boyle R, Cody JD, Mørkved S, Kernohan A, et al. Pelvic floor muscle training for preventing and treating urinary and faecal incontinence in antenatal and postnatal women. Cochrane Database Syst Rev. 2020;5(5):Cd007471.
41. Westcott WL. Resistance training is medicine: effects of strength training on health. Curr Sports Med Rep. 2012;11(4):209–16.
42. Miller JM, Sampselle C, Ashton-Miller J, Hong GR, DeLancey JO. Clarification and confirmation of the knack maneuver: the effect of volitional pelvic floor muscle contraction to preempt expected stress incontinence. Int Urogynecol J Pelvic Floor Dysfunct. 2008;19(6):773–82.
43. Rockwood TH, Church JM, Fleshman JW, Kane RL, Mavrantonis C, Thorson AG, et al. Fecal incontinence quality of life scale: quality of life instrument for patients with fecal incontinence. Dis Colon Rectum. 2000;43(1):9–16; discussion −7

44. Oakley SH, Ghodsi VC, Crisp CC, Estanol MV, Westermann LB, Novicki KM, et al. Impact of pelvic floor physical therapy on quality of life and function after obstetric anal sphincter injury: a randomized controlled trial. Female Pelvic Med Reconstr Surg. 2016;22(4):205–13.

45. Von Bargen E, Haviland MJ, Chang OH, McKinney J, Hacker MR, Elkadry E. Evaluation of Postpartum Pelvic Floor Physical Therapy on Obstetrical Anal Sphincter Injury: A Randomized Controlled Trial. Female Pelvic Med Reconstr Surg. 2021;27(5):315–21. https://doi.org/10.1097/SPV.0000000000000849. PMID: 32282525; PMCID: PMC8924744.

46. Bø K. Physiotherapy management of urinary incontinence in females. J Physiother. 2020;66(3):147–54.

47. Mørkved S, Bø K. Effect of pelvic floor muscle training during pregnancy and after childbirth on prevention and treatment of urinary incontinence: a systematic review. Br J Sports Med. 2014;48(4):299–310.

48. Mahony RT, Malone PA, Nalty J, Behan M, O'Connell PR, O'Herlihy C. Randomized clinical trial of intra-anal electromyographic biofeedback physiotherapy with intra-anal electromyographic biofeedback augmented with electrical stimulation of the anal sphincter in the early treatment of post-partum fecal incontinence. Am J Obstet Gynecol. 2004;191(3):885–90.

49. Sigurdardottir T, Steingrimsdottir T, Geirsson RT, Halldorsson TI, Aspelund T, Bø K. Can postpartum pelvic floor muscle training reduce urinary and anal incontinence?: an assessor-blinded randomized controlled trial. Am J Obstet Gynecol. 2020;222(3):247.e1–8.

50. Meyer S, Hohlfeld P, Achtari C, De Grandi P. Pelvic floor education after vaginal delivery. Obstet Gynecol. 2001;97(5 Pt 1):673–7.

51. Wilson PD, Herbison GP. A randomized controlled trial of pelvic floor muscle exercises to treat postnatal urinary incontinence. Int Urogynecol J Pelvic Floor Dysfunct. 1998;9(5):257–64.

52. Glazener CM, Herbison GP, MacArthur C, Grant A, Wilson PD. Randomised controlled trial of conservative management of postnatal urinary and faecal incontinence: six year follow up. BMJ. 2005;330(7487):337.

53. Glazener CM, MacArthur C, Hagen S, Elders A, Lancashire R, Herbison GP, et al. Twelve-year follow-up of conservative management of postnatal urinary and faecal incontinence and prolapse outcomes: ran-domised controlled trial. BJOG. 2014;121(1):112–20.

54. Glazener CM, Herbison GP, Wilson PD, MacArthur C, Lang GD, Gee H, et al. Conservative manage-ment of persistent postnatal urinary and faecal incontinence: randomised controlled trial. BMJ. 2001;323(7313):593–6.

55. Bergman I, Westergren Söderberg M, Ek M. Perineorrhaphy compared with pelvic floor muscle therapy in women with late consequences of a poorly healed second-degree perineal tear: a randomized controlled trial. Obstet Gynecol. 2020;135(2):341–51.

56. Fynes MM, Marshall K, Cassidy M, Behan M, Walsh D, O'Connell PR, et al. A prospective, randomized study comparing the effect of augmented biofeed-back with sensory biofeedback alone on fecal incon-tinence after obstetric trauma. Dis Colon Rectum. 1999;42(6):753–8; discussion 8-61.

57. Johannessen HH, Wibe A, Stordahl A, Sandvik L, Mørkved S. Do pelvic floor muscle exercises reduce postpartum anal incontinence? A randomised con-trolled trial. BJOG. 2017;124(4):686–94.

58. Frawley HC, Dean SG, Slade SC, Hay-Smith EJC. Is pelvic-floor muscle training a physical therapy or a behavioral therapy? A call to name and report the physical, cognitive, and behavioral elements. Phys Ther. 2017;97(4):425–37.

59. Moossdorff-Steinhauser HF, Albers-Heitner P, Weemhoff M, Spaanderman ME, Nieman FH, Berghmans B. Factors influencing postpartum women's willingness to participate in a preventive pelvic floor muscle training program: a web-based survey. Eur J Obstet Gynecol Reprod Biol. 2015;195:182–7.

60. Hill AM, McPhail SM, Wilson JM, Berlach RG. Pregnant women's awareness, knowledge and beliefs about pelvic floor muscles: a cross-sectional survey. Int Urogynecol J. 2017;28(10):1557–65.

61. Salmon VE, Hay-Smith EJC, Jarvie R, Dean S, Terry R, Frawley H, et al. Implementing pelvic floor muscle training in women's childbearing years: a critical interpretive synthesis of individual, pro-fessional, and service issues. Neurourol Urodyn. 2020;39(2):863–70.

Non-surgical Management of Anal Incontinence

19

Wendy Ness

Overview
Test your learning and check your understanding of this book's contents: use the "Springer Nature Flashcards" app to access questions using ▶ https://sn.pub/wqrf89. To use the app, please follow the instructions in Chap. 1.

Learning Objectives
- Understand the prevalence and different types of anal incontinence
- Understand how childbirth can affect anal continence
- Examine what lifestyle aspects can affect anal continence
- Describe the importance of a thorough assessment and establishing a differential diagnosis
- Describe how patient education can help reduce anxiety and increase understanding
- Understand what conservative measures can be offered to help restore anal continence
- Detail coping mechanisms that give a better quality of life despite having symptoms of anal incontinence

19.1 Introduction

Anal incontinence (AI) is a very taboo subject which women find very difficult to discuss; they often don't seek help for many months or years. This results in a dramatic reduction in a person's quality of life (QOL) which, in turn, restricts their activities.

The International Urogynecological Association (IUGA) and International Continence Society (ICS) Terminology document [1] provides the following definitions of anorectal incontinence symptoms:

- Anal incontinence: Complaint of involuntary loss of faeces or flatus.
- Fecal incontinence: Complaint of involuntary loss of faeces.
  (a) Solid
  (b) Liquid
- Flatus Incontinence: Complaint of involuntary loss of flatus (gas).
- Double incontinence: Complaint of both anal incontinence and urinary incontinence.
- Coital faecal (flatal) incontinence: Faecal (flatal) incontinence occurring with vaginal intercourse.
- Passive faecal leakage: Involuntary soiling of liquid or solid stool without sensation or warning or difficulty wiping clean.
- Overflow fecal incontinence: Seepage of stool due to faecal impaction.

W. Ness (✉)
Croydon University Hospital, Croydon, UK
e-mail: w.ness@nhs.net

© The Author(s), under exclusive license to Springer Nature Switzerland AG 2024
A. H. Sultan et al. (eds.), *Pelvic Floor, Perineal, and Anal Sphincter Trauma During Childbirth*,
https://doi.org/10.1007/978-3-031-43095-4_19

19.2 Prevalence of Anal Incontinence

The prevalence of AI in adults is 7% – 15% [2], and is dependent on the definition used. In fact, these numbers may underestimate the actual prevalence. Women often fail to discuss these issues and health care providers often neglect to ask about this embarrassing condition [3].Women tend to be more willing to report symptoms than men, and more studies are carried out on the female population due to its association with childbirth. AI in care homes is estimated to range from 10% to 50% [2] and AI (as well as urinary incontinence) is often the reason for going into care homes. However, the risk of AI is independently associated with older age, diabetes, loose stools and three or more bowel movements per day [4]. In 2009, it was suggested by Buckley and Lapitan [5] that there were 6.5 million adults with bowel control problems; this number is likely higher now, as more people present and seek care for the problem. Box 19.1 shows the main causes and contributing factors of AI.

Box 19.1 Main Causes and Contributing Factors of Anal Incontinence [6–9]

- Obstetric injury (most common)
- Increasing age
- Sphincter disruption from anal surgery such as haemorrhoidectomy, fistula repair, sphincterotomy
- Trauma to the anal area
- Congenital defect
- Idiopathic degeneration
- Neurological conditions such as diabetes, Parkinson's or multiple sclerosis
- Severe cognitive impairment
- Loose stools or diarrhoea from any cause (for example, inflammatory bowel disease)
- Spinal cord injury
- Faecal impaction
- Posterior wall prolapse or rectal prolapse
- Diarrhoea secondary to chronic pancreatitis, irritable bowel syndrome, and infection

---

19.3 Impact of Anal Incontinence on Women

It is well-known that women who suffer from AI have significantly decreased quality of life [10–12] as the condition is very embarrassing and often prevents women from leaving their homes. When they do go out, many do not eat anything beforehand and will take an antidiarrheal tablet before stepping outside the door. Many have had bowel accidents while in the company of others, which has been devastating for them, and the possibility of this happening again affects them physically, psychologically and socially [13]. AI is also associated with hygiene problems, as there are often no facilities to clean up after having a bowel accident. Similarly, the condition restricts employment, educational and/or leisure opportunities.

Anal incontinence is more prevalent among individuals with inflammatory bowel disease, coeliac disease, irritable bowel syndrome, and diabetes [14], as often these patients have a very loose stool which they are unable to control. In a qualitative study of the impact of Inflammatory Bowel Disease (IBD) on quality of life, Dibley and Norton [15] found that 60% avoid going away from home, 50% feel odd or different from others, 45% avoid public transport and 50% report avoiding sexual activity due to fear of incontinence. Although this study focused on patients with IBD, the same has been shown in women who have AI. For example, Cichowski et al [16] found that sexually active women with FI had poorer sexual function than those without FI. Similarly, another cross-sectional study found that while women with FI are at high risk for sexual dysfunction, the presence of FI did not impair a woman's ability to engage in sexual activity [17].

19.4 Lifestyle Aspects that Can Affect Anal Incontinence

19.4.1 Body Mass Index (BMI)

Higher BMI has been identified as a significant risk factor for the development of AI, and it has been reported that AI is 50% more prevalent in the obese population compared to those of a normal weight [18]. Observational studies suggest an association between FI and being overweight or obese [2]. Generally, people that are obese have a poorer diet which may be high in fats and carbohydrates and low in dietary fibre; this can have an effect on increasing the motility of the colon, making the stool looser. As noted above, looser stool is more difficult to control; this may be further exacerbated from a functional standpoint if weight impedes the timeliness of reaching the bathroom.

19.4.2 Smoking

Nicotine is known to be a stimulant drug which causes a surge in the release of adrenaline immediately after inhalation, therefore causing an increased contraction of the colonic and rectal muscles in the form of peristalsis leading to an increased desire to empty bowels [19].

19.4.3 Physical Exercise

Often women will complain that when they are out running, they can have bowel accidents with a very loose stool or have passive AI which makes the anal area sore. It is documented that runners, especially women, experience gastrointestinal symptoms whilst running which include diarrhoea (27%), increased urge to stool, gas, flatulence, and abdominal pain [20]. It has also been shown that high levels of physical activity may be associated with an increased risk of FI in younger athletic women [2].

Excessive exercise may also be a factor in rectal prolapse, which is also associated with AI. For example, this is seen in young women with anorexia nervosa who combine excessive exercise with extreme nutritional impairment, presumably thus compromising tissue quality. Women whose jobs involve a lot of heavy lifting are more likely to need vaginal prolapse surgery than the general population [21], but it is not known if this is also true of AI. However, many women that have rectal prolapse also have a problem with AI.

19.4.4 Assessment

To establish the aetiology of AI, a detailed initial assessment and a structured approach to management is needed, starting with addressing reversible factors [22] as noted in Box 19.2.

Box 19.2 Conditions Coexisting with AI [22]
- Impaction
- Treatable causes of diarrhoea – enteritis (viral, bacterial, parasitic)
- Warning signs of lower gastrointestinal cancer
- Rectal prolapse
- Anorectal injury – trauma, child birth or surgical intervention
- Acute disc prolapse – cauda equina syndrome

Empathetic and knowledgeable nurses in many healthcare settings can make a valuable and positive difference to patients with a comprehensive assessment and by implementing a range of strategies [23]. There are many aspects to consider when assessing a patient such as obstetric, medical and surgical history; more specific bowel related symptoms of AI and their duration also need to be elucidated. (See Box 19.3).

Box 19.3 Condition-specific Assessment Criteria [22]
- Relevant medical, surgical, neurological and obstetric history
- Psychological history including any history of abuse [24]
- Body mass index and smoking status
- Cognitive assessment – essential when assessing the older person so that an appropriate treatment or management plan can be devised [25]
- Duration of symptoms
- General and anorectal examination – must include visualisation of the anal

area for any abnormalities, digital rectal examination (DRE) which can establish strength of the internal anal sphincter (IAS) and external anal sphincter (EAS) and condition of skin

- Medication – oral and rectal, prescribed, self-administered, vitamins, herbal, creams and alternative
- Symptoms – type of incontinence (passive, urge), incomplete emptying, flatus control, abdominal pain, anal irritation, passing blood or mucus
- Evacuation difficulties
- Food diary – to establish a baseline and any triggers
- Stool diary – frequency, stool consistency, when incontinence occurs
- Mobility and toilet access – functional problem may be causing the incontinence
- Triggers
- Coping strategies

Diet and eating pattern changes should be included in the assessments for AI when developing a plan of care [26], as these can often result in a change of stool consistency, which could be misinterpreted as a change in bowel habit, one of the "red flag symptoms" of bowel cancer. Others symptoms to consider are blood mixed in with stool, increase in mucus and flatus, unintentional weight loss, excessive fatigue, anaemia and family history (especially first-degree relatives).

Apart from stool and food diaries, it is important to collect patient reported outcomes. Valuable tools are bowel and quality of life questionnaires. For example, the Faecal Incontinence Quality of Life Scale (FIQL) [27], Modified Manchester Health Questionnaire [28], the Bowel version of the International Consultation on Incontinence questionnaire (ICIQ-B) [29] and the St Mark's symptom severity score can be used [30].

19.5 Conservative Treatments

Once a thorough assessment has been carried out and a differential diagnosis has been reached, a treatment plan can be established to best treat the individual woman, focusing on what is most bothersome and how this can be improved.

19.6 Education and Empowerment

Often when patients are seen for the first time by a specialist nurse for AI, they have misconceptions about what is causing the problem. This may be secondary to scouring the internet. However, the internet may also be helpful to patients with AI. For example, in a study carried out by Leo et al [31], they concluded that the internet appears to have potential to be a useful platform for patients to learn about faecal incontinence and share information.

On occasion, patients may have had a colonoscopy to rule out cancer or inflammatory bowel disease, yet nobody has explained to them that their problem does not have an organic cause but is instead a functional one. Therefore, before starting conservative treatment, it is important to explain (with the aid of pictures, videos and other visual aids) results of investigations carried out, how the bowel and anal sphincters work and what the aim of the treatment is. This is often to manage the problem better rather than to find a cure.

19.7 Biofeedback

The theoretical basis for biofeedback is 'learning through reinforcement' or 'operant conditioning' techniques [32]. It is classed as a re-education tool, in which information concerning a normally subconscious physiological function is relayed to patients and they are actively involved in learning to change this function [33]. Biofeedback is about building a relationship of trust and care with the patient so they feel safe, enabling them to talk about their problem. It covers many aspects of conservative treatment such as education, dietary changes, pelvic floor exercise, bowel emptying techniques, medications, the use of products and low or high-volume irrigation. Biofeedback treatment programmes have been shown to not only improve faecal incontinence, but also quality of life, anxiety and depression [34]. The aim of biofeedback therapy is for the patient to improve and take control of their bowel function.

19.8 Diet and Fluids

Modification of diet and fluid consumption can help firm up stool consistency, which will, in turn, allow for improved anal continence. Therefore, using a food and fluid diary in patients' assessments can be invaluable. Similarly, simply asking the patient if they have noticed any triggers in their diet that make the problem worse can be useful.

Caffeine is known to stimulate colonic motility [35] and can increase urgency in susceptible individuals. This can be useful to enable evacuation at a chosen time, such as before leaving the house in the morning. Some patients find that restricting the amount or timing of caffeine is useful [36]. Coffee, tea and colas, especially when combined with artificial sweeteners such as sorbitol (which can cause osmotic diarrhoea), worsen symptoms. Excessive alcohol can also lead to loose stool.

Some foods seem to promote flatus production. Common culprits are onions, garlic, fatty and spicy food, brassicas and other green vegetables, beans and pulses. Although there is no way to stop flatus production completely, avoiding certain foods may help. Decreasing flatal production by definition decreases flatal incontinence.

Box 19.4 instructs patients on which foods can affect the gut motility and gives recommendations as to what to avoid or increase to optimize stool consistency.

Box 19.4 Foods and Fluids Which May Affect Gut Motility [13, 22]

- Reduce or stop coffee, as this can make the stool looser
- Have a breakfast rich in oats to add bulk to the stool
- Consume a probiotic drink or bio yogurt daily to increase the good bacteria in the bowel
- Reduce fibre because too much fibre in the diet can make the stool looser
- Avoid high fibre foods such as pears, nuts, mushrooms, onions, bran and green vegetables
- Avoid onions, garlic, mushrooms and green vegetables as these not only increase the transit time of the stool but increase flatulence
- Avoid liquorice, chocolate and dried fruit, as these act like a laxative
- Avoid spicy or foods with monosodium glutamate, as these may make the stool looser
- Consider increasing jelly, apple sauce, tapioca, white bread, pasta and rice, as they may help thicken the stool
- Stop diet fizzy drinks and avoid sugar-free products, as sorbitol can cause diarrhoea and flatulence
- Avoid chocolate, fatty foods such as bacon and gravy, dairy products such as milk, ice cream, and cheese, as these are associated with looser stools
- Determine if you may have a food intolerance such as wheat and lactose, as these can cause looser stools
- When modifying the diet, change one item at a time and beware of other food restrictions, especially if you have diabetes
- Consider also increasing dietary fibre, as it might lessen AI by increasing rectal distension, increasing sensory awareness of the need to defaecate, promoting more
- Complete elimination of faeces and leaving less in the rectum to leak, or normalising the consistency and reducing the liquidity of faeces

If simple dietary modifications haven't helped, referral to a dietician to look at following a low Fermentable Oligosaccharides Disaccharides Monosaccharides Polyols (FODMAP) diet could be initiated. This diet has been shown to reduce AI symptoms in 64% of patients [2]. As this is a very specialised and restrictive diet the patient needs to be monitored by a dietician.

19.9   Pelvic Floor Muscle Training

Pelvic floor muscle training (PFMT) should be recommended as an early intervention in the treatment of AI, based on low cost and low morbidity [2]. PFMT is commonly recommended during pregnancy and after birth for both prevention and treatment of incontinence, both urinary and faecal [37].

Pelvic floor exercises (PFE) have been shown to be effective in the treatment of AI, and the majority of women are able to carry these out with little effort if taught by a competent healthcare practitioner (HCP). These can be taught during a rectal examination and using biofeedback can inform the patient if what they are doing is correct. It is also possible during anal manometry using the THD Anopress device (Fig. 19.1) to, at the same time, use this as a biofeedback tool.

How pelvic floor exercises are taught differs with the HCP. When teaching these, visual aids are useful. Also it is important to ensure a leaflet is given to take away as a reminder of how to do the exercises at home. It is also imperative to explain the aim of the exercises, the importance of doing them 3–5 times every day, and to set expectations to keep patients motivated.

Box 19.5 Sample of PFMT patient leaflet

Box 19.5 Pelvic Floor Exercises

This leaflet explains how to carry out the pelvic floor exercises that have previously been explained to you by a nurse specialist

1. Sit down in a comfortable but supportive chair and relax for a few moments.
2. Now imagine that you are going to pass wind and it is not convenient. Squeeze your anal muscles to stop it and then relax it.
3. There are two types of exercises that you will need to carry out.
4. *Type one* = squeeze your anal/vaginal muscle as hard as you can and then relax it. This is called a fast contraction.
5. *Type two* = squeeze your anal/vaginal muscle and hold the squeeze for a couple of seconds (number shown below) and then relax. This is called a slow contraction. It is important that you relax for the same amount of time as you squeeze.
6. It is important that you carry out these exercises correctly and try to keep to the amount described below.
7. You may find that when you start doing these exercises your anal/vaginal muscle will ache. This is because you are using a muscle you don't often use.
8. Your exercises can be done sitting in a supportive chair, lying down or standing. If you do them standing it may help if you turn your feet in (toes together and heels apart)- unless you have had a hip replacement- as this helps to reduce you using your buttocks or thighs
9. Spread the number of times you do these (as suggested below) throughout the day.

Ways to help you remember; —

- Do them with something you do every day, meals etc.
- Put small stickers around the home or office so that every time you see one you will think "exercises"
- Do them whilst sitting on the bus, sitting at traffic lights, whilst brushing your teeth or after you have emptied your bladder (do not stop and start during passing urine as this is not good for your bladder)
- If you forget to do the anal/vaginal exercises do not try to do them all at the end of the day as the anal muscle will be tired. Instead, just do one set and start a fresh the following day.
- Download the NHS Squeezy App

Your nurse specialist will go over these exercises and make sure you are doing them correctly. If you want to check this when at home, this can be done by sitting on the toilet or in the bath; merely put your finger on your back passage or in the vagina. When you squeeze, you should feel tightening and upward motion. Your buttock and thigh muscles should hardly move.

The tailored programme of exercises exists especially for you

Each session is made up of the two types of exercises as described above

Number of sessions to be spread throughout the day: 3–5

Number of fast contractions (type one): 10. Be sure you feel the muscle relax between each squeeze as taught.

Number of slow contractions (type two): 5. Squeeze for ___ seconds, then relax

For ___ seconds.

19.10 Defaecatory Dynamics

Showing the patient how to empty their bowel correctly can help in reducing AI. This is especially useful in post defecatory passive AI, as this is mainly caused by a weak internal sphincter and subsequent incomplete and incorrect emptying of the rectum. This is often made worse by a trapping rectocele where stool gets stuck. This necessitates certain manoeuvres to empty, such as digitating vaginally or supporting the perineum between the anus and vagina.

Figure 19.2 illustrates the best position to promote emptying and includes having knees higher than hips, leaning forward, and putting elbows on knees, bulging out the abdomen and straightening the spine.

This position straightens the anorectal junction and improves rectal emptying.

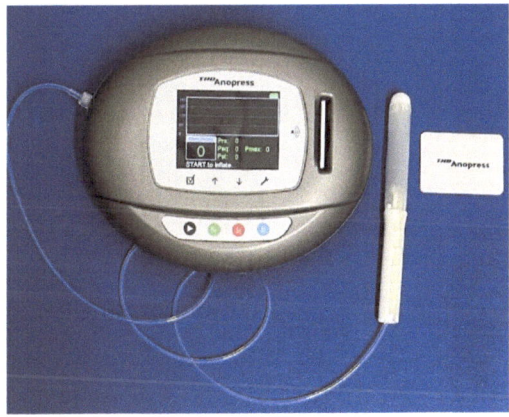

Fig. 19.1 THD Anopress Device

Fig. 19.2 Correct position for bowel emptying. (Reproduced and distributed with the kind permission of the co-authors, including Wendy Ness, Colorectal Nurse Specialist. Produced as a service to the medical profession by Norgine Ltd. ©2017 Norgine group of companies.)

Correct position for opening your bowels

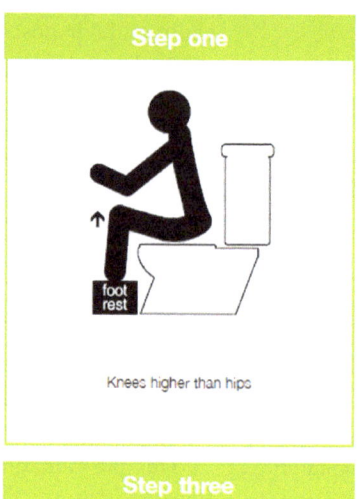

Step one

Knees higher than hips

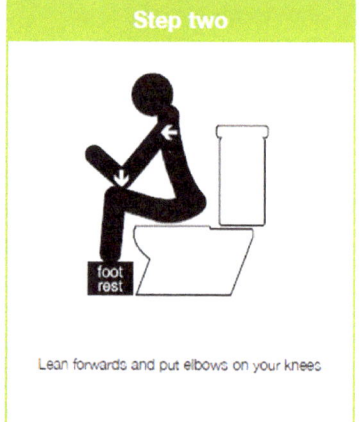

Step two

Lean forwards and put elbows on your knees

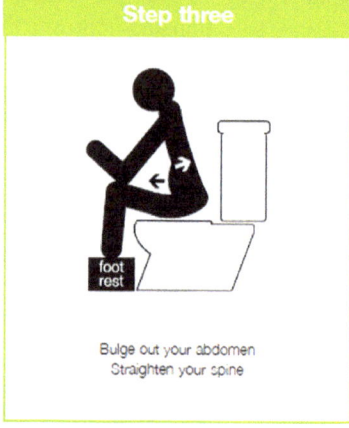

Step three

Bulge out your abdomen
Straighten your spine

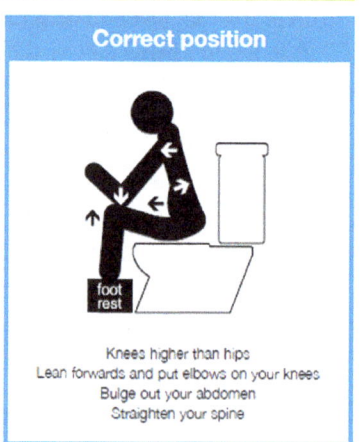

Correct position

Knees higher than hips
Lean forwards and put elbows on your knees
Bulge out your abdomen
Straighten your spine

19.11 Femmeze

This is a device that was invented by Sharon Eustace, a Nurse Consultant for continence Cornwall Foundation NHS Trust. The FEMMEZE® Vagina Trainer is a single user medical device that removes the need to use fingers to splint and assists women to safely, simply and easily realign the rectum for passing stool. The device can be purchased online (see Fig. 19.3).

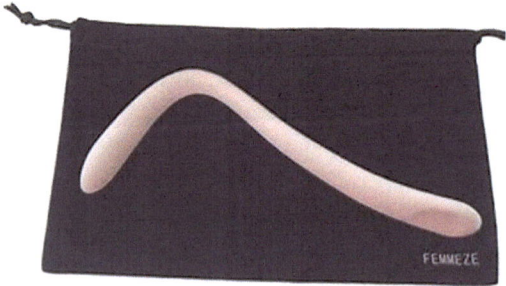

Fig. 19.3 Femmeze

19.12 Suppositories

Suppositories have a mild stimulant affect when they come in contact with the rectal mucosa, which then encourages rectal emptying. If the rectum is empty, then the passive AI is less likely to happen. The patient is advised to use these following defecation to empty the rectum, rather than using before defecation as would be advised for constipation. The most commonly used suppository is glycerine but a stronger stimulant suppository such as Bisacodyl can also be used.

19.13 Low Volume Irrigation

Some women require more than suppositories to empty the rectum, especially if they have a rectocele. Low volume irrigation can be used easily to administer water into the rectum and normally works within 5 minutes. There are many different products on the market, and the one used is based on patient preference (Fig. 19.4). An audit carried out on the use of the Qufora mini-irrigation sys-

tem in 50 patients (48 female, 2 male) with passive faecal incontinence and/or evacuation problems showed that 70% who irrigated found it comfortable and 74% rated the system as good or acceptable. Of these, two-thirds believed symptoms were improved and would wish to continue using the system [38].

19.14 High Volume Irrigation

The rationale for high volume trans-anal irrigation is that by emptying the descending colon, there is a reduction in the likelihood of incontinence. It also allows for increased control of timing and frequency of defaecation [39]. If bowel continence cannot be achieved by medication, changes to diet and other conservative measures, long-term management strategies such as trans anal irrigation should be considered [40]. The patient is advised to use it daily to alternate days. There are many different devices available, and the clinician needs to discuss with the patient ensuring patient choice [40] (Fig. 19.5).

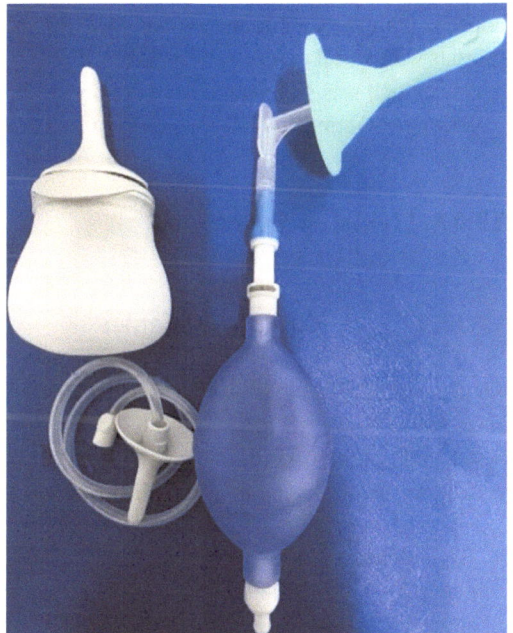

Fig. 19.4 Two different types of low volume irrigation

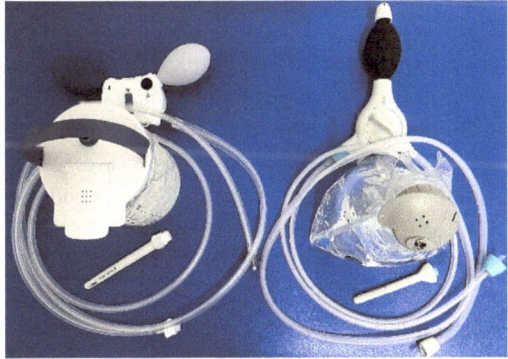

Fig. 19.5 Two different types of high volume trans anal irrigation

19.15 Medication Management

A large number of prescribed and over the counter medications can have an effect on the bowel. Therefore, it is important as part of the patient's assessment that their current medications are reviewed. For example, one of the most common medications used in diabetic patients is metformin, which causes very loose stools.

If AI is secondary to soft or loose stool and modifying the diet has not helped, using medication to firm or bulk the stool is recommended. For example, loperamide liquid can be easily titrated. A small amount can be very effective; 0.5 mg – 1 mg (1/2 – 1tsp) a day is often enough [22]. Other useful medications include antispasmodics (to reduce the pressure in the bowel and reduce fecal urgency), acidophilus (for bowel health to introduce good bacteria), and bulk forming agents (to give more bulk to a loose stool).

19.16 Posterior Tibial Nerve Stimulation

If other forms of conservative treatment have not helped, percutaneous tibial nerve stimulation (PTNS) could be considered. PTNS is a minimally invasive, low risk neuromodulation procedure carried out in a nurse or physiotherapy led outpatient service.

The aim of PTNS is to achieve a neuromodulator effect similar to that of sacral nerve stimulation through a less invasive route, but its exact mechanism of action is unclear. A fine gauge needle is inserted percutaneously, just above and medial to the ankle, next to the posterior tibial nerve, and a surface electrode is placed near the arch of the foot. The needle and electrode are connected to a low-voltage stimulator (Fig. 19.6). Stimulation of the posterior tibial nerve produces a motor (plantar flexion or fanning of the toes) and/or sensory (tingling in the ankle, foot or toes) response [41]. Initial treatment consists of 12 sessions lasting 30 minutes each, either over a 6 (twice a week) or 12 (once a week) week period. Following this one off "top up" sessions are offered every 6–8 weeks to maintain the efficacy.

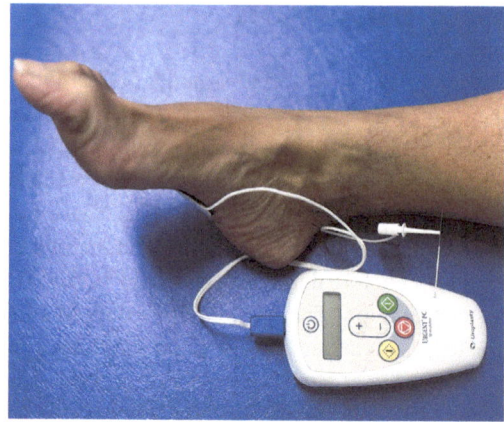

Fig. 19.6 Placement of PTNS needle

However, in a recent randomised control trial that compared PTNS to sham stimulation in women with FI concluded that although symptom reduction after 12 weeks of PTNS met a threshold of clinical importance, it did not differ from sham stimulation [42]. Therefore, it did not support the use of PTNS for the treatment of FI in women. However, Panel et al [43] showed that PTNS in conjunction with regular counselling from a specialist practitioner in pelvic floor disorders can improve both the symptoms and quality of life of patients with faecal urgency and mild faecal incontinence which was maintained for up to 5 years.

Sacral nerve stimulation is described in Chap. 20.

19.17 Living with Anal Incontinence

19.17.1   Coping Strategies

As it is not always possible to cure AI, individuals need to be taught coping strategies to help better manage their AI [8].

Coping strategies include the following:

- Best cleaning techniques – do not use dry paper to wipe; instead use a moist cloth or shower the area or use a bidet
- Perineal skin care – clean, moisturise and protect the individual's skin therefore avoiding skin breakdown

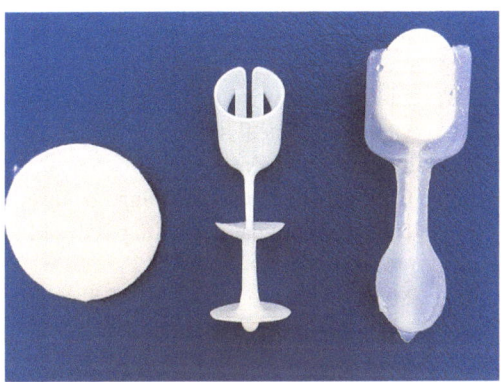

Fig. 19.7 Cotton wool pad, and inserts (Renew and Navina) from left to right

Use of cotton wool pads or inserts (Fig. 19.7) – mainly used for patients with passive FI to stop the leakage
- Pad usage – most pads are designed for urinary incontinence rather than FI so it is important that the pad fits correctly
- Spare skincare kits – these could contain spare underclothes, moisture cloths, disposable bag etc. and can be used when the individual is out and has a bowel accident
- Strategies for traveling – Imodium could be taken before going on a long journey
- RADAR key access to locked toilets and toilet "urgent" cards

19.18 Conclusions

Anal incontinence is an embarrassing and debilitating condition for many women following sphincter trauma. It affects them physically, psychologically, sexually and socially. AI impacts quality of life by preventing women from going out, toilet mapping when they do, becoming isolated due to fear of having a bowel accident in public, and becoming depressed. A thorough assessment to establish the aetiology of AI needs to be carried out. Following this, once a differential diagnosis has been established, an individual treatment plan should be implemented, focusing on improving symptoms and quality of

life. It is hoped that with more awareness of the problem being publicised in social media, television programs, newspaper and magazine articles, more women will come forward and seek help. Less will suffer in silence.

Take Home Messages

- Anal incontinence is a devastating and embarrassing problem for many women following childbirth.
- AI is often overlooked by the healthcare professionals who don't ask the right questions following childbirth.
- Under reporting of AI by women due to embarrassment and hiding of this problem for many years is common.
- Performing an assessment is critical in being able to establish an individualised plan of care.
- There is an imperative need for the healthcare professional to establish a relationship of trust and care with the patient so they feel safe, enabling them to talk about their problem.
- That the aim of conservative treatment is to improve the woman's symptoms and thereby improving her quality of life.

Appendix: MCQ

Questions

1. Regarding definitions of bowel incontinence which of the following statements is false?
   (A) Anal incontinence (AI) is the involuntary loss of flatus and faeces and/or mucus.
   (B) Faecal incontinence (FI) is the involuntary loss of faeces.
   (C) Flatus (or Flatal) incontinence is the involuntary loss of rectal gas or flatus.
   (D) Faecal incontinence (FI) is the voluntary loss of faeces
   (E) Mucus incontinence is the involuntary loss of mucus only (without faeces)

2. Regarding the prevalence of AI which of the following statements is false?
   (A) The prevalence of AI in adults is 7% – 15%
   (B) Men tend to be more willing to report AI symptoms than women
   (C) AI in care homes is estimated to range from 10% to 50%
   (D) AI is independently associated with older age, diabetes, loose stools
   (E) More studies on AI are carried out on the female population

3. Which of the following is a condition that does not commonly coexist with AI?
   (A) Impaction
   (B) Treatable causes of diarrhoea – enteritis (viral, bacterial, parasitic)
   (C) Warning signs of lower gastrointestinal cancer
   (D) Vaginal prolapse
   (E) Anorectal injury –trauma, child birth or surgical intervention

4. Which of the following recommendations is false?
   (A) Consuming a probiotic drink or bio yogurt daily to increase the bad bacteria in the bowel is helpful
   (B) Reducing fibre in the diet is helpful, as too much fibre in the diet can make the stool looser
   (C) Avoiding high fibre foods such as pears, nuts, mushrooms, onions, bran and green vegetables can decrease AI
   (D) Avoiding onions, garlic, mushrooms and green vegetables is beneficial, as these not only increase the transit time of the stool but also increase flatulence
   (E) Avoiding liquorice, chocolate and dried fruit can be helpful, as these foods act like a laxative

5. Regarding coping strategies for AI, which of the following statements is false?
   (A) Best cleaning techniques include constantly wiping with dry paper and avoid-ing the use of a moist cloth or shower to clean the area.
   (B) Clean, moisturise and protect the individual's perineal skin, as the aim is to avoid skin breakdown.
   (C) Cotton wool pads, anal plugs or inserts can be used in patients with passive FI to stop the leakage.
   (D) Most pads are designed for urinary incontinence rather than FI, so it is important that the pad fits correctly.
   (E) Spare skincare kits could contain spare underclothes, moisture cloths, disposable bag etc and can be used when the individual is out and has a bowel accident.

Answers

1. Regarding definitions of bowel incontinence which of the following statements is false?
   (A) FALSE
   (B) FALSE
   (C) FALSE
   (D) TRUE
   (E) FALSE

2. Regarding the prevalence of AI which of the following statements is false?
   (A) FALSE
   (B) TRUE
   (C) FALSE
   (D) FALSE
   (E) FALSE

3. Which of the following is a condition that does not commonly coexist with AI?
   (A) FALSE
   (B) FALSE
   (C) FALSE
   (D) TRUE
   (E) FALSE

4. Which of the following recommendations is false?
   (A) TRUE

(B) FALSE
(C) FALSE
(D) FALSE
(E) FALSE

5. Regarding coping strategies for AI, which of the following statements is false?
(A) TRUE
(B) FALSE
(C) FALSE
(D) FALSE
(E) FALSE

References

1. Sultan AH, Monga A, Lee J, Emmanuel A, Norton C, Santoro G, Hull T, Berghmans B, Brody S, Haylen BT. An international Urogynecological association (IUGA)/international continence society (ICS) joint report on the terminology for female anorectal dysfunction. Int Urogynecol J. 2017;28(1):5–31. https://doi.org/10.1007/s00192-016-3140-3. Epub 2016 Oct 24.
2. Bliss DJ. Assessment and conservative management of faecal incontinence and quality of life in adults. In: Cardozo L, Rovner E, Wagg A, Wein A, Abrams P, editors. Incontinence, 7th; 2023. p. 1577–674.
3. Bharucha AE, Dunivan G, Goode PS. Epidemiology, pathophysiology, and classification of faecal incontinence: state of the science summary for the National Institute of Diabetes and Digestive and Kidney Diseases (NIDDK) workshop. Am J Gastroenterol. 2015;110:127–36.
4. Ditah I, Devaki P, Luma H, Ditah C, Njei B, Jaiyeoba C, et al. Prevalence, trends, and risk factors for fecal incontinence in United States adults, 2005–2010. Clin Gastroenterol Hepatol. 2014;12:636–43.e1–2.
5. Buckley BS, Lapitan MCM. Prevalence of urinary and faecal incontinence and nocturnal enuresis and attitudes to treatment and help-seeking amongst a community-based representative sample of adults in the United Kingdom. Int J Clin Pract. 2009;63(4):568–73.
6. Rao KA, Yazaki E, Evans DF, Carbon R. Objective evaluation of small bowel and colonic transit time using pH telemetry in athletes with gastrointestinal symptoms. Br J Sports Med. 2004;38(4):482–7.
7. Norton C, Chelvanayagam S. Bowel problems and coping strategies in people with multiple sclerosis. Br J Nurs. 2010;19(4):220, 221–226.
8. Ness W. Faecal incontinence: causes, assessment and management. Nurs Stand. 2012;26(42):52–60.
9. National Institute for Health and Clinical Excellence. Faecal incontinence in adults Quality standard guidance QS54; 2014.
10. Brown HW, Dyer KY, Rogers RG. Management of fecal incontinence. Obstet Gynecol. 2020;136(4):811–22.
11. Meyer I, Richter HE. Impact of fecal incontinence and its treatment on quality of life in women. Womens Health (Lond). 2015;11(2):225–38.
12. Markland AD, Greer WJ, Vogt A, Redden DT, Goode PS, Burgio KL, Richter HE. Factors impacting quality of life in women with fecal incontinence. Dis Colon Rectum. 2010;53(8):1148–54.
13. Ness W. Managing faecal incontinence. Br J Nurs. 2018;27(7):378–81.
14. Menees S, Almario C, Spiegel B, Chey W. Prevalence of and factors associated with faecal incontinence results from a population -based survey. Gastroenterology; 2018;154(6):1672–81.
15. Dibley L, Norton C. Experiences of faecal incontinence in people with inflammatory bowel disease: self-reported experiences among a community sample. Inflamm Bowel Dis. 2013;19(7):1450–62.
16. Cichowski SB, Komesu YM, Dunivan GC, Rogers RG. The association between fecal incontinence and sexual activity and function in women attending a tertiary referral center. Int Urogynecol J. 2013;24(9):1489–94.
17. Imhoff LR, Brown JS, Creasman JM, Subak LL, Van den Eeden SK, Thom DH, Varma MG, Huang AJ. Fecal incontinence decreases sexual quality of life, but does not prevent sexual activity in women. Dis Colon Rectum. 2012;55(10):1059–65.
18. Varma MG, Brown JS, Creasman JM, Thom DH, Van Den Eeden SK, Beattie MS, Subak LL. Faecal incontinence in females older than aged 40 years; who is at risk? Dis Colon Rectum. 2006;49(6):841–51.
19. Carter D. Conservative treatment for anal incontinence. Gastroenterol Rep. 2014;2(2):85–91.
20. Swora-Cwynar E, Marciniak M, Podulka D, Dobrowolska A. Gastrointestinal complaints in runners and their relationship to diets. Polish J Sports Med. 2022;38(4):227–41, 15p.
21. Jorgensen S, Hein HO, Gyntelberg F. Heavy Lifting at work and risk of genital prolapse and herniated lumbar disc in assistant nurses. Occup Med. 1994;44:47–9.
22. National Institute for Health and Clinical Excellence. Faecal incontinence: the management of faecal incontinence in adults Clinical guideline CG49; 2007.
23. Allison M. Conservative management of faecal incontinence in adults. Nurs Stand. 2010;24(26):49–56.
24. Yasuko M, Parcs D, Norton C, Vaizey C, Kamm M. Does the St. Mark's incontinence score reflect patients' perception? A review of 390 patients. Dis Colon Rectum. 2007;0:1–7.

25. Nazarko L. Faecal incontinence: diagnosis, treatment and management. Nurs Residential Care. 2011;13(6):270–5.

26. Croswell E, Bliss D, Savik K. Living adults to manage their Faecal incontinence diet and eating pattern modifications used by community. J Wound Ostomy Continence Nurs. 2010;37(6):677–82.

27. Rockwood TH, Church JM, Fleshman JW, Kane RL, Mavrantonis C, Thorson AG, et al. Fecal incontinence quality of life scale. Dis Colon Rectum. 2000;43:9–16.

28. Kwon S, Visco AG, Fitzgerald MP, Ye W, Whitehead WE. Pelvic floor disorders network. Validity and reliability of the modified Manchester health questionnaire in assessing patients with fecal incontinence. Dis Colon Rectum. 2005;48:323–34.

29. Cotterill N, Norton C, Avery KN, Abrams P, Donovan JL. Psychometric evaluation of a new patient-completed questionnaire for evaluating anal incontinence symptoms and impact on quality of life: the ICIQ-B. Dis Colon Rectum. 2011;54:1235–50.

30. Vaizey CJ, Carapeti E, Cahill JA, Kamm MA. Prospective comparison of faecal incontinence grading systems. Gut. 1999;44:77–80.

31. Leo CA, Murphy J, Hodgkinson JD, Vaizey CJ, Maeda Y, Chir G. Does the Internet provide patients or clinicians with useful information regarding faecal incontinence? An observational study. 2018;39(2):71–6. PMID: 29694304.

32. Norton C. Faecal Incontinence and Biofeedback Therapy. Gastroenterol Clin N Am. 2008;37(3):587–604.

33. Horton N. Behavioural and biofeedback therapy for evacuation disorders. In: Norton C, Chelvanaygam S, editors. Bowel continence nursing. Beaconsfield: Beaconsfield Publishers Ltd; 2004.

34. Norton C, Chelvanayagam S, Wilson-Barnett J, Redfern S, Kamm M. Randomized controlled trial of biofeedback for fecal incontinence. Gastroenterology. 2003;125:1320–9.

35. Brown SR, Cann PA, Read NW. Effect of coffee on distal colon function. Gut. 1990;31:450.

36. Norton C, Chelvanayagam S. Conservative management of faecal incontinence in adults. In: Norton C, Chelvanayagam S, editors. Bowel continence nursing. Beaconsfield: Beaconsfield Publishers; 2004. p. 114–3.

37. Woodley S, Boyle R, Cody J, Mørkved S, Jean E, Hay-Smith C. Pelvic floor muscle training for prevention and treatment of urinary and faecal incontinence in antenatal and postnatal women first published: 22 December 2017 editorial group. Cochrane Incontinence Group. 2017; https://doi.org/10.1002/14651858.CD007471.pub3.

38. Collins B, Norton C. Managing passive incontinence and incomplete evacuation. Br J Nurs. 2013;22(10) https://doi.org/10.12968/bjon.2013.22.10.575.

39. Coggrave M. Transanal irrigation for bowel management. Nurs Times. 2007;103(26):47,49.

40. National Institute for Health and Clinical Excellence. Peristeen transanal irrigation system for managing bowel dysfunction, MTG36; 2018.

41. National Institute for Health and Clinical Excellence. Percutaneous tibial nerve stimulation for faecal incontinence Interventional procedures guidance. Published: 25 May 2011 IPG395; 2011.

42. Zyczynski H, Richter H, Sung V, Lukacz E, Arya L, Rahn D, Visco A, Mazloomdoost D, Carper B, Gantz M. Percutaneous tibial nerve stimulation vs sham stimulation for faecal incontinence in women: neuromodulation for accidental bowel leakage randomized clinical trial. Am J Gastroenterol. 2022;117(4):654–67. https://doi.org/10.14309/ajg.0000000000001605.

43. Panel J, Solon A, Waudby B, O'Grady A. Percutaneous tibial nerve stimulation can improve symptoms and quality of life in selected patients with faecal incontinence – a single-Centre 5-year clinical experience. Surgeon. 2020;18(3):P154–8.

Surgical Management of Anal Incontinence

20

Gregory Thomas and Carolynne Vaizey

Overview

Test your learning and check your understanding of this book's contents: use the "Springer Nature Flashcards" app to access questions using ▶ https://sn.pub/wqrf89 To use the app, please follow the instructions in Chap. 1.

Key Learning Points

- The symptomatic burden, effect on the patient's quality of life and cause of anal incontinence, must all be considered prior to offering surgical management.
- In women with anal incontinence (AI), conservative management should usually be offered first. Several exceptions to this are those with an external rectal prolapse, an obstetric anal sphincter injury wound breakdown, and a missed cloacal type injury.
- Overlapping sphincteroplasty can be offered to a very selected group of patients with significant faecal incontinence and a documented full length sphincter injury. Most patients improve after sphincteroplasty, but the treatment efficacy decreases over time.
- Sacral neuromodulation is an effective therapy for patients with significant incontinence in whom conservative management fails. It has the advantage of allowing a therapeutic trial prior to permanent stimulator implantation.
- A colostomy may restore a more normal lifestyle and may improve quality of life. An end sigmoidostomy alone is recommended.
- Newer technologies such as regenerative medicine and the anal injectable device may offer effective treatment options in the future.

20.1 Introduction

Faecal incontinence (FI) is a life changing affliction; sadly, many patients often seek care from numerous physicians who are not equipped to treat the condition appropriately. Because of the multifactorial etiology of FI, patients should be treated in specialist centres, offering a full range of therapies. Equally, when considering treatment options, emphasis should be made on ensuring that surgical treatment does not lead to the worsening of the patient's condition. The treatment of FI must be guided by the severity of symptoms, the aetiology of the disease, and the results of diagnostic investigations. Current recommendations are based more on expert opinion than high-quality evidence. Indeed, most of the

G. Thomas (✉)
St Mark's Hospital, London, UK
e-mail: gregorythomas1@nhs.net

C. Vaizey
St Mark's Hospital, London, UK

Department of surgery and cancer, Imperial College of London, London, UK
e-mail: cvaizey@nhs.net

published literature in this field reports single series studies, and very few are large, randomised comparative studies. Faecal incontinence is a life changing affliction, with many patients being brushed off or passed from clinician to clinician.

The range of surgical options for those who have failed conservative therapies is currently quite limited. Sphincteroplasty is the direct repair of the external anal sphincter, with or without the internal anal sphincter. The use of injectable bulking agents to narrow the anal canal has limited application and poor evidence on long term outcomes. Sacral nerve stimulation/sacroneuromodulation (SNM), on the other hand, has relatively low morbidity and good long term outcomes, with widespread indications for its use. Replacement anal sphincter devices have largely been discontinued. At the end of the spectrum, a stoma should not be perceived as a failure of management, as when patients are appropriately chosen and adequately counselled, this procedure can provide a better quality of life for affected patients.

The exceptions to the rule that conservative therapy should be pursued first, are when an external rectal prolapse is present, in cases of wound breakdown in the setting of OASI, or in cases when a missed cloacal type injury is encountered. However, conservative measures should still be available along side the surgical solutions (Fig. 20.1).

20.2 Evaluation of a Patient Presenting with Fecal or Anal Incontinence

20.2.1 History

20.2.1.1 Key Points
The following are imperative data points that should be collected in gathering a patient's history with FI or AI:

- Type of FI/AI (urge, passive, or "mixed") Frequency of defaecation Stool type
- Effect on activities of daily living/ family life/ employment
- Concurrent evacuatory problems (incomplete emptying, re-visiting toilet, digitation, sensation of a blockage)
- History of pelvic organ prolapse
- Obstetric history
- Previous medical/surgical history (especially perineal/anal surgery)
- Bladder dysfunction
- "Red-flag" symptoms (weight loss, rectal bleeding, recent change in bowel habit)

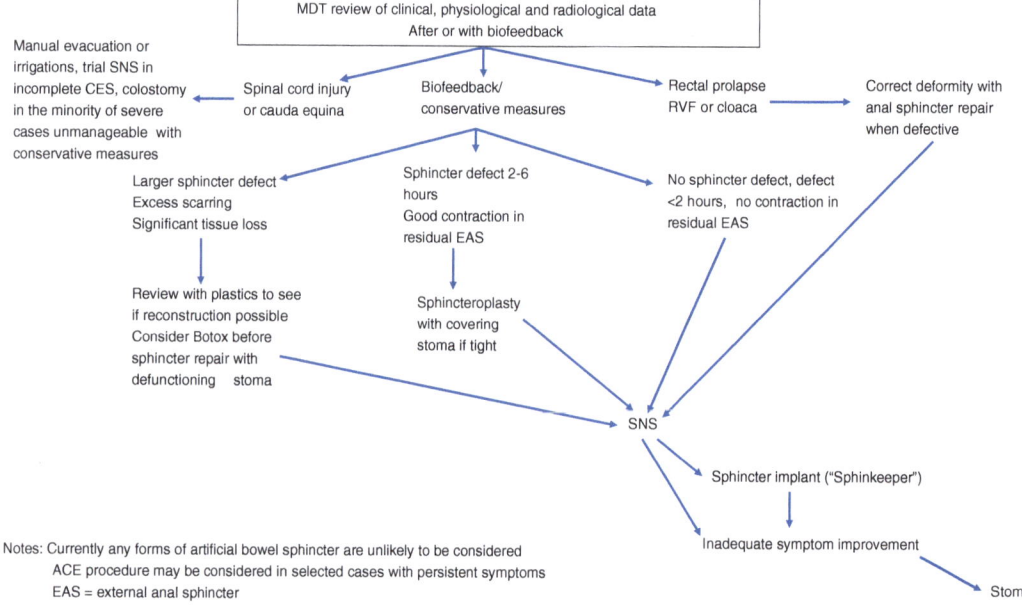

Fig. 20.1 Algorithm of surgical options for faecal incontinence

20.2.2 Investigations (See Chap. 14 and 15)

- Consider lower GI endoscopy (especially if "red-flag" symptoms present, or if chronic loose stool)
- Endoanal ultrasonography
- Anorectal physiology testing
- Consider defaecating proctography (especially if history of obstructed defecation)

20.2.3 Treatment

Conservative management: Refer to chapter on conservative management of faecal incontinence (See Chap. 19)

Surgical management

20.3 Sphincteroplasty

'Anal sphincteroplasty' typically describes a secondary or delayed repair of the anal sphincter muscles. Overlapping sphincteroplasty is the standard technique used for delayed repairs. This technique was first reported by Parks [1] in 1971. The perineum is usually deficient (Fig. 20.2a) and on palpation, a sphincter defect may be palpable. If the perineum is completely deficient, then a cloacal-like defect is seen. An inverted -U incision is made in the perineum. (Fig. 20.2b) The external sphincter ends lie medial to the ischional fat (Fig. 20.2b) The scar tissue and external sphincter muscle ends are dissected from the anal canal (Fig. 20.2b). Usually, most colorectal surgeons and obstetricians repair both the external and internal sphincters *en masse* are in an overlap repair. If there is a defect and the sphincter ends are accessible (Fig. 20.2c), the internal anal sphincter can be repaired at the same time (Fig. 20.2d) [2]. Adequate mobilisation is necessary to ensure a tension-free closure. (Fig. 20.2d). The scar tissue is then divided and the two ends are overlapped over the midline and stitched with 2/0 mattress sutures, using a delayed absorbable suture material (Fig. 20.2e, f). It is important that the perineum is reconstructed by including the disrupted superficial transverse muscles (Fig. 20.2g) and bulbospongiosus muscles (Fig. 20.2h). A small opening can be left in the centre of the wound or a Penrose/Minivac drain inserted (Fig. 20.2i). A very small study of 10 patients suggested that reinforcement of the repair with a small collagen porcine mesh may be beneficial [3]. However, this has not been investigated in larger studies and is generally not recommended.

Sphincteroplasty may confer benefit in patients with localised (from 2 to 6 hours (or 60–180 degrees) of circumference) full thickness and full length combined sphincter defects. It is our opinion that a defect of less than two hours (<60 degrees) is likely to represent scar tissue and a better apposition of the muscle ends is unlikely to be achieved with a sphincter repair. The exception to this, may be those who have an obvious "guttering" type defect. This may benefit from a repair even when the defect is less than sixty degrees. There are no established factors that predict outcome, but it is thought that those with low squeeze pressures of the residual sphincter muscle preoperatively are probably less likely to have a good result. This may be assessed by anorectal physiology testing. The young patient who attends with a cloaca type defect should be offered a sphincteroplasty and perineal reconstruction, irrespective of residual function. It is believed that restoration of the perineal anatomy will be of significant benefit to this particular patient group.

The short term outcome of sphincteroplasty suggests good to excellent results in a majority of patients (up to 80%) [4]. However, the outcome measures and patient selection in these studies are mixed. Unfortunately, in the medium to longer term, there is a demonstrable decline in the effectiveness of the repair, down to 30% [5, 6]. In a systematic review that analysed the outcome of over 900 reported repairs, the authors described good initial results; these decreased over time. Interestingly, there was a poor correlation between symptoms and quality of life, and all studies reported high satisfaction scores, despite decline in continence [7].

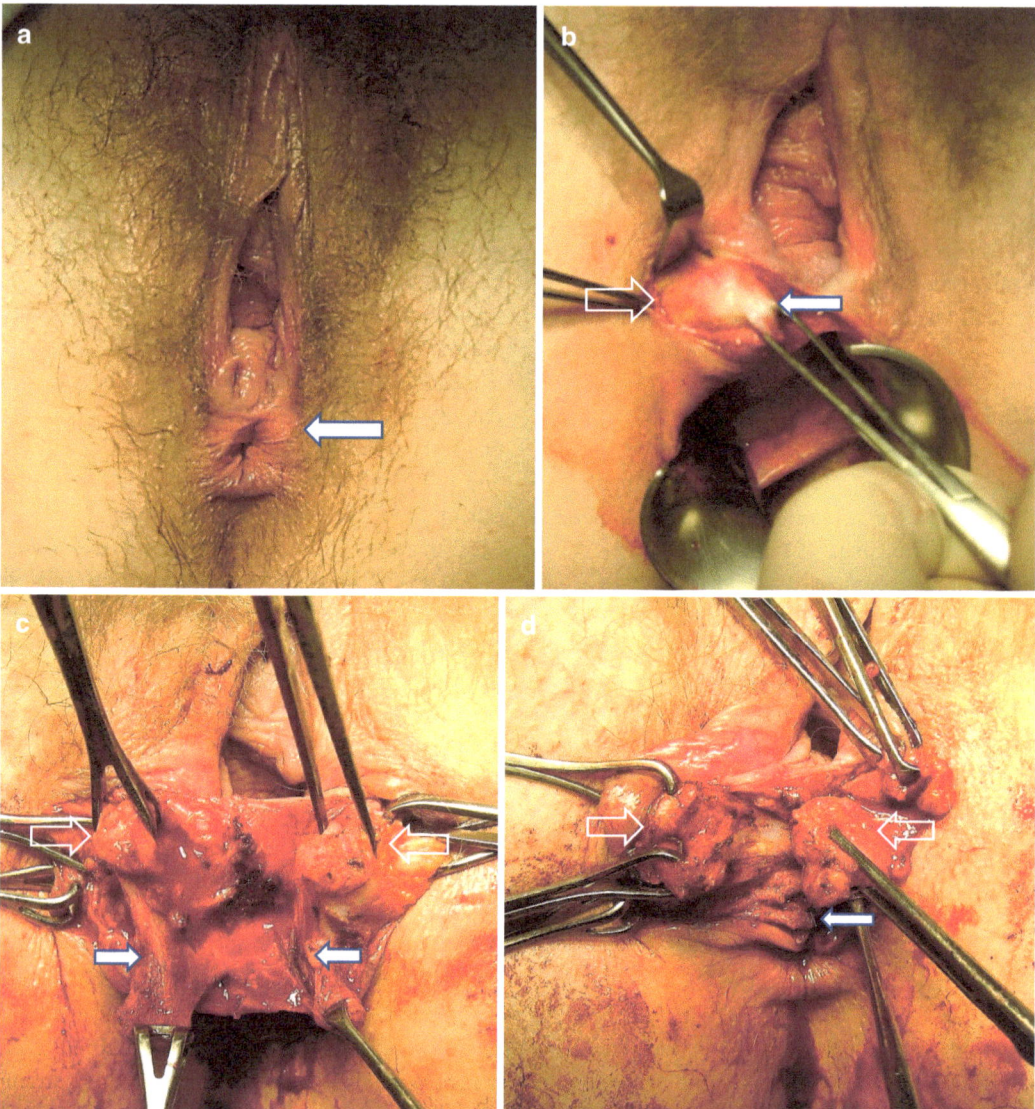

Fig. 20.2 (**a**) Photograph of perineal area in a woman complaining of faecal incontinence. A deficient perineum can be seen (white arrow). Endoanal scan of the patient showed an anterior internal and external sphincter defect. (All photographs supplied by courtesy of Abdul Sultan). (**b**) Following an inverted 'U' shaped incision, the scarred disrupted sphincter ends (filled arrow) are grasped and lie medial to the ischioanal fat (open arrow). (**c**) The separated ends of the internal sphincter can be easily seen (white arrow), lateral to which the torn external sphincter ends can be seen (unfilled arrow). (**d**) The internal sphincter has been repaired with mattress 2.0 PDS sutures (white arrow). The external sphincter ends have been grasped (unfilled arrows) in preparation for an overlap repair. (**e**) The first three sets of sutures of the overlap have been inserted the external sphincter (white arrow). (**f**) After tying the first set of sutures (white arrow), the second set of sutures have been inserted and tied (unfilled arrow) to complete the overlap repair. (**g**) The perineum is then reconstructed by ensuring that the transverse perineal muscles are brought together (arrows) followed by the Bulbospongiosus muscles (**h**) The bulbospongiosus muscles are grasped and sutured in the midline to reconstruct the perineum. (**i**) A minivac drain is then inserted and the the perineal skin is then closed in a subcuticular fashion. Note the difference in the size of the perineum when compared to Fig. 20.2a

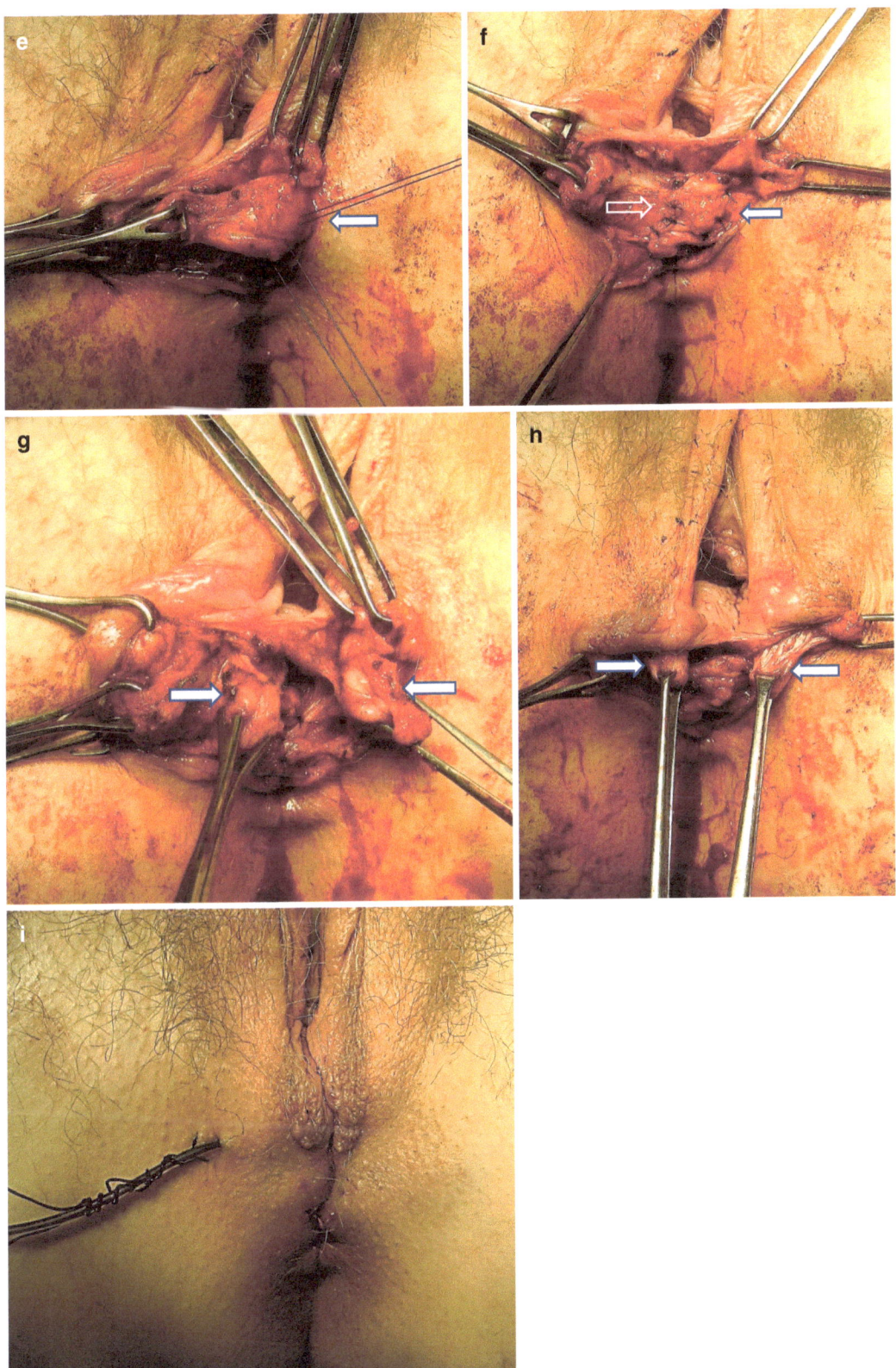

Fig. 20.2 (continued)

Pelvic floor biofeedback therapy before and after surgery may confer some improvement in quality of life and on sustaining symptomatic improvement in the longer term [8]. Previous sphincter repair has not been shown to affect the clinical outcome of a subsequent repair. In a comparative study, the outcome was similar between patients with or without a previous sphincter repair, with good results obtained in 50% and 58% of patients, respectively [5]. The long-term benefit of a repeat sphincter repair was better than for an initial repair, perhaps reflecting the improved selection of patients for this operation [6]. The role of sphincteroplasty when compared to sacral neuromodulation is currently debated [9, 10].

20.4 Sacral Neuromodulation

Sacral neuromodulation (SNM) (Figs. 20.3 and 20.4) was first described for use in urological disorders in 1983 and was not reported for use in FI until 1995 [11].

Typically, SNM consists of a *screening phase* of peripheral nerve evaluation (PNE), followed by a second, *therapeutic phase,* of permanent

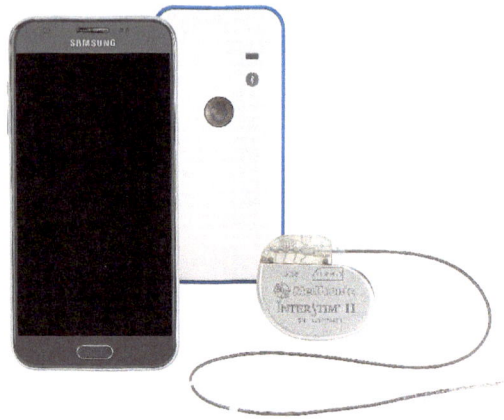

Fig. 20.4 SNM implant and patient controller

neurostimulator implantation. Both stages may be performed under either general or local anaesthesia. The patient is positioned prone, the S3 foramen is cannulated with a needle, and ultimately a lead is placed through the foramen which allows for stimulation. If performed under general anesthesia in the opetrating room, a "bellows" motor response of the pelvic floor and plantar flexion of the ipsilateral hallux will confirm correct lead placement. If performed under only local anaesthesia, then sensory stimulation around the anus or vagina will indicate correct lead placement, as eliciting motor responses can be too painful. The lead is secured in place and connected to a portable external stimulator [18]. The patient then undergoes a 1–3 week trial of stimulation while filling out a bowel-habit diary. Only patients with significant clinical improvement, which may be demonstrated by a reduction in frequency of episodes or days of faecal incontinence of at least 50%, are then selected for the *therapeutic phase*, of permanent stimulator implantation. Alternatively, patients may be asked if they feel to have improved sufficiently to move onto permanent implantation. If a PNE was performed, the lead is removed and a more advanced lead is placed in the same fashion, this time using fluoroscopic guidance. If a permanent lead was used for the test stage, then this is retained. The permanent stimulator is placed subcutaneously in the gluteal area and connected to the lead (Figs. 20.3 and 20.4). The pulse generator

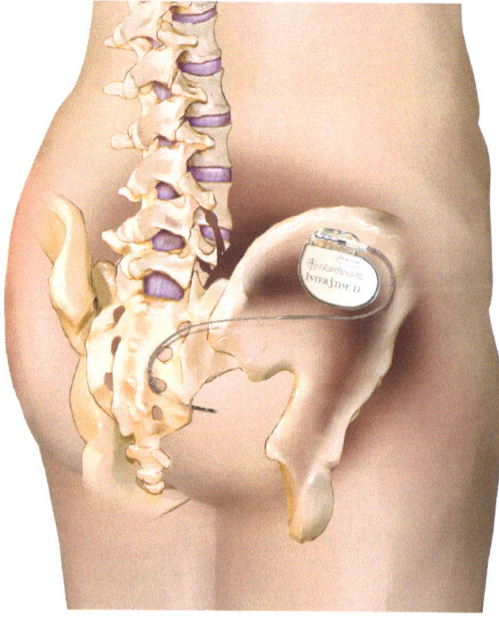

Fig. 20.3 SNM implant and lead

is activated and stimulation parameters are set by telemetry. The patient can adjust and deactivate it with a small, hand-held device.

The mechanism of action of SNM is currently unclear. There are no consistent anal or pelvic floor motor or sensory responses evident in the literature, such as changes in anal sphincter contractility or rectal sensitivity [12]. However, more recent work suggests that the device may modulate fine motor activity of the anal sphincters, particularly by optimizing or modulating the interplay between the rectum and the anal canal. There may be some effect on distal colonic motility as well, as an effect on the sensory cortex and the perception of when defaecation is desired [13]. A crossover study in 34 patients comparing active with deactivated devices demonstrated a significant improvement in incontinence symptoms during the active stage [14].

SNM is an attractive treatment because it is minimally invasive, has a low morbidity, wide application, and sustainable long-term results. In a series of 228 patients, long term improvement was seen in 71% at a median follow-up of 84 (70–113) months. The frequency of incontinence episodes per week fell from 7 to 0.5, and the St Mark's incontinence score improved from a median of 19 to 6 (both $P < 0.001$). Fifty per cent of the patients achieved complete continence [15]. It should be remembered, however, that not all patients repond well to the PNE stage. Around 80% achieve a satisfactory response. Therefore, when the number who underwent test stimulation is taken into account, on an intention-to-treat basis, full continence is achieved in between 33% and 42.6% of patients [15, 16].

Another study looked at the outcome of 101 patients at 5 years. Sixty of these patients reported a favourable outcome, and 41 reported an unfavourable outcome. Of these, 24 had their implant deactivated or removed. The authors found that age was a negative predictive factor for success. They found that both an improvement in urgency during the test stage and a good outcome at 6 months were predictive of success. This last finding may highlight the problems associated with patient-reported outcome as a way of judging success of test stimulation [17]. However, a more recent study reported a lower device explantation rate of only 14 out of 127 permanent implants at 2.7 (2–8.5) years follow up. It is difficult to clearly identify predictive factors for a good outcome of SNM. It is likely that those with defecatory urgency may have a better outcome than those with purely passive faecal leakage. However, this should not deter the latter group from being offered SNM. A physiological assessment of response, rather than patient reported outcomes, to test stimulation may go some way to better prediction of a good outcome of SNM.

More recent work has suggested that there is a sustained benefit in the even longer term, to match that seen in the early stages. Recent work from the UK and France has shown the benefits of SNM may be maintained for over 10 years [18, 19]. Reported morbidity in the literature includes implant site pain, paraesthesia, change in sensation of stimulation, and infection. A meta-analysis of 34 studies reported an overall complication rate of 15% in permanently implanted patients, with 3% requiring explantation [20]. The latter results were similarly echoed in a separate study, which reported that at a median follow-up of 33 months, 17.6% of patients required explantation of the device or discontinued treatment entirely [21]. SNM is also an expensive treatment. The UK guidance states that it should be offered only when the patient has not improved with conservative therapy.

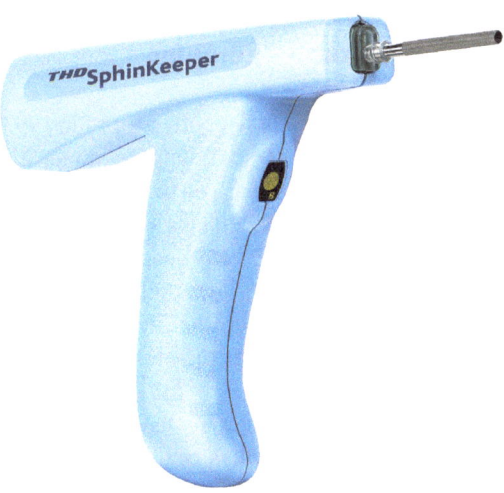

Fig. 20.5 Sphinkeeper

Contraindications to SNM include pathological conditions of the sacrum preventing adequate electrode placement, skin disease at the area of implantation, pregnancy, bleeding risk, psychological instability, low mental capacity and the presence of a cardiac pacemaker (relative contraindication) or implantable defibrillator.

SNM may be used in those with an anal sphincter defect. A systematic review of the available literature which included 119 patients, reported that the average number of incontinent episodes per week improved from 12.1 to 2.3, and the Cleveland Clinic Incontinence Score (CCIS) improved from 16.5 to 3.8 [22]. It is the authors' opinion that those with a full length defect of the external anal sphincter and with reasonable retained muscular activity, could be considered for a sphincter repair before SNM is offered.

SNM may be effective for incontinence associated with low anterior resection syndrome (LARS). A meta-analysis of ten studies in 2019 [23] described an overall median improvement in Cleveland Clinic Incontinence Score and Low Aneterior Resection Syndrome (LARS) score of 67% (35–88%). Further work in this area is needed.

A standardised approach to lead placement has been described [16]. This may have a beneficial affect on outcomes. More recently, rechargeable and MRI compatible SNM systems have become available [24].

20.5   Injectable Therapies

Anal injectables were first reported for FI in 1993 [25]. The injected material is supposed to have a bulking effect on the anal canal; there may be subsequent fibrosis and collagen deposition following implantation which may add further bulking. Materials are usually injected into either the anal canal submucosa or the intersphincteric space. Ultrasound guidance may be used to optimize placement.

A variety of fluid materials have been used, including polytetrafluorethylene (Teflon), autologous fat, glutaraldehyde cross-linked collagen (Contigen™), pyrolytic carbon beads (Durasphere™), polyacrylamide (Bulkamid), synthetic calcium hydroxyapatite (Coaptite), dextranomer/hyaluronic acid copolymer (Defux) and silicone biomaterial (PTQ™). The absorption and migratory properties of these injectables has been variable, unfortunately with most failing to maintain any bulk with time.

A Cochrane review of the published literature [26] reported on five randomised trials with the outcome of 382 patients. The review concluded that four of the five studies were at an uncertain or high risk of bias. The authors reported some benefit from the use of dextranomer in stabilised hyaluronic acid compared to placebo, but this was offset by a greater number of adverse events such as infection, implant migration and erosion. The available data suggest that the effects of bulking agents appear to be short-lived and of limited efficacy.

Another possible therapy is implantation of the SphinKeeper device. Ten expandable polyacrylamide rods are placed in the intersphincteric space using a delivery device (Fig. 20.5). In this moist environment, they shorten and expand. This creates a physical bulking effect around the anal canal (see Fig. 20.6). In 2020, a published series reported on 27 patients, who received the SphinKeeper device. All had passive FI. Postoperative endoanal ultrasonography showed that

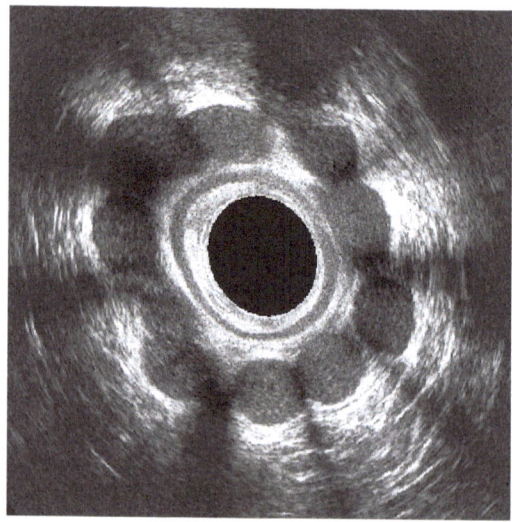

Fig. 20.6 Sphinkeeper implants

a median of seven of the original 10 implants (0–10) were seen in each patient, with a median of only five (0–10) postioned in the intended interpshincteric position. Despite this, the St Mark's FI score improved by a median of 6 points, and 14 patients (52%) achieved a greater than 50% improvement in symptoms. This success rate did not appear to be related to implant position [27]. However, there are concerns that the implants may migrate with time.

20.6 Historical Repairs

Different types of pelvic floor repairs have been described in the past [9]. For example, the aim of the postanal repair [28] was to plicate the anal sphincter muscle and levator ani, increase the length of the anal canal, restore the anorectal angle and recreate the flap valve mechanism all of which, were thought to be essential for maintaining faecal continence. Despite initial improvements in some, the long-term results of postanal repair or total pelvic floor repair for FI were too poor to recommend this approach. Similarly, non-stimulated [29] and stimulated muscle transpositions [12] were devised to reinforce the anal sphincter when local repair was not possible or had failed. Transposition of one or both gluteal muscles (*gluteoplasty*) has been reported, as well as transposition of the gracilis muscle, which is wrapped around the anus to form a neosphincter (*graciloplasty*). Improved results were noted when an implantable electrical stimulator was applied to the transposed gracilis muscle – known as a dynamic graciloplasty [29]. However, this benefit was not maintained in the medium to longer term. Considerable postoperative morbidity and need for re-operation were reported in many patients. As such, again, these techniques are generally of historical interest only.

In the past, artificial sphincters were used. Initially, these were silicone, pressure-regulated devices which aimed to restore continence through an inflatable cuff placed around the lower rectum or upper anal canal. Most of the published literature was on the Acticon Neopshincter™ (American Medical Systems (AMS), Minnetonka, MN, USA)

artificial bowel sphincter (ABS). It was comprised of a fluid-filled cuff that encircled and compressed the anal canal. A pressure-regulating balloon was implanted in the retropubic space of Retzius. A pump was then placed in the labia majora or scrotum, which was accessible to the patient and controlled the system. To initiate defaecation, squeezing the pump emptied the cuff by transferring fluid into the balloon, permitting passage of stool. The cuff then refilled automatically from pressure built up in the balloon. Very few of these are implanted currently, since the device is no longer commercially available. The withdrawal from the market was due to concerns about the high complication rate, late mechanical failure, and the availability of less invasive treatments. Whilst the most recent data had described the long-term outcome of these devices in single expert centres with satisfactory results [30], the ABS in its present state has little, role in the management of severe FI, because it has been superseded by less invasive treatments. Similarly, the magnetic anal sphincter (MAS; FENIX®, Torax Medical Inc., Shoreview, MN, USA), a novel device designed to augment the native anal sphincter, was previously available. It consisted of a series of titanium beads with magnetic cores, interlinked with titanium wires to form a flexible ring that encircles the external anal sphincter. Early trials suggested promise [31]. However, it is no longer manufactured, and this treatment is not available.

More recently, a transobturator placed polypropylene sling placed around the posterior anal canal has been investigated. The authors reported the outcome of 152 patients who had failed to improve with conservative treatment. At 24.9 months follow up, 69% had achieved a greater than 50% reduction in the frequency of Fi episodes and 19% achieved complete continence. No device erosion, extrusion or revisions were reported [32].

20.7 Regenerative Medicine

The use of regenerative medical therapies in humans for FI have been reported in a small number of papers. With regards to direct cell based therapy, in 2010, Frudinger and colleagues reported the outcome of autologous myoblast cell injection into the anal sphincters of ten women with faecal incontinence secondary to obstetric injury. At 1 year follow up, improvements in quality of life scores and a 13.7 point (CI 16.3–11.2) improvement in the Wexner faecal incontinence scores were reported [33]. Improvement was maintained at 5 year follow up [34]. Further promising work was reported in 2018. Twenty four patients were randomized to receive either placebo or autologous derived skeletal myoblast anal sphincter injections. At 12 months, there were significant improvements in Wexner FI score in the treatment arm (6.5 vs. 15 p = 0.006), when compared to baseline and not in the placebo arm (14 vs. 15 p = 0.35) [34].

There may be benefit in manipulation of the surrounding environment, rather than direct application of pluripotent stem cells. For example, the cytokine CXCL12, or stromal derived growth factor 1, has a role in vivo by attracting stem cells and progenitor cells to the site of injury and stimulate tissue regeneration. A rodent model suggested that the use of CXCL 12, without additional cell based therapy may be all that is needed for anal sphincter regeneration [35]. Further work is needed to investigate this approach.

It should be remembered that is many cases of FI, there is no clear muscular injury. Rather, symptoms may have occurred due to disruption of the local physiological reflexes between the anal canal and rectum, or even from direct nerve damage; the pudendal nerve is particularly vulnerable. As such, simply restoring sphincter structure may not be enough to restore normal function.

20.8 Stoma Formation

20.8.1 Antegrade Continence Enema

The antegrade continence enema procedure (ACE) was first described in 1990 [36]. The premise of the procedure is to irrigate the colon in an antegrade fashion in order to aid colonic and rectal emptying. Initially, the appendix was used to create a continent stoma, an '*appendicostomy*', by invaginating the tip of the appendix into the caecum to create a one-way valve. The base of the appendix was then brought out to the abdominal wall, and the patient could then introduce antegrade enemas. It is now more usual to bring the appendix up to the skin without invagination, and to maintain patency with an indwelling tube such as a gastrostomy tube. In the absence of an appendix, the caecum can be used to form a tube [37]. ACE procedures have been shown to be safe and beneficial for both paediatric and adults patients, and a proportion of patients will continue to use it in the longer term. However, patient selection should be done with care. It could be argued that there is little advantage over full irrigation techniques. Also, patients may also suffer morbidities including infection, discharge from the ostomy site, and pooling of the irrigation fluid in the right colon. In such cases, the ACE may need to be closed.

20.8.2 End Stoma

A stoma may be appropriate for patients with severe FI in which all other available treatments have failed, other treatments are inappropriate because of comorbidities, or when a stoma is preferred by the patient. While a stoma can change body image and may be associated with significant psychosocial issues and stoma-related complications, it may also allow the patient to resume normal activities and improve quality of life. For example, in a survey of patients who had a colostomy created to manage their faecal incontinence, 83% reported a significant improvement in lifestyle and 84% would choose to have the stoma again [38]. A loop end sigmoid colostomy without proctectomy is usually recommended as a procedure of choice for patients who elect to have an end stoma. Alongside stoma-specific problems, issues such as diversion proctitis and rectal mucus leakage may arise, which may necessitate a proctectomy; this is usually avoidable if expectations are managed pre-operatively. The use of minimally invasive surgery has reduced the morbidity associated with this procedure.

20.9 Conclusions

A patient with FI requires an individualised approach to their management, undertaken within a specialised Pelvic Floor Centre, offering the entire range of therapies, so as to avoid unnecessary delays and referrals. Treatment options should take into account patients' needs and preferences. In the majority of cases, conservative therapies should be offered first. Sacral neuromodulation offers an effective treatment for these patients. It is now the preferred option over older "physical barrier" centered treatments such as sphincteroplasty and the mostly defunct sphincter augmentation techniques. Further work is needed to determine the mechanism of action of SNM. Newer therapies such as regernative medicine may be of benefit in the future.

Take Home Messages

- In most cases, conservative treatment should be offered first to those with faecal incontinence.
- Those with an OASI, an external rectal prolapse, or a missed cloacal defect should be offered surgery at an early stage.
- If symptoms fail to improve with conservative measures, a small number of patients may benefit from anal sphincter repair.
- For those not suitable for this, sacral neuromodulation should be offered. This has a sustainable benefit in the long term for the majorty of those receiving this treatment.
- Newer anal sphincter injectables may be of benefit.
- Some patients will benefit from a colostomy. The impact of this on those with severe, refractory FI, should not be underestimated.
- Future work in the neuromodulation and regenerative medicine are likely to bring about new treatment modalities in the future.

Appendix: MCQ

Mark each item TRUE or FALSE

Questions

1. Anal incontinence is
   (A) More common in men
   (B) Linked to significant obstetric trauma
   (C) Always best managed with surgery
   (D) Often associated with other pelvic floor disorders
   (E) Likely to have a significant impact on quality of life of those affected

2. Regarding assessment and management of anl incontinence:
   (A) A rectal prolapse found at presentation may be left for conservative treatment
   (B) Lower GI endoscopy is indicated if rectal bleeding and/or a recent change in bowel habit is reported
   (C) Chronic loose stool should be investigated and corrected in the early stages of treatment
   (D) Endoanal ultrasonography may help determine what treatment may be offered
   (E) Biofeedback/ pelvic floor nursing therapy is unhelpful in most cases

3. Secondary anal sphincter repair:
   (A) May be offered for any type of sphincter defect
   (B) Maintains good outcomes in the long term for the majority
   (C) Requires prior endoanal ultrasonography and assessment of sphincter function
   (D) A covering colostomy should be used for all cases
   (E) May be combined with a soft tissue flap in the presence of significant perineal tissue loss

4. Sacral neuromodulation
   (A) Has a clearly defined mechanism of action

(B)   May be performed under local anaesthesia

(C)   Can be offered to those with a sphincter defect

(D)   Typically has a test stage

(E)   Once the device has been implanted, the patient may be discharged without the need for follow up

5. Regarding other surgical options for anal incontinence
    (A)   There are a wide range of artificial anal sphincter devices currently available
    (B)   Antegrade colonic enemas (ACE) are well tolerated in adults, with few complications
    (C)   The "Sphinkeeper" anal injectable requires endoanal ultrasonography to achieve optimal device placement
    (D)   A diverting colostomy should always be considered a "last resort" for those with severe faecal incontinence
    (E)   Mucus leakage may persist after a colostomy

Answers

1. Anal incontinence is
    (A)   FALSE
    (B)   TRUE
    (C)   FALSE
    (D)   TRUE
    (E)   TRUE

2. Regarding assessment and management of anl incontinence:
    (A)   FALSE
    (B)   TRUE
    (C)   TRUE
    (D)   TRUE
    (E)   FALSE

3. Secondary anal sphincter repair:
    (A)   FALSE
    (B)   FALSE
    (C)   TRUE
    (D)   FALSE
    (E)   TRUE

4. Sacral neuromodulation
    (A)   FALSE
    (B)   TRUE
    (C)   TRUE
    (D)   TRUE
    (E)   FALSE

5. Regarding other surgical options for anal incontinence
    (A)   FALSE
    (B)   FALSE
    (C)   TRUE
    (D)   FALSE
    (E)   TRUE

References

1. Parks AG, McPartlin JF. Late repair of injuries of the anal sphincter. Proc R Soc Med. 1971;64(12):1187–9.
2. Djusad S, Kouwagam AD. Repair of old total perineal rupture: a case series. J Surg Case Rep. 2023;2023(1):rjac628.
3. Zutshi M, Ferreira P, Hull T, Gurland B. Biological implants in sphincter augmentation offer a good short-term outcome after a sphincter repair. Color Dis. 2012;14(7):866–71.
4. Engel AF, Kamm MA, Sultan AH, Bartram CI, Nicholls RJ. Anterior anal sphincter repair in patients with obstetric trauma. Br J Surg. 1994;81(8):1231–4.
5. Malouf AJ, Norton CS, Engel AF, Nicholls RJ, Kamm MA. Long-term results of overlapping anterior anal-sphincter repair for obstetric trauma. Lancet. 2000;355(9200):260–5.
6. Halverson AL, Hull TL. Long-term outcome of overlapping anal sphincter repair. Dis Colon Rectum. 2002;45(3):345–8.
7. Glasgow SC, Lowry AC. Long-term outcomes of anal sphincter repair for fecal incontinence: a systematic review. Dis Colon Rectum. 2012;55(4):482–90.
8. Cerdan, Santacruz C, Cerdan Santacruz DM, Milla Collado L, Ruiz de Leon A, Cerdan Miguel J. Multimodal Management of Fecal Incontinence Focused on Sphincteroplasty: long-term outcomes from a single center case series. J Clin Med. 2022;11(13):3755.
9. Ong K, Bordeianou L, Brunner M, Buntzen S, Collie MHS, Hanly A, et al. Changing paradigm of sacral neuromodulation and external anal sphincter repair for faecal incontinence in specialist centres. Color Dis. 2021;23(3):710–5.
10. Lehur PA, Christoforidis D. Commentary on 'Changing paradigm of sacral neuromodulation and external anal sphincter repair for faecal

incontinence in specialist centres'. Color Dis. 2021;23(3):716–7.

11. Matzel KE, Stadelmaier U, Hohenfellner M, Gall FP. Electrical stimulation of sacral spinal nerves for treatment of faecal incontinence. Lancet. 1995;346(8983):1124–7.

12. Carrington EV, Knowles CH. The influence of sacral nerve stimulation on anorectal dysfunction. Color Dis. 2011;13(Suppl 2):5–9.

13. Knowles CH, de Wachter S, Engelberg S, Lehur P, Matzel KE, Zirpel L, et al. The science behind programming algorithms for sacral neuromodulation. Color Dis. 2021;23(3):592–602.

14. Leroi AM, Parc Y, Lehur PA, Mion F, Barth X, Rullier E, et al. Efficacy of sacral nerve stimulation for fecal incontinence: results of a multicenter double-blind crossover study. Ann Surg. 2005;242(5):662–9.

15. Altomare DF, Giuratrabocchetta S, Knowles CH, Munoz Duyos A, Robert-Yap J, Matzel KE, et al. Long-term outcomes of sacral nerve stimulation for faecal incontinence. Br J Surg. 2015;102(4):407–15.

16. Boyle DJ, Murphy J, Gooneratne ML, Grimmer K, Allison ME, Chan CL, et al. Efficacy of sacral nerve stimulation for the treatment of fecal incontinence. Dis Colon Rectum. 2011;54(10):1271–8.

17. Maeda Y, Lundby L, Buntzen S, Laurberg S. Outcome of sacral nerve stimulation for fecal incontinence at 5 years. Ann Surg. 2014;259(6):1126–31.

18. Desprez C, Damon H, Meurette G, Mege D, Faucheron JL, Brochard C, et al. Ten-year evaluation of a large retrospective cohort treated by sacral nerve modulation for fecal incontinence: results of a French multicenter study. Ann Surg. 2022;275(4):735–42.

19. Leo CA, Thomas GP, Bradshaw E, Karki S, Hodgkinson JD, Murphy J, et al. Long-term outcome of sacral nerve stimulation for faecal incontinence. Color Dis. 2020;22(12):2191–8.

20. Tan E, Ngo NT, Darzi A, Shenouda M, Tekkis PP. Meta-analysis: sacral nerve stimulation versus conservative therapy in the treatment of faecal incontinence. Int J Color Dis. 2011;26(3):275–94.

21. Maeda Y, Lundby L, Buntzen S, Laurberg S. Suboptimal outcome following sacral nerve stimulation for faecal incontinence. Br J Surg. 2011;98(1):140–7.

22. Ratto C, Litta F, Parello A, Donisi L, De Simone V, Zaccone G. Sacral nerve stimulation in faecal incontinence associated with an anal sphincter lesion: a systematic review. Color Dis. 2012;14(6):e297–304.

23. Huang Y, Koh CE. Sacral nerve stimulation for bowel dysfunction following low anterior resection: a systematic review and meta-analysis. Color Dis. 2019;21(11):1240–8.

24. De Wachter S, Knowles CH, Elterman DS, Kennelly MJ, Lehur PA, Matzel KE, et al. New technologies and applications in sacral Neuromodulation: an update. Adv Ther. 2020;37(2):637–43.

25. Shafik A. Polytetrafluoroethylene injection for the treatment of partial fecal incontinence. Int Surg. 1993;78(2):159–61.

26. Maeda Y, Laurberg S, Norton C. Perianal injectable bulking agents as treatment for faecal incontinence in adults. Cochrane Database Syst Rev. 2013;(2):CD007959.

27. Leo CA, Leeuwenburgh M, Orlando A, Corr A, Scott SM, Murphy J, et al. Initial experience with SphinKeeper intersphincteric implants for faecal incontinence in the UK: a two-Centre retrospective clinical audit. Color Dis. 2020;22(12):2161–9.

28. Setti Carraro P, Kamm MA, Nicholls RJ. Long-term results of postanal repair for neurogenic faecal incontinence. Br J Surg. 1994;81(1):140–4.

29. Baeten C, Spaans F, Fluks A. An implanted neuro-muscular stimulator for fecal continence following previously implanted gracilis muscle. Report of a case. Dis Colon Rectum. 1988;31(2):134–7.

30. Wong MT, Meurette G, Wyart V, Glemain P, Lehur PA. The artificial bowel sphincter: a single institution experience over a decade. Ann Surg. 2011;254(6):951–6.

31. Sugrue J, Lehur PA, Madoff RD, McNevin S, Buntzen S, Laurberg S, et al. Long-term experience of magnetic anal sphincter augmentation in patients with fecal incontinence. Dis Colon Rectum. 2017;60(1):87–95.

32. Mellgren A, Zutshi M, Lucente VR, Culligan P, Fenner DE, Group TS. A posterior anal sling for fecal incontinence: results of a 152-patient prospective multicenter study. Am J Obstet Gynecol. 2016;214(3):349 e1–8.

33. Frudinger A, Kolle D, Schwaiger W, Pfeifer J, Paede J, Halligan S. Muscle-derived cell injection to treat anal incontinence due to obstetric trauma: pilot study with 1 year follow-up. Gut. 2010;59(1):55–61.

34. Frudinger A, Pfeifer J, Paede J, Kolovetsiou-Kreiner V, Marksteiner R, Halligan S. Autologous skeletal-muscle-derived cell injection for anal incontinence due to obstetric trauma: a 5-year follow-up of an initial study of 10 patients. Color Dis. 2015;17(9):794–801.

35. Sun L, Kuang M, Penn M, Damaser MS, Zutshi M. Stromal cell-derived factor 1 plasmid regenerates both smooth and skeletal muscle after anal sphincter injury in the long term. Dis Colon Rectum. 2017;60(12):1320–8.

36. Malone PS, Ransley PG, Kiely EM. Preliminary report: the antegrade continence enema. Lancet. 1990;336(8725):1217–8.

37. Thomas K, Bassuini M. Laparoscopic caecodivision ACE (antegrade continence enema) procedure. Tech Coloproctol. 2008;12(1):65–7.

38. Norton C, Burch J, Kamm MA. Patients' views of a colostomy for fecal incontinence. Dis Colon Rectum. 2005;48(5):1062–9.

Obstetric Rectovaginal Fistulas

Brittany Roberts, Gifty Kwakye, Dee Fenner,
and Rebecca G. Rogers

Overview
Test your learning and check your understanding of this book's contents: use the "Springer Nature Flashcards" app to access questions using ▶ https://sn.pub/wqrf89 To use the app, please follow the instructions in Chap. 1.

Learning Points
- Review the historical evaluation, management, and treatment of rectovaginal fistulas, with an emphasis on rectovaginal fistulae of obstetrical origin.
- Discuss the etiologies and classification of rectovaginal fistulas.
- Review patient evaluation of rectovaginal fistulas.
- Review surgical management and outcomes following repair of rectovaginal fistulas.

B. Roberts · R. G. Rogers (✉)
Department of Obstetrics and Gynecology, Albany
Medical Center, Albany, NY, USA
e-mail: robertb5@amc.edu; rogersr2@amc.edu

G. Kwakye
Department of Surgery, Division of Colorectal
Surgery, University of Michigan, Brighton, MI, USA
e-mail: Gkwakye@med.umich.edu

D. Fenner
Department of Obstetrics and Gynecology, University
of Michigan, Ann Arbor, MI, USA
e-mail: deef@med.umich.edu

21.1 Introduction

"There are few afflictions unattended with danger to life, which give rise to greater anxiety or produce more disagreeable results than cases of rectovaginal fistula [1]."
- TH Tanner,1855.

A rectovaginal fistula is defined as a communication between the rectum and the vagina. Although rare, quality of life impact of this condition on patients may be profound. Causes of rectovaginal fistulas include traumatic, congenital, inflammatory, neoplastic, and iatrogenic processes (See Table 21.1). While estimates vary, the most common cause of rectovaginal fistulas is thought to be secondary to obstetrical complications, followed by inflammatory and neoplastic disorders [2]. Fistulas that occur as the result of congenital malformations are beyond the scope of discussion in this chapter; only the presentation and repair of acquired fistulas with particular emphasis on those that occur due to obstetrical trauma will be presented.

Of particular importance to the practicing obstetrician gynecologist are rectovaginal fistulas that occur as a complication of vaginal birth. Symptoms of a rectovaginal fistula may include fecal or flatal incontinence, pain, skin or mucosal irritation, or dyspareunia. In rectovaginal fistula evaluation, the patient's history and physical examination are important. Whenever a postpartum patient presents with complaints of fecal or flatal incontinence, rectovaginal fistula should be included in the differential diagnosis. Fistulas of obstetrical origin are

Table 21.1 Etiology of rectovaginal fistula

Category	Condition	Mechanism
Traumatic		
Obstetric	Prolonged 2nd stage of labor	Pressure necrosis of rectovaginal septum
	Midline episiotomy	Extension directed into rectum
	Perineal lacerations	
Foreign body	Vaginal pessaries	Pressure necrosis
	Violent coitus	Mechanical perforation
	Sexual abuse	Mechanical perforation
Iatrogenic	Hysterectomy	Injury to anterior rectal wall
	Stapled colorectal anastomosis	Staple line includes vagina
	Transanal excision of anterior rectal tumors	Deep margin of resection into vagina
	Enemas	Mechanical perforation
	Anorectal surgery such as incision and drainage of intramural abscesses intramural abscesses	Mechanical perforation
Inflammatory	Crohn's disease	Transmural inflammation
Perforation	Pelvic radiation	Early-tumor necrosis
	Pelvic abscess	Late-transmural inflammation
	Perirectal abscess	
Neoplastic	Rectal tumors	Local tumor growth into neighboring structure
	Cervical tumors	
	Uterine tumors	
	Vaginal tumors	
	Primary or recurrent tumors	

Modified from: Atlas of clinical gynecology. Stenchever and Benson, eds. New York: McGraw-Hill, 2000 [64]

epithelial lined communications between the rectum and/or anus and the vaginal canal. A rectovaginal fistula tract occurring between the dentate line and the inside of the vaginal fourchette are classified as "low." A fistula occurring above the dentate line to the upper vagina is classified as "high." The terms "low rectovaginal fistula" and "anovaginal fistula" may be used interchangeably [3].

21.2 Historical Background

Obstetrical fistulas have plagued women for millennia as proven by the discovery of a large fistula in a mummy of an ancient Egyptian woman. Avicenna, an Arabo-Persian physician, was the first to describe fistulas because of difficult labors [4]. The history of the surgical treatment of rectovaginal fistulas lies in the evolution of the treatment of vesicovaginal fistulas. The first attempts at surgical repairs of vesicovaginal fistulas were made by H van Roonhuyse in 1676, who placed patients in lithotomy, exposed the fistula with a speculum and denuded the edges of the fistula before suturing it together [5]. The first cure of a rectovaginal fistula is credited to Barton in 1840 with the use of a seton [6]. In the late nineteenth century, several surgeons introduced innovations to the repair of vesicovaginal fistulas that were then popularized by James Marion Sims. In a series of surgical experiments on three slave women over 6 years with over 40 failed procedures, Sims ultimately managed to surgically close a vesicovaginal fistula. He attributed his success to the use of silver suture and the exposure of the operative site that he achieved with positioning the patient in the knee-chest position and the use of a speculum. Although he claimed credit for all these innovations, others had utilized silver suture for the repair of fistulas prior to his publication [4].

Rectovaginal fistulas, which occur less commonly than vesicovaginal fistulas, are also less commonly referred to in historical reports. The first treatise on the treatment of rectovaginal fistula was most likely written by a student and successor of Sims, Thomas Addis Emmet, who published a book "Vesicovaginal fistula from parturition and other causes: with cases of rectovaginal fistula" in 1868 [7]. Emmet greatly expanded the work of his mentor and introduced many surgical innovations and principles of fistula repair that are still followed today. For example, he insisted on preoperative preparation so that "not only the vaginal walls but also the hypertrophied and indurated edges of the fistula have attained a natural color and density" prior to taking the woman to surgery. The repairs were done without anesthesia, in the left lateral position, and began with release of tension on the scarred edges of the fistula. Repairs were often staged to fully close the fistula. Emmet advocated the use of scissors to achieve wide dissection of the tissues surrounding the fistula, and, for vesicovaginal fistulas, continual bladder drainage following the repair. These innovations were novel. Emmet was a meticulous surgeon and scientific investigator and is probably the true father of gynecological reconstructive surgery [8]. Further advancements in the repair of rectovaginal fistulas in the late nineteenth century included the adaptation of Tait's technique of perineorraphy at the time of fistula repair. Until then, fistula repairs were limited to splitting apart the perineum and allowing the perineum to heal by granulation, often with poor functional results [9].

21.3 Incidence

Although the exact incidence of rectovaginal fistulas is unknown, the most common etiology in the developed world is thought to be obstetrical [10]. The incidence of rectovaginal fistulas among patients who sustain a fourth-degree laceration is 0.5%. Infection of the perineal wound following birth may contribute to fistula occurrence in these cases [11].

Fistulas secondary to obstructed labor are rare in the developed world, but common worldwide. The exact prevalence of fistulas secondary to obstructed labor is unknown: in 1989, the World Health Organization estimated that more than two million girls and women had either a rectovaginal or vesicovaginal fistula, estimates that probably *underestimate* the extent of the disease as they are based on women who actually present for care [12]. Isolated incidence rates for rectovaginal fistula do not exist, however, rates of vesicovaginal fistulae in the sub-Saharan Africa may reach up to 350 women per 100,000 live births [13]. These fistulas differ from direct obstetrical trauma associated with a severe perineal laceration at the time of delivery because they are accompanied by widespread tissue destruction and

necrosis. While rectovaginal fistulas occur more rarely than vesicovaginal fistulas as a result of obstructed labor, approximately 17% of fistulas seen at a large fistula center in Addis Addaba, Ethiopia were either isolated rectovaginal fistulas or combined rectovaginal and vesicovaginal fistulas [14]. Another series by Ayhan reported that 19% of 182 vesicovaginal fistula patients also had intestinal fistulas [15]. Double fistulas (rectovaginal and vesicovaginal) are indicative of a poorer prognosis for surgical cure [15, 16] probably because double fistulas are a marker for widespread damage to the vaginal and rectal tissues.

21.4 Classification

Various classification schemes have been proposed for rectovaginal fistulas. No standardized system has been adopted, which has limited the ability to compare results from surgical series or to define the incidence of disease. One system divides fistulas into "simple "and "complex". Simple fistulas occur in the low or midvaginal septum, are less than 2.5 cm in diameter, and are the result of trauma or infectious causes. Complex fistulas occur high in the vaginal septum, are greater than 2.5 in diameter, and may occur from inflammatory bowel disease, irradiation or other neoplastic causes [17]. Fistulas that have failed prior repair or result from prolonged obstructed labor should probably be classified as "complex fistulas" regardless of where the location of communication between rectum and vagina occurs [8, 14]. Other classification schemes divide fistulas by anatomic descriptions: "high," "middle," and "low." "High" fistulas occur in the upper third of the vagina (where the vagina is covered only by peritoneum near the level of the cervix), while "low" fistulas occur where the vagina and the anal canal are separated by the perineal body at or below the level of the dentate line; "middle" fistulas occur in between [18].

Classification of inflammatory perianal fistulas divide them into five main types: superficial, intersphincteric, transsphincteric, suprasphincteric, and extrasphincteric [19]. This classification scheme helps to dictate the approach to surgical management. Other classification schemes have included combinations of the above as well as the addition of horseshoe fistulas [20]. Each of the above categories for perianal fistulas have multiple variations; fistulas of these types may be very extensive involving the entire pelvis.

21.5 Pathophysiology

The pathophysiology of rectovaginal fistulas varies by etiology including obstetrical and other traumatic causes, sexual trauma, inflammatory bowel disease, infectious etiologies and neoplastic processes. In this chapter, our focus is on obstetrical fistulae.

21.5.1 Obstetrical Fistulas

Obstetrical fistulas can occur as the result of direct trauma or as part of more global damage to the tissues of the pelvic floor. Obstetrical fistulas in the developed world are thought to occur through direct trauma to the rectovaginal septum and perineal body. Risk factors for third and fourth degree lacerations of the anal sphincter are also thought to increase the risk for fistula formation and include episiotomy, operative vaginal birth, as well as secondary infection of a repaired laceration [21, 22].

Failure to recognize injuries and inadequate repair have also been implicated in the etiology of rectovaginal fistulas [23]. Repair of obstetrical lacerations is often performed under sub optimal conditions with poor lighting, in an operative field contaminated by fecal material, and with lack of analgesia and surgical assistance. Identification and exposure of severe lacerations is paramount to effective repair and may require moving a patient from the delivery room to the operating room to perform an exam under anesthesia to determine the full extent of lacerations after a delivery. A rectal exam with adequate lighting and analgesia is indicated to adequately detect lacerations to the posterior rectovaginal septum. In evaluation of obstetric anal sphincter injuries (OASIs), a rectal buttonhole tear should be considered as well. A rectal buttonhole tear is a defect of the anal epithelium or rectal mucosa that does not penetrate the anal sphincter complex[24]. Both the rectal buttonhole tear and OASI may be present in the absence of a perineal laceration, making an adequate digital rectal exam imperative for diagnosis [24, 25]. One study has determined that a second observer increased the detection rates for severe lacerations by 15%, indicating that determining the extent of pelvic floor damage following birth may be difficult under poor operative conditions with a single examiner [26]. Careful documentation of the extent of the laceration, the repair performed, as well as the type of suture used should also be recorded. Following repair, a rectal examination should be repeated to ensure no suture has been inadvertently placed into the rectum [27].It is preferred to not have sutures in the rectum. If suture is identified on exam, the repair should be taken down and the suture removed. If the suture is not identified and removed, tissue necrosis may occur with a resultant rectovaginal fistula. These typically present 7–10 days following repair [28].

Trauma to the anal sphincter complex should be evaluated by physical exam at the time of birth as well as in the patient who presents remote from birth with a rectovaginal fistula. The 1998–2010 United States Nationwide Inpatient Sample reported a third-degree laceration rate of 3.3% and fourth-degree laceration rate of 1.1% for women who underwent a vaginal birth [29].

Rectovaginal fistulas resulting from obstetrical trauma typically occur immediately following the birth or 7–14 days postpartum secondary to a wound infection [30]. Risk factors for wound complications include smoking, increased body mass index, fourth degree laceration, and operative deliveries [31]. Rates of sphincter disruption can probably be assumed to be even higher in women with rectovaginal fistulas. The rates of preoperative anal incontinence had been reported as high as 48% in a series of 52 patients with rectovaginal fistulas [32]. Further evaluation of the anal sphincter complex may include ultrasound, manometry or neurological studies [21].

Fistulas that occur as the result of obstructed labor form after "sloughing" of vaginal tissue that has become necrotic from pressure from the fetal head. Typically, the sloughing occurs a week after the birth of the fetus after a prolonged labor lasting more than 2 days. A fistula "field injury" including rectovaginal and/or vesicovaginal fistula, global pelvic floor dysfunction and foot drop has been described and is indicative of widespread pelvic tissue and neurological damage. Part of the "field injury" includes the massive social displacement of the fistula patient from their families and communities [14].

21.6 Evaluation

Evaluation of a patient begins with a history to identify potential risk factors associated with fistulas as described above. Equally important is conducting an appropriate physical examination to determine the size, location, and etiology of the rectovaginal fistula. Women with very distal fistulas may be largely asymptomatic, while women with fistulas that are large and involve the anal sphincter complex may have frank loss of stool. Women with small fistulas may only have a purulent discharge and complain of pain without loss of bowel contents.

A thorough perineal exam, including observation of the anal opening as well as the perineal skin is warranted. Perianal dimpling and/or a "dovetail sign" (which consists of perianal folds posterior to the anal opening with smooth mucosa anteriorly) may indicate a disrupted anal sphincter, as well as the presence of a fistula. Observation of the perineal skin for fecal material as well as noting loss of flatus during an exam warrants further inquiry and investigation on the part of the provider. Women with loss of fecal material have proven reluctant to seek help or acknowledge the condition. In a prospective cohort study of 94 women, only a few of the 38% with symptoms of anal incontinence had sought evaluation due to embarrassment, socioeconomic reasons or lack of knowledge of where to obtain help [33]. An observant and sensitive provider can enable woman to seek care for this disabling condition.

Often the fistula can be visualized on rectovaginal exam. A rectal examination is also important to determine the integrity of the anal sphincters, the quality of the tissues surrounding the fistula, and to palpate for abscesses and other masses. If the fistula is not easily identified, placing methylene blue dyed lubricant in the rectum, massaging the rectovaginal septum and observing the posterior vaginal wall for extravasation can help to identify the fistula. This is demonstrated in Figs. 21.1 and 21.2.

A similar method can be performed with a tampon in the vagina with instillation of methylene blue into the rectum. The tampon is then removed and evaluated for the presence of blue

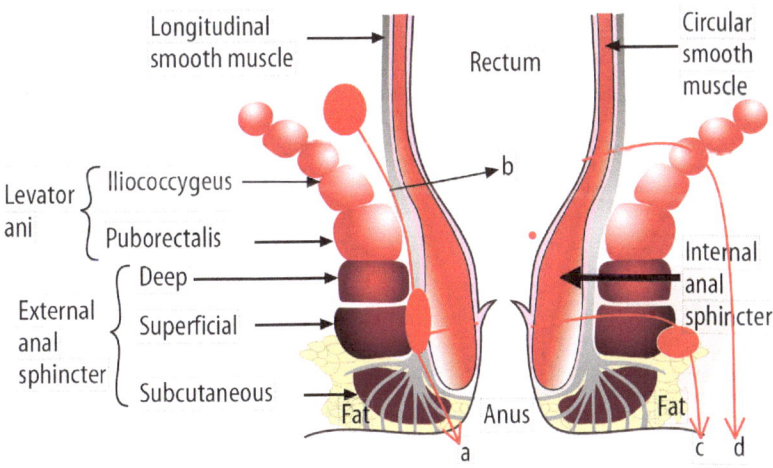

Fig. 21.1 Diagrammatic representation of types of fistula. (**a**) Intersphincteric, (**b**) Suprasphincteric, (**c**) Trans-sphincteric, (**d**) Extrasphincteric. (Courtesy of A Sultan and R Thakar)

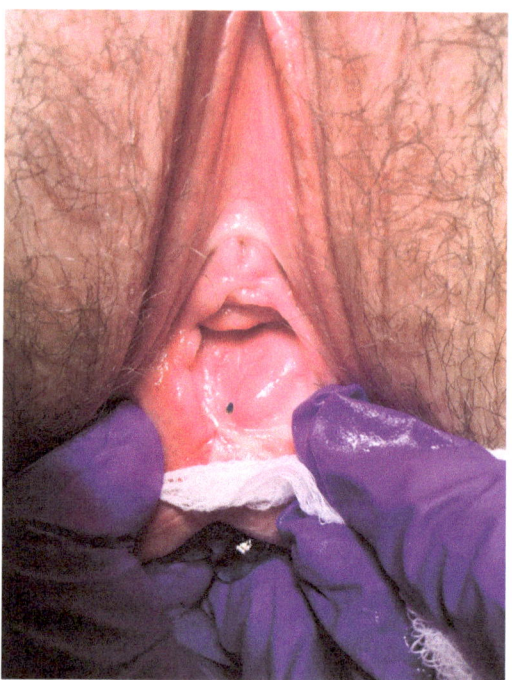

Fig. 21.2 Small rectovaginal fistula demonstrated by methylene blue dyed lubricant in the rectum

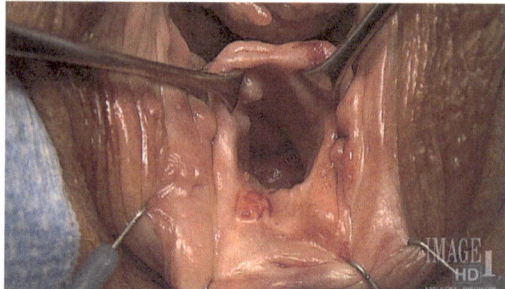

Fig. 21.4 Large Rectovaginal fistula with Allis clamps demarcating the anterior border

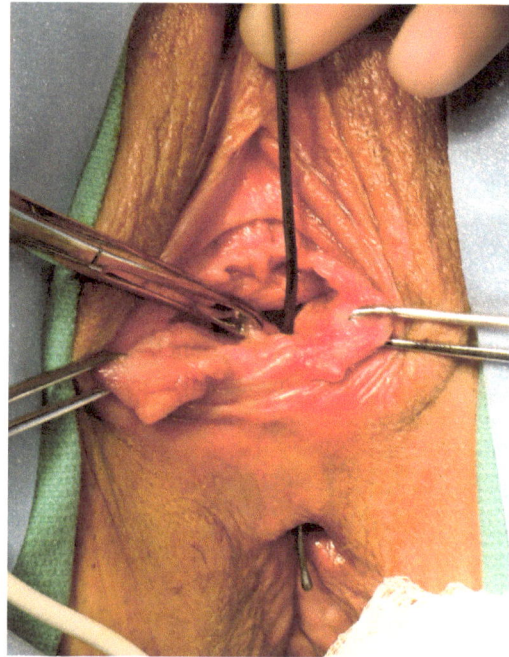

Fig. 21.5 Rectovaginal fistula with a uterine sound demonstrating the fistula tract

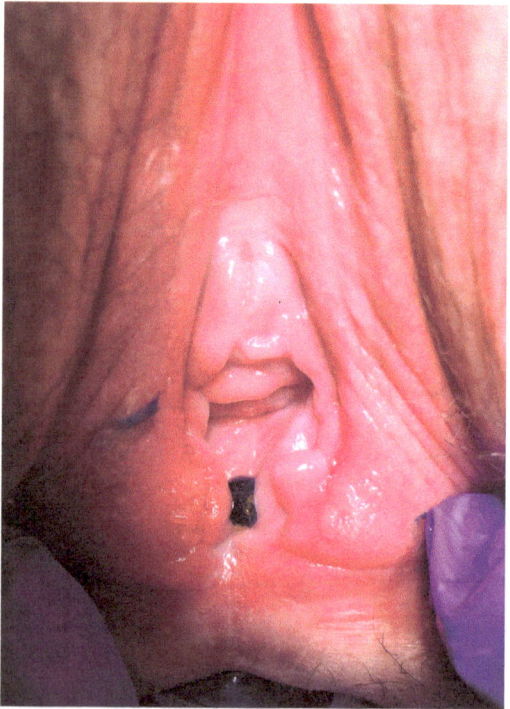

Fig. 21.3 Larger Rectovaginal Fistula Demonstrated with Methylene Blue Test

staining. Other techniques include the instillation of methylene blue stained fluid into the rectum via a large Foley catheter with a 30 cc balloon that can be used to occlude the anal canal. The rectum can also be insufflated with air, while the vagina is filled with water or saline. Bubbling may indicate the fistula site. The use of barium enemas, contrast material placed vaginally, and the use of hydrogen peroxide injected into the fistulous tract with an angiocath may help to define the exit or entrance to the tract [34] (Figs. 21.3, 21.4 and 21.5).

In general, a mature epithelized fistula that is not infected is not painful on digital examination. If the exam in the office is not successful in locating the fistula or is too painful for the patient, she should be taken to the operating room for an exam under anesthesia. Office anoscopy or proctoscopy may also help to evaluate the surrounding tissues. In women where inflammatory bowel disease is suspected by history or physical exam, colonoscopy is warranted. Biopsy of the fistulous tract is indicated in women in whom neoplastic processes are suspected.

Diagnostic imaging may be useful for diagnosis of rectovaginal fistulas not easily identified on physical examination. Endoanal ultrasound and magnetic resonance imaging (MRI) are the most useful modalities, with MRI preferred due to more widespread availability and ability to identify other disease processes within the pelvis [35, 36]. In a study of 20 patients with anorectal fistulae, endoanal MRI was able to identify the fistula in 100% of patients [37]. Vaginography has also been shown to have a high sensitivity for detection of rectovaginal fistulas [38]. Transperineal ultrasound has also demonstrated utility in detecting fistulas. This may be practiced when MRI and endoanal ultrasound are not available [39].

21.7   Surgical Technique

The approach to repair of rectovaginal fistulas should be dictated by the complexity of the fistula, its size and location, as well as its cause. For example, high fistulas are probably better addressed by abdominal procedures, while distal fistulas are better addressed by transvaginal, transperineal or transrectal procedures. The tenets of repair of obstetrically related rectovaginal fistulas date back to the innovations and recommendations made nearly 135 years ago: repair without tension, an operative field free from infection or inflammation, wide mobilization of the tissue surrounding the fistulous tract, excision of the tract if possible, and care to avoid strain on the repair in the immediate postoperative period. Although the exact management of a dehisced OASI is unclear, most authors state that the fistula needs to be completely free from inflammation or induration, with waits as long as 3–6 months suggested before repair of obstetrical fistulas be undertaken [40, 41]. This delayed approach is associated with a reduction in a patients' quality of life prior to repair [42]. In a case series and review of the literature 96 women undergoing early secondary sphincter repair demonstrated that most patients have a satisfactory postoperative recovery with few complications [43]. In a series of 1716 obstetrical vesicovaginal fistulas treated with early closure, the primary closure rate was 92%, with low rates of postoperative infection. Twelve percent of these women also had rectovaginal fistulas [44]. This study further supports the principal of early intervention and demonstrates the application to rectovaginal and vesicovaginal fistulas. Rarely, if the local tissues have active infection and continued fecal contamination that does not respond to local measures or the patient has a complex recurring fistula, a diverting colostomy is indicated until the tissue is suitable for repair [45]. Historically, mechanical and antibiotic treatments, accompanied by a restricted diet for 1–3 days prior to surgery were often recommended, although no randomized data support these practices. A Cochrane review of six randomized trials evaluating bowel anastomosis surgery compared patients undergoing mechanical bowel preparation to those with no preparation and found no difference wound infection rates (44/595 vs. 35/609, OR 1.34 95% CI .85–2.13) or other parameters measured, and may indicate that these practices in regard to repair of rectovaginal fistulas may need to be revisited [46].

In general, distal rectovaginal fistulas are repaired transvaginally (as preferred by gynecologists), transrectally (as preferred by colorectal surgeons), or transperineally. All three repair methods have similar reported success rates. Adherence to the basic tenets of fistula repair noted above are probably more important than surgical approach to the success of the intervention.

Transvaginal repair methods include conversion of the fistula to a complete fourth degree laceration followed by excision of the fistulous tract and a layered closure. In the case of a fistula that is not accompanied by anal sphincter disruption, this entails damaging an intact sphincter. Given poor rates of success with sphincteroplasty at long-term follow-up [47–50] this practice may not be in the patient's best interest. Other transvaginal repairs include inversion of the fistulous tract, followed by a layered closure. These methods will spare an intact sphincter complex. The Latzko technique is a variation of this where the anterior and posterior walls of the vagina are joined to invert the fistula into the rectum. This closes off a portion of the upper vagina and is suitable for high fistulas. A transvaginal approach is favored in patients with active Crohn's disease. Alternative techniques are described in the literature involving coring out the fistula tract, freshening the edges, creating a flapless transvaginal rectovaginal repair with healing rate of 67% in 15 patients [51]. Transvaginal repair of rectovaginal fistulas secondary to obstructed labor is influenced by the size of these fistulas (on average 2.3 by 2.5 cm) and the fact that the fistulas exist in a bed of severely damaged tissue. Excision of the fistulous tract may be impossible because of the size of the fistula and many authors introduce healthier tissue in the form of a Martius graft or flap of thigh tissue to ensure adequate blood supply to the area.

The transperineal approach starts with a curved incision on the perineum, through which the vagina and rectum are separated. The fistula is then divided and both the vaginal and rectal sides of the fistula are closed in layers in opposing directions so that the lines of the repair do not directly overlie one another [9].

Transrectal repairs generally involve the development of rectal mucosal flaps, mobilized to cover the excised fistula tract. In these repairs, the rectal mucosa, submucosa with or without portion of the rectovaginal septum and internal anal sphincter are mobilized. The fistula is excised and the flap is sutured over the previous site of the fistula. Proponents of this method of repair state that the high-pressure side of the fistula is in the rectum and that this approach focuses the repair on the rectal side. The vaginal side may be closed or left open to drain.

The best suture material for repair of fistulas has not been studied. Most series report the use of a delayed-absorbable suture, such as a 3–0 polysorb, or polyglycolic acid on all layers. Permanent suture is not used. The use of either a Martius fat pad, or gracilis flap to bring well-vascularized tissue to the fistula site is widely recommended for the repair of complex fistulas [52]. The Martius flap is harvested from the labia majora and includes fat and the bulbocavernosus muscle. Figures 21.6, 21.7 and 21.8 depict the steps of developing a martius flap. The posterolateral vascular pedicle which originates from a branch off the internal pudendal artery is preserved, and the flap is rotated and interposed between the cut and closed edges of the rectovaginal fistula. Success rates range from 60–100% [53, 54]. For the Gracilis flap, the Gracilis muscle is harvested from the thigh then passed through a tunnel from the proximal aspects of the thigh toward the perineum and then positioned between the rectum and vagina. Success rates are reported from 53% to 92% [55, 56].

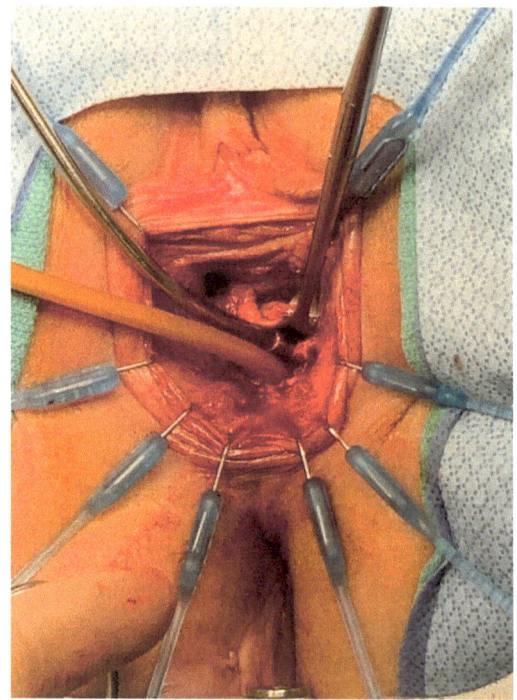

Fig. 21.6 Lonestar retractor in place with a 12 french Foley catheter transiting the fistula [1]

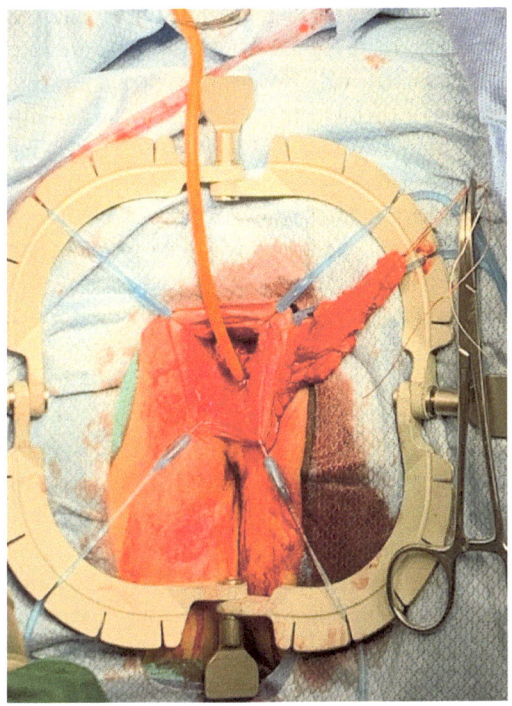

Fig. 21.7 Complete mobilization of the labial fat pad

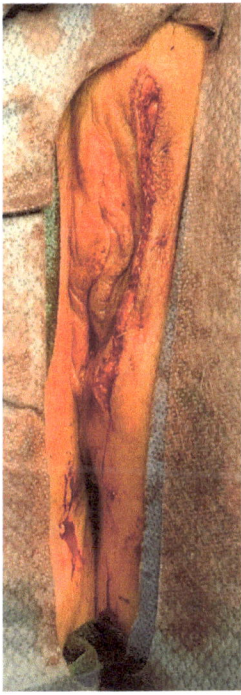

Fig. 21.8 Completed Martius flap

Postoperative management of fistula repair has not been extensively studied, however, many surgeons recommend a restrictive diet including 3 days of clear liquids followed by a low-residue diet as well as the continuation of broad-spectrum antibiotics. A single randomized study of 54 patients undergoing other anorectal reconstructive surgery found no benefit to dietary restriction [57]. Local care including sitz baths, followed by drying with a heat lamp or blow dryer on a low setting is commonly recommended to keep the operative site clean and dry [36].

21.8   Outcomes

Reports of success rates for rectovaginal fistula repair are limited to the success of closure of fistula, with little description of quality of life changes or functional outcomes. The literature is also limited by small retrospective series of patients with limited follow-up, inclusion of patients with different etiologies for the fistula, and lack of a standardized classification schema to make comparisons between reports. A thorough evaluation of the anal sphincter complex with associated sphincter repair may greatly influence surgical cure rates. If the fistula is closed, but the sphincter non-functional, the outcome may be less than desired for the patient. Reports of sexual function following fistula repair are limited to descriptions of the effect of a Martius graft on function. For example, Elkins reported on 6 patients with rectovaginal fistulas who were repaired with grafts, one of which complained of mild dyspareunia [52]. Others have reported up to a 38% incidence of pain at the site of graft harvest in small series [58]. In a study investigating sexual activity among Nigerian women following vesicovaginal and rectovaginal fistula repairs, 22.5% of women reported not being able to engage in penetrative vaginal intercourse. However, of the 102 patients involved in the study, only 9.8% of patients underwent a rectovaginal fistula repair [59].

Repair success rates of simple rectovaginal fistulas range from 40% to 86% [32]. A recent study demonstrated that non-obstetric rectovaginal fistulas have a nearly fourfold increased risk of repair failure in comparison to obstetric related rectovaginal fistulas [60]. Cure rates for more complex obstetrically related rectovaginal fistulas secondary to obstructed labor are lower than reported rates for vesicovaginal fistulas: 78% (for either combined vesicovaginal and rectovaginal fistula or rectovaginal fistula), versus a widespread reported cure (or closure) rate of 90% for isolated vesicovaginal fistula [61]. Nearly all the literature describing the treatment of these complex fistulas is retrospective in nature and because of geographical barriers, most follow-up is limited to hospital discharge. All of these reports focus on the repair of vesicovaginal fistulas. Arrowsmith et al. reported on 98 vesicovaginal fistula patients of which 9/98 had combined fistulas, however, he does not further describe the outcomes of this small cohort of combined rectovaginal and vesicovaginal fistulas [62]. Another series of 182 patients, Ayhan found 19% were reported to have intestinal fistulas; the overall success rate for this series of patients was 91%, with no further evaluation of the effect of rectovaginal fistula on surgical cure rates. Both surgical and obstetrical fistulas were represented in this cohort, however the majority of the fistulas (76%) were obstetrical in origin [15]. A series by Kelly et al. reports a similar cure rate of 85%, with approximately 20% of patients having either isolated or combined rec-

tovaginal and vesicovaginal fistulas. Again, the impact of rectovaginal fistulas on the cure rate was not analyzed. However, even among this series of difficult fistulas, the authors did classify rectovaginal fistulas as "complex" [61]. Elkins reported a series of fistula patients that he followed for 6 months, and women with combined vesicovaginal and rectovaginal fistulas had poorer outcomes than women with vesicovaginal fistulas alone, with success rates of the former with primary closure rates of 3/6(50%) versus an overall primary closure rate of 78/82 (95%) for vesicovaginal fistulas. Despite repair, 46/78 (59%) of women were found to have serious complications following successful closure of their fistula with continued complaints of either urinary or anal incontinence [16].

A single series has examined the outcome of future pregnancies following vesicovaginal repair and concluded that women who were repaired had better obstetrical outcomes than those who were not repaired, and that prenatal planning resulted in more of the women undergoing the recommended cesarean birth than those that were not scheduled for birth [63]. Presumably, the same outcomes may be applicable to women who sustain rectovaginal fistulas, given that the overall reported prognosis for these fistulas is poorer than that for vesicovaginal fistulas. Unfortunately, many of women who sustain fistulas secondary to obstructed labor are infertile as part of the "field injury" (Table 21.2).

Table 21.2 Classification of rectovaginal fistulas and perianal fistulas

Low	Tract is at the dentate line with the vaginal opening inside the vaginal fourchette
Middle	In between low and high
High	Defect is to the higher in the vagina at the level of the cervix
Simple	Low communication, <2.5 cm, occurring from trauma or infection
Complex	High communication, >2.5 cm, result from radiation, cancer, or complications of pelvic Surgical procedures, failed prior repair, prolonged obstructed labor
Superficial	Does not crossing any sphincter or muscle
Intersphincteric	Tract between the internal anal sphincter and external anal sphincter
Transsphincteric	Crosses the external anal sphincter
Suprasphincteric	Penetrates through the Intersphincteric space through the levator muscle
Extrasphinteric	Tract outside the external anal sphincter

Modified from [65]
Panés and Rimola [66]

21.9   Conclusions

Rectovaginal fistulas are a devastating condition for patients and although rare in the developed world, obstetrical fistulas are of epidemic proportion worldwide. Repair of the fistula with restoration of continence can be challenging and requires a detailed knowledge of the entire continence mechanism. Repair or other treatment of these fistula can restore patients to a healthy productive life.

Take Home Messages
- The most common etiology of rectovaginal fistulas is due to obstetrical trauma.
- Risk factors for fistula formation include episiotomy, operative vaginal birth, and secondary infection of a repaired laceration.
- Identification and exposure of severe lacerations is paramount to effective repair and failure to recognize injuries and inadequate repair are implicated in development of rectovaginal fistulas.
- Although the delayed approach has been performed historically, there is emerging evidence that early intervention has satisfactory outcomes and few complications.
- When identified and managed appropriately, obstetric related rectovaginal fistulas have favorable outcomes.

Appendix: MCQ

Mark each item TRUE or FALSE

Questions

1. The incidence of rectovaginal fistulas among patients who sustain a fourth-degree laceration is:
   (A)   <5%
   (B)   5–9%
   (C)   10–15%
   (D)   16–30%
   (E)   Greater than 30%

2. Simple fistulas
   (A)   Are greater than 2.5 cm
   (B)   Are located in the low or mid vaginal septum
   (C)   Occur secondary to inflammatory bowel disease
   (D)   Have failed prior repair
   (E)   May occur after radiation

3. Failure to recognize rectovaginal fistulas following delivery may be secondary to the following:
   (A)   Many fistulas are small and are lost in the scars from perineal lacerations
   (B)   Fistulas can only be diagnosed with advanced imaging techniques such as ultrasound and MRI
   (C)   Patients rarely present with accidental bowel leakage
   (D)   Most fistulas that form heal by themselves prior to presentation to a provider

4. A "dovetail sign":
   (A)   Consists of perianal folds posterior to the anal opening with smooth mucosa anteriorly
   (B)   May indicate an intact anal sphincter
   (C)   Indicates there is no fistula present
   (D)   Does not warrant further investigation
   (E)   Is characteristic for an intact external anal sphincter and a disrupted internal anal sphincter

5. The two most useful imaging modalities in the diagnosis of rectovaginal fistula are:
   (A)   Vaginography and Transperineal Ultrasound
   (B)   Endoanal Ultrasound and MRI
   (C)   Transperineal Ultrasound and MRI
   (D)   CT scan and Transperineal Ultrasound
   (E)   MRI and Vaginography

Answers

1. The incidence of rectovaginal fistulas among patients who sustain a fourth-degree laceration is:
   - (A) TRUE
   - (B) FALSE
   - (C) FALSE
   - (D) FALSE
   - (E) FALSE

2. Simple fistulas
   - (A) FALSE
   - (B) TRUE
   - (C) FALSE
   - (D) FALSE
   - (E) FALSE

3. Failure to recognize rectovaginal fistulas following delivery may be secondary to the following:
   - (A) TRUE
   - (B) FALSE
   - (C) FALSE
   - (D) FALSE

4. A "dovetail sign":
   - (A) TRUE
   - (B) FALSE
   - (C) FALSE
   - (D) FALSE
   - (E) FALSE

5. The two most useful imaging modalities in the diagnosis of rectovaginal fistula are:
   - (A) FALSE
   - (B) TRUE
   - (C) FALSE
   - (D) FALSE
   - (E) FALSE

References

1. Russell TR, Gallagher DM. Low rectovaginal fistulas. Am J Surg. 1977;134:13–8.
2. Das B, Snyder M. Rectovaginal Fistulae. *Clin Colon Rectal Surg.* 2016;29:50–6.
3. Vogel JD, Johnson EK, Morris AM, Paquette IM, Saclarides TJ, Feingold DL, Steele SR. Clinical practice guideline for the Management of Anorectal Abscess, fistula-in-Ano, and rectovaginal fistula. Dis Colon Rectum. 2016;59(12):1117–33.
4. Rock JA. Historical development of pelvic surgery. Telinde's Operative Gynecol. 1992:3–9.
5. Thompson JD. Vesicovaginal fistulas. Telinde's Operative Gynecol. 1992:787.
6. Barton JR. A rectovaginal fistula –cured. Am J Med Sci. 1840;26:305–6.
7. Emmet TA. Vesico-vaginal fistula from parturition and other causes: with cases of rectovaginal fistula, vol. 57. Samuel S and William Wood; 1868. p. 220.
8. Wall LL. Thomas Addis Emmet, the vesicovaginal fistula, and the origins of reconstructive gynecologic surgery. Int Urogynecol J. 2002;13:145–55.
9. Wiskind AK, Thompson JD. Transverse transperineal repair of rectovaginal fistulas in the lower vagina. Am J Obstet Gynecol. 1992;107(3):694–9.
10. Aronson MP, Lee RA. Anal incontinence and rectovaginal fistulas. Te Linde's Operative Gynecol. 2008;10:994–1030.
11. Goldaber KG, Wendel PJ, McIntire DD, Wendel GD. Postpartum perineal morbidity after fourth degree perineal repair. Am J Obstet Gynecol. 1993;168(2):489–93.
12. Murray C, Lopez A. Health dimensions of sex and reproduction. WHO; 1998.
13. Donnay F, Well L. Obstetric fistula: the international response. Lancet. 2004;363:71–2.
14. Arrowsmith S, Hamlin EC, Wall LL. Obstructed labor injury complex: obstetric fistula formation and the multifaceted morbidity of the maternal birth trauma in the developing world. Obstet Gynecol Surv. 1996;51(9):568–74.
15. Ayhan A, Tuncer ZS, Dogan L, Pekin S, Kisnisci HA. Results of treatment in 182 consecutive patients with genital fistulas. Int J Gynecol Obstet. 1995;48:43–7.
16. Elkins TE. Surgery for the obstetric vesicovaginal fistula: a review of 100 operations in 82 patients. Am J Obstet Gynecol. 1994;170(4):1108–18.
17. Rothenberger DA, Goldberg SM. The management of rectovaginal fistulae. Surg Clin N Am. 1983;63(1):61–79.
18. Rosenshein NB, Genadry RR, Woodruff JD. An anatomic classification of rectovaginal septal defects. Am J Obstet Gynecol. 1980;137(4):439–42.
19. Parks AG, Gordon PH, Hardcastle JD. A classification of fistulo in ano. Br J Surg. 1976;63:1–12.
20. Judge TA, Lichtenstein GR. Treatment of fistulzing Crohn's disease. Gastroenterol Clin N Am. 2004;33:421–54.
21. Tsang CBRD. Rectovaginal fistulas therapeutic options. Surg Clin North Am. 1997;77(1):95–114.
22. Stern HS, Dreznik Z. Rectovaginal fistula. Adv Surg. 1987;21:245–62.

23. Thompson JD. Relaxed vaginal outlet, rectocele, fecal incontinence and rectovaginal fistula. Telinde's Operative Gynecol. 1992;10:967–9.

24. Sultan AH, Kettle C. Diagnosis of perineal trauma. In: Sultan AH, Thakar R, Fenner D, editors. Perineal and anal sphincter trauma. London: Springer; 2007. p. 13–9.

25. Gurol-Urganci I, Bidwell P, Sevdalis N, et al. Impact of quality improvement project to reduce the rate of obstetric anal sphincter injury: a multi-Centre study with a stepped-wedge design. BJOG. 2020;128:584–92.

26. Groom KM, Patterson-Brown S. Third degree tears:Are they clinically underdiagnosed? Gastroenterol Int. 2000;13(2):76.

27. Sultan AH, Thakar R. Third and fourth degree tears. In: Sultan AH, Thakar R, Fenner D, editors. Perineal and anal sphincter trauma. London: Springer; 2007. p. 33–51.

28. Roper JC, Thakar R, Sultan AH. Isolated rectal buttonhole tears in obstetrics: case series and review of the literature. Int Urogynecol J. 2021;32(3):745.

29. Friedman AM, Ananth CV, Prendergast E, D'Alton ME, Wright JD. Evaluation of third-degree and fourth-degree laceration rates as quality indicators. Obstet Gynecol. 2015;125:927–37.

30. Abulafi AM, Sultan AH. Rectovaginal Fistulae. In: Pelvic floor disorders: a multidisciplinary textbook. Cham: Springer International Publishing; 2021. p. 975–94.

31. Stock L, Basham E, Gossett D, Lewicky-Gaupp C. Factors associated with wound complications in women with obstetric anal sphincter injuries (OASIS). Am J Obstet Gynecol. 2013;208(4):327–327.e6.

32. Tsang CBS, Madoff RD, Wong WD, Rothenberger DA, Finne CO, Singer D, Lowry AC. Anal sphincter integrity and function influences outcome in rectovaginal fistula repair. Dis Colon Rectum. 1998;41(9):1141–6.

33. Tetzschner T, Sorensen M, Lose G, Christionsen J. Anal and urinary incontinence in women with obstetric anal sphincter rupture. Br J Obstet Gynaecol. 1996;103(10):1034–40.

34. Song AH, Advincula AP, Fenner DE. Common gastrointestinal problems in women and pregnancy. Gastroenterology. 2004;6(3):755–73.

35. Narayanan PNM, Reynolds KM, Sahdev A, Reznek RH, Rockall AG. Fistulas in malignant gynecologic disease: etiology, imaging, and management. Radiographics. 2009;29(4):1073–83.

36. VanBuren WM, Lightner AL, Kim ST, Sheedy SP, Woolever MC, Menias CO, et al. Imaging and surgical management of anorectal vaginal fistulas. Radiographics. 2018;38(5):1385–401.

37. Dwarkasing S, Hussain S M, Hop W C, Krestin G P. Anovaginal fistulas: evaluation with endoanal MR imaging. Radiology. 2004;231:123–128.

38. Giordano P, Drew PJ, Taylor D, Duthie G, Lee PW, Monson JR. Vaginography – investigation of choice for clinically suspected vaginal fistulas. Dis Colon Rectum. 1996;39(5):568–72.

39. Maconi G, Sandro A, Salvatore G, Radice E, Bezzio C, Bianchi PG. Transperineal ultrasound in the detection of perianal and rectovaginal fistulae in Crohn's disease. Am J Gastroenterol. 2007;102(10):2214–9.

40. Cunningham FGW, Whitridge J. Puerperal infection. In: al GCFe, editor. Williams obstetrics. 19th ed. Norwalk: Appleton and Lange; 1993.

41. Fang DT, Nivatvongs S, Vermeulen FD, Herman FN, Goldberg SM, Rothenberger DA. Overlapping sphincteroplasty for acquired anal incontinence. Dis Colon Rectum. 1984;27(11):720–2.

42. Phillips R, Brown T. Surgical management of anal incontinence part a. secondary anal sphincter repair. In: Sultan AHTR, Fenner DE, editors. Perineal and anal sphincter trauma: diagnosis and clinical management. London: Springer. 2007; p. 144–53.

43. Okeahialam NA, Thakar R, Sultan AH. Early secondary repair of obstetric anal sphincter injuries (OASIs): experience and a review of the literature. Int Urogynecol J. 2021;32:1611–22.

44. Waaldijk K. The immediate management of fresh obstetrical fistulas. Am J Obstet Gynecol. 2004;191:795–9.

45. Fu J, Liang Z, Zhu Y, et al. Surgical repair of rectovaginal fistulas: predictors of fistula closure. Int Urogynecol J. 2019;30:1659–65.

46. Guenaga KF, Matos D, Castro AA, Atallah AN, Wille-Jorgensen P. Mechanical bowel preparation for elective colorectal surgery. Cochrane Library. 2011.

47. Gutierrez AB, Madoff R, Lowry AC, Parker SC, Buie WD, Baxter NN. Long-term results of anterior sphincteroplasty. Dis Colon Rectum. 2004;47:727–32.

48. Malouf AJ, Norton CS, Engel AF, Nicholls RJ, Kamm MA. Long-term results of overlapping anterior anal-sphincter repair for obstetric trauma. Lancet. 2000;355:260–5.

49. Karoui S, Leroi AM, Koning E, Menard JF, Michot F, Denis P. Results of sphincteroplasty in 86 patients with anal incontinence. Dis Colon Rectum. 2000;43(6):813–20.

50. Halverson AL, Hull TL. Long-term outcome of overlapping anal sphincter repair. Dis Colon Rectum. 2002;45(3):345–8.

51. Bhome R, Monga A, Nugent KP. A transvaginal approach to rectovaginal fistulae for the colorectal surgeon: technical notes and case series. Tech Coloproctol. 2018;22(4):305–11.

52. Elkins TE, DeLancey JO, McGuire EJ. The use of modified Martius graft as an adjunctive technique in vesicovaginal and rectovaginal fistula repair. Obstet Gynecol. 1990;75(4):727–33.

53. Pitel S, Lefevre JH, Parc Y, Chafai N, Shields C, Tiret E. Martius advancement flap for low rectovaginal fistula: short- and long-term results. Color Dis. 2011;13(6):112–5.

54. Songne K, Scotte M, Lubrano J, Huet E, Lefebure B, Surlemont Y, et al. Treatment of anovaginal or rectovaginal fistulas with modified Martius graft. Color Dis. 2007;9(7):653–6.

55. Wexner SD, Ruiz DE, Genua J, Nogueras JJ, Weiss EG, Zmora O. Gracilis muscle interposition for the treatment of rectourethral, rectovaginal, and pouch-vaginal fistulas: results in 53 patients. Ann Surg. 2008;248(1):39–43.

56. Furst A, Schmidbauer C, Swol-Ben J, Iesalnieks I, Schwandner O, Agha A. Gracilis transposition for repair of recurrent anovaginal and rectovaginal fistulas in Crohn's disease. Int J Color Dis. 2008;23(4):349–53.

57. Nessim A, Wexner SD, Agachan F, et al. Is bowel confinement necessary after anorectal reconstructive surgery? A prospective, randomized, surgeon-blinded trial. Dis Colon Rectum. 1999;92(1):16–23.

58. Tunuguntla HSGR, Gousse AE. Female sexual dysfunction following vaginal surgery: myth or reality? Curr Urol Rep. 2004;5:403–11.

59. Anzaku SA, Lengmang SJ, Mikah S, Shephard SN, Edem BE. Sexual activity among Nigerian women following successful obstetric fistula repair. Int J Gynecol Obstet. 2017;137(1):67–71.

60. Karp NE, Kobernik EK, Berger MB, Low CM, Fenner DE. Do the surgical outcomes of rectovaginal fistula repairs differ for obstetric and nonobstetric fistulas? A retrospective cohort study. Female Pelvic Med Reconstr Surg. 2019;25(1):36–40.

61. Kelly J. Vesico-vaginal and recto-vaginal fistulae. J Royal Soc Med. 1992;85:257–8.

62. Arrowsmith SD. Genitourinary reconstruction in obstetric fistulas. J Urol. 1994;152:403–6.

63. Emembolu J. The obstetric fistula: factors associated with improved pregnancy outcome after successful repair. Int J Gynecol Obstet. 1992;39:205–12.

64. Atlas of clinical gynecology. New York: McGraw-Hill; 2000.

65. Rothenberger DA, Goldberg SM. The management of Rectovaginal Fistulae. *Surg Clin N Am*. 1983;63(1):61–79.

66. Panés J, Rimola J. Perianal fistulizing Crohn's disease: pathogenesis, diagnosis and therapy. Nat Rev Gastroenterol Hepatol. 2017;14:652–64.

Patient Reported Outcomes After Childbirth

22

J. Oliver Daly

Overview
Test your learning and check your understanding of this book's contents: use the "Springer Nature Flashcards" app to access questions using ▶ https://sn.pub/wqrf89. To use the app, please follow the instructions in Chap. 1.

Learning Objectives
To provide a resource for identifying, selecting, and using appropriate childbirth-related pelvic floor trauma (CBRPFT) patient reported outcomes and measures (PRO/Ms) by developing an understanding of:

- The role of patient reported outcomes and measures (PRO/Ms) in research and clinical settings
- The context, development, and validation of PRO/Ms
- The domains of PRO/Ms
- Commonly used and validated PRO/Ms

22.1 Introduction

Patients are key stakeholders in determining the quality of maternity care, including the relative effectiveness of interventions to prevent and treat CBRPFT, and their recovery from such trauma within their own pregnancy experience. As such, when we assess the impact of trauma and associated interventions, we need to consider which outcomes are important to patients and can be reported by patients, using valid tools that accurately measure those outcomes.

CBRPFT can have short and long-term effects on pelvic floor function, symptoms, and health-related quality of life. In the case of longer-term consequences such as incontinence and pelvic organ prolapse, a range of non-obstetric related longitudinal factors e.g. genetics and age, can have an impact [1]; this can make it challenging to determine the *direct* effect of obstetric trauma and perinatal interventions on the patient reported outcome. As such, the scope of this chapter will focus on short-term PROMs, their general use in research and clinical settings, and evidence for specific PROMS in the evaluation of interventions and care for women who experience CBRPFT.

J. O. Daly (✉)
Department of Obstetrics and Gynaecology, Western Health, Melbourne, Australia

22.2 Patient Reported Outcomes (PRO) and Measures (PROM)

22.2.1 Defining PROMs

One of the key aims of healthcare is to improve outcomes important to patients and their experience, both in quality and satisfaction [2]. As such, PROs should be evaluated equally alongside clinical, quality of life (QOL), health resource utilization, and utility outcomes when evaluating healthcare interventions.

Patient Reported Outcomes (PROs) are defined as an outcome or observation that "comes directly from the patient about the status of particular aspects of, or events related to, a patient's health condition". PROs are recorded without amendment or interpretation of the patient's response by a clinician or other observer [3]. The PROM instrument or tool can be recorded by the patient directly or recorded by an interviewer, in a manner acceptable to the patient [3]. To provide a true translation of the qualitative patient experience from an outcome that is not directly observable (e.g. patient symptoms, impact of symptoms on QOL), into a quantitative score that can be analysed and compared [4], the PROM needs to be validated as a reliable and accurate measure of the outcome it intends to measure [3].

22.2.2 Types of PROMs

PROMs measure Health-related Quality of Life (HRQOL), a multidomain concept representing the patient's perception of the effect of illness and treatment on various aspects of life including physical, psychological, and social aspects. PROMs can be categorised as: [5, 6]

- *Generic*: These are PROMs that measure outcomes in broad populations including healthy and unwell individuals. These instruments are generally multidimensional, and assess the physical, social and emotional dimensions of life. These may be better for *comparing responses* from different groups, however are not sufficiently specific to identify symptoms or the impact on quality of life (QoL) for a specific group, or

- *Condition/population specific*: These are PROMs that measure outcomes specific for a medical condition or population being studied. They may be more appropriate for *diagnostic purposes* and provide increased sensitivity to change, while also minimising data collection burden.

22.2.3 PROM Validation

A range of validation methods are used to evaluate the fidelity of a PROM to ensure it measures what it intends. Validation is important because PROMs with poor or unknown psychometric properties may *overestimate* treatment effects in clinical trials [7]. Psychometric validation includes evaluating the reliability, validity, and responsiveness properties of the PROM within a cultural context [6, 8–10], as summarised in Table 22.1. For those developing a PROM, it is recommended that the Patient-Reported Outcomes Measurement Information System (PROMIS®) instrument development and validation scientific standards methodology is utilized [11].

PROMs that are validated in one language or cultural group may require adaptation in others, and readability must be at or below a sixth-to-eighth grade reading level [8], as per the National Institute of Health and Center for Disease Control recommendations. Unfortunately, many pelvic floor questionnaires are written at a higher level [11]. To assist those evaluating/selecting PROMs, researchers should publish validation studies in accordance with the Consensus-based Standards for the selection of health Measurement Instruments (COSMIN) reporting guidelines [13].

22.2.4 Evaluation and Selection of a PROM

When selecting a PROM, the first consideration is whether it will be used in a clinical or research context, followed by the patient population, condition, intervention and outcome being measured. Factors to consider when selecting a PROM, include [6]:

Table 22.1 PROM Psychometric Validation Properties [6, 8]

Validation property/ definition	Description of method	Parameters with statistical validity threshold if stated
Reliability: Ability of a measure to produce similar results when assessments are repeated. Change detected by the measure is due to the treatment or intervention and not due to measurement error or variability [10].		
Test-retest of same subject group	Results can be reproduced with repeated testing, when no change is expected. To test, patient completes the questionnaire more than once, at baseline and again after a period of time during which the impact of symptoms is unlikely to change	Spearman's correlation and Intraclass Coefficient (ICC): $r > 0.70, p > 0.05$
Internal consistency	Extent to which items within a PROM measure the same concept	Cronbach-α: $c > 0.70$
Inter-rater reliabilility	How well scores correlate when a measure is administered by different interviewers or when multiple observers rate the same phenomenon	Percentage agreement, Cohen's kappa, or Intraclass Coefficient [12]
Validity: Ability of an instrument to measure the outcome and condition for which it was intended as evaluated by the following methods: • Construct: whether quantitative relationships between the condition, groups of patients and scores conform with hypothesised conceptual framework • Content: qualitative assessment of whether the questionnaire items capture the range of the content it is intended to measure. • Criterion: correlation with gold standard measure, or another accepted measure if no standard exists		
Construct	Multi-trait scaling, confirmatory factor analysis: consistency with hypothesized measurement model	Factor loadings >0.6
	Convergence: degree to which the proposed scale correlates with another assessment tool assessing the same concept	Spearman's correlation coefficient: $r > 0.70$
	Divergence: degree to which scale does not correlate with a tool assessing and unrelated concept	Spearman's correlation coefficient: $r < 0.30$
	Discriminative: ability to distinguish between different patient groups	Spearman's correlation and Intraclass Coefficient (ICC): $r > 0.70, p > 0.05$
Content	Condition/domain captured by questions	Present or absent
Criterion	Concurrent validity against standard	Spearman's correlation coefficient: $r > 0.70$
	Predictive validity, predictive regression models	Spearman's correlation coefficient: $r > 0.70$
Responsiveness Ability to detect change, better or worse, in a patient's condition, over time or following an intervention. It is also important to evaluate the Minimal Important Difference (MID) i.e. whether that change is meaningful for the patient. This may help differentiate a statistically significant change from a clinically significant difference.		
Sensitivity to change	Comparison of scores before and after an intervention	Spearman's correlation and Intraclass Coefficient (ICC): $r > 0.70, p > 0.05$
Minimal important difference	Smallest change in a PRO questionnaire score that would be considered meaningful or important to a patient with no specific parameter or cutoff to determine MID. May use anchor-based methods comparing the measure score to another clinically relevant measures (anchors) or using statistical distributions of the data e.g. effect size, one-half standard deviation, and standard error of measurement [6, 11].	No standard cutoff for MID, determined by method.

- Relevance
- Validation
- Acceptability
- Cultural appropriateness
- Language validation
- Length/number of questions
- Simplicity-Readability

When evaluating psychometric validity, the original published validation study should be used to assess its robustness and appropriateness within the researcher or clinician's work [14]. Recognised rating schema such as the COSMIN checklist, may be of assistance [14, 15]. The International Consultation on Incontinence (ICI) also uses a grading system for PROM recommendations with stringent criteria that allow categorization as (A) Highly recommended, (B) Recommended and (C) Potential. These grades have been applied to a number of pelvic floor PROMs [6].

Of note, PROMs are validated for use as a *whole* instrument. Therefore, *selective* use (e.g. using only parts of the PROM, changing wording or using the tool in patient groups, conditions or languages for which it hasn't been validated), may limit the fidelity of outcomes reported.

The use of validated PROMs also allows for standardisation of clinical information provided to clinicians from the patient's perspective, versus the traditional clinician-oriented method of obtaining a clinical history [16]. For example, the use of PROMs eliminates the clinician's underestimation of the degree of patient bother, which can occur in up to one-third of encounters [17]. Routine use of PROMs leads to improved communication and decision making between doctors and patients [18], as well as in improved HRQOL outcomes [19]. However, embedding systematic use of PROMs into routine clinical practice can be complex. Consideration needs to be given to the method of PRO/M administration (e.g. phone, paper or electronic), and establishing a culture of using PRO/M data in real time as part of clinical care. This requires high levels of organisational support [20, 21]. Patients may also need free text options to capture other concerns, not captured by the PROM [22].

22.3 Domains of Patient Reported Outcomes Associated with Childbirth-Related Pelvic Floor Trauma (CBRPFT)

CBRPFT may result in a range of adverse outcomes. In considering which CBRPFT PRO domains to utilize, a systematic review of PRO/Ms used in perineal trauma intervention randomized controlled trials (RCTs) [17], found 47 trials reporting 51 PROs, grouped into 4 themes and 12 domains, based on the Core Outcome Measures in Effectiveness Trials (COMET) Core Outcome Set taxonomy (Table 22.2):

The most common PROMs used were the Visual Analogue Score (VAS) [21] (100 mm and 0–10 numerical), the Cleveland Clinic Continence (Wexner) score [23], Fecal Incontinence Quality-of-Life (FIQOL) score [24], and McGill Pain Questionnaire [25]. However, there was significant heterogeneity in the use of validated and unvalidated PROMs. As such, the authors recommend that a core outcome set (COS) and core outcome measures set (COMS) be developed for trials investigating CBRPFT interventions [17].

Table 22.2 Themes and Domains used to categorise patient reported outcomes using the COMET Taxonomy [17]

Theme	Domain
Clinical	Pregnancy, puerperium and perinatal symptoms
	Gastrointestinal symptoms
	General outcomes including sexual function
	Urinary symptoms
Life impact	Quality of life
	Physical functioning
	Social functioning
	Emotional functioning and mental health
	Delivery of care
Resource usage	Need for intervention
	Societal burden
Adverse events	Adverse events/effects

22.4 Commonly Used and Validated PROMs

There are a large number of PROMs validated for female pelvic floor dysfunction (PFD) [17, 21], however, very few are validated in the postpartum population [20, 22]. The following is a summary of validated and/or commonly used PROMs across the spectrum of postpartum domains.

22.4.1 Bowel Function

Bowel function is one of the most important outcomes of CBRPFT, including storage and defecatory symptoms [26], as well as the impact on associated HRQOL. Anal incontinence (AI) is reported in up to 38% of women following birth [27, 28], up to 25% in later life and increasing to >50% in those with a previous anal sphincter injury [29]. Over two-thirds of women do not seek care [30]. AI significantly impacts quality of life [31], with women experiencing anxiety about resolution, thus affecting their choices about future pregnancies [32]. Similarly, choice of subsequent mode of birth may be associated with symptoms [33, 34]. In the early recovery phase, defecatory symptoms such as dyschezia, anal fissures and haemorrhoids may also cause considerable bother [35], with constipation being a significant contributor [36].

While there are a large number of pelvic floor PROMs assessing bowel function [21], validated PROMs should be used preferentially, as they identify higher rates of AI and have high response rates of 92–100% up to 6 weeks postnatal [16]. As such, they are the most suitable candidate PROMs for consideration in *routine* clinical practice. A systematic review of methods for identifying AI in postpartum women identified 14 validated PROMs [16], with three predominantly measuring the type and frequency of storage symptoms: the Cleveland Clinic Incontinence (Wexner) Score [23], Pescatori Anal Incontinence Score [37] and Fecal Incontinence Questionnaire (FIQ) [38]. The Fecal Incontinence Quality of Life (FIQoL) score focuses on QOL, while PROMs such as the Modified Manchester Health Questionnaire (MMHQ) [39] measure both symptoms and impact on qual-

ity of life. The importance of measuring impact is highlighted by the finding that alterations in lifestyle, as a result of AI, is significantly associated with bother, even with low Wexner scores [40]. When considering defecation symptoms related to haemorrhoids and anal fissures, the HEMO-FISS-QoL PROM has been validated for use in the general population, including reproductive age women, in research and routine clinical settings [41]. It includes the dimensions of physical disorders and function, psychological and social impact, defecation and sexuality.

22.4.2 Urinary Function

Of those reporting postpartum urinary incontinence (UI), 63% experience stress urinary incontinence (SUI), 12% urgency urinary incontinence (UUI), and 22% mixed urinary incontinence (MUI) [42]. Postnatally, mean prevalence rates of UI at 3 months are reported in up to 33%, with 25% of women overall experiencing SUI and UUI in 15% [43]. Prevalence estimates do vary depending on the study population, type of study, UI definition and threshold, method and timing of data collection and questionnaire type [44].

While CBRPFT is associated with pelvic floor dysfunction, the impact of such trauma on UI is unclear, as most UI resolves by one year [45]. In the short term, SUI is associated with the following: UI during pregnancy, an instrumental vaginal birth, episiotomy, tears, and constipation. However, in the longer term, only UI during pregnancy remains a significant risk factor for SUI [46]. Levator avulsion does not appear to be a risk factor for SUI [47]. but SUI *is* associated with anal sphincter injury [48]. There is no reported association between CBRPFT and UUI.

Overt postpartum urinary retention has an incidence of 5% [49], but carries a widely reported range of 1–45% depending on the definition used [50]. It is associated with CBRPFT including levator avulsion [51], anal sphincter injury, prolonged second stage of labour, instrumental birth, episiotomy, degree of perineal pain, and fetal birth weight [52]. There is also a strong association with transient factors such as epidural analgesia.

Only one Grade A PROM has been validated in a perinatal cohort: the International Consultation on Incontinence Questionnaire-Urinary Incontinence Short Form (ICIQ-UI SF) [53]. This PROM measures UI frequency, volume, impact on quality of life, and perceived cause of incontinence [54]. The Assessment of Pelvic Floor Disorders and Their Risk Factors During Pregnancy and Postpartum Questionnaire (APFDQ), has also been validated perinatally. It includes storage and voiding symptoms, pain, as well as impact on daily life and bother [55]. As such, *either* questionnaire could be used in research or clinical contexts.

22.4.3 Pelvic Organ Prolapse (POP) and Vaginal Symptoms

In the long term, CBRPFT related to levator ani avulsion is associated with a higher stage of pelvic organ prolapse (POP) [56] and risk of recurrent POP [57]. There are a number of Grade A recommended POP PROMs that have been used in studies of perinatal cohorts. These include [20]:

- International Consultation of Incontinence Questionnaire-Vaginal Symptoms (ICIQ-VS) [58]
- Pelvic Floor Distress Inventory 20 (PFDI-20) [59]
- Pelvic Floor Impact Questionnaire (PFIQ-7) [59]

While, not yet graded, the Australian Pelvic Floor Questionnaire (APFDQ) is the only PROM validated in the perinatal period [55].

22.4.4 Sexual Health

Sexual health is defined as a state of physical, emotional, mental and social well-being in relation to sexuality, with the possibility of having pleasurable and safe sexual experiences [60]. The World Health Organization (WHO) recommends women are asked about sexual intercourse resumption and dyspareunia when reviewed postnatally [61]. While postpartum sexual dysfunction is reported in as many as 60% of women at 6 months postnatal, only 15% discuss such

problems with a health professional [62]. Sexual dysfunction is associated with physical, hormonal and psychosocial factors [63], delays resumption of sexual activity, affects all sexual domains [64], and QoL. CBRPFT is strongly associated with dyspareunia [65], and diminished sexual function.

Several validated female sexual function PROMs exist, however, none have been fully validated in the perinatal cohort. The most commonly used is the Female Sexual Function Index (FSFI) [66], but has only a single question about dyspareunia [67]. Others PROMs include:

- Pelvic Organ Prolapse Urinary Incontinence Sexual Questionnaire (PISQ) [68]
- PISQ-12 [69]
- Pelvic Organ Prolapse Urinary Incontinence Sexual Questionnaire, International Urogynecological Association Revised (PISQ-IR) [70]
- International Consultation of Incontinence Questionnaire-Vaginal Symptoms (ICIQ-VS)

22.4.5 Global Pelvic Floor Dysfunction PROMs

CBRPFT can adversely affect global pelvic floor function and several validated PROMs evaluating *multiple or all PFD* domains exist. A recent systematic review identified nine validated PROMs that have been used in the postpartum period:

- International Consultation of Incontinence Questionnaire - Vaginal Symptoms (ICIQ-VS)
- Pelvic Floor Distress Inventories (PFDI-20 and 46 [71])
- Pelvic Floor Impact Questionnaires (PFIQ-7 and 31 [71])
- Pelvic Floor Bother Questionnaire (PFBQ [72])
- Australian Pelvic Floor Questionnaires (APFQ [73] and APFDQ)
- electronic Personal Assessment Questionnaire-Pelvic Floor (ePAQ-PF [74])

Of these, the PFDI-20, PFIQ-7, and ICIQ-VS have a grade A ICI recommendation [6]. The only questionnaire validated in a postpartum population is the APFDQ. It has so far been validated in German [55], Italian [75], Turkish [76], and Brazilian Portuguese [77].

22.4.6 Pain

CBRPFT is associated with pain in up to 90% of women [78], and may become chronic in up to 10% of postpartum women following vaginal birth [79]. Chronic pain related to trauma is defined as pain that develops after a tissue injury, involving any trauma, and persists at least 3 months after the trauma [80]. It may be associated with postpartum depression and postpartum physical function, psychosocial wellbeing, sleep, breastfeeding success, and maternal-neonatal bonding [81]. A number of pain PROMs have been used in the postpartum cohort, the most common being the unidimensional Visual Analogue Scales (VAS) scales [81]. The McGill Pain Questionnaire (MPQ) and the Brief Pain Inventory (BPI) [82] have been widely used in postpartum studies, and have a Grade B recommendation [6]. The Short-form Brief Pain Inventory (SF-BPI) [83] is the one multi-dimensional PROM with a grade A recommendation, however, it requires further perinatal validation [81].

22.4.7 Birth Experience and Perception of Trauma

A traumatic birth has been defined as "the emergence of a baby from its mother in a way that involves events or care that cause deep distress or psychological disturbance, which may or may not involve physical injury, but resulting in psychological distress of an enduring nature" [84], with up to 45% of women experience childbirth as a traumatic event [85]. When a complication does occur, birth is more likely to be associated with a negative experience and dissatisfaction [86, 87]. This may be further exacerbated in those women who have experienced birth interventions or other complications [88] that may also be associated with CBRPFT. Secondary tokophobia, (fear of childbirth following a previous negative or traumatic experience of childbirth [89]) may be one such outcome that either delays future childbearing [90], and/or affect future mode of birth.

Measuring the direct effect of CBRPFT on trauma related to birth experience is challenging, as no validated scales exist [91]. While more than 17 PROMs have been developed to measure women's and/or their partner's satisfaction with maternity care (e.g. Birth Satisfaction Scale-Revised [92]), these instruments have been validated in healthy women with low-risk pregnancies [93]. It is recommended that existing instruments be evaluated in the CBRPFT cohorts before developing new PROMs [94].

22.4.8 Emotional Functioning and Mental Health

Antenatal mental health issues are associated with negative birth experiences [95], and negative experiences during pregnancy and childbirth trauma are significant risk factors for developing mood disorders in the perinatal period [91]. A recent systematic review identified 76 mood disorder screening tools used in the perinatal cohort [96]; of the validated tools, those used most frequent were the:

- Edinburgh Postnatal Depression Scale (EPDS) [97]
- Beck's Depression Inventory (BDI) [98]
- Patient Health Questionnaire (PHQ) [99]

However, there are gaps in the validation of tools screening for anxiety, post-trauma stress disorder and bipolar affective disorders. In general, the clinical use of mental health screening tools requires careful consideration of the psychological, social and cultural risk factors in the respective perinatal cohort and health system [96].

22.4.8.1 Post-Traumatic Stress Disorder (PTSD)

PTSD is a trauma and stressor-related disorder defined as significant distress or impaired functioning persisting for greater than 1 month following an event, either directly experienced, or experienced by a close family member/friend. There may be avoidance, associated negative thoughts or mood, and/or marked reactivity related to similar events [100]. PTSD is experienced by up to 4% of women [101], but may be as high as 19% in high-risk groups, such as those experiencing a difficult birth [102]. Important factors that may contribute to postpartum PTSD include negative subjective birth experiences, obstetric interventions, lack of support, dissociation [103], as well as perception of poor care [104].

Three PTSD PROMs have been validated for use in peripartum cohorts:

- Traumatic Event Scale [105]
- Perinatal PTSD Questionnaire [106]
- City Birth Trauma Scale (City BiTS) [107]

Only the City BiTS has been developed to measure all DSM-5 PTSD diagnostic criteria [107]. As a screening tool, it has been shown to be sensitive to type of birth, gestational age and perception of birth trauma related to fear of death or injury [108]. A partner version of the City BiTS has also been developed, but requires further validation [109].

22.5 Postpartum Recovery

An emerging area of research has been that of postpartum recovery, with a recent systematic review [110] and focus group study, including patients, midwives/nurses, obstetricians and anaesthetists. This review proposes a conceptual model consisting of 13 domains for assessing inpatient and outpatient postpartum recovery [111]. This body of work focuses of the development of a global set of PRO/Ms for up to six weeks post-partum. The initial study observed a difference between the rankings of issues *perceived to be significant,* prior to birth, versus those issues *reported to affect recovery,* subsequent to birth, indicating a shift in priorities prior to and follow-

ing birth. Evaluation of the conceptual model did not include physical trauma or traumatic birth as risk factors, so there is still a need to validate the recovery model in the CBRPFT cohort [112].

22.6 Generic Pregnancy and Childbirth-Specific PROMs

A number of generic pregnancy and childbirth-related PROMs have been developed and used [113], yet few have been validated in the CBPRFT cohort. A standard set of PROMS for measuring pregnancy outcomes and QoL has been proposed by the International Consortium for Health Outcomes Measurement (ICHOM) [114, 115]. It was developed in a case-mix of patients across 14 outcome domains, but other than mode of birth, did not include specific indicators of CBRPFT. However, it does include measures that may be directly related to CBRPFT; urinary and bowel incontinence using the ICIQ-SF and Wexner scores, respectively, and pain during intercourse, using an item from the PROMIS Sexual Function and Satisfaction Measures (SexFS) tool [116]. Unfortunately, only the ICIQ-SF is validated in perinatal cohorts. An implementation feasibility study concluded that while patients and clinicians found the ICHOM set of PROMs feasible, implementation considerations included the need for information technology support as well as a change in professionals' responsibilities in noticing, discussing, and acting upon responses and outcomes [117].

There are a number of resources available to search for, and identify relevant PROMs as per Table 22.3.

Table 22.3 Resources for identifying and assessing PRO/Ms.

Resource name	Description
The National Institute of Health (NIH) Patient-Reported Outcome Measurement Information System (PROMIS) [118]	Provides access to standardised PRO measures calibrated and referenced to the US general population, including generic and condition- specific PROMs
The ICHOM Set of Patient-Centered Outcome Measures for Pregnancy And Childbirth [115]	Recommendation of outcomes that matter most to pregnant women
Consensus-based standards for the selection of health measurement instruments (COSMIN) [14, 15]	Provides a database of systematic reviews of health measurement instruments
Patient-Reported Outcomes and Quality of Life Instruments Database (PROQOLID) [119]	Provides documentation of the measurement properties for over 1000 PROs
Patient Reported Outcome Measures, International Consultation on Incontinence [6]	Comprehensive review of PRO/Ms. for the evaluation of pelvic floor dysfunction and Quality of Life impact to guide the selection and use of instruments by clinicians and researchers, including PROM quality grading recommendations
Patient-reported outcomes, Cochrane handbook for systematic reviews of interventions [120]	A step-by-step approach to the evaluation of PRO/Ms. used in randomised trials when conducting systematic reviews and meta-analyses, and a useful guide for those considering PRO/Ms. in intervention studies

22.7 Conclusions

There are number of considerations that need to be considered when evaluating, selecting, and implementing measures for outcomes in women with CBRPFT. These include assessing the following:

- Suitability in the respective patient cohort
- Validation within the study context and cohort
- Feasibility to ensure the PROMs are completed by patients and either incorporated into clinical practice, or able to measure effectiveness of interventions in clinical trials

While not providing specific guidance on which PROM to use, we hope the information provided in this chapter assists clinicians and researchers with the principles, knowledge, and resources to identify PROMs most suitable to their context to support improving patient care.

Take Home Messages
- Childbirth and related pelvic floor trauma impact the physical, psychological, and social wellbeing of women and their families, and their recovery from such experiences.
- To evaluate interventions and provide care, we need to consider outcomes that are important

to and can be reported by patients, using valid tools that accurately measure those outcomes.
- The relevant domains for assessing CBRPFT include the following:
  - Pelvic floor function - bowel, urinary, pelvic organ prolapse and sexual function
  - Pain
  - Emotional wellbeing and mental health
  - Postpartum recovery
- Validated PROMs should be used to evaluate the above domains.
- PROM selection depends on the research or clinical context and requires careful evaluation with respect to the relevance, psychometric validation, cultural and language validation, acceptability, length, and readability. A range of resources are available to assist researchers and clinicians.

Appendix: MCQ

Mark each item TRUE or FALSE

Questions

1. Which of the following is a psychometric property of a PROM?
   (A) Responsiveness

(B) Reactivity
(C) Validity
(D) Accuracy
(E) Reliability

2. Benefits of the use of PROMs include:
   (A) Documentation of the clinician's observation in the patient's words
   (B) Are flexible in being able to use parts of PROM as required
   (C) Documentation of patient's response without interpretation by the clinician
   (D) Replaces the need for clinical assessment
   (E) Can translate qualitative into quantitative outcomes

3. Considerations when assessing a PROM include:
   (A) Readability
   (B) Clinical setting
   (C) Relevance to the condition
   (D) Method of administration
   (E) Number of questions

4. The following is an example of a PROM validated in a perinatal cohort:
   (A) Visual Analogue Scale
   (B) ICIQ Urinary Incontinence Short Form
   (C) Pelvic Floor Distress Inventories (PFDI-20)
   (D) Female Sexual Function Index
   (E) Edinburgh Postnatal Depression Scale

5. When using PROMs in clinical practice, considerations include:
   (A) Organisational support
   (B) Languages spoken
   (C) Method of administration
   (D) Adjusting PROM to measure unit outcomes
   (E) Culture of collecting PROMs

Answers

1. Which of the following is a psychometric property of a PROM?
   (A) TRUE

(B) FALSE
(C) TRUE
(D) FALSE
(E) TRUE

2. Benefits of the use of PROMs include:
   (A) FALSE
   (B) FALSE
   (C) TRUE
   (D) FALSE
   (E) TRUE

3. Considerations when assessing a PROM include:
   (A) TRUE
   (B) TRUE
   (C) TRUE
   (D) FALSE
   (E) TRUE

4. The following is an example of a PROM validated in a perinatal cohort:
   (A) FALSE
   (B) TRUE
   (C) FALSE
   (D) FALSE
   (E) TRUE

5. When using PROMs in clinical practice, considerations include:
   (A) TRUE
   (B) TRUE
   (C) TRUE
   (D) FALSE
   (E) TRUE

References

1. Deprest JA, Cartwright R, Dietz HP, et al. International Urogynecological Consultation (IUC): pathophysiology of pelvic organ prolapse (POP). Int Urogynecol J. 2022; https://doi.org/10.1007/s00192-022-05081-0.
2. Berwick DM, Nolan TW, Whittington J. The triple aim: care, health, and cost. Health Aff. 2008;27:759–69.
3. Velentgas P, Dreyer NA, Nourjah P, Smith SR, Torchia MM. Developing a protocol for observa-

tional comparative effectiveness research: a user's guide. Rockville (MD): Agency for Healthcare Research and Quality (US); 2013.

4. Krogsgaard MR, Brodersen J, Christensen KB, Siersma V, Kreiner S, Jensen J, Hansen CF, Comins JD. What is a PROM and why do we need it? Scand J Med Sci Sports. 2021;31:967–71.

5. About PROMs | Australian Commission on Safety and Quality in Health Care. https://www.safetyandquality.gov.au/our-work/indicators-measurement-and-reporting/patient-reported-outcomes/about-proms. Accessed 26 Mar 2022.

6. Abrams P, Cardozo L, Wagg A, Wein A. Patient reported outcome assessment. In: Incontinence, vol. 1. 6th ed. Bristol, UK: International Continence Society; 2016. p. 541–98.

7. Gagnier JJ, Johnston BC. Poor quality patient reported outcome measures bias effect estimates in orthopaedic randomized studies. J Clin Epidemiol. 2019;116:36–8.

8. Lee JT, Madoff RD, Rockwood TH. Quality-of-life measures in fecal incontinence: is validation valid? Dis Colon Rectum. 2015;58:352–7.

9. Food and Drug Administration (2009) Patient reported outcome measures: use in medical product development to support labelling claims. In: (CDER) CfDEaRFaDA, editor. Silver Spring, MD: US Dept of Health and Human Services Food and Drug Administration.

10. Deshpande P, Bl S, Rajan S, Abdul Nazir C. Patient-reported outcomes: a new era in clinical research. Perspect Clin Res. 2011;2:137.

11. PROMIS® Instrument Development and Validation Scientific Standards, Version 2.0 (revised May 2013). p. 72.

12. Alavi M, Biros E, Cleary M. A primer of inter-rater reliability in clinical measurement studies: pros and pitfalls. J Clin Nurs. 2022;31:e39–42.

13. Gagnier JJ, Lai J, Mokkink LB, Terwee CB. COSMIN reporting guideline for studies on measurement properties of patient-reported outcome measures. Qual Life Res. 2021;30:2197–218.

14. Mokkink LB, Prinsen CA, Patrick DL, Alonso J, Bouter LM, de Vet HC, Terwee CB (2019) COSMIN Study Design checklist for Patient-reported outcome measurement instruments. Amsterdam, The Netherlands. pp. 1–32.

15. Checklists for Assessing Study Qualities. COSMIN. In: COSMIN. https://www.cosmin.nl/tools/checklists-assessing-methodological-study-qualities/. Accessed 31 Mar 2022.

16. Gray TG, Vickers H, Jha S, Jones GL, Brown SR, Radley SC. A systematic review of non-invasive modalities used to identify women with anal incontinence symptoms after childbirth. Int Urogynecol J. 2019;30:869–79.

17. Doumouchtsis SK, Loganathan J, Fahmy J, Falconi G, Rada M, Elfituri A, Haddad JM, Pergialiotis V, Betschart C, CHORUS: An International Collaboration for Harmonising Outcomes, Research and Standards in Urogynaecology and Women's Health. Patient-reported outcomes and outcome measures in childbirth perineal trauma research: a systematic review. Int Urogynecol J. 2021;32:1695–706.

18. McCormack HM, Horne DJDL, Sheather S. Clinical applications of visual analogue scales: a critical review. Psychol Med. 1988;18:1007–19.

19. Cockell SJ, Oates-Johnson T, Gilmour DT, Vallis TM, Turnbull GK. Postpartum flatal and fecal incontinence quality-of-life scale: a disease- and population-specific measure. Qual Health Res. 2003;13:1132–44.

20. Suzuki Zuchelo LT, Pinheiro Bezerra IM, Marcial Da Silva AT, Menezes Gomes J, Soares JM Jr, Chada Baracat E, de Abreu LC, Esposito Sorpreso IC. Questionnaires to evaluate pelvic floor dysfunction in the postpartum period: a systematic review. IJWH. 2018;10:409–24.

21. Gray TG, Vickers H, Krishnaswamy P, Jha S. A systematic review of English language patient-reported outcome measures for use in urogynaecology and female pelvic medicine. Int Urogynecol J. 2021;32:2033–92.

22. Grigoriadis T, Athanasiou S, Rizk D. Female pelvic floor dysfunction questionnaires: the modern Tower of Babel? Int Urogynecol J. 2020;31:1059–61.

23. Jorge MJN, Wexner SD. Etiology and management of fecal incontinence. Dis Colon Rectum. 1993;36:77–97.

24. Rockwood TH, Church JM, Fleshman JW, Kane RL, Mavrantonis C, Thorson AG, Wexner SD, Bliss D, Lowry AC. Fecal incontinence quality of life scale: quality of life instrument for patients with fecal incontinence. Dis Colon Rectum. 2000;43: 9–16.

25. Melzack R. The McGill Pain Questionnaire: major properties and scoring methods. Pain. 1975;1:277–99.

26. LaCross A, Groff M, Smaldone A. Obstetric anal sphincter injury and anal incontinence following vaginal birth: a systematic review and meta-analysis. J Midwifery Womens Health. 2015;60:37–47.

27. Sideris M, McCaughey T, Hanrahan JG, Arroyo-Manzano D, Zamora J, Jha S, Knowles CH, Thakar R, Chaliha C, Thangaratinam S. Risk of obstetric anal sphincter injuries (OASIS) and anal incontinence: a meta-analysis Eur J Obstetr Gynecol Reprod Biol. 2020;252:303–12.

28. Guise J-M, Morris C, Osterweil P, Li H, Rosenberg D, Greenlick M. Incidence of fecal incontinence after childbirth. Obstetr Gynecol. 2007;109(2 Part 1):8.

29. Wegnelius G, Hammarström M. Complete rupture of anal sphincter in primiparas: long-term effects and subsequent delivery: sphincter rupture and subsequent delivery. Acta Obstetr Gynecol Scand. 2010;90(3):258–63.

30. Brown HW, Wexner SD, Lukacz ES. Factors associated with care seeking among women with acci-

dental bowel leakage. Female Pelvic Med Reconstr Surg. 2013;19:66–71.

31. Keighley MRB, Perston Y, Bradshaw E, Hayes J, Keighley DM, Webb S. The social, psychological, emotional morbidity and adjustment techniques for women with anal incontinence following obstetric anal sphincter injury: use of a word picture to identify a hidden syndrome. BMC Pregnancy Childbirth. 2016;16:275.

32. Darmody E, Bradshaw C, Atkinson S. Women's experience of obstetric anal sphincter injury following childbirth: An integrated review. Midwifery. 2020;91:102820.

33. Fitzpatrick M, Cassidy M, Barassaud ML, Hehir MP, Hanly AM, O'Connell PR, O'Herlihy C. Does anal sphincter injury preclude subsequent vaginal delivery? Eur J Obstetr Gynecol Reprod Biol. 2016;198:30–4.

34. Woolner AM, Ayansina D, Black M, Bhattacharya S. The impact of third- or fourth-degree perineal tears on the second pregnancy: a cohort study of 182,445 Scottish women. PLoS One. 2019;14:e0215180.

35. Abramowitz L, Sobhani I, Benifla JL, Vuagnat A, Darai E, Mignon M, Madelenat P. Anal fissure and thrombosed external hemorrhoids before and after delivery. Dis Colon Rectum. 2002;45:650–5.

36. Ferdinande K, Dorreman Y, Roelens K, Ceelen W, De Looze D. Anorectal symptoms during pregnancy and postpartum: a prospective cohort study. Color Dis. 2018;20:1109–16.

37. Pescatori M, Anastasio G, Bottini C, Mentasti A. New grading and scoring for anal incontinence. Dis Colon Rectum. 1992;35:482–7.

38. Reilly WT, Talley NJ, Pemberton JH, Zinsmeister AR. Validation of a questionnaire to assess fecal incontinence and associated risk factors. Dis Colon Rectum. 2000;43:146–53.

39. Kwon S, Visco AG, Fitzgerald MP, Ye W, Whitehead WE. Validity and reliability of the modified Manchester Health Questionnaire in assessing patients with fecal incontinence. Dis Colon Rectum. 2005;48:323–34.

40. Jangö H, Langhoff-Roos J, Rosthøj S, Sakse A. Wexner score and quality of life in women with obstetric anal sphincter injury. Int Urogynecol J. 2020;31:1115–21.

41. Abramowitz L, Bouchard D, Siproudhis L, Trompette M, Pillant H, Bord C, Senejoux C, Favreau-Weltzer C, Berdeaux G, Zkik A. Psychometric properties of a questionnaire (HEMO-FISS-QoL) to evaluate the burden associated with haemorrhoidal disease and anal fissures. Color Dis. 2019;21:48–58.

42. Moossdorff-Steinhauser HFA, Berghmans BCM, Spaanderman MEA, Bols EMJ. Prevalence, incidence and bothersomeness of urinary incontinence in pregnancy: a systematic review and meta-analysis. Int Urogynecol J. 2021;32:1633–52.

43. Thom DH, Rortveit G. Prevalence of postpartum urinary incontinence: a systematic review. Acta Obstet Gynecol Scand. 2010;89:1511–22.

44. Langeland S, Hunskaar S, Rortveit G. Epidemiology of urinary incontinence in pregnancy and postpartum. In: Urinary incontinence. Rijeka: InTech; 2012. https://doi.org/10.5772/33742.

45. Fritel X, Ringa V, Quiboeuf E, Fauconnier A. Female urinary incontinence, from pregnancy to menopause: a review of epidemiological and pathophysiological findings: Female urinary incontinence, from pregnancy to menopause. Acta Obstet Gynecol Scand. 2012;91:901–10.

46. Hage-Fransen MA, Wiezer M, Otto A, Wieffer-Platvoet MS, Slotman MH, Nijhuis-van der Sanden MW, Pool-Goudzwaard AL. Pregnancy-and obstetric-related risk factors for urinary incontinence, fecal incontinence, or pelvic organ prolapse later in life: a systematic review and meta-analysis. Acta Obstet Gynecol Scand. 2021;100:373–82.

47. Smeets CFA, Vergeldt TFM, Notten KJB, Martens FMJ, Kuijk SMJ. Association between levator ani avulsion and urinary incontinence in women: a systematic review and meta-analysis. Int J Gynecol Obstet. 2021;153:25–32.

48. Scheer I, Andrews V, Thakar R, Sultan AH. Urinary incontinence after obstetric anal sphincter injuries (OASIS)—is there a relationship? Int Urogynecol J Pelvic Floor Dysfunct. 2008;19:179–83.

49. Yip S-K, Sahota D, Pang M-W, Chang A. Postpartum urinary retention. Acta Obstet Gynecol Scand. 2004;83(10):881–91.

50. Mulder F, Hakvoort R, Schoffelmeer M, Limpens J, Van der Post J, Roovers J. Postpartum urinary retention: a systematic review of adverse effects and management. Int Urogynecol J. 2014;25:1605–12.

51. Gonzalez-Díaz E, Biurrun GP. Levator ani muscle avulsion: a risk factor for persistent postpartum voiding dysfunction. Int Urogynecol J. 2020;31:2327–35.

52. Mohr S, Raio L, Gobrecht-Keller U, Imboden S, Mueller MD, Kuhn A. Postpartum urinary retention: what are the sequelae? A long-term study and review of the literature: Int Urogynecol J; 2022. https://doi.org/10.1007/s00192-021-05074-5.

53. Avery K, Donovan J, Peters TJ, Shaw C, Gotoh M, Abrams P. ICIQ: a brief and robust measure for evaluating the symptoms and impact of urinary incontinence. Neurourol Urodyn. 2004;23:322–30.

54. Slavin V, Gamble J, Creedy DK, Fenwick J. Perinatal incontinence: psychometric evaluation of the international consultation on incontinence questionnaire—urinary incontinence short form and Wexner scale. Neurourol Urodyn. 2019;38:2209–23.

55. Metz M, Junginger B, Henrich W, Baeßler K. Development and validation of a questionnaire for the assessment of pelvic floor disorders and their risk factors during pregnancy and post partum. Geburtshilfe Frauenheilkd. 2017;77:358–65.

56. Dietz H, Simpson J. Levator trauma is associated with pelvic organ prolapse. BJOG Int J Obstet Gynaecol. 2008;115:979–84.

57. Friedman T, Eslick GD, Dietz HP. Risk factors for prolapse recurrence: systematic review and meta-analysis. Int Urogynecol J. 2018;29:13–21.

58. Price N, Jackson S, Avery K, Brookes S, Abrams P. Development and psychometric evaluation of the ICIQ Vaginal Symptoms Questionnaire: the ICIQ-VS. BJOG Int J Obstet Gynaecol. 2006;113:700–12.

59. Barber M, Walters M, Bump R. Short forms of two condition-specific quality-of-life questionnaires for women with pelvic floor disorders (PFDI-20 and PFIQ-7). Am J Obstet Gynecol. 2005;193:103–13.

60. World Health Organisation (2006) Defining sexual health. https://www.who.int/teams/sexual-and-reproductive-health-and-research/key-areas-of-work/sexual-health/defining-sexual-health. Accessed 1 May 2022.

61. World Health Organization. Postnatal care of the mother and newborn. Geneva: World Health Organization; 2013.

62. Barrett G, Pendry E, Peacock J, Victor C, Thakar R, Manyonda I. Women's sexual health after childbirth. BJOG. 2000;107:186–95.

63. Leader-Cramer A, Kenton K, Dave B, Gossett DR, Mueller M, Lewicky-Gaupp C. Factors associated with timing of return to intercourse after obstetric anal sphincter injuries. J Sex Med. 2016;13:1523–9.

64. Roos A-M, Speksnijder L, Steensma AB. Postpartum sexual function; the importance of the levator ani muscle. Int Urogynecol J. 2020;31:2261–7.

65. Gutzeit O, Levy G, Lowenstein L. Postpartum female sexual function: risk factors for postpartum sexual dysfunction. Sexual Med. 2020;8:8–13.

66. Brown RC, Heiman J, Leiblum S, Meston C, Shabsigh R, Ferguson D, D'Agostino R. The Female Sexual Function Index (FSFI): a multidimensional self-report instrument for the assessment of female sexual function. J Sex Marital Ther. 2000;26:191–208.

67. López-Lapeyrere C, Serna-Gómez N, Hernández-López AB, Pérez-García MF, Tejeda-Esteban A, Solís-Muñoz M. The development and validation of a new postpartum sexual function and dyspareunia assessment tool: the Carol scale. Midwifery. 2018;58:27–36.

68. Rogers RG, Kammerer-Doak D, Villarreal A, Coates K, Qualls C. A new instrument to measure sexual function in women with urinary incontinence or pelvic organ prolapse. Am J Obstet Gynecol. 2001;184:552–8.

69. Rogers RG, Coates KW, Kammerer-Doak D, Khalsa S, Qualls C. A short form of the pelvic organ prolapse/urinary incontinence sexual questionnaire (PISQ-12). Int Urogynecol J. 2003;14:164–8.

70. PISQ-IR Questionnaire. https://www.iuga.org/resources/pisq-ir. Accessed 18 Mar 2023.

71. Barber MD, Kuchibhatla MN, Pieper CF, Bump RC. Psychometric evaluation of 2 comprehensive condition-specific quality of life instruments for women with pelvic floor disorders. Am J Obstet Gynecol. 2001;185:1388–95.

72. Peterson TV, Karp DR, Aguilar VC, Davila GW. Validation of a global pelvic floor symptom bother questionnaire. Int Urogynecol J. 2010;21:1129–35.

73. Baessler K, O'Neill SM, Maher CF, Battistutta D. A validated self-administered female pelvic floor questionnaire. Int Urogynecol J. 2010;21:163–72.

74. Radley S, Jones G, Tanguy E, Stevens V, Nelson C, Mathers N. Computer interviewing in urogynaecology: concept, development and psychometric testing of an electronic pelvic floor assessment questionnaire in primary and secondary care. BJOG Int J Obstet Gynaecol. 2006;113:231–8.

75. Palmieri S, Cola A, Ceccherelli A, Manodoro S, Frigerio M, Vergani P. Italian validation of the German Pelvic Floor Questionnaire for pregnant and postpartum women. Eur J Obstet Gynecol Reprod Biol. 2020;248:133–6.

76. Koyuncu K, Sakin O, Akalın EE, Akalın M, Anğın AD, Aboalhasan Y, Sönmezer E. Translation, cultural adaptation, and validation and reliability of assessment of pelvic floor disorders and their risk factors during pregnancy and postpartum questionnaire in Turkish population. Ginekol Pol. 2020;91:12.

77. da Silva Vieira RCM, da Silva JB, de Carvalho CR, Driusso P. Validation and cross-cultural adaptation of the Brazilian Portuguese version of the questionnaire for the assessment of pelvic floor disorders and their risk factors during pregnancy and postpartum. Int Urogynecol J. 2022; https://doi.org/10.1007/s00192-022-05101-z.

78. Andrews V, Thakar R, Sultan AH, Jones PW. Evaluation of postpartum perineal pain and dyspareunia—a prospective study. Eur J Obstet Gynecol Reprod Biol. 2008;137:152–6.

79. Vermelis JM, Wassen MM, Fiddelers AA, Nijhuis JG, Marcus MA. Prevalence and predictors of chronic pain after labor and delivery. Curr Opin Anaesthesiol. 2010;23:295–9.

80. Treede R-D, Rief W, Barke A, et al. A classification of chronic pain for ICD-11. Pain. 2015;156:1003–7.

81. Sultan P, Ando K, Sultan E, et al. A systematic review of patient-reported outcome measures to assess postpartum pain using Consensus Based Standards for the Selection of Health Measurement Instruments (COSMIN) guidelines. Br J Anaesth. 2021;127:264–74.

82. Brief Pain Inventory (BPI). In: MD Anderson Cancer Center. https://www.mdanderson.org/research/departments-labs-institutes/departments-divisions/symptom-research/symptom-assessment-tools/brief-pain-inventory.html. Accessed 19 Mar 2023.

83. Atkinson TM, Mendoza TR, Sit L, Passik S, Scher HI, Cleeland C, Basch E. The Brief Pain Inventory and its "pain at its worst in the last 24 hours" item: clinical trial endpoint considerations. Pain Med. 2010;11:337–46.

84. Watson K, White C, Hall H, Hewitt A. Women's experiences of birth trauma: A scoping review. Women Birth. 2021;34:417–24.

85. Ertan D, Hingray C, Burlacu E, Sterlé A, El-Hage W. Post-traumatic stress disorder following childbirth. BMC Psychiatry. 2021;21:155.

86. Molyneux R, Fowler G, Slade P. The effects of perineal trauma on immediate self-reported birth experience in first-time mothers. J Psychosom Obstet Gynecol. 2022;43(2):228–34.

87. Falk M, Nelson M, Blomberg M. The impact of obstetric interventions and complications on women's satisfaction with childbirth a population based cohort study including 16,000 women. BMC Pregnancy Childbirth. 2019;19:494.

88. Crookall R, Fowler G, Wood C, Slade P. A systematic mixed studies review of women's experiences of perineal trauma sustained during childbirth. J Adv Nurs. 2018;74:2038–52.

89. Nilsson C, Hessman E, Sjöblom H, Dencker A, Jangsten E, Mollberg M, Patel H, Sparud-Lundin C, Wigert H, Begley C. Definitions, measurements and prevalence of fear of childbirth: a systematic review. BMC Pregnancy Childbirth. 2018;18:28.

90. Gottvall K, Waldenstrom U. Does a traumatic birth experience have an impact on future reproduction? BJOG. 2002;109:254–60.

91. Chen Y, Ismail F, Xiong Z, Li M, Chen I, Wen SW, Xie R. Association between perceived birth trauma and postpartum depression: a prospective cohort study in China. Int J Gynecol Obstet. 2022;157(3):598–603.

92. Martin CJH, Martin CR. Development and psychometric properties of the Birth Satisfaction Scale-Revised (BSS-R). Midwifery. 2014;30:610–9.

93. Alfaro Blazquez R, Corchon S, Ferrer Ferrandiz E. Validity of instruments for measuring the satisfaction of a woman and her partner with care received during labour and childbirth: systematic review. Midwifery. 2017;55:103–12.

94. Nilvér H, Begley C, Berg M. Measuring women's childbirth experiences: a systematic review for identification and analysis of validated instruments. BMC Pregnancy Childbirth. 2017;17:203.

95. McKelvin G, Thomson G, Downe S. The childbirth experience: a systematic review of predictors and outcomes. Women Birth. 2021;34:407–16.

96. Sambrook Smith M, Cairns L, Pullen LSW, Opondo C, Fellmeth G, Alderdice F. Validated tools to identify common mental disorders in the perinatal period: a systematic review of systematic reviews. J Affect Disord. 2022;298:634–43.

97. Cox JL, Holden JM, Sagovsky R. Detection of postnatal depression: development of the 10-item Edinburgh Postnatal Depression Scale. Br J Psychiatry. 1987;150:782–6.

98. Beck CT, Gable RK. Comparative analysis of the performance of the Postpartum Depression Screening Scale with two other depression instruments. Nurs Res. 2001;50:242–50.

99. Spitzer RL, Williams JB, Kroenke K, Hornyak R, McMurray J, Patient Health Questionnaire Obstetrics-Gynecology Study Group. Validity and utility of the PRIME-MD patient health questionnaire in assessment of 3000 obstetric-gynecologic patients: the PRIME-MD Patient Health Questionnaire Obstetrics-Gynecology Study. Am J Obstet Gynecol. 2000;183:759–69.

100. American Psychiatric Association Diagnostic and Statistical Manual of Mental Disorders: DSM-5.

101. Cook N, Ayers S, Horsch A. Maternal posttraumatic stress disorder during the perinatal period and child outcomes: a systematic review. J Affect Disord. 2018;225:18–31.

102. Yildiz PD, Ayers S, Phillips L. The prevalence of posttraumatic stress disorder in pregnancy and after birth: a systematic review and meta-analysis. J Affect Disord. 2017;208:634–45.

103. Ayers S, Bond R, Bertullies S, Wijma K. The aetiology of post-traumatic stress following childbirth: a meta-analysis and theoretical framework. Psychol Med. 2016;46:1121–34.

104. Creedy DK, Shochet IM, Horsfall J. Childbirth and the development of acute trauma symptoms: incidence and contributing factors. Birth. 2000;27:104–11.

105. Wijma K, Söderquist J, Wijma B. Posttraumatic stress disorder after childbirth: a cross sectional study. J Anxiety Disord. 1997;11:587–97.

106. Callahan JL, Borja SE, Hynan MT. Modification of the Perinatal PTSD Questionnaire to enhance clinical utility. J Perinatol. 2006;26:533–9.

107. Ayers S, Wright DB, Thornton A. Development of a measure of postpartum PTSD: the city birth trauma scale. Front Psych. 2018;9:409.

108. Dobson H, Malpas C, Kulkarni J. Measuring posttraumatic stress disorder following childbirth. Australas Psychiatry. 2022;30(4):476–80. https://doi.org/10.1177/10398562221077900.

109. Webb R, Smith AM, Ayers S, Wright DB, Thornton A. Development and validation of a measure of birth-related PTSD for fathers and birth partners: the City Birth Trauma Scale (partner version). Front Psychol. 2021;12:596779.

110. Sultan P, Sadana N, Sharawi N, et al. Evaluation of domains of patient-reported outcome measures for recovery after childbirth: a scoping and systematic review. JAMA Netw Open. 2020;3:e205540.

111. Sultan P, Jensen S, Taylor J, El-Sayed Y, Carmichael S, Cella D, Angst M, Gaudilliere B, Lyell D, Carvalho B. Proposed domains for assessing postpartum recovery: a concept elicitation study. BJOG. 2022;129:9–20.

112. Landau R. Deconstructing current postpartum recovery research—the need to contextualize patient-reported outcome measures. JAMA Netw Open. 2021;4:e2111689.

113. Dickinson F, McCauley M, Smith H, van den Broek N. Patient reported outcome measures for use in

pregnancy and childbirth: a systematic review. BMC Pregnancy Childbirth. 2019;19:155.

114. Nijagal MA, Wissig S, Stowell C, et al. Standardized outcome measures for pregnancy and childbirth, an ICHOM proposal. BMC Health Serv Res. 2018;18:953.

115. Pregnancy And Childbirth—ICHOM Connect. https://connect.ichom.org/patient-centered-outcome-measures/pregnancy-and-childbirth/. Accessed 27 Mar 2022.

116. Weinfurt KP, Lin L, Bruner DW, Cyranowski JM, Dombeck CB, Hahn EA, Jeffery DD, Luecht RM, Magasi S, Porter LS. Development and initial validation of the PROMIS® sexual function and satisfaction measures version 2.0. J Sex Med. 2015;12:1961–74.

117. Depla AL, Ernst-Smelt HE, Poels M, Crombag NM, Franx A, Bekker MN. A feasibility study of implementing a patient-centered outcome set for pregnancy and childbirth. Health Sci Rep. 2020;3:e168.

118. PROMIS Health Measures site.

119. Mapi Research Trust PROQOLID, the Patient-Reported Outcome and Quality Of Life Instruments Database. https://www.qolid.org/. Accessed 19 Mar 2023.

120. Johnston BC, Patrick DL, Devji T, Maxwell LJ, Bingham CO III, Beaton DE, Boers M, Briel M, Busse JW, Carrasco-Labra A. Patient-reported outcomes. In: Cochrane handbook for systematic reviews of interventions. Wiley-Blackwell; 2022. p. 479–92.

Education and Training in OASIS

23

Joanna C. Roper, Ranee Thakar, and Abdul H. Sultan

Overview

Test your learning and check your understanding of this book's contents: use the "Springer Nature Flashcards" app to access questions using ▶ https://sn.pub/wqrf89. To use the app, please follow the instructions in Chap. 1.

Learning Objectives

- To be able to recognise the importance of training in the diagnosis and repair of OASIs
- To be cognisant of differences in the availability of hands-on and simulation training for obstetrical providers
- To understand the variations in teaching methods for education in OASIs diagnosis and repair

23.1 Introduction

Education and training in the clinical environment are continuous processes. As new healthcare professionals begin their clinical work, they must be trained in current, evidence-based practices. As new techniques are implemented, all clinicians should be able to benefit from continuing medical education courses and retraining, as continuing professional development and revision of clinical practice forms an important part of education for all healthcare professionals. The responsibility of offering training often falls on the experts in various fields, but the onus of accessing that training lies with the healthcare professionals themselves. With regards to education and training in obstetric anal sphincter injuries (OASIs), this responsibility falls on doctors and midwives.

Best practice dictates that diagnosis and classification of OASIs should take place immediately after birth by performing a systematic combined digital rectal and vaginal examination after every vaginal birth [1, 2]. It is important for all healthcare professionals who assist in a vaginal birth, and the subsequent assessment and diagnosis of perineal trauma, to be aware of the anatomy of the perineum. This knowledge is required to correctly diagnose, classify and repair any injury. Therefore, all doctors and midwives who practice within the scope of obstetrics must be adequately trained in diagnosing and classifying OASIs. In 1993, Sultan described OASIs that were unrecognised at birth and instead identified on ultrasound 6 weeks after birth; these were deemed 'occult' injuries because it was assumed that the injuries were not visible clinically at the time of birth [3]. However, in a subsequent study

J. C. Roper (✉)
Department of Obstetrics and Gynecology, Croydon University Hospital, Croydon, Surrey, UK

Croydon University Hospital, Thornton Heath, UK
e-mail: jo.roper@doctors.org.uk

R. Thakar · A. H. Sultan
Croydon University Hospital, London, UK

by Andrews et al. in 2003, 241 women were re-examined after delivery by an experienced research fellow with endoanal ultrasound (EAUS) performed immediately and again at 6 weeks after birth. This study revealed that the previously believed "occult" injuries were actually missed tears in nearly all cases. The prevalence of OASIs increased from 11% to 24.5% when women were re-examined; only 3 women (1.2%) suffered an occult/missed OASI, detected only on EAUS [4]. Not surprisingly, in a matched retrospective cohort study by Taithongchai et al., women with missed OASIs were found to have significantly worse symptoms of anal and urinary incontinence when compared to women with recognised OASIs [5]. A study in 2016 comparing diagnosis of OASIs by clinical examination with 3D trans-perineal ultrasound (TPUS) found only 1% of OASIs detected on TPUS were not detected clinically by doctors [6]. In this same study, midwives missed 80% of OASIs and doctors missed 12.5% . This is comparable to Andrews et al. in 2005 who found 87% of OASIs were missed by midwives [4]. Despite the 13-year gap between these studies, there appears to have been no discernible improvement among midwives, which highlights the need for structured, hands-on training programs to be mandated in midwifery training programs and a shift in practice, such as two midwives examining the patient after every vaginal birth. By contrast, the rate of missed OASIs amongst doctors reduced by more than half from 28% to 12.5% after this 13-year time period reflecting the effect of the ongoing hands-on workshops initiated in 2000 (www.perineum.net).

23.2 History of Education in OASI

Before the year 2000, education in the diagnosis and repair of OASIs was unstructured and undertaken on an *ad-hoc* basis in labour wards across the country. In 2000, the Croydon OASI course was introduced and subsequently, many other national and international courses have been initiated. Over time, the courses have been refined and developed to incorporate perineal tears, episiotomy and even prevention methods of OASI, such as manual perineal protection. Following each Croydon OASI course, the organisers review the feedback from attendees and re-appraise the content and delivery of the course.

23.3 Importance of Classification and Repair

OASIs not identified and repaired at the time of delivery can lead to long term consequences, such as anal incontinence [5, 7–9]. Classification of OASIs using the Sultan Classification (first described in 1999) [10], is now recommended by most national OASI guidelines [11]. Before 2000, textbooks were inconsistent in the classification and grading of OASIs [12]. Classification of perineal trauma with a universally accepted system ensures a systematic and thorough evaluation of the injury and thereby allows for appropriate repair of the trauma [11]. It also provides a standardised record of perineal trauma, which can be interpreted by all clinicians, allowing for an audit of outcomes. If a tear is under-classified as, for example, a 3c tear (complete external anal sphincter (EAS) and internal anal sphincter (IAS) tear) is diagnosed as a 3b tear (IAS intact), this would result in an inadequate repair. Subsequently, this results in a persistent defect in the IAS, which can be seen on endoanal ultrasound (EAUS). A prospective observational study, looking at under-classified OASIs based on EAUS at follow up, found that 11.36% of 1056 women with a diagnosis of a 3a or 3b tear were actually found to have a defect greater than the original diagnosis at the time of birth [13]. It was also found that women with a 3c tear diagnosed as a 3b tear had significantly worse St Mark's incontinence scores [13].

The importance of recognising IAS injury was also highlighted by Mahony et al. They investigated 500 women 3 months following OASI repair [14]. IAS injury was found to be significantly related to the presence of faecal incontinence and an IAS defect was predictive of severe incontinence [14].

A United Kingdom (UK) national survey, in 2002, of obstetricians (consultants and trainees) and coloproctologists also found that obstetric doctors (33% of consultants and 22% of trainees) were incorrectly classifying a complete or partial EAS tear as a second-degree tear [15]. These studies all highlight the importance of training in the diagnosis and repair of OASIs, to improve outcomes for women.

23.4 National Guidelines on OASIs

Guidelines are defined by the Institute of Medicine as 'statements that include recommendations intended to optimise patient care, that are informed by a systematic review of evidence and an assessment of the benefits and harms of alternative care options' [16]. The Royal College of Obstetricians and Gynaecologists (RCOG) published a 'Green-top' guideline in 2015 with recommendations for the management of OASIs [17]. This guide-

line has been referenced as a key document for the development of many other national guidelines on OASI management [11]. Guidelines are an essential part of training and maintaining education because they can be used as a reference at any time. However, it is important that healthcare professionals correctly interpret and use guidelines, exercising awareness of the process of their development, timing, and the available evidence included [11]. Roper et al. [11] performed a literature review of 13 national OASI guidelines (Table 23.1). This review evaluated the methodological rigour of development and comparison of recommendations regarding the management and prevention of OASI [11]. There was wide variation in the development and scope of the included guidelines. The variation in included recommendations can be seen in Table 23.2. It is interesting to note that some guidelines found evidence to support certain recommendations, whereas others felt there was insufficient evidence, as in the example of pre-

Table 23.1 Available national guidelines on OASIs included in the evaluation by Roper et al. (cited with permission under creative commons (https://creativecommons.org/licenses/by/4.0/) [11]

Name of guideline	Country of origin	Publication date
Government of South Australia- south Australian perinatal practice guideline. Third and fourth degree tear management	Australia	June 2018
Queensland clinical guidelines- perineal care	Australia	June 2018
Austria Urogynaecology working group- guidelines for the management of third and fourth degree tears after vaginal birth.	Austria	2013
Society of obstetrics and Gynaecology of Canada- clinical practice guideline, number 330. OASIs: Prevention, recognition and repair.	Canada	December 2015
Forebyggelse af sphincterruptur (prevention of sphincter rupture)	Denmark	December 2015
Sphincterruptur: Diagnostik, behandling og opfolgning (OASI: Diagnosis, treatment and follow up)	Denmark	2019
German society of Gynaecology and obstetrics – Management of third and fourth degree tears after vaginal birth	Germany	October 2014
Institute of obstetricians and Gynaecologists- clinical practice guideline- management of OASIs	Ireland	April 2014
Prevencion, diagnostico y tratamiento de episiotomia complicada (prevention, diagnosis and treatment of complicated episiotomy)	Mexico	2014
Dutch Society of Obstetrics and Gynaecology: Risk factors for and interventions that reduce the risk of a total rupture during childbirth.	The Netherlands	May 2013
Saudi Society of Obstetrics and Gynaecology, policy and procedure- PERINEAL TRAUMA	Saudi Arabia	July 2016
Royal college of obstetrics and Gynaecology -green-top guideline no.29. Management of third and fourth degree perineal tears.	UK	June 2015
American College of Obstetrics and Gynaecology- Practice Bulletin Number 198. Prevention and management of obstetric lacerations at vaginal delivery	USA	September 2018

Table 23.2 Mapped recommendations from national OASI guidelines evaluation by Roper et al.[a] (cited with permission under creative commons (https://creativecommons.org/licenses/by/4.0/) [11]

	Australia-South	Australia-Queensland	Austria	Canada	Denmark 2015	Denmark 2019	Germany	Ireland	Mexico	The Netherlands	Saudi Arabia	UK	USA
Classification of perineal trauma	✓	✓	✓	✓	✓	✓	✓	✓	✓	N	✓	✓	✓
Buttonhole tears	✓	✓	N	✓	N	N	✓	N	N	N	✓	✓	N
Risk factors for OASI	✓	✓	✓	✓	✓	✓	✓	N	✓	✓	✓	✓	✓
Prevention- perineal protection	N	i	i	i	✓	N	i	N	✓	✓	✓	✓	i
Prevention- mediolateral episiotomy for instrumental delivery	N	✓	N	✓	✓	(✓)	(✓)	N	✓	i	✓	✓	i
Prevention- warm compress	N	✓	N	✓	✓	N	i	✓	✓	✓	✓	✓	✓
Diagnosis- examination with digital rectal examination	(✓)	✓	✓	(✓)	✓	✓	(✓)	✓	N	(✓)	N	✓	(✓)
Repair- in theatre with regional analgesia	(✓)	✓	✓	✓	N	✓	✓	✓	✓	✓	✓	✓	✓
Repair- trained person doing repair	✓	✓	✓	✓	N	✓	✓	✓	✓	N	N	✓	✓
Repair – Mucosa continuous or interrupted, position of knots	N	✓	N	✓	N	✓	N	N	N	N	N	✓	✓
Repair- IAS separately if torn	✓	✓	✓	✓	N	✓	✓	✓	N	(✓)	✓	✓	(✓)
Repair- full thickness EAS end to end or overlap	✓	✓	✓	✓	N	✓	✓	✓	N	N	✓	✓	✓
Suture materials	✓	✓	✓	✓	N	✓	✓	✓	✓	N	N	✓	✓
Post repair PR	✓	N	✓	✓	N	✓	✓	✓	✓	N	N	✓	✓
Broad-spectrum antibiotics at time of repair	✓	✓	✓	✓	N	✓	✓	✓	N	N	N	✓	✓
Post repair antibiotics	✓	(✓)	✓	N	N	i	✓	i	N	N	N	i	N
Recommend physiotherapy	N	✓	✓	(✓)	N	✓	✓	✓	✓	✓	N	✓	✓
Post repair use of laxatives	✓	✓	✓	✓	N	✓	✓	i	✓	N	N	✓	✓
Risk of OASI recurrence quoted	✓	✓	✓	✓	N	✓	✓	✓	✓	N	N	✓	✓
Follow up- endoanal ultrasound recommended	N	✓	N	N	N	N	i	N	N	(✓)	N	✓	N
Episiotomy at subsequent delivery	i	i	i	N	N	N	i	N	✓	i	N	i	i
Advise caesarean section for symptomatic women in subsequent pregnancy	✓	✓	✓	✓	N	✓	✓	✓	✓	N	N	✓	✓

[a] ✓ = included and recommended, (✓) = recommended with restrictions, i = Insufficient evidence for recommendation, N = not mentioned

vention of OASIs with warm compresses. This may reflect the timing of when guidelines were written and when evidence was published. The suggestion of a universal guideline was proposed to reduce variation in clinical practice and interpretation of available evidence [11]. Similar findings were reported by Nygaard et al. [18] and Tsakiridis et al. [19] in their smaller reviews of national guidelines on perineal trauma and OASIs respectively. In the UK, the RCOG guideline [17] is easily available online and can be accessed at any time; however, its target audience is mainly doctors and not midwives.

23.5   Training for Doctors

Education in the diagnosis and repair of OASIs for doctors in the UK is a mandatory part of training in Obstetrics and Gynaecology. All doctors in the speciality training programme must attend a Perineal and OASI Repair course in their second year [20]. They must also demonstrate competence in repairing OASIs during their hands-on training. This is assessed by a senior obstetrician observing the trainee performing the repair. By the end of the fourth training year, they must have completed three objective structured assessments of technical skills (OSATS) [20]. These must be on three separate occasions observed by a senior doctor, with only one assessment required to be by a consultant. This is the only clinical assessment of skills that are required to achieve competence [20]. The 'Training Matrix' states that they must repair a 'third-degree tear' [19]. Therefore, a doctor may pass the OSATS and be declared competent, having only repaired a grade 3a or 3b tear, without ever repairing a grade 3c or fourth-degree tear. This highlights an important deficiency in the curriculum that needs reappraisal.

Given the rarity of OASIs and the pressures of time for doctors in training (such as the European Working Time Directive), it can be difficult to gain the clinical experience needed to feel confident in the diagnosis and repair of OASIs. It is therefore essential that training courses include simulation to supplement the clinical experience that doctors have.

In 1995, an audit in the UK of 75 doctors and 75 midwives reported their experience of training in obstetric perineal trauma [21]. Less than 20% of doctors and less than 48% of midwives described their training in perineal anatomy, perineal repair and recognition of OASIs to be a 'good' standard [21]. By 2002, a national practice survey by Fernando et al., reported that 64% of consultants ($n = 672$) and 64% of trainees ($n = 148$) felt they had either 'a lack of' or 'unsatisfactory' training in the management of OASIs [15].

Interestingly, quite some time later in 2020, a survey of 302 obstetric doctors in the UK found 69.2% of respondents described their training in obstetric tears as 'good' or 'excellent' [22]. Most (65.1%) junior doctors (non-consultant level) had received training in the previous 5 years. 10.4% of had not received training for over 10 years, perhaps indicating their knowledge may be dated. When asked to classify tears from descriptive text or standardised images, doctors were very good at identifying tears (91–100% correctly classified standardised images of tears, and 80–99% correctly classified tears from descriptive text). This implies that the general level of theoretical training in OASIs for UK doctors has improved over time and is very good. Still, it is imperative that the training for doctors in OASIs management is regularly revisited to ensure the practice is up to date.

Similar surveys have been conducted in Spain, America, New Zealand and Australia [23–25]. In 2021, an American survey of obstetrician-gynaecologists found that only 33% of participants had had formal training in perineal injuries. However, when asked to classify standardised descriptions and images, 81–100% correctly classified standardised images of tears (first-fourth degree tears), and 70–95% correctly classified tears from the descriptive text (first-fourth degree tears) [23]. Interestingly, 17% of doctors classified an image of a 3c tear as a 'fourth-degree tear' and 25% of doctors classified a description of a second-degree tear with exposure of an intact anal sphincter as a 'third-degree tear'. The study concluded that improved training in perineal trauma identification is needed for American doctors. This echoes the suggestion by Hickmann and Propst of ongoing education and training in the diagnosis and management of OASIs at all levels of practice [26].

In 2018, a Perineal Care Bundle, aimed at reducing OASIs and improving identification and repair was introduced in Australia [27]. It consisted of five care elements: warm compresses, perineal support, episiotomy technique, assessing and grading of perineal tears [27]. A national standard also recommended that registrars should be supervised by a senior clinician until they have completed their 'Assessment of Procedural Skills' or equivalent [27]. A 2019 survey of 132 trainees in obstetrics and gynaecology in Australia and New Zealand found that only 62% of respondents reported a credentialing process at their training site and 23% felt their training at the time of first unsupervised OASI repair was suboptimal [24]. 76% of respondents had attended a workshop on OASIs, but 86% expressed that a workshop would be valuable at the time of survey completion. Ultimately, this study concluded that additional structured training is needed to improve outcomes. Finally, a 2011 survey of 46 Spanish residents (trainees) revealed that 98% of respondents felt there was a need for a theoretical-practical training course in pelvic floor anatomy and repair of its injuries [25].

Training courses provide a safe environment for learning and practicing skills which are essential for sound, evidence-based, clinical work. A study looking at participant confidence across key obstetric skills before and after attending a simulation training day showed a significant increase in confidence for participants when assessed on a Likert scale [28].

23.6 Training for Midwives

Training for midwives in the diagnosis of OASIs is essential, as they may be the only healthcare professional to examine a woman after birth. Roper et al. [1] highlighted the importance of a thorough examination, including rectal examination, to ensure that OASI and buttonhole tears are identified. In the UK, training for midwives is less structured than for doctors. The 'Standards of Proficiency for Midwives', from the Nursing and Midwifery Council (NMC), simply state that midwives must demonstrate at qualification, the skill to 'undertake repair of 1st and 2nd-degree perineal tears, and refer additional trauma' [29]. At UK Universities, midwifery courses vary in their content; training on the diagnosis of perineal trauma may be only mentioned by the midwives on placement (a student midwife will work, voluntarily, alongside a qualified midwife as part of their university training), therefore resulting in a huge variation in experience. In the UK, there are some training courses in OASIs available to midwives (www.perineum.net), but they are not mandatory.

In 2007 a UK survey showed that more than 90% of midwives felt inadequately prepared to assess perineal trauma [30]. Unfortunately, in a more recent survey in 2020, 61% ($n = 149$) described their training (experience and knowledge) in obstetric tears as 'adequate', 'poor' or 'very poor' [31]. Most respondents (52.7%) said their lack of training was due to a lack of available courses. However, when asked to classify tears from descriptive text and standardised images respondents were generally accurate (79–99% correctly classified perineal tears (first-fourth degree) from standardised images, 45–92% correctly classified perineal tears (first-fourth degree) from descriptive text). Given the small number of respondents to the survey, this study may not be truly generalisable.

In a survey of American midwives, 63% of respondents said their ability to identify third-degree tears was 'good' or 'excellent', and 66% correctly identified a standardised image of a third-degree tear [32]. However, one-third incorrectly identified this as a fourth-degree injury. They concluded, given that certified 'nurse-midwives' core competencies only include first- and second-degree repair, that training needs to be revised and expanded. The findings of these surveys support the concept that training in OASIs for midwives should be more widely available, with a standardised approach to assessment.

23.7   Training Courses

In response to the audit of training in 1995, the first UK hands-on workshop was initiated in Croydon, London in 2000 (www.perineum.net) where Sultan and Thakar introduced the pig anal sphincter repair (Fig. 23.1) and the Sultan model (Fig. 23.2). There are now many perineal trauma training courses available in the UK. Most are only available for doctors. The content of these courses is not very variable, with most courses focused on the anatomy and physiology of the anal sphincters, classification of OASIs, and the standardised approach to repair (in keeping with the RCOG guideline [17]). Most have a practical element that involves simulating the repair of OASIs, using an animal tissue (pig) model. The Croydon hands-on course is internationally renowned, with over 190 courses completed. Studies in the UK and Palestine have shown a significant improvement in knowledge and clinical practice after training [33–35]. In 2005, Andrews et al. requested midwives and doctors in the UK to complete a questionnaire before and 8 weeks after, attending a perineal repair course [33]. They reported a significant improvement in the correct classification of OASIs after attending the course ($p < 0.001$). In yet another study by Andrews et al. in 2008, doctors completed a questionnaire before and 8 weeks after training [35]. After the course, participants classified OASIs more accurately and changed to evidence-based practice.

Palestinian doctors and midwives from 6 hospitals were asked to complete a questionnaire before and 3 months after a hands-on training course conducted by Sultan and Thakar [34]. At 3 months, significant improvement in many training aspects including accuracy of perineal anatomy (doctors: 11.4% vs 78.85%, $p < 0.001$, midwives: 9.8% vs 54.2%, $p < 0.001$), rectal examination, and anal sphincter repair techniques were reported.

Internationally, other training courses have been described [24, 34, 36, 37]. Another study in Palestine looked at the effect of a series of training programmes [38]. The study included an expert workshop followed by three phases: pre-

clinical training observation (phase 1), a training intervention for 15 weeks (phase 2) and post-intervention observation (phase 3). Using OASI rates as a measure of OASI recognition, the increase (0.5% to 2.8% in phase 2 ($p < 0.001$) and 3.1% in phase 3 ($p < 0.001$) was assumed to be due to improved detection secondary to the training [38].

23.8   Training Models and Resources

Many of the training courses use fresh bovine or porcine tissue models for demonstration and hands-on repair of OASIs (see Fig. 23.1).

Other courses use synthetic models that have been designed specifically for training in the diagnosis and repair of OASIs. For example, the Sultan Anal Sphincter Repair Trainer, with a central replaceable block, has been designed for hands-on training (Fig. 23.2).

A modified model is now available that allows for the repair of an episiotomy in the same model (www.limbsandthings.com). Another similar anatomical silicone training model was designed by a Canadian team, Team Broken Earth [36] (Fig. 23.3). In 2018, the team used the model in a training programme in Bangladesh. They also conducted an evaluation survey which found the models were considered superior to current training methods, which involved textbook education and hands-on learning in emergency birthing scenarios by non-medically trained attendants [36].

For individuals seeking personal improvement and updating of their skills, there is a video series which includes education on the anatomy of the perineum and anal sphincter, diagnosis of third and fourth-degree tears and repair using the Sultan model, pig sphincter and a postpartum woman (www.perineum.net). All these resources are very useful, not only for personal training and development, but also for ensuring a standardising of techniques and training courses. Finally, there are many other reports of 'homemade' models used for teaching repair of OASIs. Knobel et al. describe a low-cost simulator using a condom, bovine meat and cotton tissue (Fig. 23.4)

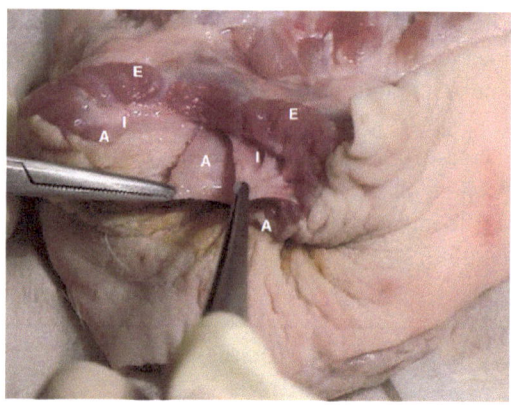

Fig. 23.1 Pig Anal sphincter. A- anal mucosa, I- IAS, E-EAS [35]

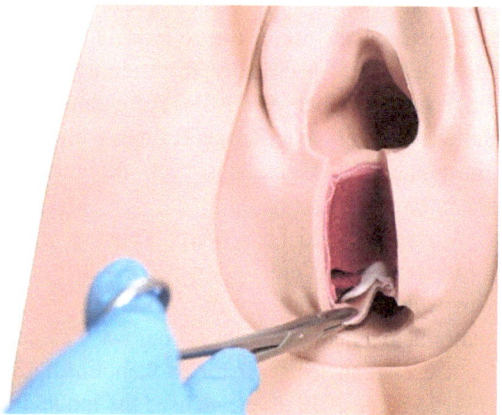

Fig. 23.2 The original Sultan anal sphincter repair trainer [35]

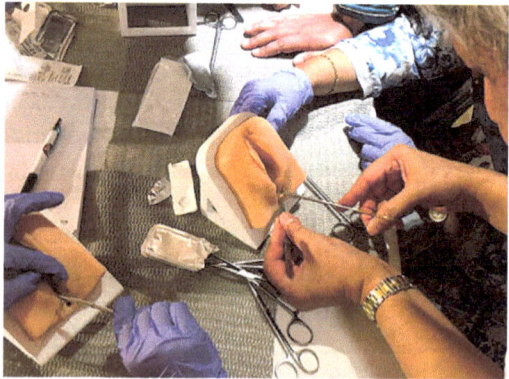

Fig. 23.3 Silicone training model designed by Team Broken Earth [36]. (cited with permission under creative commons (https://creativecommons.org/licenses/by/4.0/)

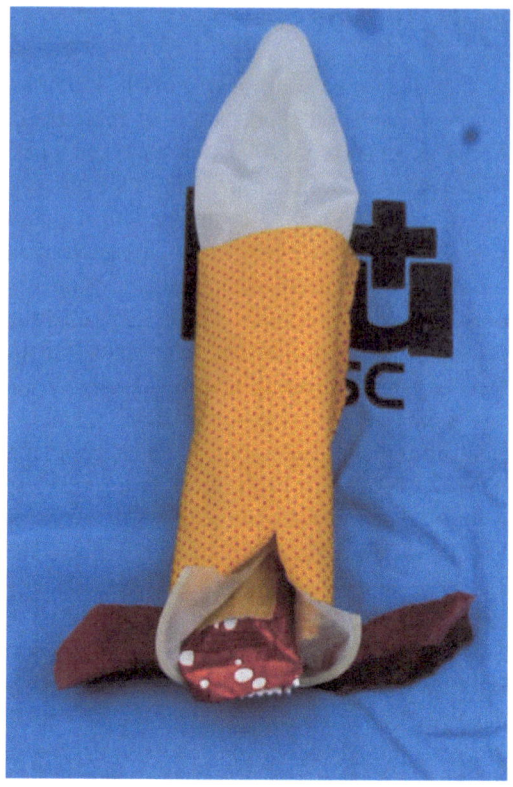

Fig. 23.4 A low-cost simulator for teaching OASI repair [39] (cited with permission under creative commons (https://creativecommons.org/licenses/by/4.0/)

[39]. This model is particularly useful in settings where other models are not available or affordable.

Another model described by Illston et al. uses a beef tongue and chicken leg muscles [40]. This requires some preparation, but is a good and useful low-cost option.

In an American study, 16 obstetrics and gynaecology doctors' knowledge, confidence, technical skill and preference for two training models (sponge [41] versus beef tongue [42]) were compared; a significant improvement was found with the use of both models, with no difference between the two [42]. Unfortunately, there are no studies comparing all available models, therefore one model's superiority over others cannot be concluded. Yet, it should be noted that all synthetic models provide an opportunity for practice in a safe environment with time for teaching; this is essential for all who are learning a new technique. However, those models lack the advantage of using animal tissue, which most closely resemble the anatomy and muscle texture to the actual live repair of OASIs.

23.9   Online Training Programmes

The benefit of online training programs include availability and accessibility. A study in America looked at the training of labour and delivery nurses in OASIs. A set of 10 knowledge-based questions were used to compare pre and post-test scores of participants after they completed a computer-based learning module. A significant improvement in knowledge was noted after completing the learning module [43].

There is a perineal repair training programme that is available online from https://gynzone. com. This has been created by Sara Kinderg and Karl Moller Bek from Denmark. Founded in 2008, the programme has a database of videos including live surgical patients, medical models and computer-generated animations. The modules include diagnosis and repair of first, second-, third- and fourth-degree tears, buttonhole repairs and episiotomy, and labial repair using models, pig tissue and clinical videos. This online learning platform is a very useful tool and could be used as a wonderful refresher course for any healthcare professional. Gynzone has also developed a silicone training model which they use for hands-on teaching (Fig. 23.5).

Through the International Urogynecological Association (IUGA), another OASI training program is available to all doctors, midwives and allied healthcare professionals, called PROTECT (Prevention and Repair Of perineal Trauma Episiotomy through Co-ordinated Training) (www.iuga.org/education/protect). This is a 'train the trainer' program, to promote knowledge globally in the management of perineal trauma and episiotomy. The intention of the programme is that graduates will use the knowledge and skills gained to then train others, particularly in their own country and in their native language

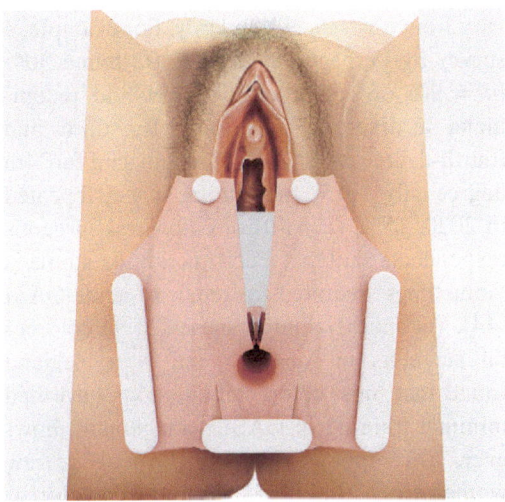

Fig. 23.5 Silicone anal sphincter repair model, © Gynzone

so that they can reach out to practitioners and traditional birth attendants.

To become a PROTECT certified trainer 4-steps must be completed:

1. Complete the electronic theoretical test.
2. Attend the OASIs Hands-on Workshop at the IUGA Annual Meeting or one conducted by a PROTECT-trained trainer.
3. Attend the IUGA PROTECT Workshop within 2 years of completing Step 2. Training must include teaching episiotomy repair.
4. Upload personal videos demonstrating your live surgical technique within 2 years of completing Step 2.

This online course is easily accessible globally. In 2022, there were 17 individuals from 12 different countries who have completed the program and the courses they have conducted are described (IUGA.org).

23.10   Colorectal Involvement in the Repair of OASIs

There has been an ongoing debate about the role of colorectal surgeons in the repair of acute OASIs. In the acute setting of birth trauma, their management has been reported to vary from obstetrical standards. For example, a survey by Fernando et al. in 2002 found 30% (n = 90) of coloproctologists would recommend a diverting colostomy for third and fourth-degree tears (83% of whom said for '4th degree only') [15]. In a similar survey repeated in 2020, 15%, (n = 40) of colorectal surgeons respondents said that a de-functioning stoma is 'sometimes' required for repair of acute OASI [44]. Yet another similar survey of 94 colorectal surgeons in Australia and New Zealand found that most colorectal surgeons have had minimal training in OASI management, however, 70% reported that they routinely review women with OASIs [45]. Fortunately, colorectal surgeons are more likely to be involved in OASIs in the non-acute setting [45]. The evidence for successful acute repair, as described by the RCOG [17], is sufficient, but there could be situations when assistance from colorectal surgeons may be useful and this is discussed in Chap. 5.

23.11 Conclusion

Over the last two decades, there has been a dramatic improvement in training and education of recognition and repair of OASIs. This has been reflected in improved outcomes for women who sustain these injuries. However, there is still room for improvement, particularly in implementing a structured programme in the education of midwives, to ensure all OASIs are recognised. Various simulation models exist and should be utilised to augment training. In low resource countries, this information needs to be dispersed to traditional birth attendants so that women can be timely referred to the nearest hospital. Admittedly, due to staff shortages and rotation of trainees, OASIs continue to go unrecognised, and there is a compelling argument to introduce a program whereby every woman who undergoes a vaginal birth should be re-examined by a second trained doctor or midwife to exclude OASIs. Given the availability of resources and training packages, suboptimal diagnosis and repair should no longer be acceptable.

Take-Home Messages
- Education in the diagnosis and classification of OASIs is essential for all healthcare professionals attending vaginal births.
- All trainee doctors must attend a hands-on workshop on OASIs, but continuing education in updated diagnosis and management of OASIs is imperative.
- Midwives' training in OASIs is variable and should be standardised and formally assessed.
- There is still room for improvement in the availability and frequency of training and use of simulation models to ensure all OASIs are recognised and correctly managed.

Appendix: MCQ

Mark each item TRUE or FALSE

Questions

1. Regarding OASIs:
   (A) Women with missed OASIs have significantly worse anal incontinence symptoms.
   (B) Occult sphincter injuries are common.
   (C) Trans-perineal ultrasound is often used to diagnose OASIs.
   (D) There has been little improvement in midwives knowledge of OASIs (according to studies) over the last decade.
   (E) Doctors have demonstrated significant improvement (according to studies) in the knowledge of OASIs over the last decade.

2. Regarding guidelines:
   (A) The UK national guideline for OASIs is the Royal College of Obstetricians and Gynaecologists Green Top Guideline number 29.
   (B) All guidelines include details on management of rectal buttonhole tears.
   (C) All guidelines recommend post-repair antibiotics for OASIs.
   (D) Most guidelines found insufficient evidence for the use of episiotomy for subsequent deliveries after OASIs.

(E) Some guidelines recommend the prevention of OASIs with warm compresses, while other guidelines found insufficient evidence for this practice.

3. Regarding training:
   (A) Training for doctors in the UK in OASIs is mandatory.
   (B) Doctors are required to be observed on five separate occasions repairing OASIs to be competent.
   (C) Observation by a consultant only has to occur once for competency.
   (D) Doctors must be observed repairing all subgroups of third degree tear for competency.
   (E) The Australian 'Perineal Care Bundle' comprised of warm compresses, perineal support, episiotomy technique, assessing and grading of perineal tears.

4. Regarding midwifery training:
   (A) UK Midwives are only required to 'undertake repair of 1st and 2nd-degree perineal tears, and refer additional trauma'.
   (B) A 2007 UK survey found 50% of midwives felt inadequately trained to assess perineal trauma.
   (C) In a 2020 survey of midwives more than 50% said they lack training in OASIs due to lack of courses.
   (D) An American survey of midwives found one third incorrectly identified a third degree tear as a fourth degree tear.
   (E) The first UK hands-on perineal repair course started in 2000.

5. Regarding training for the care of OASIs:
   (A) Many training courses use porcine models to demonstrate repair of OASIs.
   (B) A study comparing sponge and beef tongue models found beef tongue to be superior for training.
   (C) PROTECT stands for Prevention and Repair Of perineal Trauma Episiotomy through Co-ordinated Training.
   (D) A survey in 2002 found that 30% of coloproctologists would recommend a colostomy in the management of acute OASIs.

(E) Colorectal surgeons are more likely to be involved in non-acute OASIs.

Answers

1. Regarding OASIs:
   (A) TRUE
   (B) FALSE
   (C) FALSE
   (D) TRUE
   (E) TRUE

2. Regarding guidelines:
   (A) TRUE
   (B) FALSE
   (C) FALSE
   (D) TRUE
   (E) TRUE

3. Regarding training:
   (A) TRUE
   (B) FALSE
   (C) TRUE
   (D) FALSE
   (E) TRUE

4. Regarding midwifery training:
   (A) TRUE
   (B) FALSE
   (C) TRUE
   (D) TRUE
   (E) TRUE

5. Regarding training for the care of OASIs:
   (A) TRUE
   (B) FALSE
   (C) TRUE
   (D) TRUE
   (E) TRUE

References

1. Roper JC, Sultan AH, Thakar R. Diagnosis of perineal trauma: getting it right first time. Br J Midwifery. 2020;28:710–7.

2. Sultan AH, Kettle C. Diagnosis of perineal trauma. In: Perineal and anal sphincter trauma. London: Springer; 2007. p. 13–20.

3. Sultan AH, Kamm MA, Hudson CN, Thomas JM, Bartram CI. Anal-sphincter disruption during vaginal delivery. N Engl J Med. 1993;329:1905–11.

4. Andrews V, Sultan AH, Thakar R, Jones PW. Occult anal sphincter injuries—myth or reality? BJOG. 2006;113:195–200. Occult anal sphincter injuries—myth or reality?

5. Taithongchai A, Veiga SI, Sultan AH, Thakar R. The consequences of undiagnosed obstetric anal sphincter injuries (OASIS) following vaginal delivery. Int Urogynecol J. 2019;31:635–41. https://doi.org/10.1007/s00192-019-04033-5.

6. Wong KW, Thakar R, Sultan AH, Andrews V. Can transperineal ultrasound improve the diagnosis of obstetric anal sphincter injuries? Int Urogynecol J. 2022;33:2809–14.

7. Sioutis D, Thakar R, Sultan AH. Overdiagnosis and rising rate of obstetric anal sphincter injuries (OASIS): time for reappraisal. Ultrasound Obstet Gynecol. 2017;50:642–7.

8. Andrews V, Shelmeridine S, Sultan AH, Thakar R. Anal and urinary incontinence 4 years after a vaginal delivery. Int Urogynecol J. 2013;24:55–60.

9. Ramage L, Yen C, Qiu S, Simillis C, Kontovounisios C, Tan E, Tekkis P. Does a missed obstetric anal sphincter injury at time of delivery affect short-term functional outcome? Ann Royal College Surg Engl. 2018;100:26–32.

10. Sultan AH. Editorial: obstetrical perineal injury and anal incontinence. AVMA Med Legal J. 1999;5:193–6.

11. Roper JC, Amber N, Wan OYK, Sultan AH, Thakar R. Review of available national guidelines for obstetric anal sphincter injury. Int Urogynecol J. 2020;31:2247–59.

12. Sultan AH, Thakar R. Lower genital tract and anal sphincter trauma. Best Pract Res Clin Obstet Gynaecol. 2002;16:99–115.

13. Roper JC, Thakar R, Sultan AH. Under-classified obstetric anal sphincter injuries. Int Urogynecol J. 2022;33:1473–9. https://doi.org/10.1007/s00192-021-05051-y.

14. Mahony R, Behan M, Daly L, Kirwan C, O'Herlihy C, O'Connell PR. Internal anal sphincter defect influences continence outcome following obstetric anal sphincter injury. Am J Obstet Gynecol. 2007;196:217.e1–5.

15. Fernando RJ, Sultan AH, Radley S, Jones PW, Johanson RB. Management of obstetric anal sphincter injury: a systematic review & national practice survey. BMC Health Serv Res. 2002;2:9.

16. Institute of Medicine (US) Committee on Standards for Developing Trustworthy Clinical Practice Guidelines. Clinical practice guidelines we can trust. Washington (DC): National Academies Press (US); 2011.

17. Royal College of Obstetricians and Gynaecologists. Management of third and fourth degree perineal tears. MIDIRS. 2015;2:9. Greentop Guideline

18. Nygaard CC, Tsiapakidou S, Pape J, Falconi G, Betschart C, Pergialiotis V, Doumouchtsis SK. Appraisal of clinical practice guidelines on the management of obstetric perineal lacerations and care using the AGREE II instrument. Eur J Obstet Gynecol Reprod Biol. 2020;247:66–72.

19. Tsakiridis I, Mamopoulos A, Athanasiadis A, Dagklis T. Obstetric anal sphincter injuries at vaginal delivery: a review of recently published National Guidelines. Obstet Gynecol Surv. 2018;73:695–702.

20. The Royal College of obstetricians and gynaecologists (2020) Matrix of progression 2020–2021.

21. Sultan AH, Kamm MA, Hudson CN. Obstetric perineal trauma: an audit of training. J Obstet Gynaecol. 1995;15:19–23.

22. Roper JC, Thakar R, Hurt KJ, Sultan AH Diagnosis, management, and training in perineal trauma: A UK National survey of obstetricians. Int Urogynecol J. 2023 Jul 27. Epub ahead of print.

23. Bunn J. Obstetric anal sphincter injuries (OASIs) and other delivery trauma: a US National survey of obstetrician-gynaecologists. Int Urogynecol J. 2022;33(6):1463–72.

24. Young R, Nippita TAC. Training in obstetric anal sphincter injuries in Australia and New Zealand: a survey of Royal Australian and New Zealand College of Obstetricians and Gynaecologists trainees. Aust N Z J Obstet Gynaecol. 2022;62(2):250–4.

25. Cornet A, Porta O, Piñeiro L, Ferriols E, Gich I, Calaf J. Management of obstetric perineal tears: do obstetrics and gynaecology residents receive adequate training? Results of an anonymous survey. Obstet Gynecol Int. 2012;2012:316983. https://doi.org/10.1155/2012/316983.

26. Hickman LC, Propst K. Accurate diagnosis and repair of obstetric anal sphincter injuries: why and how. Am J Obstetr Gynecol. 2020;222(6):580-e1.

27. Women's Healthcare Australasia Reducing harm from perineal tears [Internet].

28. Metcalfe R, Patrick K, Ferguson E. A before and after study of the impact of simulation training on practitioner confidence in complex operative deliveries. J Obstet Gynaecol. 2022;42(7):2746–52.

29. Nursing and Midwifery Council (2019) Standards of proficiency for midwives.

30. Mutema EK. 'A tale of two cities': auditing midwifery practice and perineal trauma. Br J Midwifery. 2007;15:511–3.

31. Roper J, Thakar R, Hurt KJ, Sultan AH A national survey of UK midwives regarding diagnosis, management, and training in perineal trauma. Br J Midwifery. 2023 May 31.

32. Diko S, Sheeder J, Guiahi M, Nacht A, Reeves S, Connell KA, Hurt KJ. Identification of obstetric anal sphincter injuries (OASIs) and other lacerations: a national survey of nurse-midwives. Int Urogynecol

J. 2020;32:1745–53. https://doi.org/10.1007/s00192-020-04304-6.

33. Andrews V, Thankar R, Sultan AH, Kettle C. Can hands-on perineal repair courses affect clinical practice? Br J Midwifery. 2005;13:562–6.

34. Zimmo K, Laine K, Vikanes Å, Fosse E, Zimmo M, Ali H, Thakar R, Sultan AH, Hassan S. Diagnosis and repair of perineal injuries: knowledge before and after expert training—a multicentre observational study among Palestinian physicians and midwives. BMJ Open. 2017;7:e014183.

35. Andrews V, Thakar R, Sultan AH. Structured hands-on training in repair of obstetric anal sphincter injuries (OASIS): an audit of clinical practice. Int Urogynecol J. 2009;20:193–9.

36. Goudie C, Gill A, Shanahan J, Furey A, Dubrowski A. Development of an anatomical silicone model for simulation-based medical training of obstetric anal sphincter injury repair in Bangladesh. Cureus. 2019;11:e3991.

37. Sara K, Karl MB Gynzone. Denmark.

38. Ali-Masri H, Hassan S, Ismail K, Zimmo K, Zimmo M, Fosse E, Vikanes Å, Laine K. Enhancing recognition of obstetric anal sphincter injuries in six maternity units in Palestine: an interventional quality improvement study. BMJ Open. 2018;8:e020983.

39. Knobel R, Volpato L, Gervasi L, Viergutz R, Trapani A. A simple, reproducible and low-cost simulator for teaching surgical techniques to repair obstetric anal sphincter injuries. Rev Bras Ginecol Obstet. 2018;40:465–70.

40. Illston JD, Ballard AC, Ellington DR, Richter HE. Modified beef tongue model for fourth-degree laceration repair simulation. Obstet Gynecol. 2017;129:491–6.

41. Sparks RA, Beesley AD, Jones AD. "The sponge perineum:" an innovative method of teaching fourth-degree obstetric perineal laceration repair to family medicine residents. Fam Med. 2006;38:542–4.

42. Dancz CE, Sun V, Moon HB, Chen JH, Özel B. Comparison of 2 simulation models for teaching obstetric anal sphincter repair. Simul Healthc. 2014;9:325–30.

43. Trowbridge ER, Subbarao S, Melanson M, Childress RM, Hullfish KL, Vaughan M. Self-assessment of nursing preparedness and knowledge in the care of patients with obstetric anal sphincter injuries and utilization of a computer-based learning module for continued nursing education in the United States. Midwifery. 2022;115:103483.

44. Roper JC, Thakar R, Sultan AH Management of acute obstetric anal sphincter injuries: a UK national survey of colorectal surgeons. Colorectal Disease 2023.

45. Oh D, Wright C, Young CJ. Management of obstetric anal sphincter injury: colorectal surgeons' perspectives in Australia and New Zealand. Aust N Z J Obstet Gynaecol. 2021;61:16–21.

Litigation After Pelvic Floor and Anal Sphincter Injuries

24

Michael Mylonas KC and Shivi Nathan

Overview

Test your learning and check your understanding of this book's contents: use the "Springer Nature Flashcards" app to access questions using ▶ https://sn.pub/wqrf89. To use the app, please follow the instructions in Chap. 1.

Learning Objectives

- Understand what a Claimant must prove in order to succeed in a clinical negligence claim.
- Understand what the test is for negligence.
- Learn how the Montgomery case changed the test for negligence in obtaining informed consent.
- Learn how to reduce the risk of being involved in a claim for negligence arising out of an OASI.

24.1 Introduction

This chapter is written from the perspective of Leading Counsel and a Partner in a national firm of solicitors specialising in medical cases and with particular experience acting and advising in connection with claims where a woman has suffered an obstetric anal sphincter injury ("OASI").

OASI injuries are frequently devastating and life-changing for the patient, her family and children; the consequences of the psychological symptoms are often reported to have a similar or even greater impact than the physical symptoms. The social impact of OASI may mean that the patient cannot return to their pre-morbid work[1] and, in some cases, cannot return to any form of work.

The first edition of this textbook was published in 2007. Despite the work that had been done prior to that to increase the rates of identification and repair of OASIs, the rates of recorded OASIs among primiparous women had tripled in the NHS (National Health Service) from 1.8% 2000 to 5.9% by 2011.[2] However, this increase has been attributed to improved recognition of OASIs, rather than an increase in the rate. Since

---

[1] Although if there is any dividend from the Covid-19 pandemic, it includes the fact that "working from home" is now commonly accepted and may assist victims of OASI make a partial return to their previous type of work (if not to their previous place of work).

[2] RCM release [2019]: OASI Care Bundle to be rolled out in more maternity units.

M. Mylonas KC (✉)
Serjeants Inn Chambers, London, UK
e-mail: MMylonasKC@serjeantsinn.com

S. Nathan
Partner, Medical Negligence, Fieldfisher, London, UK
e-mail: Shivi.Nathan@fieldfisher.com

© The Author(s), under exclusive license to Springer Nature Switzerland AG 2024
A. H. Sultan et al. (eds.), *Pelvic Floor, Perineal, and Anal Sphincter Trauma During Childbirth*,
https://doi.org/10.1007/978-3-031-43095-4_24

the Supreme Court's 2015 decision in the *Montgomery* case (detailed below), there has been a four fold increase in claims brought alleging a failure to obtain fully informed consent.[3]

Happily, there is also good news to report. Since 2007, there have been further advances in the training of medical professionals that have already resulted in a reduction in the number of OASIs. For example, the OASI Care Bundle ("OASI-CB") was produced in a collaborative effort between the RCOG (Royal College of Obstetricians and Gynaecologists) and the RCM (Royal College of Midwives) and was first rolled out as a pilot scheme in 2016. Early indications point to a substantial improvement in clinical outcomes, with a 20% reduction in the risk of OASI in a cohort of 55,600 singleton, live vaginal births.[4] And, while the OASI-CB continues to be rolled out in more maternity units in England and Wales, nevertheless, there will still be cases where claims are brought arising out of an OASI. How are those cases handled by the Courts? What standards are imposed on clinicians? How are the claims valued? Most importantly, what advice can the lawyers provide to bring down the number of claims, thereby benefitting both patients and clinicians? This chapter aims to answers those questions.

24.2   Why Do Patients Bring a Claim?

The first and most obvious answer is that patients bring a claim because they have sustained injury. As a result, they have suffered loss; this includes the pain and suffering associated with the injury as well as any financial loss.

The second answer to this question is that patients bring claims because they feel they have been betrayed. In one example, a claim was brought against a consultant obstetrician and gynaecologist operating in a private capacity. Following the primiparous mother's first delivery, he failed to advise her or record anywhere that she had suffered a third degree tear. Even the Summary of Labour failed to record the OASI in the relevant section. There was also no evidence of any repair or attempt at repair. Furthermore, the patient was not given discharge instructions on wound management or what to expect following the repair. When she returned complaining of bleeding and discomfort, the surgeon again failed to disclose the severity of the tear and suggested instead that there had been a breakdown of the episiotomy repair. The mother was referred to a surgeon. It was only in the referral letter that the consultant obstetrician accurately described her OASI. The case proceeded to trial, but breach of duty was eventually admitted. The value of the claim was disputed. The Defendant offered £800,000. The Claimant—a successful investment banker who had suffered significant lost earnings – offered to settle for a discounted sum of £900,000. The Defendant rejected that offer. At trial, the Claimant recovered in excess of £1.5 m, the majority of which was compensation for her lost earnings. In addition—having comprehensively "beaten" her own offer to settle for £900,000 she was awarded a further £75,000[5] by the Court together with her costs, assessed on a preferential basis.

24.3   What Do Claimants Need to Establish to Obtain Damages?

There are three key elements to any successful claim:

– *Breach of Duty:* The Claimant must establish that they were owed a duty of care and a breach of this care by the clinician or treating team occurred; and

---

[3] The effect of the Montgomery judgment on settled claims against the National Health Service due to failure to inform before giving consent to treatment: Wald et al. 2020: https://pubmed.ncbi.nlm.nih.gov/32188990/.

[4] The OASI care bundle quality improvement project: lessons learned and future direction, Jurczuk et al. [2021]. https://link.springer.com/article/10.1007/s00192-021-04786-y/metrics.

[5] This was awarded pursuant to the Civil Procedure Rules – specifically CPR36.14(3)(d) – a provision that was drafted with the intention of encouraging the parties to make realistic offers to settle proceedings and avoid the costs of litigation.

- *Causation:* that the identified breach of duty has caused some injury; and finally
- *Quantum:* the Claimant must prove the amount of her loss.

24.4 Burden & Standard of Proof

The Court will assess the evidence before it with respect to the above three elements by referencing the following basic principles. First, the **burden** of establishing each element is on the Claimant at all times. Second, in establishing whether the Claimant has succeeded in establishing their case, the **standard of proof** is the "balance of probabilities". For example, in relation to breach of duty issues, the Claimant must show that it was "probable" or "more likely than not" that the treatment provided was negligent; in other words, that that there was more than a 50% probability that the treatment was negligent.

We turn now to the individual steps the Claimant must take to establish a claim.

24.5 Breach of Duty in Relation to Treatment

How does one define the standard expected of a clinician in treating a patient? Regardless of whether the claim is brought in contract against a private provider or in tort against the NHS, the test for breach of duty is the same. With the single, important exception of consenting a patient (see below), the starting point in establishing a standard of care is the test first set out in *Bolam v Friern Hospital* in 1957:

A man need not possess the highest expert skill; it is well established law that it is sufficient if he exercises the ordinary skill of an ordinary competent man exercising that particular art ... in the case of a medical man, negligence means failure to act in accordance with the standards of reasonably competent medical men at the time.

Thus, in order to successfully defend a claim, a Defendant will only need to persuade the Court that there is a reasonable body of competent medical professionals (exercising the same skills as those whose treatment is the subject of the dispute) who would have treated the patient in the same manner in which

the treating clinician or team did. It should also be noted that in order to avoid liability, the treatment decisions made do not need to be supported by a majority of responsible clinicians. Instead, it is sufficient for the treatment to be supported by a minority of responsible professionals in that specialist area. This being said, the minority view must be able to withstand logical analysis. For example, in *Bolitho v City & Hackney Health Authority*, the Court of Appeal confirmed in 1998 that:

The use of these adjectives—responsible, reasonable and respectable—all show that **the court has to be satisfied that the exponents of the body of opinion relied upon can demonstrate that such opinion has a logical basis**. In particular in cases involving, as they so often do, the weighing of risks against benefits, the judge (before accepting a body of opinion as being responsible, reasonable or respectable), will need to be satisfied that, in forming their views, the experts have directed their minds to the question of comparative risks and benefits and have reached a defensible conclusion on the matter.[6]

In assessing breach of duty, published or known guidelines are very important. Although by their very nature guidelines are not mandatory, a doctor will need to be able to identify very good reasons—supported by a reasonable, responsible group of their peers—for not following any relevant guidance. For example, in 2007, Sultan and Thakar produced definitive guidance on the performance of a systematic examination to ensure that sphincter injury and buttonhole tears were not missed. Where there is evidence that the Claimant has suffered a tear that was not identified, the claim will be immensely difficult to defend if the clinician concerned cannot prove that they carried out a systematic examination in accordance with the Sultan and Thakar guidance.

24.6 The Montgomery Decision and Informed Consent

Gone are the days when it was thought that, on becoming pregnant, a woman lost, not only their capacity, but also their right to act as a genuinely autonomous human being.[7]

---

[6]Lord Browne-Wilkinson.
[7]Montgomery v Lanarkshire HA, [2015] SC, Baroness Hale at §116.

Until 2015, the test of whether a clinician had obtained informed consent from a patient was judged by the standard of a reasonable, responsible body of peers as identified in *Bolam* (noted above). This standard (applied in 1957 and for many decades thereafter) was determined by obstetric consultants, the overwhelming majority of whom were male. To put this into context, in 1992 –some 35 years after the *Bolam* decision— female registrars still accounted for only a little over 30% of obstetric registrars. That figure increased to around 50% by 2000 and to around 75% in 2013.[8] Thus, insofar as the obtaining of consent was concerned, the Bolam standard test has repeatedly—and rightly—been referred to as paternalistic. On the 11th of March 2015, the Supreme Court gave judgment in the landmark decision of *Montgomery v Lanarkshire Health Board.* The position relating to informed consent changed fundamentally. We set out below §81–2 and 87 of the judgment (with our emphasis):

81. **The social and legal developments which we have mentioned point away from a model of the relationship between the Doctor and the patient based on medical paternalism. They also point away from a model based on a view of the patient as being entirely dependent on information provided by the Doctor. What they point towards is an approach to the law which, instead of treating patients as placing themselves in the hands of their doctors (and then being prone to sue their doctors in the event of a disappointing outcome), treats them so far as possible as adults who are capable of understanding that medical treatment is uncertain of success and may involve risks, accepting responsibility for the taking of risks affecting their own lives, and living with the consequences of their choices.**

82. In the law of negligence, **this approach entails a duty on the part of doctors to take reasonable care to ensure that a patient is aware of material risks of injury that are inherent in treatment**. This can be understood, within the traditional framework of negligence, as a duty of care to avoid exposing a person to a risk of injury which she would otherwise have avoided, but it is also the counterpart of the patient's entitlement to decide whether or not to incur that risk. The existence of that entitlement, and the fact that its exercise does not depend exclusively on medical considerations, are important. **They point to a fundamental distinction between, on the one hand, the Doctor's role when considering possible investigatory or treatment options and, on the other, her role in discussing with the patient any recommended treatment and possible alternatives, and the risks of injury which may be involved.**

87. The correct position, in relation to the risks of injury involved in treatment, can now be seen to be substantially that adopted *(citing previous decisions).* **An adult person of sound mind is entitled to decide which, if any, of the available forms of treatment to undergo, and her consent must be obtained before treatment interfering with her bodily integrity is undertaken. The Doctor is therefore under a duty to take reasonable care to ensure that the patient is aware of any material risks involved in any recommended treatment, and of any reasonable alternative or variant treatments. The test of materiality is whether, in the circumstances of the particular case, a reasonable person in the patient's position would be likely to attach significance to the risk, or the Doctor is or should reasonably be aware that the particular patient would be likely to attach significance to it.**

This more collaborative, shared approach had been trailed both in the GMC's 2013 edition of Good Medical Practice[9] and much earlier in a 2008 document: "Consent: patients and doctors making decisions together".[10] However, it was only with the decision in *Montgomery* that the Court confirmed the requirement that when obtaining consent, one must enter into discussions with the patient and identify what was relevant specifically and subjectively to that patient.

---

[8]The Health and Social Care Information Centre. NHS Hospital and Community Health Services: 2013 Workforce Statistics in England. London: Department of Health, 2013.

[9]Which included under the heading "The duties of a doctor registered with the GMC" the advice that they: "Work in partnership with patients. Listen to, and respond to, their concerns and preferences. Give patients the information they want or need in a way they can understand. Respect patients' right to reach decisions with you about their treatment and care."

[10]See §5: "The doctor explains the options to the patient, setting out the potential benefits, risks, burdens and side effects of each option, including the option to have no treatment. The doctor may recommend a particular option which they believe to be best for the patient, but they must not put pressure on the patient to accept their advice. The patient weighs up the potential benefits, risks and burdens of the various options as well as any non-clinical issues that are relevant to them. The patient decides whether to accept any of the options and, if so, which one."

24.7   Urgent Situations

Does the duty imposed by *Montgomery* still apply when there is time pressure in an urgent situation? This issue may arise in any area of treatment, but is more acutely realised in obstetric practice and is specifically relevant to those clinicians taking decisions where delivery is imminent. For example, the mother may be exhausted following a lengthy labour, she may be medicated with concerns about the impact of medication upon her decision making and she may be in considerable pain. Even further, there is the burden of identifying and explaining clearly to her the risks and benefits of different options, whilst not delaying delivery which may compromise her and her fetus's outcome. The burden on the treating team is already very substantial. Despite those difficulties, however, in *CNZ v Royal Bath Hospitals*,[11] the Judge held that the duty imposed by *Montgomery* did extend to the delivery room and specifically to the period between the delivery of the first twin (by vaginal birth) and delivery of the second twin, when the mother requested a C-section.

The complexity of the assessment that must be performed by the clinician in the delivery room is brought into sharp focus by the earlier decision of the High Court in *ML v Guy's and St Thomas'* [2018] where the Court was concerned with a request for a C-section made in the delivery room by a mother who was in pain. At §90, the Judge said this:

> I regard it as significant that, in her statement of 1 November 2010, SL referred to feeling "Much more coherent" after she had been given the epidural. This is a tacit admission that, before the epidural and given the pain she was in, she was less than coherent and I suspect this will be the case for many women undergoing labour for the first time or, indeed, not for the first time. **It would in fact be impossible to have the kind of discussion of risk and benefit envisaged by Mr Forbes and the NICE (National Institute for Health and Care Excellence) guidelines with a woman who is not wholly coherent and thinking straightforwardly and logically because of the extreme pain she was in and it could be regarded as irresponsible for a midwife or obstetrician to attempt to have such a discussion with a woman before her pain**

> had been addressed. It seems to me that this situation is qualitatively different to the situation in the ante-natal clinic where a request for a caesarean section is made.

In the more recent case of *CNZ*, the Judge found that there was a duty to take into account the mother's expressly stated view, despite the urgency of the situation and the potential difficulties involved in a late move to the theatre for the C-section to be performed. This case arose out of a delivery that occurred in 1996 and the requirements imposed by *Montgomery* were still deemed to apply.

24.8   What About More Junior Staff?

Does the law recognise a different standard of care for those with less experience in a role? The question before the Court is always whether in each case a specific professional (or group of professionals) has provided treatment which would be supported by a reasonable, responsible group of professionals *in that post*. Therefore, if a Registrar is acting up in a Consultant's role, they will be judged against the standards of a Consultant.[12] Earlier decisions had referred to the example of a driver who had passed a driving test. The driving standards are not reduced for a newly qualified driver; similarly, standards are not higher for one who has been driving for many years. Simply put, all drivers are to be judged by reference to the standard expected of a reasonable, responsible driver. There is, however, an important caveat to this conclusion. Although a junior doctor may avoid individual liability for the reasons identified above (because for example the standard of care expected of an Foundation Year 1 (FY1) doctor is lower than that expected of a Consultant), that may not always provide a Defence when a claim is against an NHS Trust where it may be alleged that there was a failure to involve senior clinical input early on in the treatment.

---

[11] Judgment handed down in January 2023.

[12] See *Wilsher v Essex AHA* [1987] 1 QB 730 & FB v Princess Alexandra Hospital NHS Trust [2017] EWCA Civ 334.

24.9 Will a Failure to Identify a Tear Always Establish Breach of Duty?

There have been recent attempts by Defendants to avoid liability by arguing that a competent examination was conducted, but the tear was "non-negligently" missed despite a systematic examination. Those arguments, however, face an evidential difficulty, as the literature demonstrates the relative rarity with which a Grade 3c tear is missed. For example, in 2022, Roper et al.[13] published a prospective collected dataset of 1271 women between 2012 and 2020. Although 14.8% of 3c tears were missed overall as confirmed by endoanal ultrasound, the rate of missed 3c injuries fell significantly from 12% to 7.4% during the time periods 2012–2015 and 2016–2019 respectively. This fall is likely a reflection of the benefits and efficacy of training and hands-on workshops. The Claimant must only show "on the balance of probabilities" either (i) that no examination was performed at all; or (ii) that if an examination was undertaken then it was not effective. Given the available literature, it will be challenging—albeit not impossible—for a clinician to establish that a tear was missed despite a systematic examination. The prospects of successfully defending a claim will be improved if:

(a) there was evidence of the clinician having attended relevant recent courses and hands-on workshops; and

(b) the fact, nature and extent of the examination was carefully documented; and

(c) the clinician had significant documented experience of carrying out systematic examinations and had successfully identified tears in the past.

---

[13] Roper JC, Thakar R, Sultan AH. Under-classified obstetric anal sphincter injuries. Int Urogynaecology J 2022;33(6): 1473–9.

24.10 Causation

To establish a right to damages, it is not sufficient merely to establish that treatment has been negligent. The Claimant must prove (again, on the balance of probabilities), that the deficient treatment "caused" injury. Questions of causation can be legally complex and space does not permit a detailed explanation of the different issues relating to causation. For the purposes of this chapter, it is sufficient to discuss briefly the "but for" test of causation. This test, in our experience, is the most likely to be relevant in relation to OASIs.

As the name implies, the "but for" test means that a Claimant will have established a causal link if they can show, on the balance of probability, that "but for" the Defendant's negligence they would either (a) not have suffered any injury; or (b) would have suffered a reduced level of injury. Consider the example of a case where it was alleged that the treating team had failed to identify and repair an OASI. The Claimant mother would provide:

– A witness statement setting out the bowel symptoms from which she was suffering (typically involving urgency, leakage of stool, lack of control of flatus); and
– Expert evidence detailing:
    (1) what surgery would have been carried out if the tear had been identified; and
    (2) how much better the current and future functional outcome would have been if the tear had been identified and repaired in a timely fashion.

In those circumstances, the Claimant's causation argument would be that "but for" the failure to identify and repair the tear earlier, she would have been left with either no bowel symptoms or bowel symptoms that affected her to a lesser degree than she presently suffers.

24.11 Quantum

Quantum is essentially the exercise the parties go through in order to establish the value of the compensation that should be paid to the Claimant. In summary, it is made up of two main "heads of claim", one of which may contain multiple sub-headings.

24.11.1 First Head of Claim: Pain, Suffering and Loss of Amenity ("PSLA")

The Court awards a sum (referred to either as "general damages" or the "PSLA" award) in respect of the specific injury sustained by the Claimant and its current and future impact on their life. That award is made principally by reference to the Judicial College (JC) Guidelines and to reported judgements in cases involving comparable injuries.

For ease of reference, we set out below the JC Guidelines with respect to bowel injury. The Guidelines are updated approximately every two years by reference to Retail Price Index (RPI); the most recent edition (the 16th) was updated in September 2021 (Fig. 24.1).

The Guidelines are simply guidelines and figures will be adjusted depending on the specific symptoms of each Claimant. PSLA awards in OASI cases are most likely to fall into category (c) with awards around £80,000. However, those awards will be increased where there is a risk of colostomy and they will be increased significantly if there is a probability or certainty of colostomy. As OASIs can leave victims with significant psychological symptoms as well, the JC Guidelines include a separate category for these (Fig. 24.2).

Section (I) - Bowels
(a) Cases involving double incontinence namely total loss of natural bowel function and complete loss of urinary function and control, together with other medical complications: **Up to £184,200**
(b) Total loss of natural function and dependence on colostomy, depending on age: **Up to £150,110**
(c) Faecal urgency and passive incontinence persisting after surgery and causing embarrassment and distress, typically following injury giving birth: **In the region of £79,920**
(d) Severe abdominal injury causing impairment of function and often necessitating temporary colostomy (leaving disfiguring scars) and/or restriction on employment and on diet: **£44,590 - £69,730**
(e) Penetrating injuries causing some permanent damage but with an eventual return to natural function and control: **£12,590 to £24,480**

Fig. 24.1 JC Guidelines 16th edition

Section (A) - Psychiatric Damage Generally
The factors to be taken into account in valuing claims of this nature are as follows: (i)the injured person's ability to cope with life, education, and work; (ii)the effect on the injured person's relationships with family, friends, and those with whom he or she comes into contact; (iii)the extent to which treatment would be successful; (iv)future vulnerability; (v)prognosis; (vi)whether medical help has been sought.
(a) Severe In these cases the injured person will have marked problems with respect to factors (i) to (iv) above and the prognosis will be very poor: **£54,830 to £115,730**
(b) Moderately Severe: In these cases there will be significant problems associated with factors (i) to (iv) above but the prognosis will be much more optimistic than in (a) above. While there are awards which support both extremes of this bracket, the majority are somewhere near the middle of the bracket. Cases involving psychiatric injury following a negligent stillbirth or the traumatic birth of a child will often fall within this bracket. Cases of work-related stress resulting in a permanent or long-standing disability preventing a return to comparable employment would appear to come within this category: **£19,070 to £54,830**
(c) Moderate: While there may have been the sort of problems associated with factors (i) to (iv) above there will have been marked improvement by trial and the prognosis will be good: **£5,860 to £19,070**
(d) Less Severe: The level of the award will take into consideration the length of the period of disability and the extent to which daily activities and sleep were affected. Cases falling short of a specific phobia or disorder such as travel anxiety when associated with minor physical symptoms may be found in the Minor Injuries chapter: **£1,540 to £5,860**

Fig. 24.2 Chap. 4: Psychiatric and psychological damage

24.11.2 Second Head of Damages: Special Damages

Special Damages are those past and future financial losses that the Claimant can establish they have or are likely to suffer in future. Typically in OASI cases the Special Damages claim will include separate claims for:

- Lost earnings and pension (see below)
- Additional required care (for example, the mother requires assistance with childcare and/

or future anticipated care with possible colostomy)
- Medical treatment including the cost of investigations, treatment and surgery such as biofeedback, sacral nerve stimulation, colostomy, pain management and any reviews or scanning that are required.
- If the Claimant can establish that these services will be sought privately (rather than under the NHS), then the full private cost will be recoverable.

24.11.2.1 Lost Earnings and Pension Claims

These claims deserve special mention because they frequently form the largest part of a financial claim. If a Claimant can return to some, albeit limited, employment, then credit must be given for their residual earnings. Lost earnings claims may be substantial if the Claimant was a higher earning professional and cannot return to work either at all or at her previous level of earning. If the evidence supports the contention that they would have been promoted and received a higher salary, bonus or pension then that will all form part of the award.

Given the current predictions for life expectation, pensions claims can be very significant for those who enjoyed generous pension provision in employment that they can no longer maintain. For example, in one recent claim on behalf of a senior doctor, the earnings and pensions claims were in the order of £1 m and £950 k respectively.

24.12 OASI Claims in Practice

Above, we have set out the legal framework within which OASI claims will be heard by the Court. Below we set out the circumstances in which OASI claims typically arise. By providing the list below identifying those "hot spots" for litigation, we hope clinicians can avoid any personal experience of the litigation process.

1. **Failure to identify a tear:** This was a frequently reported cause of injury. The hope is that with mandatory training in examination, the number of instances where a tear is missed will drop significantly. *Litigation Avoidance Advice:* Perform a systematic examination and document the same. Keep up training in the performance of systematic examinations.
2. **Failure to identify the nature and extent of a tear:** This is less frequently reported, but still identified. Please keep in mind that it is occasionally argued that a tear can be "non-negligently" missed despite a examination. *Litigation Avoidance Advice:* Perform a sys-tematic examination and document the same. Keep up training in the performance of systematic examinations.
3. **Failure to properly repair tears that have been identified:** Again, a less frequently reported cause of complaint but can be associated with a failure to identify the extent of the tear. *Litigation Avoidance Advice:* Perform a systematic examination and document the same. Keep up training in the performance of systematic examinations.
4. **Failure to identify an increased risk of tear:** This is usually advanced alongside a claim that the mother was not properly consented about mode of delivery. The claims are usually advanced where there was a material risk that the baby would be big and therefore a material risk of perineal trauma. In those circumstances, *Montgomery* consent requires clear discussion of the risks and benefits of vaginal delivery and caesarean section. Historically these claims have been brought in relation to risks that were identifiable (e.g. gestational diabetes and the risk of macrosomia) or because the fetal growth scans showed a baby that was large for dates. However, following the decision in *CNZ v Royal Bath Hospitals* (January 2023 as above), we anticipate claims will be made in future where there was no early indication of macrosomia and the fact of a large baby was only identified late in the pregnancy—perhaps only during labour. *Litigation Avoidance Advice:* Patients should be counselled during their pregnancy about the risks and benefits of vaginal versus Caesarean modes of birth and a plan made prior to the onset of labour.
5. **Performing a midline episiotomy:** We identified in the introduction to this chapter a case where the obstetrician appeared deliberately to have hidden from the mother the fact that she had suffered a third degree tear. That injury was sustained after he had performed a midline episiotomy. Although midline episiotomies were no longer supported in England and Wales, the case was initially defended on the basis that they were acceptable in the United States. Liability was admitted before the case

came to trial. We have not seen a case since then where a midline episiotomy was performed and assume that this was an outlying example. Certainly it is very likely indeed that negligence will be established if a midline episiotomy is performed without there being both some extenuating circumstance. *Litigation Avoidance Advice:* A full explanation to the patient of the comparative risks and benefits of midline and medio-lateral incisions followed by explicit patient choice should be done.

24.13 Midwifery Care and OASI

Special mention should be made of the litigation situation amongst midwives. Midwives are only trained to repair first and second degree tears. In responding to a survey in two district general hospitals, 90% of midwives felt inadequately prepared to assess perineal trauma. That lack of confidence was underlined by a relative lack of experience in carrying out rectal examinations as well; 18% in one hospital and less than 30% in a second hospital were carrying out examinations as recommended.[14] By 2020, a survey of midwives revealed that more than 50% considered they had insufficient training in OASIs due to a lack of courses. That was despite the first hands-on course for perineal repair being provided in 2000.

24.14 Avoiding Litigation while Providing Appropriate Treatment

Litigation is stressful, time consuming and expensive. Avoiding litigation can most easily be achieved by maintaining high standards of clinical practice. Most of the cases brought by Claimants for OASI arise because of basic and

inadvertent failures, all of which can easily be avoided:

1. Throughout the pregnancy, properly assess the risk of a larger fetus and counsel patients about the risks of perineal injury and various modes of delivery. Carefully document those continuing assessments, all counseling given and the patient's ultimate choice for delivery mode.
2. Should fetal macrosomia present late in the pregnancy, offer and document as above. In cases of extreme urgency or unsuspected macrosomia, make retrospective notes, explaining carefully when those notes were made and why they were not made at the time (e.g. the urgency of the situation).
3. Perform a systematic examination to identify and/or exclude a tear after the delivery. Document the examination and your findings.
4. Perform a systematic examination after the repair has been performed. Document the examination and your findings.

Maintain training in avoiding and identifying perineal trauma. Ensure training is documented.

24.15 Case Law Update and the Updated Situation in the United States

The previous edition of this work included a summary of the situation in the United States. The basis of claim for medical malpractice in the US originally derived from the English common law but the tests to establish breach of duty are not yet harmonised throughout the US. At the time of preparing this update to the law in England and Wales, we are not aware of any significant developments in the relevant US law since the previous edition but we will provide and make available online an update both of:

– Any significant developments in the US law; and
– Any relevant case law in England and Wales that may be of assistance to clinicians.

---

[14] Mutema EK. 'A tale of two cities': auditing midwifery practice and perineal trauma. Brit J Midwifery. 2007;15:(8)511–513. https://doi.org/10.12968/bjom.2007.15.8.24394.

24.16 Conclusions

OASIs do arise despite the best care and, absent some confounding feature (such as a midline episiotomy), a clinician will not incur liability simply because a mother has suffered an OASI. However, a clinician who fails to identify an OASI, fails to correctly identify the nature and extent of an OASI, or fails to carry out an early and proper repair places themselves in unnecessary jeopardy when defending a claim. There are two critical steps in either avoiding a claim or, where a claim is brought, in successfully defending it. The first is the performance of a systematic examination as recommended by Sultan, Thakar et al. The second step is the careful documentation of that examination. In the Courts, evidence is all. The clinician is in a uniquely advantageous position because they are under a duty to keep a record and should therefore have the evidence to establish that they have conducted a satisfactory examination.

Take Home Messages
- Clinicians must perform systematic examinations as recommended by Sultan, Thakar et al. after delivery. A failure to do so is likely to be regarded as negligent.
- Clinicians should ensure they have recent training in and have hands on experience of identifying OASIs.
- Clinicians should keep an up to date log of all training in identifying OASIs.
- Clinicians should ensure all discussions with patients are Montgomery compliant and documented.

Appendix: MCQ

Mark each item TRUE or FALSE

Questions

1. What is the correct legal test to determine breach of duty?
   - (A) Bolam is the only test used to determine breach of duty
   - (B) Beyond all reasonable doubt is the only test
   - (C) The Bolam test requires a majority of clinicians to agree
   - (D) On the balance of probabilities means more than a 50% chance
   - (E) The only requirement for a successful clinical negligence claim is to establish causation

2. Which of the following did the Montgomery test establish?
   - (A) That doctors should take reasonable care to ensure that a patient is aware of material risks of injury that are inherent in treatment
   - (B) That it is the duty on the part of doctors to take reasonable care to ensure that a patient is aware of material risks of injury that are inherent in treatment
   - (C) That a doctor does not have to ensure that the patient is aware of any material risks involved in any recommended treatment, and of any reasonable alternative or variant treatments
   - (D) That when obtaining consent, one must enter into discussions with the patient and identify what was relevant specifically and subjectively to that patient
   - (E) That the duty does not apply in an urgent situation

3. Which of the following is true regarding compensation in a medical negligence case?
   - (A) An award for pain, suffering and loss of amenity is also known as a General Damages Award
   - (B) A Claimant cannot claim for both physical and psychiatric injury as a result of birth trauma
   - (C) In most claims, the potential loss of earnings claim will attract the largest financial award
   - (D) Evidence is required to support any financial claim
   - (E) A Claimant cannot claim for private medical treatment

4. OASI claim hotspots include:
   - (A) A failure to correctly identify the level of tear

(B)   A failure to identify the correct level of tear
(C)   Failure to properly repair tears that have been identified
(D)   Failure to identify an increased risk of tear
(E)   Performing a mediolateral episiotomy

5. Regarding Midwifery training:
   (A)   UK Midwives are only required to undertake repair of 1st and 2nd-degree perineal tears, and refer additional trauma
   (B)   A 2007 UK survey found 50% of midwives felt inadequately trained to assess perineal trauma
   (C)   In a 2020 survey of midwives more than 50% said they lack training in OASIs due to lack of courses
   (D)   An American survey of midwives found one third incorrectly identified a third degree tear as a fourth degree tear
   (E)   The first UK hands-on perineal repair course started in 2000

Answers

1. What is the correct legal test to determine breach of duty?
   (A)   FALSE
   (B)   FALSE
   (C)   FALSE
   (D)   TRUE
   (E)   FALSE

2. Which of the following did the Montgomery test establish?
   (A)   TRUE
   (B)   TRUE
   (C)   FALSE
   (D)   TRUE
   (E)   FALSE

3. Which of the following is true regarding compensation in a medical negligence case?
   (A)   TRUE
   (B)   FALSE
   (C)   TRUE
   (D)   TRUE
   (E)   FALSE

4. OASI claim hotspots include:
   (A)   TRUE
   (B)   TRUE
   (C)   TRUE
   (D)   TRUE
   (E)   FALSE

5. Regarding Midwifery training:
   (A)   TRUE
   (B)   FALSE
   (C)   TRUE
   (D)   TRUE
   (E)   TRUE

Index